DIETARY AGEs AND THEIR ROLE IN HEALTH AND DISEASE

DIETARY AGEs AND THEIR ROLE IN HEALTH AND DISEASE

EDITED BY

Jamie Uribarri

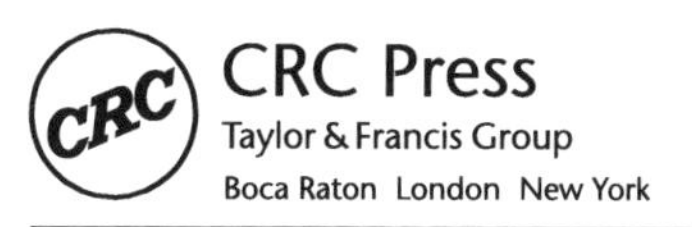

CRC Press is an imprint of the
Taylor & Francis Group, an **informa** business

CRC Press
Taylor & Francis Group
6000 Broken Sound Parkway NW, Suite 300
Boca Raton, FL 33487-2742

Printed on acid-free paper

International Standard Book Number-13: 978-1-4987-2151-6 (Hardback)

Library of Congress Cataloging-in-Publication Data

Names: Uribarri, Jaime, editor.
Title: Dietary AGEs and their role in health and disease / edited by Jaime Uribarri.
Description: Boca Raton, Florida : CRC Press, [2018] | Includes bibliographical references and index.
Identifiers: LCCN 2017022981| ISBN 9781498721516 (hardback : alk. paper) | ISBN 9781315120041 (e-book) | ISBN 9781498721523 (e-book) | ISBN 9781351646352 (e-book) | ISBN 9781351636810 (e-book)
Subjects: | MESH: Glycosylation End Products, Advanced--adverse effects | Glycosylation End Products, Advanced--metabolism | Glycosylation End Products, Advanced--drug effects | Diet--adverse effects
Classification: LCC QP606.G6 | NLM QU 55.5 | DDC 572.792--dc23
LC record available at https://lccn.loc.gov/2017022981

Visit the Taylor & Francis Web site at
http://www.taylorandfrancis.com

and the CRC Press Web site at
http://www.crcpress.com

Contents

Section IV Therapeutic Alternatives to Deal with Dietary AGEs

Preface

Modern "Western" society has brought with itself profound changes in lifestyle but at the same time a much greater prevalence of chronic diseases such as cardiovascular disease, metabolic syndrome, insulin resistance, obesity, and type-2 diabetes mellitus. All these diseases seem to have in common elevated levels of markers of inflammation and oxidative stress. Of the many components of modern lifestyle, which alone or in combination may play a role increasing inflammation and oxidative stress, diet is a prominent one. Of the many dietary factors that may be associated with inflammation and oxidative stress, we have been particularly interested in a specific group of food-derived pro-inflammatory and pro-oxidant compounds, the so-called advanced glycation end products (AGEs). AGEs represent a large heterogeneous group of compounds, which has made it difficult to standardize their measurement. Although endogenous AGEs have been widely recognized as important factors in the pathogenesis of diabetic complications, the importance of AGEs of dietary origin as a factor in human disease has been largely unappreciated until recently. Over the past two decades, several clinical trials have tested the effects of a low-AGE dietary intervention on a variety of conditions. These trials demonstrate that a simple low-AGE dietary intervention decreases circulating levels of AGEs, markers of inflammation and oxidative stress in healthy, chronic kidney disease, and diabetic patients, and improves insulin resistance in type 2 diabetes patients. These data have generated a new paradigm of disease, widely unrecognized, suggesting that excessive consumption of dietary AGEs secondary to a "Western lifestyle" represents an independent risk factor for inappropriate chronic oxidative stress and inflammation during life, which over time facilitates the emergence of the chronic diseases of the modern world, especially diabetes and cardiovascular disease. Moreover, the data also show that reducing AGE content of common foods by simple changes in culinary techniques is a feasible, safe, and easily applicable intervention in both health and disease.

This book presents most of the data that have been accumulated in the past two decades on the role of food-derived AGEs in causing chronic human disease. The book starts with a general definition of the compounds passing through all the clinical diseases that have been associated with them and finally offers different therapeutic options to deal with the problem. I have been extremely lucky to have the participation of a selected group of national and international experts in the field to develop these concepts at a highly academic level. I have also left room for presentation by scholars who may not fully agree with the concept that dietary AGEs are toxic to the body. I am very indebted to all these collaborators. My hope is that this book provides the basis to initiate a serious academic conversation about the real role of dietary AGEs in human disease.

Jaime Uribarri, MD
Icahn School of Medicine at Mount Sinai
New York, NY

Editor

Dr. Jaime Uribarri is a physician and clinical investigator. He was born in Chile and received his medical degree from the University of Chile School of Medicine. He did all his postgraduate training in the United States. He has been in the Icahn School of Medicine at Mount Sinai, NY, since 1990, where he is currently professor of medicine and director of the Renal Clinic and the Home Dialysis Program at the Mount Sinai Hospital.

In parallel with his clinical activities, Dr. Uribarri has been very active in clinical investigation for the past 30 years. His main areas of research have been on acid-base and fluid and electrolytes disorders as well as nutrition in chronic kidney disease and diabetic patients. Dr. Uribarri, working together with Dr. Helen Vlassara, were among the first to explore the role of food-derived advanced glycation end products (AGEs) and their negative effects in healthy persons as well as in those with diabetes or with kidney disease from different causes. This teamwork for more than 10 years was instrumental in establishing the first food AGE database and its application in the form of practical guidelines for everyone, which is now widely used. He has published over 150 peer-reviewed papers and written many chapters in books. He has lectured extensively on these research topics in New York City as well as in national and international meetings. He serves as an ad hoc referee for numerous nutrition, medical, and other scientific journals and he is an active member of several health organizations and professional associations, including the American Society of Nephrology, the American Society of Nutrition, the International Society of Nephrology, The New York Academy of Sciences, The Maillard Society, etc.

Contributors

Latifa Abdennebi-Najar, PhD
Société Francophone pour la recherche et l'éducation sur les origines développementales, environnementales et épigénétiques de la santé et des maladies (SF-DOHaD)
Chatillon, France

Carolina Añazco
Biomedical research Laboratories
Medicine Faculty, Catholic University of Maule
Talca, Chile

Estifanos Baye, BSc, MPH
Monash Centre for Health Research and Implementation
School of Public Health and Preventive Medicine
Monash University
Clayton, VIC, Australia

Michal Schnaider Beeri, PhD
The Joseph Sagol Neuroscience Center Tel Hashomer
Ramat Gan, Israel
and
Department of Medicine
Icahn School of Medicine at Mt Sinai
New York, NY
and
Interdisciplinary Center (IDC) Herzliya
School of Psychology
Herzliya, Israel

Stig Bengmark, MD, PhD, FRACS (Hon), FRCPS (Hon)
Division of Surgery & Interventional Science
University College London
London, United Kingdom

Guido Bosch, PhD
Animal Nutrition Group
Wageningen University
Wageningen, The Netherlands

Dipshikha Chakravortty, PhD
Department of Microbiology and Cell Biology
Indian Institute of Science
Bangalore, India
and
Center for Biosystems Science and Engineering
Indian Institute of Science
Bangalore, India

Kasturi Chandra
Department of Microbiology and Cell Biology
Indian Institute of Science
Bangalore, India

Laura C. Cogoi
Universidad de Buenos Aires
Facultad de Farmacia y Bioquímica
Departamento de Farmacología.
and
CONICET-Universidad de Buenos Aires
Instituto de Química y Metabolismo del Fármaco (IQUIMEFA)
Buenos Aires, Argentina

Alma Rosa Corrales Escobosa, PhD
Chemistry Department
University of Guanajuato
Guanajuato, Mexico

Barbora de Courten, MD, PhD, MPH, FRACP
Monash Centre for Health Research and Implementation
School of Public Health and Preventive Medicine
Monash University
Clayton, VIC, Australia
and
Diabetes and Vascular Medicine Unit
Monash Health
Clayton, VIC, Australia

Cristina Delgado-Andrade, PhD
Department of Physiology and Biochemistry of Animal Nutrition
Estación Experimental del Zaidín (EEZ-CSIC)
Granada, Spain

Evanthia Diamanti-Kandarakis, MD, PhD
Department of Endocrinology and Metabolism
Hygeia Hospital
Athens, Greece

Ghada Elmhiri
PRP-HOM/SRBE/LRTOX
Laboratoire de Radiotoxicologie Expérimentale
Fontenay-aux-Roses, France

Rosana Filip, PhD
Universidad de Buenos Aires
Facultad de Farmacia y Bioquímica
Departamento de Farmacología.
and
CONICET-Universidad de Buenos Aires
Instituto de Química y Metabolismo del Fármaco (IQUIMEFA)
Buenos Aires, Argentina

Victoria J. Findlay, PhD
Department of Pathology & Laboratory Medicine
Hollings Cancer Center
Medical University of South Carolina
Charleston, SC

Josephine M. Forbes, PhD
Glycation and Diabetes, Mater Research Institute
University of Queensland, Translational Research Institute
Woolloongabba, Australia
and
School of Biomedical Sciences
University of Queensland
St Lucia, Australia
and
Mater Clinical School
University of Queensland
St Lucia, Australia
and
Department of Medicine
The University of Melbourne
Austin Hospital
Heidelberg, Australia
and
Baker IDI Heart and Diabetes Institute
Melbourne, Australia

Amelia K. Fotheringham
Glycation and Diabetes, Mater Research Institute
University of Queensland, Translational Research Institute
Woolloongabba, Australia
and
School of Biomedical Sciences
University of Queensland
St Lucia, Australia

Linda A. Gallo, PhD
Glycation and Diabetes, Mater Research Institute
University of Queensland, Translational Research Institute
Woolloongabba, Australia

Ma. Eugenia Garay-Sevilla, MD, PhD
Department of Medical Science
Division of Health Science
University of Guanajuato Campus León
León, México

Mayuri Gogoi
Department of Microbiology and Cell Biology
Indian Institute of Science
Bangalore, India

Armando Gómez-Ojeda, PhD
Department of Medical Science
Division of Health Science
University of Guanajuato Campus León
León, México

Ileana Gonzalez
Biomedical research Laboratories
Medicine Faculty, Catholic University of Maule
Talca, Chile

Alejandro Gugliucci, MD, PhD
TGlycation Oxidation and Disease Laboratory Department of Research
Touro University College of Osteopathic Medicine
Vallejo, CA

Weidun Alan Guo, MD, PhD
Department of Surgery
University at Buffalo
Buffalo, NY

Anshu Gupta, MBBS, MS
Department of Pediatrics
Children's Hospital of Richmond
Virginia Commonwealth University
Richmond, VA

Kristian F. Hanssen, MD, PhD
Department of Endocrinology,
Morbid obesity and Preventive Medicine
Oslo University Hospital and Institute of Clinical Medicine
University of Oslo
Oslo, Norway

John C. He, MD, PhD
Division of Nephrology
Department of Medicine
Icahn School of Medicine at Mount Sinai
New York, NY

Wouter Hendriks, PhD
Animal Nutrition Group
Wageningen University
Wageningen, The Netherlands
and
Faculty of Veterinary Medicine
Utrecht University
Utrecht, The Netherlands

Sarahi Jaramillo Ortiz, PhD
Chemistry Department
University of Guanajuato
Guanajuato, Mexico

Eleni A. Kandaraki, MD, PhD, MRCP(UK)
Unit of Endocrinology and Metabolism
Third Department of Internal Medicine
Medical School of Athens University
Athens, Greece

Kapudeep Karmakar
Department of Microbiology and Cell Biology
Indian Institute of Science
Bangalore, India

Roni Lotan, MSc
The Nutrition and Brain Health Laboratory
The Institute of Biochemistry, Food and Nutrition Science
Robert H. Smith Faculty of Agriculture, Food and the Environment
The Hebrew University of Jerusalem
Rehovot, Israel
and
The Joseph Sagol Neuroscience Center Tel Hashome
Ramat Gan, Israel

Claudia Luevano-Contreras, PhD
Department of Medical Science
Division of Health Science
University of Guanajuato Campus León
León, México

Michael Murkovic, PhD
Graz University of Technology
Institute of Biochemistry
Graz, Austria

Delminda Neves, PhD
Department of Biomedicine—Experimental Biology Unit
Faculty of Medicine of the University of Porto, Al. Prof. Hernâni Monteiro
Porto, Portugal
and
Instituto de Investigação e Inovação em Saúde (I3S) Rua Alfredo Allen
Porto, Portugal

Melinda M. Nugent, MD
Division of Nephrology
Department of Medicine
Icahn School of Medicine at Mount Sinai
New York, NY

Julie Ottosen, MD
Department of Surgery
University of Minnesota
Minneapolis, MN

Marisa Passarelli, PhD
Lipids Laboratory (LIM10)
University of Sao Paulo Medical School
Sao Paulo, SP, Brazil

Silvia Pastoriza, PhD
Departamento de Nutrición y Bromatología
Facultad de Farmacia
Universidad de Granada
Granada, Spain

Franco Pedreschi, PhD
Departamento de Ingeniería Química y Bioprocesos
Pontificia Universidad de Católica de Chile
Santiago de Chile, Chile

Melpomeni Peppa, MD
Endocrine and Bone Metabolic Disorders Unit
2nd Department of Internal Medicine Propaedeutic
Research Institute and Diabetes Center
National and Kapodistrian School of Athens
Attikon University Hospital
Athens, Greece

Sergio Pérez-Burillo
Departamento de Nutrición y Bromatología
Facultad de Farmacia
Universidad de Granada
Granada, Spain

Tasnim Rahman, BS
Virginia Commonwealth University
Richmond, VA

Armando Rojas, PhD
Biomedical research Laboratories
Medicine Faculty
Catholic University of Maule
Talca, Chile

José Ángel Rufián-Henares, PhD
Departamento de Nutrición y Bromatología
Facultad de Farmacia
Universidad de Granada
Granada, Spain

Katarina Šebeková, MD, DSc
Institute of Molecular Biomedicine
Medical Faculty, Comenius University
Bratislava, Slovakia

Halyna Semchyshyn, PhD
Department of Biochemistry and Biotechnology
Vasyl Stefanyk Precarpathian National University
Ivano-Frankivsk, Ukraine

Peter Smit, MD
Department of Cardiothoracic Surgery
Wake Forest University
Winston-Salem, NC

Ovidiu Alin Stirban, MD
Department of Diabetes and Endocrinology
Sana Klinikum and MVZ Sana Artzpraxen
Remscheid, Germany

Kari Anne Sveen, MD, PhD
Department of Endocrinology
Morbid Obesity and Preventive Medicine
Oslo University Hospital and Institute of Clinical Medicine
University of Oslo
Oslo, Norway

Katarina Brouder Šebeková, MD
Intensive Care Unit
John Radcliffe Hospital
Oxford, United Kingdom

Masako Toda, PhD
Paul-Ehrlich-Institut
Langen, Germany

Aron M. Troen, DPhil
The Nutrition and Brain Health Laboratory
The Institute of Biochemistry, Food and Nutrition Science
The Robert H. Smith Faculty of Agriculture Food and the Environment
The Hebrew University of Jerusalem
Rehovot, Israel

David P. Turner, PhD
Department of Pathology & Laboratory Medicine
Hollings Cancer Center
Medical University of South Carolina
Charleston, SC

Jaime Uribarri, MD
Icahn School of Medicine at Mount Sinai
New York, NY

Katarzina Wrobel, PhD
Chemistry Department
University of Guanajuato
Guanajuato, Mexico

Rabi Yacoub, MD
Department of Internal Medicine
Jacobs School of Medicine and Biomedical Sciences
University at Buffalo
Buffalo, NY

Sho-ichi Yamagishi, MD, PhD
Department of Pathophysiology and Therapeutics of Diabetic Vascular Complications
Kurume University School of Medicine
Kurume, Japan

Section I

What Are AGEs?

1

What Are AGEs, Their Chemical Structure, and How Can They Be Measured?

Katarzyna Wrobel, Kazimierz Wrobel, Sarahi Jaramillo Ortiz, and Alma Rosa Corrales Escobosa
University of Guanajuato
Guanajuato, Mexico

CONTENTS

KEY POINTS

- N^{ε}-(carboxymethyl)-L-lysine (CML), N^{ε}-(carboxyethyl)-L-lysine (CEL), and pentosidine—three advanced glycation end products generally accepted as biomarkers of *in vitro* and *in vivo* glycation processes.
- Analytical chemistry procedures for the determination of advanced glycation end products (AGEs) provide high selectivity, sensitivity, and detection power demanded in clinical studies.
- Liquid chromatography–tandem mass spectrometry is a gold standard for the determination of known AGEs in clinical samples and in food products.
- Proteomic-based mass spectrometry tools are required for full characterization of AGE structures and their role in human aging and diseases.

1.1 Formation and Structural Diversity of AGEs

Advanced glycation end products (AGEs) are formed in a branched chain of nonenzymatic reactions that start by condensation of free amino groups present in a given biomolecule with carbonyl group of reducing sugars or other related chemical species. Initially, these processes had been referred to as Maillard reaction and were studied within the context of food processing. Since mid-1950s, when glycated hemoglobin (HbA1c) was first described, the research interest has partially moved to *in vivo* glycation processes.

Despite inevitable formation of AGEs in physiological conditions and their gradual accumulation during normal aging, today there is no doubt that the excess of glycation products is harmful and is associated with several health disorders including diabetes and its complications. In this regard, contribution of endogenously formed and exogenous AGEs has to be considered.

During the last decades, extensive studies have been carried out in order to elucidate molecular mechanisms underlying glycation processes and to understand their role in human diseases and aging. The detailed description of currently known glycation pathways can be found in several comprehensive reviews [1–4]; a simplified scheme elaborated for the purposes of this chapter is presented in Figure 1.1. The already mentioned amine-carbonyl reaction yields imine group in the condensed labile compound, generically called Schiff base. Although at this early stage glycation is reversible, Shiff base is slowly rearranged to a more stable open-chain ketoamine—still an intermediate glycation product (Amadori product). In the classic pathway, Amadori products undergo dehydration, fragmentation, oxidation, and cyclization reactions, which ultimately lead to the formation of irreversible AGEs.

Among reducing sugars, glucose itself is a relatively weak glycation agent, especially as compared to the small alpha-dicarbonyl compounds produced from glucose auto-oxidation, from polyol pathway, from degradation of Amadori products, from intermediates of glycolysis, and also from lipids peroxidation. As shown in Figure 1.1, glyoxal (GO), methylglyoxal (MGO), and 3-deoxyglucosone

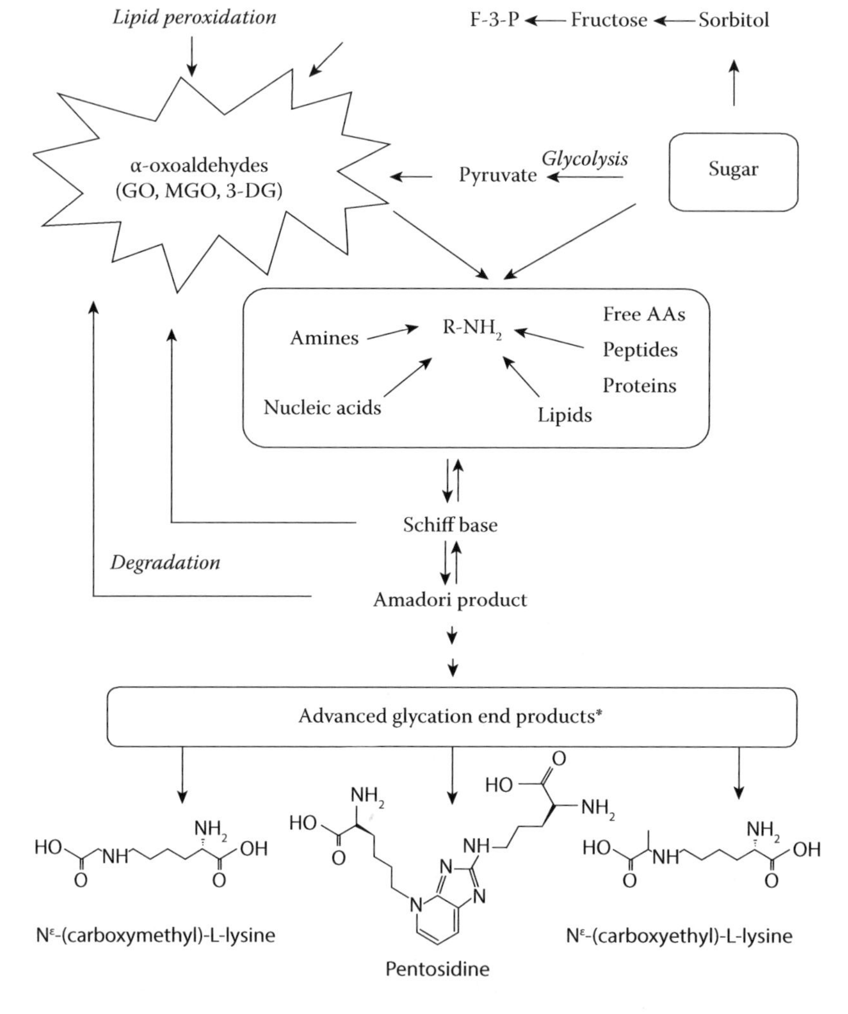

FIGURE 1.1 Simplified scheme of glycation pathways, highlighting the role of alpha-dicarbonyl compounds and the formation of three often determined AGEs: CML, CEL, and pentosidine.

(3-DG) are the key metabolites that act as intermediates of glycation processes as well as the precursors and propagators of AGEs.

It should be stressed that actual physicochemical conditions play a critical role in the formation and progression of AGEs; in particular, alkaline pH favors initial Schiff base formation, whereas rearrangement to Amadori products occurs preferentially at physiological pH. Furthermore, transition metal ions, complex redox equilibria, and, more generally, the increased oxidative stress exert catalytic effect of AGEs generation.

The main feature of AGEs is their structural diversity and their ability for cross-linking the biomolecules. Consequently, relatively few individual compounds have been fully characterized and even fewer have proved their utility as biomarkers of glycation processes or related diseases. Three important compounds from the latter group are N^{ε}-(carboxymethyl)-L-lysine (CML), N^{ε}-(carboxyethyl)-L-lysine (CEL), and pentosidine; their structures are shown in Figure 1.1. On the contrary, glycation processes are capable of modification of proteins, nucleic acids, and lipids (advanced lipoxidation end products, ALEs). Unfortunately, majority of AGEs' cross-links still remain unknown which at least in part is due to their high stability and resistance to typical hydrolysis procedures. In relation to proteins, explorative studies employing proteomics tools are in use for the full characterization of glycation sites and their specific biological roles [5,6]. Finally, the intrinsic aspect of AGE biochemistry is their role in prooxidant and proinflammatory signaling; in this regard, AGE receptors present on the cell surface (RAGE) have been characterized and extensively studied [7]. The discovery of soluble circulating receptors (sRAGE) and their potential in counterbalancing RAGE signaling has triggered new directions in studies of AGEs [8].

1.2 Endogenous and Exogenous AGEs

Maillard reactions take place during food heating that is usually applied for processing, conservation, or may occur during storage of food [9]. A wide range of compounds (MRPs, Maillard reaction products) is generated in the course of heating, depending on the "cooking intensity," specific raw product, water content, pH conditions, etc. [10]. Due to the variety of sugars present in foods, their degradation products, and also different sources of amine groups, structural/functional complexity of MRP is higher as compared to the glycation products generated *in vivo*, specifically when concerning low molecular mass compounds. Food multiple reaction monitoring (MRM) may have positive or negative health effects [11,12]. In particular, unsaturated heterocyclic nitrogenous compounds denominated as melanoidins confer antioxidant and antimicrobial properties and are responsible for the brown color of processed products [13,14]. Food aroma is determined by volatile MRP generated from fragmentation/degradation of sugars (furans, pyrones, and carbonyls) and amino acids (aldehydes and sulfur compounds); these products are further converted in pyrazines and alkylpyrazines [15,16]. On the contrary, some of the MRPs are classified as prooxidant, toxic, and even carcinogenic agents; such is the case of acrylamide [17]. Finally, Maillard reactions in food produce the same AGEs as are generated *in vivo*—among them CML, CEL, and pentosidine [18].

Food AGEs deteriorate bioavailability of free amino acids (lysine, arginine, and histidine) and cause protein cross-linking, thereby affecting the food texture and its digestibility. Furthermore, consumption of AGE-rich diets has been associated with an increase in circulating AGEs and with progression of AGE-related clinical conditions. Noteworthy, it has been demonstrated that restriction of dietary AGEs is helpful in the prevention of diabetes, and vascular and kidney disorders [19].

Based on the above discussion, there is a clear need for the determination of AGEs in food, principally in order to control/lower their daily intake. On the contrary, determination of AGEs that are common for food products and for *in vivo* conditions is highly demanded for the elucidation of the putative role that exogenous AGEs might play in aging, diabetes, and other chronic degenerative diseases [1,18,20]. The three AGEs most studied within this context have been CML, CEL, and pentosidine.

N^{ε}-(carboxymethyl)-L-lysine is produced directly by binding the epsilon amine group of lysine to the electrophilic carbonyl moiety of GO and by the subsequent reduction/oxidation. Owing to the variety of possible sources of GO *in vivo* and during thermal treatment of food and also because CML can be derived from any stage of glycoxidation or from lipoxidation processes, this specific compound has been accepted as a versatile biomarker of formation/accumulation of endogenous and exogenous AGEs. In this regard, extensive database of CML content in a variety of food items had been obtained by means of enzyme-linked immunosorbent assay (ELISA) [19]. It should be highlighted that CML in clinical and food-related samples is present in free form and as bound to proteins, both of which are important and need to be quantitatively evaluated in studies focused on the biological role of AGEs.

When glyoxal is substituted by methylglyoxal in the reaction with lysine, CEL is generated. There are many sources of MGO *in vivo*; it is formed by enzymatic and nonenzymatic reactions from intermediates of glycolysis, during the metabolism of amino acids (glycine and threonine), during lipolysis, and also as an intermediate of glycation reactions. In foods, MGO is formed from sugars, from the intermediates of Maillard reactions, and from lipids. Microbial fermentation applied in food processing or undesirably occurring during storage is an additional source of MGO. CEL is considered as endogenous and exogenous AGE, and it has been determined both in foods and in clinical samples.

Pentosidine is the third AGE often reported in foods and in human tissues; this compound is generated from linking arginine and lysine via pentose molecule, and it is indicative of protein cross-linking by glycation processes.

In the following sections, an overview of the existing determination methodologies is presented with an emphasis on CML, CEL, and pentosidine as the target compounds.

1.3 Determination of AGEs

Measurement of AGEs can be carried out by several approaches, depending on the number of target compounds, their identity, required selectivity, expected concentration, and chemical composition of the sample. The existing methods can be grouped as follows: (1) assays enabling estimation of AGEs based on their native fluorescence, (2) immunochemical methods; (3) determination of individual compounds by highly selective analytical procedures; and (4) explorative studies focused on the structural characterization of new compounds or AGEs cross-links. Procedural tools currently available for the determination of known AGEs are schematically presented in Figure 1.2 and briefly discussed below.

1.3.1 Simple Assays for Fluorescent AGEs

Structural rigidity of AGEs cross-links (mainly via lysine and arginine) is responsible for fluorescent properties of several compounds such as pentosidine, GOLD (glyoxal-derived lysine dimer), MOLD (methylglyoxal-derived dimer), and argypirimidine, pyrraline. Direct fluorimetric measurements provide useful information of cumulative tissue damage by AGEs, but they are unable to quantify individual compounds. On the contrary, these assays are simple with no need for any sophisticated instrumentation or trained analyst, and they can be adopted in routine laboratory control, especially when performed in

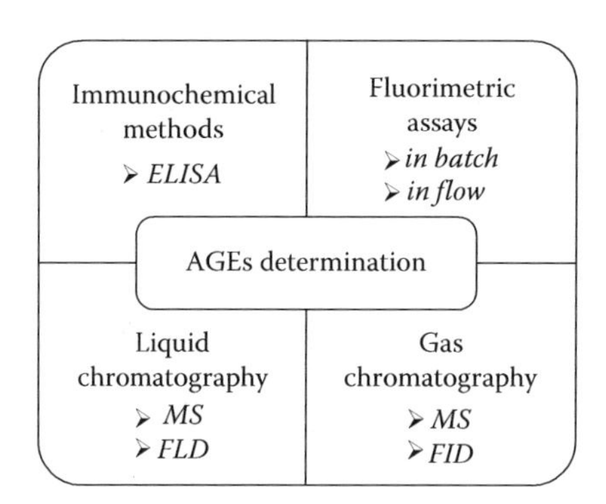

FIGURE 1.2 Currently available tools for measurement of known AGEs.

a flow system or directly in exposed skin. Typically, excitation wavelengths in the range of 350–390 nm are used with fluorescence emission measurement at 440–470 nm; it is recommended to remove lipids from the analyzed sample and potential interferences from naturally fluorescent peptides/protein can be eliminated by signal normalization using sample absorbance acquired at 280 nm [21]. Fluorimetric assays have been preferentially used to assess endogenous AGEs in serum, saliva, or skin [22]. While analyzing biological fluids, AGEs can be evaluated in low and high molecular mass fractions after protein precipitation with trichloroacetic or perchloric acid [21,23,24]. Commercially available AGE reader from DiagnOptics B.V. (Groningen, The Netherlands) was designed for noninvasive measurement of skin auto-fluorescence; relative skin reflectance is also measured by this device in order to compensate for differences in skin pigmentation [25].

Despite obvious convenience of fluorescence assays, it remains uncertain what units should be used to express AGE content, what AGEs are measured, what calibrator should be applied, and how to assure analytical reliability of the obtained results.

1.3.2 Immunochemical Methods

The most common biochemical approach to AGE measurement is based on the ELISA. It had been generally accepted that CML would be the dominant epitope recognized by AGE antibodies (especially those that are polyclonal) [26]; however, over the past two decades, several studies have reported production of antibodies against other specific compounds (MGO-glycated albumin, CEL, pentosidine, among others) that proved their feasibility in the analysis of clinical samples and food items [19,27–29]. Commercial ELISA kits are also available from several international (e.g., OxiSelect™ from Cell Biolabs) or local suppliers. These kits are preferentially used in clinical studies or more generally, when large sample series have to be run and when accurate/precise quantification is not required. Although quite popular and easy to use, ELISA kits present several drawbacks that have often been highlighted in scientific literature [26]. The main problems include uncertain specificity and possible cross-reactivity of the applied antibodies, and a lack of universal and reliable quantification method, which in consequence will hamper the highly demanded direct comparisons of the results obtained in different studies. Furthermore, the assessment of bound AGEs or cross-link structures requires protein digestion. Noteworthy, ELISA results have often been validated by analytical procedures based on chromatographic separation and mass spectrometry detection [18,26,30–32].

1.3.3 Analytical Methods Based on Liquid Chromatography Separations

The principal strength of analytical chemistry procedures relies on their high specificity toward individual compounds and ability for precise and exact determination. The results obtained are expressed directly as the mass of analyte per unit of mass or volume of the initial sample or per protein content; such a quantitative approach is extremely important when concentrations of specific compounds are to be compared among experimental groups, among different analytical procedures or clinical trials, in dose–response studies, and also in the evaluation of dietary intake of exogenous AGEs.

Sample pretreatment is the critical step in AGE analysis. As aforementioned, data regarding free-, bound-, and total AGE content are of interest, and for the second and the third contents, acid or enzymatic protein hydrolysis has to be performed [33]. Typical protocol involves extractive elimination of lipids (hexane and chloroform), reduction in sodium borohydride necessary to prevent artifacts from being oxidatively formed during hydrolysis, protein precipitation, recovery of the pellet, and finally acid or enzymatic hydrolysis [34–38]. For further protection of the samples from oxidation, especially during chemically harsh acid hydrolysis, the tubes are often flushed with nitrogen before being sealed [32]. Finally, the supernatant after protein precipitation can be used for the determination of free AGEs [32,39–41].

For the determination of various compounds in a single analytical run and also for enhanced selectivity, chromatographic separation is usually coupled to a convenient detection system [42,43]. Because AGEs are nonvolatile and individual compounds differ in polarity, high performance liquid chromatography (HPLC) has been preferentially used with the reversed phase- or ion-pair reversed phase separation mode. Several representative examples of HPLC applications in the analysis of clinical and food samples are briefly summarized below and in Table 1.1.

Fluorimetric detection (FLD) with the excitation/emission wavelengths tuned for specific compound(s) offer high selectivity and sensitivity; this detection system is of special interest in the analysis of fluorescent AGEs, such as pentosidine or argypirimidine [44]. Several methods for the determination of these two compounds in blood plasma, urine, human tissues, and food products can be found in the literature. Ion-pair reversed phase separation with mobile phases containing trifluoroacetic acid or heptafluorobutyric acid has usually been reported, and the excitation/emission wavelengths were in the range of 320–330 and 378–385 nm, respectively [44–49]. On the contrary, fluorimetric detection has proved its utility for nonfluorescent AGEs after their suitable pre-column derivatization. Noteworthy, derivatization reaction not only confers a fluorescent tag but also alters physicochemical properties of the original compounds facilitating their chromatographic separation; hence, the selection of derivatizing agent is an important issue. In this regard, ortho-phthal-aldehyde (OPA) is typically used for primary amines with excitation/emission detection wavelengths of 340/455 nm [43], respectively. Another derivatizing agent is 6-aminoquinolyl-N-hydroxysuccinimidyl-carbamate (AQC); it binds to both primary and secondary amines and allows for fluorimetric detection at 230–245/395 nm [50,51]. HPLC-FLD systems have been used for the determination of CML and CEL in clinical and food samples as described in several research articles [43,51–55].

With the advent of instrumental and methodological development of mass spectrometry (MS), liquid chromatography coupled with tandem MS is the gold standard in all areas referred for AGE determination [18,42,56]. Owing to the exceptional selectivity and detection capability of MS, baseline chromatographic separation of the target compounds and their pre-column derivatization are not necessary in this technique. Typically, column effluent is directly introduced to the soft electrospray ionization (ESI) source, and suitable parent ion formed for each compound is selected and fragmented enabling for quantification in MRM or selective reaction monitoring (SRM) mode. Once specific ion transition is established for each analyte, and quantification is based on the intensity of fragment (product) ion. Although product intensity is lower as compared to that of parent ion, the great advantage of MRM relies on the enhanced selectivity toward target species and efficient removal of spectral background with obvious benefits for accuracy and precision. Of note, MRM is especially apposite for routine clinical practice because it can be carried out using triple quadrupole (TQ) or ion trap spectrometers that present low susceptibility to variation of chromatographic conditions, are easy to operate, and allow for ion fragmentations.

Additional strength of MS detection is the use of isotopically enriched target compounds as internal standards (IS). For a given compound, up to eight atoms of less abundant stable isotope of hydrogen (^{2}H), carbon (^{13}C), or nitrogen (^{15}N) can be introduced to the molecule and such prepared IS during the entire procedure behaves identically as the analyte, although it is detected as a separate species. In such an approach, any imprecision committed during sample manipulation is efficiently eliminated as also any ionization suppression/enhancement problem. Typical MRM conditions for CML analysis involve ion transition m/z 205→84 or 205→130 (207→84 for d_2-CML and 209→88 for d_4-CML); ion transitions used for CEL are 219→130 or 219→84 (223→88 for d_4-CML); for pentosidine, 379→135 transition is applied; in each case, mass precision would depend on the resolution capability of a specific instrument [32–41,57–62]. The IS technique not only assures enhanced accuracy and precision but also enables for higher robustness and for the adoption of nonrigorous protocols, an important issue in routine analysis of large series of biological/clinical samples.

Several applications of liquid chromatography—tandem mass spectrometry are briefly summarized in Table 1.1. Pentosidine is a cationic species, CML and CEL are polar compounds, so retention/separation of these AGEs on the reversed phase columns has often been achieved in the presence of ion-pair reagent, typically nonafluoropentanoic acid (NFPA) [32,35–38,40,57,59, 62]. Alternatively, hydrophilic interaction chromatographic columns (HILIC) or silica columns modified with amino groups can also be applied [41,58,61]. Finally, ultra performance liquid chromatography should be mentioned as the effective separation technique in terms of speed, sensitivity, and resolution, which makes it well suited for MS detection [34,35,38,40].

TABLE 1.1

Selected Examples of High Performance Liquid Chromatography-Tandem Mass Spectrometry Procedures (HPLC-MS/MS) for the Determination of Typical AGEs in Clinical and Food Samples

Sample Type	Analytes	Sample Pretreatment	F,B,T	Instrumental Set-up	Quantification	Results	Ref.
Variety of foods	CML CEL MG-H1	R: NaBH4, pH 9.2, 2 hours, room temp. PP: TFA or $CHCl_3$:MeOH (2:1) H: 6N HCl, 24 hours, 110°C Derivatization: 1-butanol:HCl (3:1), 90 minutes, 70°C	B	UPLC-ESI(+)-TQMS/MS	MRM IS: d_2-CML, d_4-CEL, d_3-MG-H1	High-AGEs items: 20–50 mg/kg CML 20–70 mg/kg CEL 0.15–0.60 g/kg MG-H1	[34]
Infant formula, milk, biscuits soybean	Furosine CML CEL	H: 6N HCl, 20 hours, 110°C SPE on HLB cartridge	T	HPLC-ESI(+)-TQMS (ion-pair separation, core shell column)	MRM IS: d_2-CML, d_4-CEL, d_4-Lys	CML: 1.3–44; CEL: 0.3–46; furosine: 10-–639, as mgAGE/100 mg protein	[33]
Processed food, China	CML CEL	LE: n-hexane R: NaBH4, pH 9.2, 12 hours, 4°C PP: TCA H: 6N HCl, 24 hours, 110°C SPE on HLB cartridge with addition of NFPA as ion-pair agent Derivatization: 9-fluorenyl-methyl chloroformate	B	UPLC-ESI(+)-TQMS (ion-pair reversed phase separation)	MRM IS: d_4-CML, d_4-CEL	CML: 2.29–480 mg/kg food CEL: 0.56–107 mg/kg food (Results also presented as mg per kg of protein and mol of Lys).	[38]
Infant gruels	CML CEL	Free water:MeOH (1:3), NFPA addition (pH < 2), centrifugation, SPE on PCX cation exchange cartridge activated with NFPA. H: 6N HCl, 20 hours, 110°C (flushed with N_2), SPE as above.	F, T	HPLC-ESI(+)-TQMS (reversed phase column, no NFPA added)	SRM IS: d_4-CML, d_4-CEL	T CML: 103–408 mg/kg protein; F CML 1,000 × lower. T CML about 3× higher than T CEL.	[32]
Western-style diet	CML	R: NaBH4, pH 9.2, 12 hours, 4°C PP: $CHCl_3$:MeOH (2:1) H: 6N HCl, 20 hours, 110°C SPE on C18 cartridge	B	UPLC-ESI(+)-TQMS (ion-pair reversed phase separation, NFPA)	MRM IS: d_2-CML, d_4-Lys	Data expressed as mg CML per kg of proteins, mol Lys, 100 g food, and per average edible portion	[35]
Raw and cooked meat	pentosidine	PP: TCA Centrifugation and addition of ion-pair agent (heptafluorobutanoic acid)	F	HPLC-ESI(+)-LTQ Orbitrap MS (ion-pair reversed phase separation)	MRM No IS for pentosidine	Pentosidine was not detected in any sample; carnosine, anserine, and homocarnosine determined	[39]

(Continued)

TABLE 1.1 ***(Continued)***

Selected Examples of High Performance Liquid Chromatography-Tandem Mass Spectrometry Procedures (HPLC-MS/MS) for the Determination of Typical AGEs in Clinical and Food Samples

Sample Type	Analytes	Sample Pretreatment	F,B,T	Instrumental Set-up	Quantification	Results	Ref.
Chocolate-flavored drink mixes	CML	Delipidation was not needed R: NaBH4, pH 9.5, 4 hours, room temp. H: 6N HCl, 20 hours, 110°C Clean-up by SPE was not needed	B	HPLC-ESI(+)-LTQMS (porous graphitic carbon stationary phase, NFPA as an ion-pair agent)	MRM IS: d_2-CML	CML: 8.1–131.9 mg/kg powder or 95–3527 mg/kg protein	[36]
Raw and roasted almonds	CML CEL pentosidine pyralline argypirimidine	Free: water extraction of ground almonds, NFPA addition, SPE on Strata-X cartridge preconditioned with NFPA Total: LE with hexane, Hydrolysis with a cocktail of proteolytic enzymes compared with acid hydrolysis (6N HCl, 20 hours, 110°C)	F, T	HPLC-ESI(+)-TQMS (ion-pair reversed phase separation, NFPA)	MRM IS: d_2-CML	Roasted almonds contained higher CML, CEL, and pyralline; the latter accounted for 64.4% of total AGEs. Argypirimidine and pentosidine were not detected.	[57]
Blood plasma	CML	PP: TCA	F	HPLC-ESI(+)-QTMS (NH_2-modified silica column)	MRM IS: d_2-CML	CML in healthy subjects: 10.1–32.6 ng/mL; in diabetic patients: 13.0–44.4 ng/mL	[41]
Human serum (healthy, diabetics)	CML pentosidine	H: 6N HCl, 20 hours, 110°C For pentosidine: SPE on Strata-X cartridge	T	HPLC-ESI(+)-TQMS (HILIC column for CML, PFP column for pentosidine)	MRM IS: d_3-MG-H1, d_2-CML	Mean CML: 0.38 and 2.45 mmol/mol Lys in healthy and diabetic patients; respective values for pentosidine: 1.99 and 2.45 µmol/mol Lys	[58]
Human serum (healthy)	CML CEL	Stabilization cocktail treatment evaluated R: NaBH4, pH 9.2, 12 hours, 4°C PP: TCA H: 6N HCl, 24 hours, 110°C	B	UPLC-ESI(+)-QTMS (ion-pair reversed phase separation, NFPA)	MRM IS: d_2-CML, d_4-CEL	Stabilization/storage did not affect AGEs concentration; CML: 0.135–0.140 mmol/mol Lys; CEL: 56–60 µmol/mol Lys.	[40]
Urine, Feces (young volunteers)	CML	R: NaBH4, pH 9.2, 12 hours, 4°C H: 6N HCl, 24 hours, 110°C	T	HPLC-ESI(+)-LTQMS (ion-pair reversed phase separation, NFPA)	MRM IS: d_2-CML	The results confirmed that CML absorption and fecal excretion is highly influenced by dietary CML levels.	[62]

(Continued)

TABLE 1.1 ***(Continued)***

Selected Examples of High Performance Liquid Chromatography-Tandem Mass Spectrometry Procedures (HPLC-MS/MS) for the Determination of Typical AGEs in Clinical and Food Samples

Sample Type	Analytes	Sample Pretreatment	F,B,T	Instrumental Set-up	Quantification	Results	Ref.
Abdominal skin	CML	Protein extraction buffer contained urea, dithiothreitol, 2-(N-cyclo- hexylamino)-ethanesulfonic acid (pH 9.3, 1 hour, 70°C). H: 6N HCl, 20 hours, 110°C.	T	HPLC-ESI(+)-TOFMS (HILIC column)	none	The technique was used for CML identification in skin proteins.	[61]
Human and rat blood, tissues, urine	Fructosyllysine, MG-H1, G-H1, MOLD, GOLD, DOLD, CEL, CML, Argpyrimidine pentosidine	Free: filtration of plasma and urine Bound: enzymatic digestion of rat tissues, human cells, and blood plasma	F, B	HPLC-ESI(+)-TQMS (two porous graphitized carbon columns in series)	MRM IS: $^{15}N_2$-MG-H1, $^{15}N_2$-3DG-H, $^{15}N_2$ -G-H1, $^{15}N_2$-argpyrimidine d_8-GOLD, d_8-MOLD d_8-DOLD $^{13}C_6$-CEL, $^{13}C_6$-CML, $^{13}C_6$-pentos	Results obtained in different sample types for control and diabetic subjects were comparatively discussed.	[60]
Exhaled breath condensate	CML	A commercial breath condenser was used; after evaporation, the residue was dissolved in water:methanol containing NFPA	F	HPLC-ESI(+)-TQMS (ion-pair reversed phase separation, NFPA)	MRM Synthesized IS: d_4-CML	CML range: 35–110 pg/mL	[59]
Blood plasma	CML CEL	R: NaBH4, pH 9.2, 2 hours, room temp. H: 6N HCl, 20 hours, 110°C	B	HPLC-ESI(+)-TQMS (ion-pair reversed phase separation, NFPA)	MRM IS: d_4-CML, d_4-CEL	Healthy: CML 2.1-3.4 mol/L, CEL 0.5-1.2 mol/L; in dialyzed patients, both AGEs were increased.	[37]

Note: F, free AGE; B, bound AGE; T, total AGE; R, reduction; PP, protein precipitation; H, hydrolysis; LE, lipids extraction; SPE, solid phase extraction; HPLC/UPLC, high/ultra performance liquid chromatography; HILIC, hydrophilic interaction chromatography; PFP, pentafluorophenyl; ESI, electrospray ionization; TQ, triple quadrupole; LTQ, linear ion trap quadrupole; MRM/SRM, multiple/selective reaction monitoring; IS, internal standard; CML, N^{ε}-(carboxymethyl)-L-lysine; CEL, N^{ε}-(carboxyethyl)-L-lysine; MG-H1, N^{δ}-(5-hydro-5-methyl-4-imidazolon-2-yl)-ornithine; G-H1, N^{δ}-(5-hydro-4-imidazolon-2-yl)-ornithine; NFPA, nonafluoropentanoic acid.

1.3.4 Analytical Methods Based on Gas Chromatography Separations

Gas chromatography is an attractive technique due to the simplicity of separation mechanism/conditions, high resolution power, and high tolerance to sample matrix; however, AGEs need to be converted to volatile and thermostable compounds prior to their on-column introduction. There have been only few studies using gas chromatography for the determination of AGEs; food or clinical sample is usually prepared in a similar manner as for liquid chromatography and then free or released AGEs are chemically derivatized. When methanol/thionyl chloride is used under strong acidic conditions, esterification of carboxylic groups by methanol takes place [30,32,63]. At elevated temperature (65°C–70°C), *N-tert*-butyldimethylsilyl-*N*-methyltrifluoroacetamide (MTBSTFA) is reactive toward active hydrogen in functional groups and yields volatile *N-tert*-butyldimethylsilyl (tBDMSi) derivatives of AGEs such as CML or CEL [64]. Alternatively, trifluoroacetyl methyl ester (TFAME) derivatives of CML and CEL can be obtained [65,66]. In some applications, flame ionization detector has been used [64]; however, tandem mass spectrometry with quantification by MRM [30] or by selected ion monitoring (SIM) [63,65,66] offers undisputed advantages.

1.4 MS Tools in Explorative Studies of Glycation Processes

Full understanding of the molecular mechanisms determining the role of AGEs in human aging and diseases calls for the identification/characterization of glycation sites and structures in biomolecules. In this regard, MS-based proteomics techniques are in use owing to their exceptional capability of structural characterization and of quantitative evaluation of such modifications [6,67]. Typically, peptide modifications are detected/characterized in protein digest by means of liquid chromatography coupled via ESI to the high resolution MS, most often using quadrupole-time of flight mass analyzer (HPLC-ESI-QTOFMS) [68] or peptide mapping by matrix-assisted laser desorption/ionization mass spectrometry (MALDI-TOFMS) [69]. Analysis of intact proteins in a top-down approach has also been explored by using high mass accuracy and resolution instruments such as QTOF, Orbitrap, or Fourier transform-ion cyclotron resonance mass spectrometers [70].

Substantial progress has been achieved for individual proteins glycated *in vitro*. Serum albumin, as an abundant and relatively long-lived circulating protein, is an important target of glycation with 59 lysines found to be modified by fructosyllysine/Amadori products or AGEs [71]. Using alpha-dicarbonyl compounds as glycant agents, several AGEs have been identified as modifications of lysine or arginine, among them methylglyoxal-derived N^{δ}-(5-hydro-5-methyl-4-imidazolon-2-yl)-ornithine, glyoxal-derived N^{δ}-(5-hydro-4-imidazolon-2-yl)-ornithine (G-H1); 3-deoxyglucosone-derived N_{ε}-[5-(2,3,4-trihydroxybutyl)-5-hydro-4-imidazolon-2-yl]ornithine (3-DG-H1), CEL, CML [69,71]. Modifications of guanidine group of arginine residues such as tetrahydropyrimidine (THP) or argpyrimidine have also been reported [71,72].

Analysis of protein glycation in the real-world samples is less straightforward because low abundant glycated proteins/peptides have to be separated from the sample. To this end, intact proteins can be analyzed by two-dimensional gel electrophoresis and the glycated protein spots can be in-gel digested prior to LC-MS of MALDI-TOFMS analysis [70]. Otherwise, glycated proteins/peptides can be separated/concentrated by submitting properly prepared sample to boronic acid affinity chromatography; in this technique, retention of glycated species occurs by interaction of tetrahedral anion formed from boronic acid at alkaline pH with 1,2-*cis*-diol groups of modified peptides [6,73].

Comparative evaluation of modification sites/structures found in subjects at different clinical conditions is highly demanded and particularly useful for discovery of new biomarkers for early diagnostics of diabetes and related diseases [73,74]. As an example of relatively simple and high-throughput approach, a mass shift $\Delta m/z = 162$ or its multiplication detected in intact proteins by MALDI-TOFMS is indicative of a single or multiple modification by Amadori product (due to glucose condensation on the protein) and has been used to compare the extent of early glycation in healthy subjects versus those at different stages of diabetes progression [67,75]. Similar MALDI-TOFMS system has also been used to study modifications of hemoglobin in diabetic patients; the results revealed that both β-globin (*m/z* 15866) and α-globin (*m/z* 15126) fractions become glycated and glyco-oxidated [76], which seems to be an additional argument that HBA1c is far from being a perfect biomarker of glucose control in diabetes.

Neutral loss of labile glycation tags can be promptly detected by tandem mass spectrometry; this method has been often used to analyze peptide glycation and to compare the amount of glycated moieties between different clinical samples. With such an approach, modifications of human serum albumin had been examined in healthy individuals, and the reported products were 3DG-H1(the most abundant), G-H1, CML, CEL, pentosidine, and MOLD; the amount of these modifications tended to increase in renal failure patients [60,71].

Despite their crucial importance in human pathologies, structures/sites responsible for protein cross-linking have been studied to a lesser extent as compared to linear AGE modifications such as CML, CEL, G-H1, MG-H1, 3DG-H1, 3-deoxygalactosone-derived hydroimidazolone, and THP. Such studies usually rely on the enzymatic protein digestion, MALDI-TOFMS, or LC-ESI-QTOF tandem mass spectrometry followed by bioinformatic data analysis. As an example, mass-to-charge values corresponding to the sum of two peptides cross-linked by pentosidine, 3-deoxyglucosone-derived imidazolium, and glucosepane-containing species have been detected *in vitro* and in protein extracts from diabetic rats [77,78].

A more detailed description of MS applications in the analysis of protein glycation and comprehensive survey over the real-world applications can be found elsewhere [5,71].

1.5 Conclusions and Future Trends

Accelerated formation, accumulation, and adverse health effects of AGEs have been associated with aging, diabetes, and other degenerative human diseases. AGE measurement is required in clinical practice centered at prevention of related pathologies, their early diagnosis, in the follow-up of patients, and to evaluate the efficiency of the applied therapy/treatment. In this regard, preference has been given to relatively simple, robust, and high-throughput procedures such as fluorimetric assays and ELISA kits. On the contrary, a clear trend of moving toward more reliable, accurate, and precise analytical procedures—specifically those based on liquid chromatography-tandem mass spectrometry—can be noted. It should be stressed that analytical procedures are very effective in the analysis of individual AGEs providing sensitivity and detection power demanded in clinical studies.

Within the context of current discussion regarding possible role of exogenous AGEs in health and disease, these compounds (principally CML) need to be determined in food items. Quantitative data serve for controlling AGE dietary intake and also to establish food processing protocols suitable to obtain healthy products. Similarly as for clinical samples, ELISA kits are mainly in use, but their uncertainty and need for quality control of the results is now widely recognized.

Further progress in the actual knowledge of specific impact of AGEs in humans at least in part relies on structural characterization of glycated biomolecules; in this regard, different techniques and protocols based on MS are gaining strength. In particular, proteomic tools provide identification of specific glycation sites, their chemical structures, as well as enable for their absolute or comparative quantification when comparing different groups/samples.

In future development, commercial production of improved or new simple devices for AGE measurements can be expected. Validation of ELISA results and the use of AGE antibodies produced by unified protocols would be very helpful in both clinical practice and in food control. More emphasis will be given to the explorative studies characterizing nonenzymatic glycation of biomolecules *in vivo*.

ACKNOWLEDGMENT

The financial support from CONACYT (Mexico) projects 178553 and 260373 is gratefully acknowledged.

REFERENCES

1. Singh, R., Barden, A., Mori, T. and Beilin, L. (2001). Advanced glycation end-products: A review. *Diabetologia*. **44**, 129–146.
2. Vistoli, G., De Maddis, D., Cipak, A., Zarkovic, N., Carini, M. and Aldini, G. (2013). Advanced glycoxidation and lipoxidation end products (AGEs and ALEs): An overview of their mechanisms of formation. *Free Radical Res*. **47**(Suppl.1), 3–27.

3. Tessier, J. F. (2010). The Maillard reaction in the human body. The main discoveries and factors that affect glycation. *Pathol Biol.* **58**, 214–219.
4. Gkogkolou, P. and Böhm, M. (2012). Advanced glycation end products: Key players in skin aging? *Dermato-Endocrinol.* **4**, 259–270.
5. Arena, S., Salzano, A. M., Renzone, G., D'Ambrosio, C. and Scaloni, A. (2014). Non-enzymatic glycation and glycoxidation protein products in foods and diseases: An interconnected, complex scenario fully open to innovative proteomic studies. *Mass Spectrom Rev.* **33**, 49–77.
6. Zhang, Q., Ames, J. M., Smith, R. D., Baynes, J. W. and Metz, T. O. (2009). A perspective on the Maillard reaction and the analysis of protein glycation by mass spectrometry: Probing the pathogenesis of chronic disease. *J Proteome Res.* **8**, 754–769.
7. Ott, C., Jacobs, K., Haucke, E., Navarrete Santos, A., Grune, T. and Simm, A. (2014). Role of advanced glycation end products in cellular signaling. *Redox Biol.* **2**, 411–429.
8. Fujisawa, K., Katakami, N., Kaneto, H., Naka, T., Takahara, M., Sakamoto, F., Irie, Y., et al. (2013). Circulating soluble RAGE as a predictive biomarker of cardiovascular event risk in patients with type 2 diabetes. *Atherosclerosis.* **227**, 425–428.
9. Hellwig, M. and Henle, T. (2014). Baking, ageing, diabetes: A short history of the Maillard reaction. *Angew Chem Int Ed Engl.* **53**, 10316–10329.
10. Markowicz Bastos, D. H. and Gugliucci, A. (2015). Contemporary and controversial aspects of the Maillard reaction products. *Curr Opin Food Sci.* **1**, 13–20.
11. Markowicz Bastos, D., Monaro, E., Siguemoto, E. and Séfora, M. (2012). Maillard reaction Products in processed food: Pros and Cons. In: *Food Industrial Processes: Methods and Equipment*, Valdez, B. (Ed.). *InTech.* Available from: http://www.intechopen.com/books/food-industrial-processes-methods-and-equipment/maillard-reaction-products-in-processed-food-pros-and-cons.
12. Toda, M., Heilmann, M., Ilchmann, A. and Vieths, S. (2013). The Maillard reaction and food allergies: Is there a link? *Clin Chem Lab Med.* **52**, 61–67.
13. Delgado-Andrade, C. (2013). Maillard reaction products: Some considerations on their health effects. *Clin Chem Lab Med.* **52**, 53–60.
14. Morales, F. J., Somoza, V. and Fogliano, V. (2011). Physiological relevance of dietary melanoidins. *Amino Acids.* **42**, 1097–1109.
15. Mottram, D. S. (2007). The Maillard reaction: Source of flavour in thermally processed foods. In *Flavours and Fragrances*, Berger, R.G. (Ed.), pp. 269–283. Springer, Berlin.
16. van Boekel, M. A. J. S. (2006). Formation of flavour compounds in the Maillard reaction. *Biotechnol Adv.* **24**, 230–233.
17. Lineback, D. R., Coughlin, J. R. and Stadler, R. H. (2012). Acrylamide in foods: A review of the science and future considerations. *Annu Rev Food Sci Technol.* **3**, 15–35.
18. Poulsen, M. W., Hedegaard, R. V., Andersen, J. M., de Courten, B., Bügel, S., Nielsen, J., Skibsted, L. H. and Dragsted, L. O. (2013). Advanced glycation endproducts in food and their effects on health. *Food Chem Toxicol.* **60**, 10–37.
19. Uribarri, J., Woodruff, S., Goodman, S., Cai, W., Chen, X., Pyzik, R., Yong, A., Striker, G. E. and Vlassara, H. (2010). Advanced glycation end products in foods and a practical guide to their reduction in the diet. *J Am Diet Assoc.* **110**, 911–916.
20. Lapolla, A., Traldi, P. and Fedel, D. (2005). Importance of measuring products of non-enzymatic glycation of proteins. *Clin Biochem.* **38**, 103–115.
21. Wrobel, K., Wrobel, K., Garay-Sevilla, M. E., Nava, L. E. and Malacara, J. M. (1997). Novel analytical approach to monitoring advanced glycosylation end products in human serum with on-line spectrophotometric and spectrofluorometric detection in a flow system. *Clin Chem.* **43**, 1563–1569.
22. Garay-Sevilla, M. E., Regalado, J. C., Malacara, J. M., Nava, L. E., Wrobel, K., Castro-Rivas, A. and Wrobel, K. (2005). Advanced glycosylation end products in skin, serum, saliva and urine and its association with complications of patients with type 2 diabetes mellitus. *J Endocrinol Invest.* **28**, 223–230.
23. Sharp, P. S., Rainbow, S. and Mukherjee, S. (2003). Serum levels of low molecular weight advanced glycation end products in diabetic subjects. *Diab Med.* **20**, 575–579.
24. Münch, G., Keis, R., Wessel, A., Riederer, P., Bahner, U., Heidland, A., Niwa, T., Lemke, H. D. and Schnizel, R. (1997). Determination of advanced glycation end products in serum by fluorescence spectroscopy and competitive ELISA. *Eur J Clin Chem Clin Biochem.* **35**, 669–677.

25. Mulder, D. J., Van De Water, T., Ludgers, H. L., Graaf, R., Gans, R. O., Zijlstra, F. and Smit, A. J. (2006). Skin autofluorescence, a novel marker for glycemic and oxidative stress-derived advanced glycation endproducts: An overview of current clinical studies, evidence, and limitations. *Diabetes Technol Ther.* **8**, 523–535.
26. Onorato, J. M., Thorpe, S. R. and Bayens, J. W. (1998). Immunohistochemical and ELISA assays for biomarkers of oxidative stress in aging and disease. *Ann N Y Acad Sci.* **854**, 277–290.
27. Nagai, R., Fujiwara, Y., Mera, K., Yamagata, K., Sakashita, N. and Takeya, M. (2008). Immunochemical detection of N^{ε}-(carboxyethyl)lysine using a specific antibody. *J Immunol Methods.* **332**, 112–120.
28. Sanaka, T., Funaki, T., Tanaka, T., Hoshi, S., Niwyama, J., Taitoh, T., Nishimura, H. and Higuchi, C. (2002). Plasma pentosidine levels measured by a newly developed method using ELISA in patients with chronic renal failure. *Nephron.* **91**, 64–73.
29. Makita, Z., Vlassara, H., Cerami, A. and Bucala, R. (1992). Immunochemical detection of advanced glycosylation end products *in vivo*. *J Biol Chem.* **267**, 5133–5138.
30. Chaissou, A., Ait-Ameur, L. and Birlouez-Aragon, I. (2007). Evaluation of gas chromatography/mass spectrometry method for the quantification of carboxymethyllysine in food samples. *J Chromatogr A.* **1140**, 189–194.
31. Goldberg, T., Cai, W., Peppa, M., Dardaine, V., Baliga, B. S., Uribarri, J. and Vlassara, H. (2004). Advanced glycoxidation end products in commonly consumed foods. *J Am Diet Assoc.* **104**, 1287–1291.
32. Tareke, E., Forslund, A., Lindh, C. H., Fahlgren, C. and Östman, E. (2013). Isotope dilution ESI-LC-MS/MS for quantification of free and total Ne-(1-Carboxymethyl)-L-Lysine and free Ne-(1-Carboxyethyl)-L-Lysine: Comparison of total Ne-(1-Carboxymethyl)-L-Lysine levels measured with new method to ELISA assay in gruel samples. *Food Chem.* **141**, 4253–4259.
33. Troise, A. D., Fiore, A., Wiltafsky, M. and Fogliano, V. (2015). Quantification of Ne-(2-Furoylmethyl)-L-lysine (furosine), Ne-(Carboxymethyl)-L-lysine (CML), Ne-(Carboxyethyl)-L-lysine (CEL) and total lysine through stable isotope dilution assay and tandem mass spectrometry. *Food Chem.* **188**, 357–364.
34. Scheijen, J. L. J. M., Clevers, E., Engelen, L., Dagnelie, P. C., Brouns, F., Stehouwer, C. D. A. and Schalkwijk, C. G. (2016). Analysis of advanced glycation endproducts in selected food items by ultra-performance liquid chromatography tandem mass spectrometry: Presentation of a dietary AGE database. *Food Chem.* **190**, 1145–1150.
35. Hull, G. L. J., Woodside, J. V., Ames, J. M. and Cuskelly, G. J. (2012). Nε-(carboxymethyl)lysine content of foods commonly consumed in a Western style diet. *Food Chem.* **131**, 170–174.
36. Niquet-Léridon, C. and Tessier, J. F. (2011). Quantification of Ne-carboxymethyl-lysine in selected chocolate-flavoured drink mixes using high-performance liquid chromatography–linear ion trap tandem mass spectrometry. *Food Chem.* **126**, 655–663.
37. Teerlink, T., Barto, R., ten Brink, H. J. and Schalkwijk, C. G. (2004). Measurement of N-(Carboxymethyl) lysine and N-(Carboxyethyl)lysine in human plasma protein by stable-isotope-dilution tandem mass spectrometry. *Clin Chem.* **50**, 1222–1228.
38. Zhou, Y., Lin, Q., Jin, C., Cheng, L., Zheng, X., Dai, M. and Zhang, Y. (2015) Simultaneous analysis of Nε-(carboxymethyl)lysine and Nε-(carboxyethyl)lysine in foods by ultra-performance liquid chromatography-mass spectrometry with derivatization by 9-fluorenylmethyl chloroformate. *J Food Sci.* **80**, C207–C217.
39. Peiretti, P. G., Medana, C., Visentin, S., Dal Bello, F. and Me, G. (2012). Effect of cooking method on carnosine and its homologues, pentosidine and thiobarbituric acid-reactive substance contents in beef and turkey meat. *Food Chem.* **132**, 80–85.
40. Hull, G. L. J., Woodside, J. V., Ames, J. M. and Cusk, G. J. (2013). Validation study to compare effects of processing protocols on measured Nε-(carboxymethyl)lysine and Nε-(carboxyethyl)lysine in blood. *J Clin Biochem Nutr.* **53**, 129–133.
41. Kuang, L., Jing, Z., Wang, J., Ma, L., Liu, X. and Yang, J. (2014) Quantitative determination of e-N-carboxymethyl-L-lysine in human plasma by liquid chromatography–tandem mass spectrometry. *J Pharm Biomed Anal.* **90**, 1–6.
42. Vogeser, M. and Seger, C. (2008). A decade of HPLC–MS/MS in the routine clinical laboratory—Goals for further developments. *Clin Biochem.* **41**, 649–662.
43. Ames, J. M. (2008). Determination of Nε-(Carboxymethyl)lysine in foods and related systems. *Ann N Y Acad Sci.* **1126**, 20–24.

44. Scheijen, J. L. J. M., van de Waarenburg, M. P. H., Stehouwer, C. D. A. and Schalkwijk, C. G. (2009). Measurement of pentosidine in human plasma protein by a single-column high-performance liquid chromatography method with fluorescence detection. *J Chromatogr B.* **877**, 610–614.
45. Mikulikova, K., Eckhardt, A., Kunes, J., Zicha, J. and Miksik, I. (2008) Advanced glycation end-product pentosidine accumulates in various tissues of rats with high fructose intake. *Physiol Res.* **57**, 89–94.
46. Gomes, R., Sousa Silva, M., Quintas, A., Cordeiro, C., Freire, A., Pereira, P., Martins, A., Monteiro, E., Barboso, E. and Ponces Freire, A. (2005). Argpyrimidine, a methylglyoxal-derived advanced glycation end-product in familial amyloidotic polyneuropathy. *Biochem J.* **385**, 339–345.
47. Wilker, S. C., Chellan, P., Arnold, B. M. and Nagaraj, R. H. (2001) Chromatographic quantification of argpyrimidine, a methylglyoxal-derived product in tissue proteins: Comparison with pentosidine. *Anal Biochem.* **290**, 353–358.
48. Spacek, P. and Adam, M. (2006). Pentosidine in osteoarthritis: HPLC determination in body fluids and in tissues. *Rheumatol Int.* **26**, 923–927
49. Henle, T., Schwarzenbolz, U. and Klostermeyer, H. (1997). Detection and quantification of pentosidine in foods. *Z Lebensm Unters Forsch A.* **204**, 95–98.
50. Ahmed, N., Agirov, O. K., Minhas, H. S., Cordeiro, C. A. and Thornalley, P. J. (2002). Assay of advanced glycation endproducts (AGEs): Surveying AGEs by chromatographic assay with derivatization by 6-aminoquinolyl-N-hydroxysuccinimidyl-carbamate and application to Nepsilon-carboxymethyl-lysine- and Nepsilon-(1-carboxyethyl)lysine-modified albumin. *Biochem J.* **364**, 1–14.
51. Ahmed, N. and Thornalley, P. J. (2002). Chromatographic assay of glycation adducts in human serum albumin glycated *in vitro* by derivatization with 6-aminoquinolyl-N-hydroxysuccinimidyl-carbamate and intrinsic fluorescence. *Biochem J.* **364**, 15–24.
52. Friess, U., Waldner, M., Wahl, H. G., Lehmann, R., Haring, H. U., Voelter, U. and Schleicher, E. (2003). Liquid chromatography-based determination of urinary free and total N(epsilon)-(carboxymethyl)lysine excretion in normal and diabetic subjects. *J Chromatogr B.* **794**, 273–280.
53. Chen, G. and Smith, J. S. (2015). Determination of advanced glycation endproducts in cooked meat products. *Food Chem.* **168**, 190–195.
54. Mildner-Szkudlarz, S., Siger, A., Szwengiel, A. and Bajerska, J. (2015). Natural compounds from grape by-products enhance nutritive value and reduce formation of CML in model muffins. *Food Chem.* **172**, 78–85.
55. Fujiwara, Y., Kiyota, N., Tsurushima, K., Yoshitomi, M., Mera, K., Sakashita, N., Takeya, M., et al. (2011). Natural compounds containing a catechol group enhance the formation of Nε-(carboxymethyl) lysine of the Maillard reaction. *Free Radic Biol Med.* **50**, 883–891.
56. Thornalley, P. J. and Rabbani, N. (2014). Detection of oxidized and glycated proteins in clinical samples using mass spectrometry—A user's perspective. *Biochim Biophys Acta.* **1840**, 818–829.
57. Zhang, G., Huang, G., Xiao, L. and Mitchell, A. E. (2011). Determination of advanced glycation endproducts by LC-MS/MS in raw and roasted almonds (*Prunus dulcis*). *J Agric Food Chem.* **59**, 12037–12046.
58. Kerkeni, M., Santos Weiss, I., Jaisson, S., Dandana, A., Addad, F., Gillery, P. and Hammami, M. (2014). Increased serum concentrations of pentosidine are related to presence and severity of coronary artery disease. *Thromb Res.* **134**, 633–638.
59. Gonzalez-Reche, L. M., Kucharczyk, A., Musiol, A. K. and Kraus, T. (2006). Determination of Ne-(carboxymethyl)lysine in exhaled breath condensate using isotope dilution liquid chromatography/electrospray ionization tandem mass spectrometry. *Rapid Commun Mass Spectrom.* **20**, 2747–2752.
60. Thornalley, P. J., Battah, S., Ahmed, N., Karachalias, N., Agalou, S., Babaei-Jadidi, R. and Dawnay, A. (2003). Quantitative screening of advanced glycation endproducts in cellular and extracellular proteins by tandem mass spectrometry. *Biochem J.* **375**, 581–592.
61. Kawabata, K., Yoshikawa, H., Saruwatari, K., Akazawa, Y., Inoue, T., Kuze, T., Sayo, T., Uchida, N. and Sugiyama, Y. (2011). The presence of Nε-(Carboxymethyl) lysine in the human epidermis. *Biochim Biophys Acta.* **1814**, 1246–1252.
62. Delgado-Andrade, C., Tessier, F. J., Niquet-Leridon, C., Seiquer, I. and Navarro, M. P. (2012). Study of the urinary and faecal excretion of Ne-carboxymethyllysine in young human volunteers. *Amino Acids.* **43**, 595–602.
63. Wang, J., Tian, S. L., Sun, W. H., Lin, H. and Li, Z. X. (2015). Determination of Nε-carboxymethyl-lysine content in muscle tissues of turbot by gas chromatography-mass spectrometry. *Chin J Anal Chem.* **43**, 1187–1192.

64. Bosch, L., Sanz, M. L., Montilla, A., Alegrıa, A., Farre, R. and del Castillo, M. D. (2007). Simultaneous analysis of lysine, Ne-carboxymethyllysine and lysinoalanine from proteins. *J Chromatogr B.* **860**, 69–77.
65. Ahmed, M. U., Brinkmann Frye, E., Degenhardt, T. P., Thorpe, S. R. and Baynes, J. W. (1997). Ne-(Carboxyethyl)lysine, a product of the chemical modification of proteins by methylglyoxal, increases with age in human lens proteins. *Biochem J.* **324**, 565–570.
66. Mesías, M., López Pérez, N., Guerra-Hernández, E. and García-Villanova, B. (2010). Determination of carboximetillysine in toasted and baked foods. *ARS Pharmaceutica.* **51**, 23–29.
67. Lapolla, A., Molin, L. and Traldi, P. (2013). Protein glycation in diabetes as determined by mass spectrometry. *Int J Endocrinol.* **2013**, 412103.
68. Lapolla, A., Fedele, D., Reitano, R., Aricòa, N. C., Seraglia, R., Traldi, P., Marotta, E. and Tonani, R. (2004). Enzymatic digestion and mass spectrometry in the study of advanced glycation end products/peptides. *J Am Mass Spectrom.* **15**, 496–509.
69. Barnaby, O. S., Cerny, R. L., Clarke, W. and Hage, D. S. (2011). Comparison of modification sites formed on human serum albumin at various stages of glycation. *Clin Chim Acta.* **412**, 277–285.
70. Colzani, M., Aldini, G. and Carini, M. (2013). Mass spectrometric approaches for the identification and quantification of reactive carbonyl species protein adducts. *J Proteom.* **92**, 28–50.
71. Anguizola, J., Matsuda, R., Barnaby, O. S., Hoy, K. S., Wa, C., DeBolt, E., Koke, M. and Hage, D. S. (2013). Review: Glycation of human serum albumin. *Clin Chim Acta.* **425**, 64–76.
72. Ahmed, N., Dobler, D., Dean, M. and Thornalley, P. J. (2005). Peptide mapping identifies hotspot site of modification in human serum albumin by methylglyoxal involved in ligand binding and esterase activity. *J Biol Chem.* **280**, 5724–5732.
73. Zhang, Q., Tang, N., Schepmoes, A. A., Phillips, L. S., Smith, R. D. and Metz, T. O. (2008). Proteomic profiling of nonenzymatically glycated proteins in human plasma and erythrocyte membranes. *J Proteom Res.* **7**, 2025–2032.
74. Frolov, A., Bluher, M. and Hoffmann, R. (2014). Glycation sites of human plasma proteins are affected to different extents by hyperglycemic conditions in type 2 diabetes mellitus. *Anal Bioanal Chem.* **406**, 5755–5763.
75. Lapolla, A., Fedele, D., Seraglia, R., Catinella, S., Baldo, L., Aronica, R. and Traldi, P. (2005). A new effective method for the evaluation of glycated intact plasma proteins in diabetic subjects. *Diabetologia.* **38**, 1076–1081.
76. Hempe, J. M., Gomez, R., McCarter, R. J. and Chalew, S. A. (2002). High and low hemoglobin glycation phenotypes in type 1 diabetes: A challenge for interpretation of glycemic control. *J Diabetes Complicat.* **16**, 313–320.
77. Dai, Z., Wang, B., Sun, G., Fan, X., Anderson, V. E. and Monnier, V. M. (2008). Identification of glucose-derived cross-linking sites in ribonuclease A. *J Proteome Res.* **7**, 2756–2768.
78. Shao, C. H., Capek, H. L., Patel, K. P., Wang, M., Tang, K., DeSouza, C., Nagai, R., Mayhan, W., Periasamy, M. and Bidasee, K. R. (2011). Carbonylation contributes to SERCA2a activity loss and diastolic dysfunction in a rat model of type 1 diabetes. *Diabetes.* **60**, 947–959.

2

How AGEs Cause Disease: Cellular Mechanisms

Melinda M. Nugent and John C. He
Icahn School of Medicine at Mount Sinai
New York, NY

CONTENTS

KEY POINTS

- Advanced glycation end products (AGEs) induce receptor-independent effects via cross-link formation with extracellular matrix, signaling molecules, and DNA.
- AGEs also have receptor-dependent effects that lead to activation of signaling pathways that increase cytokine secretion and generate reactive oxygen species.
- Glyoxylase I negatively regulates AGEs by removing them from cells and preventing them from modifying proteins.
- Activation of certain AGE receptors prevents AGE accumulation, but in disease conditions, activation of other types of AGE receptors activates inflammatory pathways.
- AGE–RAGE (receptor for advanced glycation end products) interaction has been implicated in the disease pathogenesis in the renal, cardiac, vascular, reproductive, and nervous systems.

2.1 Introduction

Although many studies on advanced glycation end products (AGEs) have been published, the exact cellular and molecular mechanisms of AGEs in disease pathogenesis remain unclear. AGEs can be generated extracellularly or intracellularly.[1] Their deleterious effects can be broken into two main categories: receptor-independent effects with cross-link formation or receptor-dependent effects via interaction with its receptor for advanced glycation end products (RAGE). Several intracellular signaling pathways induced by AGEs have been described, but it is unclear how AGE receptors interact with the intracellular signaling molecules. Extracellular AGEs can bind to AGE receptors to induce cellular signaling pathways while intracellular AGEs may directly modify signaling molecules in the cells. AGEs are known to activate several transcription factors including NF-κB and STAT3. Here, we will review the studies which demonstrate cellular and molecular mechanisms by which AGEs induce pathological processes that lead to amplification and maintenance of tissue injury and progression of disease in multiple organ systems (Figure 2.1).

2.2 AGE Cross-Links

2.2.1 Cross-Link with Matrix Proteins

AGE cross-links contribute to atherosclerosis, myocardial dysfunction, nephropathy, neuropathy, cataracts, and retinopathy. In addition to trapping macromolecules, AGE cross-links alter the structural and functional properties of proteins including those in the extracellular matrix and glomerular basement membranes.[2,3] Once proteins form a cross-link with AGEs, they become less susceptible to proteolytic degradation because of protease resistance and suppression of metalloproteinase expression.[4] In total, 0.1–1% of lysine and arginine residues on proteins are affected by glycation,[5,6] which leads to a change in charge that modifies protein structure and leads to protein aggregation such as in cataract formation.[7,8] Glycation also affects protein function by creating a physical hindrance when they bind amino acid residues at sites of substrate binding or allosteric regulation on enzymes.[9] For example, glycated residues in integrin-binding sites of collagen cause endothelial cell detachment because of abnormal cell–extracellular matrix interactions.[10]

2.2.2 Cross-Link with Signaling Molecules and DNA

In addition to extracellular cross-linking, AGEs modify intracellular organelles and intracellular molecules, including lipids, signaling molecules, and DNA.[11] Glycation of lipids compromises lipid membrane integrity and fluidity.[12] It can even cause lipid peroxidation, which leads to oxidative damage.[13]

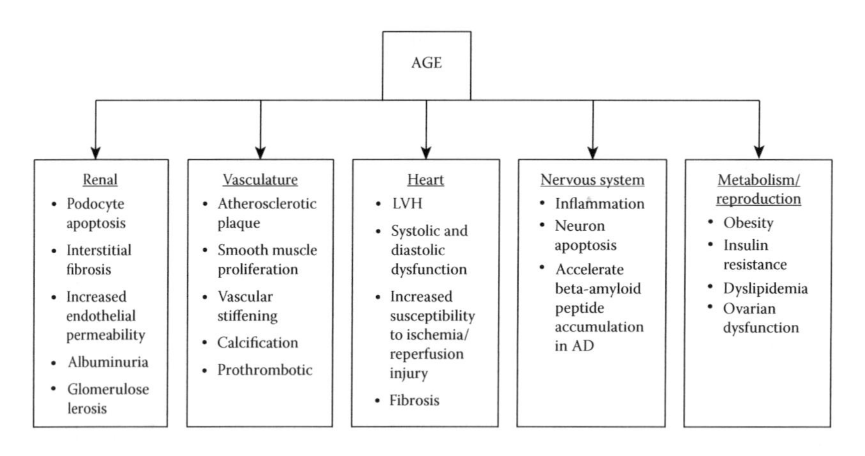

FIGURE 2.1 AGE effects on different organ systems.

DNA glycation contributes to aging and is increased in diabetics.[14] Glyoxal (G) and methylglyoxal (MG) are reactive dicarbonyl intermediates of endogenous glycation that are increased in the plasma and urine of patients with diabetes and even more so in those with diabetic nephropathy.[15,16] G and MG react with deoxyguanosine residues of DNA to form nucleotide advanced glycation end products.[17] Normally, glycated nucleosides are removed from DNA by excision repair. When there is an imbalance in glycation production and removal, the resulting glycated DNA adversely affects the genome integrity and is associated with DNA single strand breaks, unwinding of the double helix and increased mutation frequencies.[18,19–22] Glycated DNA also impairs transcription by preventing binding of transcription factors.[23]

2.3 Negative Regulators of AGE Reaction

2.3.1 Role of Glyoxalase I

Under normal conditions, antiglycation systems are enough to prevent damage due to glycation. Proteasomes and lysosomes prevent accumulation of glycated proteins[24] while nucleotide excision removes glycated nucleotides.[25] When there is an imbalance in AGE production and removal, glycation damage ensues. The role of these antiglycation systems is illuminated in studies of glyoxalase 1 (Glo1), which minimizes the DNA damage induced by G and MG by removing them from the cell.[20,26] There is decreased expression and activity of Glo1 in the kidneys of rodent models with streptozotocin-induced DM.[27–29] Knockdown of Glo1 in nondiabetic mice leads to MG modification of glomerular proteins and oxidative stress that causes kidney pathology that mirrors diabetic nephropathy.[30] Overexpression of Glo1 prevents posttranslational modification of proteins by MG and prevents hyperglycemia-induced oxidative stress in cells and mice. In diabetic mice, Glo1 overexpression prevents diabetes-induced increases in MG modification of glomerular proteins and prevents increases in oxidative stress and the development of diabetic nephropathy.[30]

There is conflicting data about the role of Glo1 in cancer and whether its upregulation in cancer is a cause of tumor growth or is a response to increased glycated DNA adducts in tumor cells. Overexpression of Glo1 correlates with multidrug-resistant tumors.[31] Upregulation of this enzyme system may allow tumor growth by preventing a rise in MG accumulation and, therefore, preventing the subsequent apoptosis from DNA glycation.[31] But studies also show that tumor cells high in Glo1 expression have higher levels of DNA glycation adducts than those with lower expression. There is a chance that Glo1 expression increases in response to the high MG levels.[18,32]

2.3.2 Role of Superoxide

The role of mitochondrial superoxide in forming intracellular AGE was underscored in a study where inhibitors of various parts of the electron transport chain were each able to prevent hyperglycemia-induced formation of intracellular AGEs.[33] Glycation within mitochondria affects the matrix, phospholipids, outer and inner mitochondrial membranes, and mitochondrial DNA. Increasing removal of AGEs by administering aminoguanidine or overexpressing Glo1 decreased glycation and oxidative damage, restored complex III activity, and improved respiration in experimental models of diabetes.[34,35] In nematodes, increasing Glo1 expression led to decreased mitochondrial levels of AGEs and increased lifespan. Conversely, inhibiting Glo1 in nematodes increased MG levels and reduced lifespan.[36] Treating isolated mitochondria from rat kidney with MG led to decreased oxygen consumption by mitochondria. Treatment of cells with MG or G decreased mitochondrial membrane potential, reduced activity of respiratory chain complexes, reduced ATP synthesis, but increased production of reactive oxygen species.[20] The mitochondrion, itself, is involved in AGE production while its components can be adversely affected by AGEs.

2.4 Receptors of AGE

Several AGE receptors or binding proteins have been identified including RAGE; AGE-R1, R2, and R3; and scavenger receptors. AGE receptors are found on vascular, renal, hematopoietic, and neuronal glial cells. They regulate AGE uptake and removal but are also involved in signal transduction that leads to production of ROS, and release of cytokines and growth factors.[37] Under healthy conditions, certain AGE receptors prevent AGE accumulation, but in disease states, other types of AGE receptors can actually contribute to the inflammatory environment.

2.4.1 Receptor for AGE

The most well-known AGE receptor is the receptor for AGE (RAGE) which is a signal-transducing peptide.[37] The RAGE gene is highly evolutionarily conserved across multiple species, including humans, pigs, rats, and mice. The human RAGE gene is on chromosome 6 in the major histocompatibility complex. It has a NF-κB site, an interferon-gamma response element, and an NF-κB interleukin-6 DNA-binding motif in the RAGE promoter. RAGE is a multi-ligand receptor that is part of the immunoglobulin superfamily of surface receptors.[38] Full length human RAGE consists of 404 amino acids and is 45–50 kilodaltons depending on its N-linked glycosylation state. It is a signal transduction receptor that contains transmembrane, cytosolic, and extracellular domains. The extracellular domain contains a signaling sequence that targets it to the cell membrane and a V-type immunoglobulin domain which is where ligand binding occurs.[39] There is a transmembrane domain with one hydrophobic helix. The intracellular domain has a 42 amino acid cytoplasmic tail that plays a significant role in RAGE-mediated signaling and RAGE function.[39,40] Some studies suggest that RAGE needs to form dimers and multimers in order for ligand binding to occur.[41,42]

In early development, RAGE is highly expressed at mRNA and protein levels, but in healthy adulthood, RAGE expression is generally downregulated in all tissues except in the lung. Unlike the majority of receptor-ligand axis feedback systems in which excess ligand leads to downregulation of receptor, AGE–RAGE interaction is actually a positive feedback loop. In disease or physiologic stress, there is an accumulation of AGE with resultant increased AGE–RAGE interaction leading to upregulation of RAGE gene expression.[43–46] This has been observed in multiple tissues and cell types, including heart; lung; skeletal muscle; vessel wall; ovaries; and immune cells such as monocytes, macrophages, and lymphocytes.[43,45–47]

In addition to interacting with AGE, RAGE also binds non-AGE ligands which are structurally distinct from one another, yet are all involved in proinflammatory pathways, thus earning its classification as a pattern-recognition receptor. One example is B-amyloid peptide which accumulates in Alzheimer's disease and binds RAGE.[48] Another ligand is amphoterin or high mobility group box 2 which binds RAGE in developing neurons and is involved in migration and outgrowth.[49] In tumor cells, amphoterin interaction with RAGE augments cell migration, invasion, and proliferation.[50] RAGE also binds S100 calgranulin proteins and B2-integrin Mac-1.[51,52] A more detailed description of RAGE is also found in another chapter of this book.

2.4.2 AGE Receptor-1

Cell-associated AGE-specific receptors (AGE-Rs) modulate cell activation and cell proliferation. AGE-R1 (OST-48) is a 48kd, type I integral membrane protein with a short extracellular N-terminal domain, a single transmembrane segment, and a cytoplasmic C-terminal domain.[37] While RAGE expression is enhanced in disease states associated with high AGE, AGE-R1 expression is suppressed in mesangial cells and inflammatory cells in diabetic mice and diabetic patients who have high AGE levels and severe nephropathy.[53] Exposure to high levels of AGEs induces MC phenotypic changes; AGE-activated MCs secrete cytokine growth factor and overproduce extracellular matrix, contributing to the progression of glomerulosclerosis.[53,54]

2.4.3 AGE Receptor-2

AGE-R2, initially called 80K-H protein, is a phosphorylation substrate for protein kinase C (PKC). Although its functions are not well understood, AGE-R2 is expressed in vascular endothelial cells and kidney cells and may play a role in diabetic complications.[55,56]

2.4.4 AGE Receptor-3

A member of the lectin family, AGE-3 was first named Mac-2 and was first found on the cell surface of activated macrophages.[57] Later, its name was changed to galectin-3. Its molecular weight is 32 kDa, and it is part of the AGE-R complex and has a high binding affinity for AGE ligands.[58,59] Binding of AGE to AGE-3's C-terminal carbohydrate recognition domain leads to the formation of a high molecular weight complex with other receptor molecules.[59] Since AGE-3 lacks a transmembrane domain, it is hypothesized that the protein secures its position on the cell surface by associating with other AGE receptors.[59] Studies suggest that AGE-R3/galectin-3 protein is involved in cell migration and adhesion, immune response modulation, and growth and differentiation.[58,59]

2.4.5 Scavenger Receptors

The scavenger receptor class A (SR-A) is made up of trimeric transmembrane glycoproteins with a molecular weight of 220 kDa, which consists of five or six different domains. There is an N-terminal cytoplasmic domain, a transmembrane domain, a spacer region, an α-helical coiled coil motif, a collagen-like triple helix, and a C-terminal domain.[60] When SR-A binds oxidized LDL or acetylated LDL, it promotes its endocytic uptake in macrophages.[61] SR-A is also an AGE-binding receptor that mediates the endocytic uptake and degradation of AGE-modified proteins that compete with LDL for binding sites.[62] Considering that foam cells come from macrophages and that SR-A are mainly expressed on these cells, the fact that their SR-As bind AGEs may be an important clue in further understanding how atherosclerosis develops. Scavenger receptor class B (SR-B) includes CD36 and SR-BI, which have also been identified as AGE receptors; in cell culture, AGE-modified BSA binding to CD36 and SR-BI led to endocytic uptake of AGEs.[63,64] Studies show that binding of AGE to SR-B1 inhibited selective HDL uptake, thus supporting the role of SR-B1 in cholesterol metabolism.[64] CD36 was described on mouse 3T3-L1 cells and human subcutaneous adipocytes, which recognized AGE-modified BSA undergoing endocytic degradation.[65] Incubation of these cells with AGE-modified BSA induced intracellular oxidative stress and led to leptin downregulation which worsened insulin sensitivity *in vivo*.[66] As an AGE receptor, there is mounting evidence that CD36 has a role in diabetic complications and atherosclerosis.

2.5 AGE-Induced Intracellular Signaling Pathway

Each of the AGE receptors is known to induce distinct intracellular signaling pathways. Downstream effects of RAGE activation include a myriad of signaling pathways involved in perpetuating inflammation and toxicity by increasing cytokine secretion and generation of reactive oxygen species (Figure 2.2). The specific pathway turned on depends on the cell type and the duration of RAGE stimulation. RAGE activation in pathologic states leads to sustained activation of NF-κB and transcription of inflammatory genes and apoptosis.[39,67,68] RAGE activation of extracellular signal-regulated kinase (ERK) 1/2 ultimately leads to medial vascular calcification as will be discussed later.[69] Transduction of signals such as NADPH oxidase, p21ras, mitogen-activated protein kinase (MAPK), ERK 1/2, p38, GTPases Cdc42, and Rac leads to activation of transcription factors to transcribe target genes[50,70–74] that include endothelin-1; vascular cell adhesion molecule-1; intercellular adhesion molecule-1; E-selectin; vascular endothelial growth factor; and proinflammatory cytokines, including IL-1alpha, IL-6, tumor necrosis factor-alpha.[75,76]

AGE-R1 may serve to protect cells from AGE toxicity as studies show that it removes AGE and negatively regulates signals that are activated by AGE.[53,77,78] Mesangial cells overexpressing AGE-R1 show suppressed AGE stimulation of NF-κB activity and MAPK p44/42 phosphorylation and do not have macrophage chemotaxis protein1 or RAGE overexpression. Accordingly, after silencing AGE-R1 in MC using siRNA, AGE-mediated MAPk/p44/p42 increased twofold compared to control.

It was demonstrated that phosphorylation of AGE-R2 (80KH) occurs on tyrosine residues and is involved in intracellular receptor signaling such as fibroblast growth factor receptor signaling.[79,80] The AGE-R2 protein is also linked to intracellular trafficking of AGEs.[81] It has been suggested that

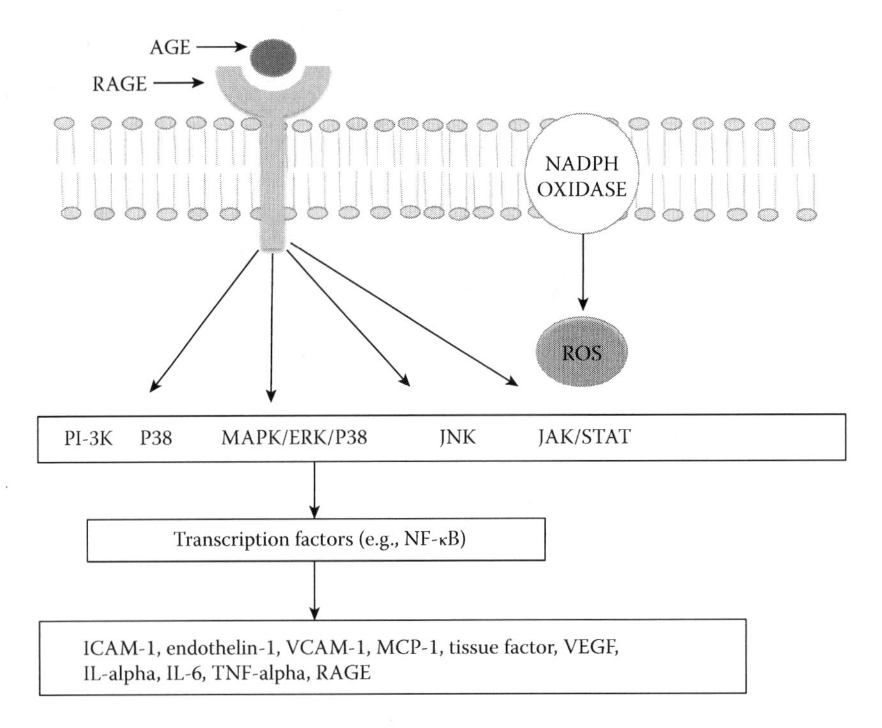

FIGURE 2.2 RAGE activation leads to oxidative stress. There is signaling via phosphatidylinositol-3 kinase (PI-3K), MAP/ERK1/ERK2, JNK,KAK/STAT, P38, activation of nuclear factor-κB (NF-κB) which leads to expression of proinflammatory mediators such as intercellular adhesion molecule-1 (ICAM-1), endothelin-1, vascular cell adhesion molecule-1 (VCAM-1), monocyte chemoattractant protein-1 (MCP-1), tissue factor, vascular endothelial growth factor (VEGF), Il-α, Il-6, TNF-α, RAGE.

the phosphorylated AGE-R2 interacts with both the PKCζ and munc18c and plays a role in the GLUT4 vesicle trafficking pathway.[82]

It has been shown that AGE-R3/galectin-3 participates in vascular osteogenesis by modulating Wnt/β-catenin signaling.[83]

The scavenger receptors are mostly involved in the uptake of AGE ligands without inducing intracellular signaling pathways themselves. However, they may affect RAGE-mediated cell signaling activation through competitive binding of the AGE ligands.

2.6 Cellular and Molecular Mechanism of AGE Effects in the Specific Organ

2.6.1 Kidney Disease

Decreased renal clearance of AGEs in kidney disease leads to toxic systemic AGE levels, but the kidney itself can also be a target of AGE damage.[84] RAGE–AGE interaction has been implicated in the pathogenesis and progression of renal disease. In the diseased kidney, RAGE is predominantly expressed in podocytes although there is some expression in endothelial cells.[46] Under pathophysiologic stress, RAGE activation in the kidney leads to increased glomerulosclerosis and derangement of glomerular function. Depending on the renal cell type, AGE-binding RAGE modulates cell proliferation, apoptosis, migration, and expression of adhesion molecules and prothrombotic/proinflammatory molecules.[18]

In vitro studies with cultured podocytes have elucidated the signaling pathways of AGE–RAGE interaction that affect podocyte gene expression. AGE stimulation of RAGE resulted in production of reactive oxygen species, activation of NF-κB, and phosphorylation of ERK.[85] RAGE activation leads to upregulation of podocyte expression of monocyte chemoattractant protein-1, which kicks off the process of mesangial activation, TGF-β production, increased oxygen radical formation, and consequent albuminuria and glomerulosclerosis.[85] Incubation of cultured podocytes with AGE from the serum of subjects with chronic kidney disease resulted in apoptosis. Other studies determined that AGEs activate apoptosis pathways in podocytes via the FOXO4 transcription factor and activation of p38 MAP kinase. Several experiments that either knocked down FOXO4 expression or inhibited p38 MAP kinase activation were able to eliminate the effects of AGE–RAGE on podocyte apoptosis.[86] Decreased RAGE expression via siRNA also suppressed AGE-mediated podocyte apoptosis.[86] *In vitro* studies in cultured renal proximal tubular epithelial cells demonstrated that RAGE activation contributes to tubulointerstitial fibrosis in the diabetic kidney by mediating epithelial-myofibroblast transdifferentiation in a TGF-B dependent manner.[87,88]

RAGE activation alters glomerular endothelial properties *in vitro* by increasing expression of vascular endothelial growth factor, which attracts and activates inflammatory cells. RAGE activation further contributes to this inflammatory milieu by changing the endothelial cell surface properties from that of an anticoagulant to a procoagulant endothelium by reducing thrombomodulin activity and increasing tissue factor expression.[89–91] When human glomerular endothelial cells were incubated with AGEs, upregulation of vascular endothelial growth factor receptor 2 (VEGFR2) resulted in decreased expression of heparan sulfate proteoglycans and reduced glomerular endothelial cell growth.[92] Another receptor-mediated effect of AGEs on diabetic vasculature is increased endothelial permeability.[89,90,93] Administration of soluble RAGE or sRAGE, a receptor that scavenges free AGE and limits its interaction with RAGE, inhibits vascular leakage in the intestine and skin of streptozotocin-treated rats.[94]

Exclusion of RAGE-mediated effects via RAGE blockade or RAGE-null mice has renal protective effects. Homozygous RAGE-null mice were protected against the albuminuria and glomerulosclerosis that is usually induced by adriamycin.[95] RAGE blockade in db/db mice prevented the expression of factors that can cause glomerular hyperpermeability and mononuclear phagocyte infiltration and activation.[45] SiRNA reduction of RAGE expression led to suppression of AGE-mediated podocyte apoptosis.[86] Anti-RAGE antibody had a beneficial effect on the course of diabetic nephropathy in murine models.[96,97] Blocking AGE–RAGE interaction using polyclonal antibodies to RAGE blocked vascular permeability in the intestine and skin of streptozotocin rats.[94]

In contrast to RAGE, AGE-R1 has a protective role in kidney disease. It was demonstrated that AGE-R1 expression is suppressed in diabetic kidney and AGE-R1 mediates anti-inflammatory and antioxidative effects in kidney cells and, therefore, protects renal cells from injury.[53,55] The expression of AGE-R1 in the peripheral blood cells was shown to be associated with kidney disease and affected by dietary AGE.[98] The role of AGE-R2 in kidney disease is unclear. It was shown that AGE-R2/Galectin-3 deficient mice developed more severe diabetic nephropathy[99] and accelerated AGE-induced glomerular disease.[100] The role of CD36 in diabetic nephropathy has been well documented.[101] However, it is less clear whether this is through interaction with AGE.[102]

2.6.2 Peripheral Vascular Disease

RAGE's vascular effects are not limited to the glomerular endothelium. Multiple studies have implicated RAGE in atherogenesis systemically. RAGE accelerates diabetes-induced vascular disease.[103] Administration of sRAGE to apoE-null STZ diabetic mice decreased markers of vascular inflammation and stabilized atherosclerotic lesions compared to mice given vehicle. This effect is likely due to sRAGE blockade of proliferation and migration of mononuclear phagocytes and smooth muscle cells.[103] In vascular injury, RAGE signaling contributes to smooth muscle proliferation in the expansion of the neointima.[40] RAGE signaling pathways in the endothelium include Jak2 and Stat, which cause upregulation of genes involved in expansion and remodeling of the extracellular matrix.[40]

The AGE–RAGE system causes vascular stiffening in a multipronged attack. AGEs form cross-links with collagen to decrease its pliability. In addition to stimulating smooth muscle cell proliferation, RAGE induces phenotypic cell changes such as stimulating osteogenic differentiation of vascular smooth muscle cells via ERK 1/2 pathways.[104–106] Studies found that AGE–RAGE interaction in vascular smooth muscle cells induced cell calcification while adding an antibody to RAGE-inhibited calcification.[104,106] Further damage to the vasculature occurs when RAGE transforms the endothelial surface into a more prothrombotic environment as discussed earlier.[89–91]

Inhibition of RAGE signaling reduces diabetes-accelerated medial calcification induced by AGE.[107] RAGE–ligand interaction increased vascular permeability and enhanced vasculopathy in diabetes. These effects were abrogated with administration of recombinant soluble RAGE, which would scavenge excess AGE and prevent AGE from binding and activating RAGE. Recombinant sRAGE used in rat/mouse models of vascular disease suppressed acceleration of atherosclerosis in diabetic and nondiabetic disease states.[94,103,108,109] RAGE is essential for the development of vascular injury. In the murine model of restenosis, there was no vascular damage in RAGE homozygous null mice.[40] In mice deficient in apolipoprotein E but also RAGE null, there was no vascular inflammation, endothelial dysfunction, or atherosclerotic plaque formation.[110]

Patients with diabetes or chronic kidney disease often have dyslipidemia and are at higher risk of developing atherosclerosis. These patients have a higher degree of AGE-modified LDL than do normal controls.[111] Mice injected with diabetic levels of AGE-modified LDL showed impaired LDL clearance, suggesting that AGE modification of LDL may contribute to dyslipidemia in patients with diabetes or renal disease. This hypothesis was further supported by the observation that the administration of the advanced glycation inhibitor aminoguanidine to diabetic patients decreased circulating LDL levels by 28%.[111]

A protective role of AGE-R1 in vascular disease has been also well documented. Mice with overexpression of AGE-R1 are resistant to inflammation, oxidative stress, and post-injury intima hyperplasia.[112] AGE-R1 was shown to attenuate vascular disease through negative regulation of oxidative stress.[113]

The SA binds to oxidized low-density lipoprotein (OxLDL) or acetylated LDL (AcLDL) as well as AGE leading to their endocytic uptake. This could lead to the intracellular accumulation of cholesterol and the formation of foam cells from macrophages in the early state of atherosclerosis.[61]

2.6.3 Heart Disease

The AGE/RAGE axis indirectly affects the heart with its changes of the systemic vasculature. As mentioned above, vessels lose their elasticity due to smooth muscle proliferation, calcification, and AGE cross-links with collagen fibers. These effects on the aorta lead to elevated systolic blood pressure and pulse pressures. The increased workload on the heart contributes to left ventricular hypertrophy, myocardial ischemia, and ultimately heart failure. This is supported in a study that showed that sRAGE levels are inversely related to LVH in chronic kidney disease patients.[114] AGE–RAGE is also responsible for myocardial inflammation. In the aging heart, AGE cross-linked collagen has been implicated in the signaling of macrophage recruitment in hypertensive myocardial fibrosis that results in deteriorating diastolic function.[115–118]

The AGE/RAGE system also has direct adverse effects on the cardiac system. There is increased RAGE expression in ischemic rat hearts. RAGE-null mice were protected from ischemia/reperfusion injury in the heart.[119] Occlusion and reperfusion of the LAD in RAGE knockout mice resulted in smaller infarct size compared to wild-type mice. Compared to wild-type mice, RAGE knockout mice had superior systolic function, smaller infarct size after ischemic injury, lower levels of plasma creatine kinase, and decreased apoptosis likely because these mice had attenuation of JNK and STAT5 phosphorylation compared to wild type.[120] Administration of sRAGE reduced ischemic injury and improved functional recovery of the myocardium.[120] Similar findings were seen in RAGE knockout mice.[121]

The AGE–RAGE signaling pathway increases oxidative stress of the ryanodine receptor, thus modifying calcium signaling which leads to a decrease in sarcoplasmic reticulum calcium content.[122] This altered reserve of sarcoplasmic reticulum calcium results in decreased systolic function and impaired myocardial relaxation.[122,123] RAGE played an integral role in diabetic cardiomyopathy in animal studies. Diabetes increased cardiac AGE and RAGE levels with increased AGE and RAGE in cardiomyocytes. Diabetes led to decreased LV contractility, which was not seen in RAGE gene knockdown mice.[114,124] RAGE expression is increased in the diabetic hearts of *db/db* mice. This increase in RAGE results in myocardial fibrosis and an altered extracellular matrix structure, causing diastolic dysfunction.[125,126] Cardiomyocyte dysfunction was prevented with RNA interference knockdown of RAGE expression.[114]

AGE cross-links increase vessel stiffness and result in decreased elasticity causing increased systolic blood pressure. AGE cross-linking with LDL and collagen contribute to atherogenesis. Alagebrium, a drug that disrupts AGE-connective tissue cross-links, attenuates LVH and cardiomyopathy in rat models of DM.[127] In aged dogs, alagebrium improved cardiac diastolic compliance with improved diastolic filling and cardiac output, reduced aortic stiffness, and restored ejection fraction.[115,128] The drug also increased left ventricular collagen solubility.

The role of AGE-R1 and scavenge receptors has not been well studied in heart disease.

2.6.4 Nervous System Disease

RAGE is expressed in neurons, microglia, and astrocytes where RAGE–ligand interaction contributes to inflammation, neuronal degeneration, and apoptosis.[129] AGE–RAGE interaction on neurons leads to increased oxidative stress and activation of NF-κB.[130,131] Persistent activation of NF-κB by RAGE is seen in multiple types of neuropathy including inflammatory demyelinating polyneuropathy, Charcot-Marie-Tooth neuropathy, alcohol-related neuropathy, B12 deficiency neuropathy, or vasculitic neuropathy.[132] This was confirmed in biopsies of neuropathic nerves that showed increased RAGE and AGE with associated increased NF-κB expression.[132] RAGE is overexpressed in the brains of amyotropic lateral sclerosis (ALS) patients.[133] These patients have glycated proteins in the neurons which promote cross-linking and contribute to the pathology of ALS.[134]

RAGE activation is prominent in multiple neurodegenerative diseases including Alzheimer's disease (AD), which is characterized by deposits of an aggregated beta-amyloid peptide in the brain and cerebrovasculature. Purified plaque fractions from AD brains have more AGE adducts per milligram of protein than parallel fractions from healthy, age-matched controls.[135] These findings are likely due to the fact that *in vivo* half-life of beta-amyloid is prolonged in AD, resulting in greater accumulation of AGE modifications which in turn promote accumulation of additional amyloid. *In vitro* studies with AGE-modified beta-amyloid peptide nucleation seeds demonstrated accelerated aggregation of soluble beta-amyloid peptide compared to nonmodified seed material.[135] Extracellular AGEs accumulate on senile plaques and induce oxidative stress and inflammation.[20] Besides the AGE deposits, RAGE signaling disrupts the tight junctions of the blood–brain barrier which contributes to the pathogenesis of AD.[136] Giving AGEs to retinal ganglion cells caused upregulation of amyloid precursor protein.[137] Increased Glo1 expression in the brains of early and mid-stage Alzheimer's patients is possibly part of an attempt to scavenge excessive alpha, beta-dicarbonyls.[138] Recent studies suggest a negative correlation between AGE-R1 expression and dementia in patients and mice with AD.[139]

2.6.5 Metabolism/Reproductive System Disease

AGEs stimulate adipogenesis, and RAGE is required for diet-induced obesity.[140] AGE–RAGE decreases the metabolic rate and energy expenditure and is associated with insulin resistance and dyslipidemia.[141] Obese patients have significantly lower sRAGE concentrations, while diet-induced weight loss can increase serum sRAGE levels by 150%.[142] AGE–RAGE is linked to insulin resistance independent of serum glucose levels, weight, and diet, making it a nontraditional risk factor for insulin resistance.[98] Mice fed a high AGE diet became dysmetabolic with impaired insulin-signaling pathways in insulin-sensitive tissues and had active inflammation in their macrophages and adipocytes. RAGE deficiency is associated with less fat mass and smaller adipocyte size compared to controls.[143] RAGE-deficient mice given a high-fat diet have less weight gain and less of an increased fasting glucose compared to wild-type mice.[141]

AGE–RAGE is implicated in obesity-related ovarian dysfunction.[144] Women with PCOS have increased AGEs and RAGE expression in theca and granulosa cell layers compared with healthy women.[145] Ovarian AGEs alter glucose metabolism and folliculogenesis. *In vitro* studies show that AGEs may be responsible for reduced glucose uptake by granulosa cells, potentially altering follicular growth. *In vitro*, AGEs interfere with luteinizing hormone leading to a sustained abnormal activation of the ERK1/2 pathway whose proper functioning is important for regulating normal follicular development and initiating the ovulation process.[146] Lysyl oxidase is an enzyme that is vital to the organization of the extracellular matrix during follicular development, regulating collagen and elastin cross-linking.[147] A study has shown that the deposition of excess collagen in PCO tissue may be due to AGE-mediated stimulation of lysyl oxidase activity.[148]

High AGE levels have a negative impact on the reproductive outcome of patients undergoing artificial reproductive technology. High levels of AGE correlated negatively with follicular growth, fertilization, and embryonic development in patients undergoing IVF.[149] Women who conceived with IVF had significantly higher sRAGE levels in the follicular fluid compared to women who did not conceive.[150] There is a positive relationship between sRAGE and ovarian response to controlled ovarian hyperstimulation manifested by oocyte quantity.[151]

AGE–RAGE's inflammatory axis makes it reasonable to hypothesize that it is involved in the menstrual irregularity and infertility seen in patients with endometriosis. Endometrial tissue of patients with endometriosis does show that there is a higher expression of RAGE compared to healthy endometrial tissue.[152]

Recent studies suggest that dietary AGE could suppress AGE-R1 expression in the peripheral mononuclear cells leading to insulin resistance and diabetes.[98] AGE-R1 expression in the peripheral mononuclear cells is also associated with metabolic syndrome in humans.[153] These studies suggest a protective role of AGE-R1 in these metabolic disorders.

2.7 Conclusions

AGEs are formed as part of the normal aging process. However, under normal physiologic conditions, there are multiple regulatory mechanisms in place to ensure that the rate of removal of AGE matches its production. In disease states, there is an imbalance which leads to AGE accumulation. AGEs can manifest their harmful effects in a receptor-independent manner by cross-linking with molecules extracellularly and intracellularly, affecting organ structure, genome integrity, and mitochondrial function. AGEs also exert receptor-dependent effects by binding different AGE receptors. AGE-R1 has protective effects in various organs through negative regulation of inflammation and oxidative stress. In contrast, RAGE mediates activation of inflammatory signaling pathways. The harmful results of AGE–RAGE engagement have been documented in various organ systems. Drugs that activate AGE-R1 or block RAGE could be developed to treat these diseases.

REFERENCES

1. Brownlee M. Negative consequences of glycation. *Metabolism* 2000;49:9–13.
2. Schmidt AM, Hori O, Chen JX, et al. Advanced glycation endproducts interacting with their endothelial receptor induce expression of vascular cell adhesion molecule-1 (VCAM-1) in cultured human endothelial cells and in mice. A potential mechanism for the accelerated vasculopathy of diabetes. *J Clin Invest* 1995;96:1395–403.
3. Schmidt AM, Hasu M, Popov D, et al. Receptor for advanced glycation end products (AGEs) has a central role in vessel wall interactions and gene activation in response to circulating AGE proteins. *Proc Natl Acad Sci U S A* 1994;91:8807–11.
4. Kuzuya M, Asai T, Kanda S, Maeda K, Cheng XW, Iguchi A. Glycation cross-links inhibit matrix metalloproteinase-2 activation in vascular smooth muscle cells cultured on collagen lattice. *Diabetologia* 2001;44:433–6.
5. Thornalley PJ, Battah S, Ahmed N, et al. Quantitative screening of advanced glycation endproducts in cellular and extracellular proteins by tandem mass spectrometry. *Biochem J* 2003;375:581–92.
6. DeGroot J, Verzijl N, Wenting-Van Wijk MJ, et al. Age-related decrease in susceptibility of human articular cartilage to matrix metalloproteinase-mediated degradation: The role of advanced glycation end products. *Arthritis Rheumat* 2001;44:2562–71.
7. Sell DR, Monnier VM. Ornithine is a novel amino acid and a marker of arginine damage by oxoaldehydes in senescent proteins. *Ann N Y Acad Sci* 2005;1043:118–28.
8. Crabbe MJ, Cooper LR, Corne DW. Use of essential and molecular dynamics to study gammaB-crystallin unfolding after non-enzymic post-translational modifications. *Comput Biol Chem* 2003;27:507–10.
9. Hamelin M, Mary J, Vostry M, Friguet B, Bakala H. Glycation damage targets glutamate dehydrogenase in the rat liver mitochondrial matrix during aging. *FEBS J* 2007;274:5949–61.

10. Dobler D, Ahmed N, Song L, Eboigbodin KE, Thornalley PJ. Increased dicarbonyl metabolism in endothelial cells in hyperglycemia induces anoikis and impairs angiogenesis by RGD and GFOGER motif modification. *Diabetes* 2006;55:1961–9.
11. Waris S, Winklhofer-Roob BM, Roob JM, et al. Increased DNA dicarbonyl glycation and oxidation markers in patients with type 2 diabetes and link to diabetic nephropathy. *J Diabetes Res* 2015;2015:915486.
12. Ravandi A, Kuksis A, Marai L, et al. Isolation and identification of glycated aminophospholipids from red cells and plasma of diabetic blood. *FEBS Lett* 1996;381:77–81.
13. Bucala R, Makita Z, Koschinsky T, Cerami A, Vlassara H. Lipid advanced glycosylation: Pathway for lipid oxidation *in vivo*. *Proc Natl Acad Sci U S A* 1993;90:6434–8.
14. Bucala R, Model P, Cerami A. Modification of DNA by reducing sugars: A possible mechanism for nucleic acid aging and age-related dysfunction in gene expression. *Proc Natl Acad Sci U S A* 1984;81:105–9.
15. Baynes JW. Role of oxidative stress in development of complications in diabetes. *Diabetes* 1991;40:405–12.
16. McLellan AC, Thornalley PJ, Benn J, Sonksen PH. Glyoxalase system in clinical diabetes mellitus and correlation with diabetic complications. *Clin Sci* 1994;87:21–9.
17. Thornalley PJ, Waris S, Fleming T, et al. Imidazopurinones are markers of physiological genomic damage linked to DNA instability and glyoxalase 1-associated tumour multidrug resistance. *Nucleic Acids Res* 2010;38:5432–42.
18. Thornalley PJ. Cell activation by glycated proteins. AGE receptors, receptor recognition factors and functional classification of AGEs. *Cell Mol Biol* 1998;44:1013–23.
19. Seidel W, Pischetsrieder M. DNA-glycation leads to depurination by the loss of N2-carboxyethylguanine *in vitro*. *Cell Mol Biol* 1998;44:1165–70.
20. Pun PB, Murphy MP. Pathological significance of mitochondrial glycation. *Int J Cell Biol* 2012;2012:843505.
21. Murata-Kamiya N, Kamiya H, Kaji H, Kasai H. Glyoxal, a major product of DNA oxidation, induces mutations at G:C sites on a shuttle vector plasmid replicated in mammalian cells. *Nucleic Acids Res* 1997;25:1897–902.
22. Pischetsrieder M, Seidel W, Munch G, Schinzel R. N(2)-(1-Carboxyethyl)deoxyguanosine, a nonenzymatic glycation adduct of DNA, induces single-strand breaks and increases mutation frequencies. *Biochem Biophys Res Commun* 1999;264:544–9.
23. Breyer V, Frischmann M, Bidmon C, Schemm A, Schiebel K, Pischetsrieder M. Analysis and biological relevance of advanced glycation end-products of DNA in eukaryotic cells. *FEBS J 2008*;275:914–25.
24. Stolzing A, Widmer R, Jung T, Voss P, Grune T. Degradation of glycated bovine serum albumin in microglial cells. *Free Radic Biol Med* 2006;40:1017–27.
25. Tamae D, Lim P, Wuenschell GE, Termini J. Mutagenesis and repair induced by the DNA advanced glycation end product N2-1-(carboxyethyl)-2'-deoxyguanosine in human cells. *Biochemistry* 2011;50:2321–9.
26. Xue M, Rabbani N, Thornalley PJ. Glyoxalase in ageing. *Semin Cell Dev Biol* 2011;22:293–301.
27. Barati MT, Merchant ML, Kain AB, Jevans AW, McLeish KR, Klein JB. Proteomic analysis defines altered cellular redox pathways and advanced glycation end-product metabolism in glomeruli of db/db diabetic mice. *Am J Physiol Renal Physiol* 2007;293:F1157–65.
28. Bierhaus A, Fleming T, Stoyanov S, et al. Methylglyoxal modification of Nav1.8 facilitates nociceptive neuron firing and causes hyperalgesia in diabetic neuropathy. *Nat Med* 2012;18:926–33.
29. Palsamy P, Subramanian S. Resveratrol protects diabetic kidney by attenuating hyperglycemia-mediated oxidative stress and renal inflammatory cytokines via Nrf2-Keapl signaling. *Biochim Biophys Acta* 2011;1812:719–31.
30. Giacco F, Du X, D'Agati VD, et al. Knockdown of glyoxalase 1 mimics diabetic nephropathy in nondiabetic mice. *Diabetes* 2014;63:291–9.
31. Thornalley PJ, Rabbani N. Glyoxalase in tumourigenesis and multidrug resistance. *Sem Cell Dev Biol* 2011;22:318–25.
32. Thornalley PJ, Edwards LG, Kang Y, et al. Antitumour activity of S-p-bromobenzylglutathione cyclopentyl diester *in vitro* and *in vivo*. Inhibition of glyoxalase I and induction of apoptosis. *Biochem Pharmacol* 1996;51:1365–72.
33. Nishikawa T, Edelstein D, Du XL, et al. Normalizing mitochondrial superoxide production blocks three pathways of hyperglycaemic damage. *Nature* 2000;404:787–90.

34. Brouwers O, Niessen PM, Ferreira I, et al. Overexpression of glyoxalase-I reduces hyperglycemia-induced levels of advanced glycation end products and oxidative stress in diabetic rats. *J Biol Chem* 2011;286:1374–80.
35. Rosca MG, Mustata TG, Kinter MT, et al. Glycation of mitochondrial proteins from diabetic rat kidney is associated with excess superoxide formation. *Am J Physiol Renal Physiol* 2005;289:F420–30.
36. Morcos M, Du X, Pfisterer F, et al. Glyoxalase-1 prevents mitochondrial protein modification and enhances lifespan in Caenorhabditis elegans. *Aging cell* 2008;7:260–9.
37. Vlassara H. The AGE-receptor in the pathogenesis of diabetic complications. *Diabet/Metab Res Rev* 2001;17:436–43.
38. Neeper M, Schmidt AM, Brett J, et al. Cloning and expression of a cell surface receptor for advanced glycosylation end products of proteins. *J Biol Chem* 1992;267:14998–5004.
39. Kislinger T, Fu C, Huber B, et al. N(epsilon)-(carboxymethyl)lysine adducts of proteins are ligands for receptor for advanced glycation end products that activate cell signaling pathways and modulate gene expression. *J Biol Chem* 1999;274:31740–9.
40. Sakaguchi T, Yan SF, Yan SD, et al. Central role of RAGE-dependent neointimal expansion in arterial restenosis. *J Clin Invest* 2003;111:959–72.
41. Xie J, Burz DS, He W, Bronstein IB, Lednev I, Shekhtman A. Hexameric calgranulin C (S100A12) binds to the receptor for advanced glycated end products (RAGE) using symmetric hydrophobic target-binding patches. *J Biol Chem* 2007;282:4218–31.
42. Ostendorp T, Leclerc E, Galichet A, et al. Structural and functional insights into RAGE activation by multimeric *S100B. EMBO J* 2007;26:3868–78.
43. Brett J, Schmidt AM, Yan SD, et al. Survey of the distribution of a newly characterized receptor for advanced glycation end products in tissues. *Am J Pathol* 1993;143:1699–712.
44. Ritthaler U, Deng Y, Zhang Y, et al. Expression of receptors for advanced glycation end products in peripheral occlusive vascular disease. *Am J Pathol* 1995;146:688–94.
45. Wendt TM, Tanji N, Guo J, et al. RAGE drives the development of glomerulosclerosis and implicates podocyte activation in the pathogenesis of diabetic nephropathy. *Am J Pathol* 2003;162:1123–37.
46. Tanji N, Markowitz GS, Fu C, et al. Expression of advanced glycation end products and their cellular receptor RAGE in diabetic nephropathy and nondiabetic renal disease. *J Am Soc Nephrol* 2000;11:1656–66.
47. Rong LL, Yan SF, Wendt T, et al. RAGE modulates peripheral nerve regeneration via recruitment of both inflammatory and axonal outgrowth pathways. *FASEB J* 2004;18:1818–25.
48. Yan SD, Chen X, Fu J, et al. RAGE and amyloid-beta peptide neurotoxicity in Alzheimer's disease. *Nature* 1996;382:685–91.
49. Hori O, Brett J, Slattery T, et al. The receptor for advanced glycation end products (RAGE) is a cellular binding site for amphoterin. Mediation of neurite outgrowth and co-expression of rage and amphoterin in the developing nervous system. *J Biol Chem* 1995;270:25752–61.
50. Taguchi A, Blood DC, del Toro G, et al. Blockade of RAGE-amphoterin signalling suppresses tumour growth and metastases. *Nature* 2000;405:354–60.
51. Hofmann MA, Drury S, Fu C, et al. RAGE mediates a novel proinflammatory axis: A central cell surface receptor for S100/calgranulin polypeptides. *Cell* 1999;97:889–901.
52. Chavakis T, Bierhaus A, Al-Fakhri N, et al. The pattern recognition receptor (RAGE) is a counter-receptor for leukocyte integrins: A novel pathway for inflammatory cell recruitment. *J Exp Med* 2003;198:1507–15.
53. Lu C, He JC, Cai W, Liu H, Zhu L, Vlassara H. Advanced glycation endproduct (AGE) receptor 1 is a negative regulator of the inflammatory response to AGE in mesangial cells. *Proc Natl Acad Sci U S A* 2004;101:11767–72.
54. Doi T, Vlassara H, Kirstein M, Yamada Y, Striker GE, Striker LJ. Receptor-specific increase in extracellular matrix production in mouse mesangial cells by advanced glycosylation end products is mediated via platelet-derived growth factor. *Proc Natl Acad Sci U S A* 1992;89:2873–7.
55. He CJ, Zheng F, Stitt A, Striker L, Hattori M, Vlassara H. Differential expression of renal AGE-receptor genes in NOD mice: Possible role in nonobese diabetic renal disease. *Kidney Int* 2000;58:1931–40.
56. Stitt AW, He C, Vlassara H. Characterization of the advanced glycation end-product receptor complex in human vascular endothelial cells. *Biochem Biophys Res Commun* 1999;256:549–56.

57. Ho MK, Springer TA. Mac-2, a novel 32,000 Mr mouse macrophage subpopulation-specific antigen defined by monoclonal antibodies. *J Immunol* 1982;128:1221–8.
58. Barondes SH, Castronovo V, Cooper DN, et al. Galectins: A family of animal beta-galactoside-binding lectins. *Cell* 1994;76:597–8.
59. Vlassara H, Li YM, Imani F, et al. Identification of galectin-3 as a high-affinity binding protein for advanced glycation end products (AGE): A new member of the AGE-receptor complex. *Mol Med* 1995;1:634–46.
60. Kodama T, Freeman M, Rohrer L, Zabrecky J, Matsudaira P, Krieger M. Type I macrophage scavenger receptor contains alpha-helical and collagen-like coiled coils. *Nature* 1990;343:531–5.
61. Bickel PE, Freeman MW. Rabbit aortic smooth muscle cells express inducible macrophage scavenger receptor messenger RNA that is absent from endothelial cells. *J Clin Invest* 1992;90:1450–7.
62. Araki N, Higashi T, Mori T, et al. Macrophage scavenger receptor mediates the endocytic uptake and degradation of advanced glycation end products of the Maillard reaction. *Eur J Biochem / FEBS* 1995;230:408–15.
63. Ohgami N, Nagai R, Ikemoto M, et al. Cd36, a member of the class b scavenger receptor family, as a receptor for advanced glycation end products. *J Biol Chem* 2001;276:3195–202.
64. Ohgami N, Nagai R, Miyazaki A, et al. Scavenger receptor class B type I-mediated reverse cholesterol transport is inhibited by advanced glycation end products. *J Biol Chem* 2001;276:13348–55.
65. Kuniyasu A, Ohgami N, Hayashi S, Miyazaki A, Horiuchi S, Nakayama H. CD36-mediated endocytic uptake of advanced glycation end products (AGE) in mouse 3T3-L1 and human subcutaneous adipocytes. *FEBS Lett* 2003;537:85–90.
66. Unno Y, Sakai M, Sakamoto Y, et al. Glycolaldehyde-modified bovine serum albumin down-regulates leptin expression in mouse adipocytes via a CD36-mediated pathway. *Ann N Y Acad Sci* 2005;1043:696–701.
67. Bierhaus A, Schiekofer S, Schwaninger M, et al. Diabetes-associated sustained activation of the transcription factor nuclear factor-kappaB. *Diabetes* 2001;50:2792–808.
68. Basta G, Sironi AM, Lazzerini G, et al. Circulating soluble receptor for advanced glycation end products is inversely associated with glycemic control and S100A12 protein. *J Clin Endocrinol Metab* 2006;91:4628–34.
69. Brodeur MR, Bouvet C, Barrette M, Moreau P. Palmitic acid increases medial calcification by inducing oxidative stress. *J Vasc Res* 2013;50:430–41.
70. Yan SD, Schmidt AM, Anderson GM, et al. Enhanced cellular oxidant stress by the interaction of advanced glycation end products with their receptors/binding proteins. *J Biol Chem* 1994;269:9889–97.
71. Schiekofer S, Andrassy M, Chen J, et al. Acute hyperglycemia causes intracellular formation of CML and activation of ras, p42/44 MAPK, and nuclear factor kappaB in PBMCs. *Diabetes* 2003;52:621–33.
72. Huttunen HJ, Fages C, Rauvala H. Receptor for advanced glycation end products (RAGE)-mediated neurite outgrowth and activation of NF-kappaB require the cytoplasmic domain of the receptor but different downstream signaling pathways. *J Biol Chem* 1999;274:19919–24.
73. Braach N, Buschmann K, Pflaum J, et al. Anti-inflammatory functions of protein C require RAGE and ICAM-1 in a stimulus-dependent manner. *Mediat Inflamm* 2014;2014:743678.
74. Lander HM, Tauras JM, Ogiste JS, Hori O, Moss RA, Schmidt AM. Activation of the receptor for advanced glycation end products triggers a p21(ras)-dependent mitogen-activated protein kinase pathway regulated by oxidant stress. *J Biol Chem* 1997;272:17810–4.
75. Boulanger E, Wautier MP, Wautier JL, et al. AGEs bind to mesothelial cells via RAGE and stimulate VCAM-1 expression. *Kidney Int* 2002;61:148–56.
76. Neumann A, Schinzel R, Palm D, Riederer P, Munch G. High molecular weight hyaluronic acid inhibits advanced glycation endproduct-induced NF-kappaB activation and cytokine expression. *FEBS Lett* 1999;453:283–7.
77. Lal MA, Brismar H, Eklof AC, Aperia A. Role of oxidative stress in advanced glycation end product-induced mesangial cell activation. *Kidney Int* 2002;61:2006–14.
78. Scivittaro V, Ganz MB, Weiss MF. AGEs induce oxidative stress and activate protein kinase C-beta(II) in neonatal mesangial cells. *Am J Physiol Renal Physiol* 2000;278:F676–83.
79. Goh KC, Lim YP, Ong SH, et al. Identification of p90, a prominent tyrosine-phosphorylated protein in fibroblast growth factor-stimulated cells, as 80K-H. *J Biol Chem* 1996;271:5832–8.

80. Stitt AW, Bucala R, Vlassara H. Atherogenesis and advanced glycation: Promotion, progression, and prevention. *Ann N Y Acad Sci* 1997;811:115–27; discussion 27–9.
81. Brule S, Rabahi F, Faure R, Beckers JF, Silversides DW, Lussier JG. Vacuolar system-associated protein-60: A protein characterized from bovine granulosa and luteal cells that is associated with intracellular vesicles and related to human 80K-H and murine beta-glucosidase II. *Biol Reprod* 2000;62:642–54.
82. Hodgkinson CP, Mander A, Sale GJ. Identification of 80K-H as a protein involved in GLUT4 vesicle trafficking. *Biochem J* 2005;388:785–93.
83. Menini S, Iacobini C, Ricci C, et al. The galectin-3/RAGE dyad modulates vascular osteogenesis in atherosclerosis. *Cardiovasc Res* 2013;100:472–80.
84. Uribarri J, Peppa M, Cai W, et al. Restriction of dietary glycotoxins reduces excessive advanced glycation end products in renal failure patients. *J Am Soc Nephrol* 2003;14:728–31.
85. Gu L, Hagiwara S, Fan Q, et al. Role of receptor for advanced glycation end-products and signalling events in advanced glycation end-product-induced monocyte chemoattractant protein-1 expression in differentiated mouse podocytes. *Nephrol Dial Transplant* 2006;21:299–313.
86. Chuang PY, Yu Q, Fang W, Uribarri J, He JC. Advanced glycation endproducts induce podocyte apoptosis by activation of the FOXO4 transcription factor. *Kidney Int* 2007;72:965–76.
87. Oldfield MD, Bach LA, Forbes JM, et al. Advanced glycation end products cause epithelial-myofibroblast transdifferentiation via the receptor for advanced glycation end products (RAGE). *J Clin Invest* 2001;108:1853–63.
88. Li JH, Wang W, Huang XR, et al. Advanced glycation end products induce tubular epithelial-myofibroblast transition through the RAGE-ERK1/2 MAP kinase signaling pathway. *Am J Pathol* 2004;164:1389–97.
89. Basta G, Schmidt AM, De Caterina R. Advanced glycation end products and vascular inflammation: Implications for accelerated atherosclerosis in diabetes. *Cardiovasc Res* 2004;63:582–92.
90. Bierhaus A, Illmer T, Kasper M, et al. Advanced glycation end product (AGE)-mediated induction of tissue factor in cultured endothelial cells is dependent on RAGE. *Circulation* 1997;96:2262–71.
91. Esposito C, Gerlach H, Brett J, Stern D, Vlassara H. Endothelial receptor-mediated binding of glucose-modified albumin is associated with increased monolayer permeability and modulation of cell surface coagulant properties. *J Exp Med* 1989;170:1387–407.
92. Pala L, Cresci B, Manuelli C, et al. Vascular endothelial growth factor receptor-2 and low affinity VEGF binding sites on human glomerular endothelial cells: Biological effects and advanced glycosilation end products modulation. *Microvasc Res* 2005;70:179–88.
93. Li J, Schmidt AM. Characterization and functional analysis of the promoter of RAGE, the receptor for advanced glycation end products. *J Biol Chem* 1997;272:16498–506.
94. Wautier JL, Zoukourian C, Chappey O, et al. Receptor-mediated endothelial cell dysfunction in diabetic vasculopathy. Soluble receptor for advanced glycation end products blocks hyperpermeability in diabetic rats. *J Clin Invest* 1996;97:238–43.
95. Guo J, Ananthakrishnan R, Qu W, et al. RAGE mediates podocyte injury in adriamycin-induced glomerulosclerosis. *J Am Soc Nephrol* 2008;19:961–72.
96. Flyvbjerg A, Denner L, Schrijvers BF, et al. Long-term renal effects of a neutralizing RAGE antibody in obese type 2 diabetic mice. *Diabetes* 2004;53:166–72.
97. Jensen LJ, Denner L, Schrijvers BF, Tilton RG, Rasch R, Flyvbjerg A. Renal effects of a neutralising RAGE-antibody in long-term streptozotocin-diabetic mice. *J Endocrinol* 2006;188:493–501.
98. Cai W, Ramdas M, Zhu L, Chen X, Striker GE, Vlassara H. Oral advanced glycation endproducts (AGEs) promote insulin resistance and diabetes by depleting the antioxidant defenses AGE receptor-1 and sirtuin 1. *Proc Natl Acad Sci U S A* 2012;109:15888–93.
99. Pugliese G, Pricci F, Iacobini C, et al. Accelerated diabetic glomerulopathy in galectin-3/AGE receptor 3 knockout mice. *FASEB J* 2001;15:2471–9.
100. Iacobini C, Menini S, Oddi G, et al. Galectin-3/AGE-receptor 3 knockout mice show accelerated AGE-induced glomerular injury: Evidence for a protective role of galectin-3 as an AGE receptor. *FASEB J* 2004;18:1773–5.
101. Susztak K, Ciccone E, McCue P, Sharma K, Bottinger EP. Multiple metabolic hits converge on CD36 as novel mediator of tubular epithelial apoptosis in diabetic nephropathy. *PLoS Med.* 2005;2:e45.
102. Sourris KC, Forbes JM. Interactions between advanced glycation end-products (AGE) and their receptors in the development and progression of diabetic nephropathy - are these receptors valid therapeutic targets. *Curr Drug Targets* 2009;10:42–50.

103. Bucciarelli LG, Wendt T, Qu W, et al. RAGE blockade stabilizes established atherosclerosis in diabetic apolipoprotein E-null mice. *Circulation* 2002;106:2827–35.
104. Ren X, Shao H, Wei Q, Sun Z, Liu N. Advanced glycation end-products enhance calcification in vascular smooth muscle cells. *J Int Med Res* 2009;37:847–54.
105. Suga T, Iso T, Shimizu T, et al. Activation of receptor for advanced glycation end products induces osteogenic differentiation of vascular smooth muscle cells. *J Atheroscler Thromb* 2011;18:670–83.
106. Tanikawa T, Okada Y, Tanikawa R, Tanaka Y. Advanced glycation end products induce calcification of vascular smooth muscle cells through RAGE/p38 MAPK. *J Vasc Res* 2009;46:572–80.
107. Brodeur MR, Bouvet C, Bouchard S, et al. Reduction of advanced-glycation end products levels and inhibition of RAGE signaling decreases rat vascular calcification induced by diabetes. *PLoS One* 2014;9:e85922.
108. Park L, Raman KG, Lee KJ, et al. Suppression of accelerated diabetic atherosclerosis by the soluble receptor for advanced glycation endproducts. *Nat Med* 1998;4:1025–31.
109. Wendt T, Harja E, Bucciarelli L, et al. RAGE modulates vascular inflammation and atherosclerosis in a murine model of type 2 diabetes. *Atherosclerosis* 2006;185:70–7.
110. Harja E, Bu DX, Hudson BI, et al. Vascular and inflammatory stresses mediate atherosclerosis via RAGE and its ligands in apoE-/- mice. *J Clin Invest* 2008;118:183–94.
111. Bucala R, Makita Z, Vega G, et al. Modification of low density lipoprotein by advanced glycation end products contributes to the dyslipidemia of diabetes and renal insufficiency. *Proc Natl Acad Sci U S A* 1994;91:9441–5.
112. Torreggiani M, Liu H, Wu J, et al. Advanced glycation end product receptor-1 transgenic mice are resistant to inflammation, oxidative stress, and post-injury intimal hyperplasia. *Am J Pathol* 2009;175:1722–32.
113. Cai W, Torreggiani M, Zhu L, et al. AGER1 regulates endothelial cell NADPH oxidase-dependent oxidant stress via PKC-delta: Implications for vascular disease. *Am J Physiol Cell Physiol* 2010;298:C624–34.
114. Leonardis D, Basta G, Mallamaci F, et al. Circulating soluble receptor for advanced glycation end product (sRAGE) and left ventricular hypertrophy in patients with chronic kidney disease (CKD). *Nutr Metab Cardiovasc Dis* 2012;22:748–55.
115. Asif M, Egan J, Vasan S, et al. An advanced glycation endproduct cross-link breaker can reverse age-related increases in myocardial stiffness. *Proc Natl Acad Sci U S A* 2000;97:2809–13.
116. Herrmann KL, McCulloch AD, Omens JH. Glycated collagen cross-linking alters cardiac mechanics in volume-overload hypertrophy. *Am J Physiol Heart Circ Physiol* 2003;284:H1277–84.
117. Kass DA, Bronzwaer JG, Paulus WJ. What mechanisms underlie diastolic dysfunction in heart failure? *Circ Res* 2004;94:1533–42.
118. Kuwahara F, Kai H, Tokuda K, et al. Hypertensive myocardial fibrosis and diastolic dysfunction: Another model of inflammation? *Hypertension* 2004;43:739–45.
119. Bucciarelli LG, Kaneko M, Ananthakrishnan R, et al. Receptor for advanced-glycation end products: Key modulator of myocardial ischemic injury. *Circulation* 2006;113:1226–34.
120. Aleshin A, Ananthakrishnan R, Li Q, et al. RAGE modulates myocardial injury consequent to LAD infarction via impact on JNK and STAT signaling in a murine model. *Am J Physiol Heart Circ Physiol* 2008;294:H1823–32.
121. Bucciarelli LG, Ananthakrishnan R, Hwang YC, et al. RAGE and modulation of ischemic injury in the diabetic myocardium. *Diabetes* 2008;57:1941–51.
122. Avendano GF, Agarwal RK, Bashey RI, et al. Effects of glucose intolerance on myocardial function and collagen-linked glycation. *Diabetes* 1999;48:1443–7.
123. Petrova R, Yamamoto Y, Muraki K, et al. Advanced glycation endproduct-induced calcium handling impairment in mouse cardiac myocytes. *J Mol Cell Cardiol* 2002;34:1425–31.
124. Ma H, Li SY, Xu P, et al. Advanced glycation endproduct (AGE) accumulation and AGE receptor (RAGE) up-regulation contribute to the onset of diabetic cardiomyopathy. *J Cell Mol Med* 2009;13:1751–64.
125. Hutchinson KR, Lord CK, West TA, Stewart JA, Jr. Cardiac fibroblast-dependent extracellular matrix accumulation is associated with diastolic stiffness in type 2 diabetes. *PLoS One* 2013;8:e72080.
126. Zhao J, Randive R, Stewart JA. Molecular mechanisms of AGE/RAGE-mediated fibrosis in the diabetic heart. *World J Diabetes* 2014;5:860–7.
127. Candido R, Forbes JM, Thomas MC, et al. A breaker of advanced glycation end products attenuates diabetes-induced myocardial structural changes. *Circ Res* 2003;92:785–92.

128. Liu J, Masurekar MR, Vatner DE, et al. Glycation end-product cross-link breaker reduces collagen and improves cardiac function in aging diabetic heart. *Am J Physiol Heart Circ Physiol* 2003;285:H2587–91.
129. Ding Q, Keller JN. Evaluation of rage isoforms, ligands, and signaling in the brain. *Biochim Biophys Acta* 2005;1746:18–27.
130. Businaro R, Leone S, Fabrizi C, et al. S100B protects LAN-5 neuroblastoma cells against Abeta amyloid-induced neurotoxicity via RAGE engagement at low doses but increases Abeta amyloid neurotoxicity at high doses. *J Neurosci Res* 2006;83:897–906.
131. Mattson MP, Camandola S. NF-kappaB in neuronal plasticity and neurodegenerative disorders. *J Clin Invest* 2001;107:247–54.
132. Haslbeck KM, Neundorfer B, Schlotzer-Schrehardtt U, et al. Activation of the RAGE pathway: A general mechanism in the pathogenesis of polyneuropathies? *Neurol Res* 2007;29:103–10.
133. Casula M, Iyer AM, Spliet WG, et al. Toll-like receptor signaling in amyotrophic lateral sclerosis spinal cord tissue. *Neuroscience* 2011;179:233–43.
134. Chou SM, Wang HS, Taniguchi A, Bucala R. Advanced glycation endproducts in neurofilament conglomeration of motoneurons in familial and sporadic amyotrophic lateral sclerosis. *Mol Med* 1998;4:324–32.
135. Vitek MP, Bhattacharya K, Glendening JM, et al. Advanced glycation end products contribute to amyloidosis in Alzheimer disease. *Proc Natl Acad Sci U S A* 1994;91:4766–70.
136. Kook SY, Hong HS, Moon M, Ha CM, Chang S, Mook-Jung I. Abeta(1)(-)(4)(2)-RAGE interaction disrupts tight junctions of the blood-brain barrier via Ca(2)(+)-calcineurin signaling. *J Neurosci* 2012;32:8845–54.
137. Lee JJ, Wang PW, Yang IH, Wu CL, Chuang JH. Amyloid-beta mediates the receptor of advanced glycation end product-induced pro-inflammatory response via toll-like receptor 4 signaling pathway in retinal ganglion cell line RGC-5. *Int J Biochem Cell Biol* 2015;64:1–10.
138. Kuhla B, Boeck K, Schmidt A, et al. Age- and stage-dependent glyoxalase I expression and its activity in normal and Alzheimer's disease brains. *Neurobiol Aging* 2007;28:29–41.
139. Cai W, Uribarri J, Zhu L, et al. Oral glycotoxins are a modifiable cause of dementia and the metabolic syndrome in mice and humans. *Proc Natl Acad Sci U S A* 2014;111:4940–5.
140. Jia X, Chang T, Wilson TW, Wu L. Methylglyoxal mediates adipocyte proliferation by increasing phosphorylation of Akt1. *PLoS One* 2012;7:e36610.
141. Song F, Hurtado del Pozo C, Rosario R, et al. RAGE regulates the metabolic and inflammatory response to high-fat feeding in mice. *Diabetes* 2014;63:1948–65.
142. Vazzana N, Guagnano MT, Cuccurullo C, et al. Endogenous secretory RAGE in obese women: Association with platelet activation and oxidative stress. *J Clin Endocrinol Metab* 2012;97:E1726–30.
143. Ueno H, Koyama H, Shoji T, et al. Receptor for advanced glycation end-products (RAGE) regulation of adiposity and adiponectin is associated with atherogenesis in apoE-deficient mouse. *Atherosclerosis* 2010;211:431–6.
144. Merhi Z, McGee EA, Buyuk E. Role of advanced glycation end-products in obesity-related ovarian dysfunction. *Minerva Endocrinologica* 2014;39:167–74.
145. Kandaraki E, Chatzigeorgiou A, Piperi C, et al. Reduced ovarian glyoxalase-I activity by dietary glycotoxins and androgen excess: A causative link to polycystic ovarian syndrome. *Mol Med* 2012;18:1183–9.
146. Diamanti-Kandarakis E, Piperi C, Livadas S, Kandaraki E, Papageorgiou E, Koutsilieris M. Interference of AGE-RAGE Signaling with Steroidogenic Enzyme Action in Human Ovarian Cells. San Francisco, CA: Endocrine Society; 2013.
147. Harlow CR, Rae M, Davidson L, Trackman PC, Hillier SG. Lysyl oxidase gene expression and enzyme activity in the rat ovary: Regulation by follicle-stimulating hormone, androgen, and transforming growth factor-beta superfamily members *in vitro*. *Endocrinology* 2003;144:154–62.
148. Papachroni KK, Piperi C, Levidou G, et al. Lysyl oxidase interacts with AGE signalling to modulate collagen synthesis in polycystic ovarian tissue. *J Cell Mol Med* 2010;14:2460–9.
149. Jinno M, Takeuchi M, Watanabe A, et al. Advanced glycation end-products accumulation compromises embryonic development and achievement of pregnancy by assisted reproductive technology. *Hum Reprod* 2011;26:604–10.
150. Malickova K, Jarosova R, Rezabek K, et al. Concentrations of sRAGE in serum and follicular fluid in assisted reproductive cycles—A preliminary study. *Clin Lab* 2010;56:377–84.

151. Ambroggio J, Casson P, Merhi Z. Soluble Receptor for Advanced Glycation End-products (sRAGE): A Potential Indicator of Ovarian Response to Controlled Ovarian Hyperstimulation. Boston, MA: American Society for Reproductive Medicine; 2013.
152. Sharma I, Dhawan V, Saha SC, Rashmi B, Dhaliwal LK. Implication of the RAGE-EN-RAGE axis in endometriosis. *Int J Gynaecol Obstet* 2010;110:199–202.
153. Uribarri J, Cai W, Woodward M, et al. Elevated serum advanced glycation endproducts in obese indicate risk for the metabolic syndrome: A link between healthy and unhealthy obesity? *J Clin Endocrinol Metab* 2015;100:1957–66.

3

AGE Clearance Mechanisms

Armando Rojas, Ileana Gonzalez, and Carolina Añazco
Catholic University of Maule
Talca, Chile

CONTENTS

KEY POINTS

- Body advanced glycation end products (AGE) pool originates from both endogenous formation and dietary intake.
- This pool is under the control of different clearance mechanisms.
- In addition to renal mechanisms, AGE clearance also proceeds by cellular receptors or enzymatic systems.
- Some receptor-mediated mechanisms are able to trigger robust cellular responses.
- More research is needed to clarify the functional link between all AGE clearance mechanisms.

3.1 Introduction

Advanced glycation end products (AGEs) are a heterogeneous, complex group of compounds that are formed mainly via the Maillard reaction. A compelling body of evidence has demonstrated that engagement by AGEs or AGE-modified proteins to cellular receptors, such as the receptor for advanced glycation end products (RAGE) triggers the activation of a complex cascade of signal transduction events, leading to a marked and sustained production of proinflammatory mediators.

Since AGEs are constantly forming under physiological conditions and not less important the daily dietary intake of AGEs, complex receptor systems have evolved to remove glycation modified molecules and/or degrade existing AGE cross-links from tissues, thereby limiting their deleterious effects.

3.2 Formation of AGEs

The formation of AGEs, by the so-called Maillard reaction, is a complex cascade of glycation reactions affecting different kinds of biomolecules including proteins, lipids, and nucleic acids. These reactions include condensations, rearrangements, fragmentations, and oxidative modifications leading to a very heterogeneous myriad of products, which are linked in a complicated network.

In the Maillard reaction, an amine moiety from amines, amino acids, peptides, or proteins reacts with a carbonyl group present not only in reducing sugars such as glucose but also in oxidized lipids. The formation of advanced glycation end products occurs through different steps, where the formation of a Schiff base, by a nonenzymatic reaction, is highly dependent on the concentrations of reducing sugars or oxidized lipids. Later, this Schiff base undergoes some chemical rearrangements leading to the formation of slowly reversed Amadori products, also known as early glycation products. These Amadori products can then be converted through complex rearrangement reactions to a chemically related group of moieties, termed AGEs, which can irreversibly bind to proteins that include fibrinogen, albumin, immunoglobulins, and collagens (Brownlee et al. 1988; Vlassara 1994; Vlassara et al. 1994).

Noteworthy, AGE formation can also occur by the autoxidation of glucose and the peroxidation of lipids into dicarbonyls derivatives such as glyoxal, methylglyoxal, and 3-deoxyglucosone, which in turn can interact with proteins, lipids, and nucleic acids to form AGEs. Furthermore, AGEs can be also generated through the polyol pathway, where glucose is enzymatically converted to sorbitol by the aldose reductase and subsequently to fructose by the action of sorbitol dehydrogenase. Finally, fructose metabolites (as fructose 3-phosphate) are then converted into α-oxaldehydes, which in turn can render AGEs (Turk 2010; Miyazawa et al. 2012; Vistoli et al. 2013).

Of note, AGE formation not only occurs endogenously. Humans are exposed to exogenous sources of AGEs, which is an important contributor to the body AGE pool (Henle 2003; Poulsen et al. 2013; Uribarri et al. 2015).

3.3 Mechanisms of AGE Clearance or Uptake

The irreversible modification of proteins by AGEs is not only restricted to long half-live molecules, but it is also observed in short half-life proteins.

The spontaneous formation and slow-rate accumulation of AGE-modified proteins at both intra cellular and extracellular compartments is a hallmark of the aging process. Furthermore, the enhanced formation and/or accumulation AGEs are linked to a variety of pathological processes or clinical entities such as a diabetes mellitus, atherosclerosis, chronic inflammation, neurodegenerative diseases, renal failure, and cancer among others

It is then obvious the imperative existence of clearance or removal mechanisms for either AGE-modified plasma proteins, AGE–low molecular weight compounds -the most abundant-, and also AGE free adducts.

An obvious mechanism to clear AGEs from the body is renal elimination, which is reviewed in another Chapter 4 of this book. In the present chapter, we intend to highlight main removal or clearance mechanisms by tissues focusing on those mediated by different receptors families or enzymatic-mediated degradation mechanisms.

3.3.1 Receptor-Mediated Degradation Mechanisms

3.3.1.1 Receptors of Advanced Glycation End Products

Several AGE-binding proteins have been identified so far where RAGE (also known as AGER) is associated with triggering proinflammatory intracellular signaling cascades once it is engaged by AGEs, leading to consistent and robust cellular responses.

RAGE is a member of the immunoglobulin protein family of cell surface molecules (Park and Boyington 2010) and shares structural homology with other immunoglobulin-like receptors (Zong et al. 2010).

First described in 1992, RAGE has attracted increasing attention due to its involvement in several pathophysiological situations associated with inflammation such as in diabetes, cancer, renal failure, heart failure, and neurodegenerative diseases (González et al. 2013).

While in the majority of healthy adult tissues, RAGE is expressed at low basal level, the upregulation of RAGE has been associated with diverse pathological events, all of them associated in some way with an inflammatory process (Schmidt et al. 1999).

Noteworthy, RAGE is highly polymorphic and several RAGE splice variants have been reported, with some of them appearing to be tightly linked to different clinical entities (González et al. 2013).

However, endogenous soluble RAGE isoforms may be generated by other mechanisms different from alternative splicing, such as the participation of membrane-associated proteases, including the sheddase A disintegrin and metalloprotease-10 (ADAM-10) and the matrix metalloproteinase-9 (MMP-9) (Raucci et al. 2008).

A key consequence of RAGE engagement is the activation of multiple signaling pathways, including reactive oxygen species (ROS), p21ras, erk1/2 (p44/p42) MAP kinases, p38 and SAPK/JNK MAP kinases, rho GTPases, phosphoinositol-3 kinase, and the JAK/STAT pathway, with important downstream inflammatory consequences such as activation of NF-κB, AP-1, and Stat-3 (Hofmann et al. 1999; Yeh et al. 2001).

In fact, the pioneer works for unraveling the role of RAGE in human physiopathology were focused on the vascular complication of diabetes where the onset of chronic inflammation is a common element (Rojas and Morales 2004; Yan et al. 2008).

However, other proteins are able to bind AGEs and play a particular role in the removal of AGEs rather than in signal transduction. Among them, the AGE receptor complex consists of three different proteins known as AGE-R1, AGE-R2, and AGE-R3 (Figure 3.1), which are localized in caveolin-rich membrane domains and are involved in endocytic uptake and degradation of AGE-modified proteins.

In 1991, the pioneer work of Vlassara's group (Yang et al. 1991) identified two proteins in rat liver membranes that specifically bound AGE, named at that time as p60 and p90. Both proteins were also later described in monocytes/macrophages. The same group reported in 1996 that these two proteins p60 and p90 were identical to OST-48 (AGE-R1) and 80K-H (AGE-R2), respectively (Li et al. 1996).

From a functional point of view, this unusual number of different receptors for AGEs involved in endocytic uptake and degradation may be linked to the diversity in their biological functions in response to the same ligands.

3.3.1.1.1 AGE-R1 (OST-48)

As already mentioned, AGE-R1 was the first cell surface receptor able to bind glucose-modified proteins in a way that functioning as a detoxifying system through an endocytosis-mediated process, and thus being responsible for the clearance of circulating AGEs in the body. This finding represented a hallmark, highlighting the presence of mechanisms devoted to counteract the deleterious actions of AGEs. This protein, also known as OST-48, was initially thought to act as a stabilizing element of the oligosaccharyltransferase (OST) (Silberstein et al. 1992). At present, AGE-R1 is considered as an integral plasma membrane protein being active in binding of AGE-modified proteins. Interestingly, the activity of AGE-R1 is not only restricted to the clearance of AGE but it also has further activities linked to counteracting the prooxidant activities of AGEs (Cai et al. 2007, 2008).

Of note, AGE-R1 is able to downregulate the expression of the prooxidant protein $p66^{shc}$ and/or suppress the phosphorylation of this protein at ser-36 position (Cai et al. 2006) and thus decrease the cell oxidant stress.

Although AGE-R1 expression has been consistently shown to be reduced on different pathological conditions associated with sustained high levels of oxidative stress, such as diabetes and aging, the restriction of either dietary AGEs or calories ingested increases AGE-R1 levels (He et al. 2000, 2001; Vlassara et al. 2009).

Recently, new evidence has shed new light on the protective role of AGE-R1 on pathophysiology. AGE-R1 transgenic mice are protected against fat-diet-induced vascular disease and abnormal glucose homeostasis, where the protective effects of AGER1 require functional SIRT1, a NAD+-dependent deacetylase and survival factor (Cai et al. 2012). This factor is implicated in the prevention of many

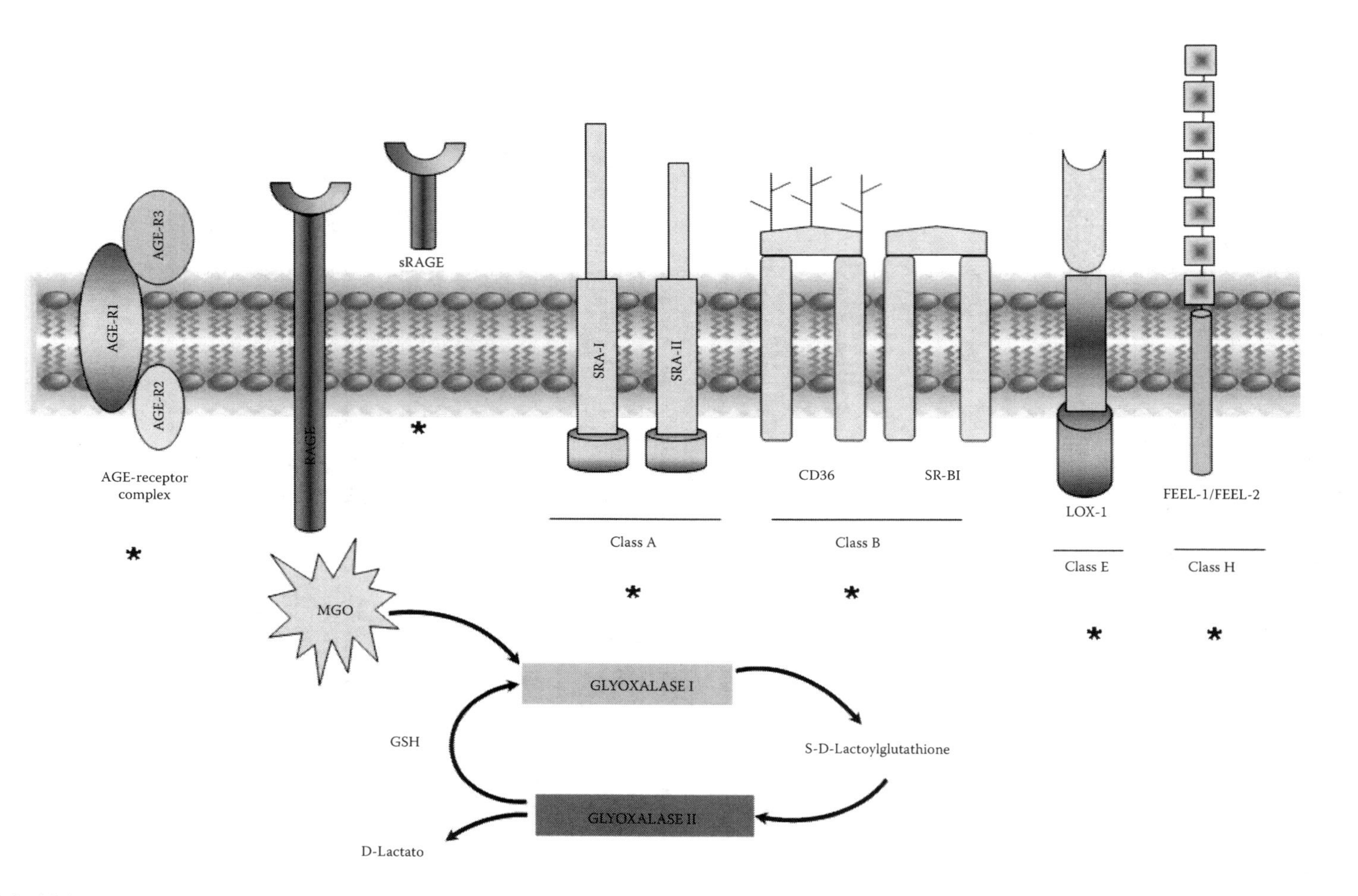

FIGURE 3.1 Main catabolic pathways for AGEs. Main receptors able to recognize and bind AGEs are depicted here. Some of these receptors belong to the scavenger receptor family. SRA-I and SRA-II are members of the class A family, CD36 and SRB-I (class B), LOX-1 (Class E), and FEEL-1 and -2 (Class H). Only those marked with (*) have been described as receptors able to bind AGEs, but their main roles are connected with removal of AGEs rather than signal transduction. In addition, the main enzymatic pathway devoted to detoxified AGEs, the glyoxalase system, is also depicted.

AGE-related diseases such as cancer, Alzheimer's disease, and type-2 diabetes, by controlling key biological processes such as DNA repair and apoptosis, circadian clocks, inflammatory pathways, insulin secretion, and mitochondrial biogenesis (Haigis and Sinclair 2010).

3.3.1.1.2 AGE-R2 (80K-H)

The second member of the AGE receptor complex is an acidic 80 kDa protein, which was first characterized as p90 and later established as a homologous to the 80K-H protein. Although this protein was initially reported as a substrate of protein kinase C, a more recent body of evidence suggests that it plays a role in the intracellular signaling of the FGF receptor (Schrijvers et al. 2004).

The biological function of 80K-H is not fully understood. A growing body of experimental data has shown that 80K-H protein has other activities than binding AGEs, such as a Ca^{2+} sensor and regulator of the epithelial Ca^{2+} channel TRPV5 (Gkika et al. 2004). Interestingly, 80K-H is also involved in GLUT4 translocation to the plasma membrane, as a part of a complex triggered by insulin (Hodgkinson et al. 2005).

3.3.1.1.3 AGE-R3 (galectin-3)

Galectin-3 is a member of the highly conserved family of soluble β-galactoside-binding lectins (Barondes et al. 1994). In 1995, it was initially reported that galectin-3 displays a high-affinity binding for ^{125}I-AGE-bovine serum albumin (BSA) with a saturable kinetic profile (Vlassara et al. 1995), and where oligomerization of galectin-3 onto the cell surface seems to be critical for its function as an AGE receptor (Nieminen et al. 2007).

In addition to binding AGEs, galectin-3 plays a role in endocytosis of modified low-density lipoproteins (LDLs), which carry both advanced lipoxidation end products (ALEs) and AGE structures (Virella et al. 2004). Compelling evidence supports the concept that galectin-3 is involved in the uptake and removal of AGE/ALE, and thus plays a protective anti-inflammatory role (Iacobini et al. 2004).

Data derived from animal models of metabolic diseases indicate that galectin-3 plays a protective role by a dual and tissue-specific modulation of RAGE expression depending on the anabolic or catabolic role of the particular tissue in the metabolism of AGEs (Pugliese et al. 2014).

3.3.1.2 Cross Talk with RAGE

RAGE is a cell surface receptor belonging to the immunoglobulin superfamily and is widely expressed in different cell types, where it is able to recognize a myriad of different ligands including AGEs. Once the receptor is engaged, the intracellular domain is essential for downstream signaling leading to the activation of different transcription factors such as NF-κB, AP-1, and STATs (Rojas et al. 2013).

Of great interest is the fact that different co-transfection approaches have demonstrated the cellular responses to the engagement of this receptor being suppressed through negative regulation of RAGE when AGE-R1 is co-expressed with RAGE (Lu et al. 2004). This negative regulation may be achieved by either the AGE-R1-dependent AGE uptake and degradation, thereby reducing the extracellular bioavailability of AGEs to bind RAGE, or by inhibiting the AGE-mediated ROS-dependent signaling promoted by RAGE engagement, particularly through the suppression of p66shc expression and its phosphorylation, which in turn decrease the oxidant stress both *in vitro* and *in vivo* (Cai et al. 2007, 2006).

Concordant with this hypothesis, AGE-R1 expression/function is reduced in conditions generally associated with high oxidative stress, such as diabetes and aging, whereas restriction of dietary AGEs increases AGER1 levels (He et al. 2001; Uribarri et al. 2011).

Finally, a potential cross talk between galectin-3 and RAGE has also been reported from data raised through *in vivo* studies, where, as a consequence of *galectin-3* ablation, the levels of AGE/ALE in tissue are increased and consequently RAGE is overexpressed (Pugliese et al. 2014).

3.3.1.2.1 sRAGE as a Decoy Receptor

At present, it is well known that the RAGE gene undergoes extensive alternative splicing to produce a variety of transcripts with diverse functions. In this context, soluble variants include a secreted isoform RAGE v1 (previously named as sRAGE, secretory C-truncated RAGE, esRAGE, hRAGE sec, or sRAGE1/2/3) and a N-terminally truncated isoform RAGE v2 (previously named Nt-RAGE, N-RAGE, or N-truncated RAGE) (González et al. 2013). However, endogenous soluble RAGE isoforms are also generated by other mechanisms involving membrane-associated proteases, including the sheddase A disintegrin and metalloprotease-10 (ADAM-10) and the matrix metalloproteinase-9 (MMP-9) (Raucci et al. 2008; Zhang et al. 2008).

At present, sRAGE is thought to function as a decoy receptor, thus preventing the interaction with the membrane-anchored full-length RAGE. In this context, a large body of evidence supports the fact that sRAGE may contribute to the removal/detoxification of AGEs.

Thus, the decoy function of sRAGE suggests the presence of a regulatory negative feedback mechanism in which it can serve to prevent the activation of cell surface RAGE (Bowman and Schmidt 2013; Gugliucci and Menini 2014). However, there are many questions yet to be answered for a full understanding of the biological and clinical significance of soluble RAGE (Schmidt 2015).

3.3.1.3 Scavenger Receptor Family

The scavenger receptor family was initially described by the pioneering work of Goldstein et al. (1979), as a group of receptors able to recognize and mediate the uptake and degradation of modified proteins like oxidized- (ox-LDL) or acetylated-LDL (acetyl-LDL). These receptors are extracellular glycoproteins, classified as pattern recognition receptors (PRRs), which mediate phagocytosis of negatively charged ligands, not only ox-LDL and acetyl-LDL but also AGE and pathogen-associated molecular patterns (PAMPs) (Martínez et al. 2011). At present, a large number of different scavenger receptors has been identified and are classified according to their structural properties. Next, we are going to focus only on the members of the family that have been described as receptors for AGEs.

3.3.1.3.1 Class A Macrophage Scavenger Receptors (SR-A) Type I and Type II

The scavenger receptor Class A (SR-A) are homotrimeric transmembrane glycoproteins with a relative molecular weight of 220 kDa consisting of five (SR-AII) or six (SR-AI) different domains. All have a short cytoplasmatic domain, a single transmembrane region, and a large extracellular domain, responsible for ligand recognition. These receptors, abundantly expressed in monocytes/macrophages, dendritic cells, and endothelial cells, were the first identified members of the scavenger receptor family (Kodama et al. 1990; Rohrer et al. 1990).

The SR-AI/II function as AGE receptor was initially reported in *in vitro* studies using SR-A-overexpressing CHO cells, where the degradation capacity for AGE–BSA was increased in parallel with that observed for acetyl-LDL. Conversely, peritoneal macrophages derived from SR-A-knockout mice showed a markedly reduced degradation of AGE–BSA (Araki et al. 1995; Suzuki et al. 1997).

Of note, an SR-A-dependent mechanism has been reported to drive glomerular migration of macrophages in diabetic SR-A-knockout mice, thus supporting the role of these receptors in the pathogenesis of diabetic nephropathy (Horiuchi et al. 2005).

The existence of a new cross talk between SR-A and RAGE has been recently reported, where the overexpression of SR-A suppressed RAGE signaling, whereas RAGE activation favored macrophages polarization toward a proinflammatory (M1) phenotype in the absence of SR-A in diabetic retinopathy (Ma et al. 2014).

3.3.1.3.2 Class B Macrophage Scavenger Receptors

These two receptors belong to the scavenger receptors Class B. They are mainly located at caveolae-like domains on the cell surface. Both receptors have been described to bind and mediate endocytic uptake and subsequent intracellular degradation of AGE-modified proteins, by the classical approach using CHO cell overexpressing CD36 or SR-B1 (Ohgami et al. 2000, 2001).

3.3.1.3.2.1 CD36 and SR-B1 CD36 is a highly glycosylated protein present in different cell types including mononuclear phagocytes, adipocytes, hepatocytes, platelets, myocytes, and some epithelial cells. In addition to AGE-modified proteins, it also binds numerous ligands such as ox-LDL, collagen, thrombospondin, fatty acids, and anionic phospholipids (Febbraio et al. 2001).

CD36 has been reported as one of the major ox-LDL receptors and is upregulated in macrophages and smooth muscle cell–derived foam cells in human atherosclerotic lesions. Of note, the binding domain of CD36 to AGE–BSA might overlap the binding domain of CD36 to ox-LDL. This finding is particularly interesting in the pathogenesis of diabetic macrovascular complications and diabetic dyslipidemia, considering the high availability of AGE-modified proteins generated *in situ* (Ohgami et al. 2001).

Recently, it has been reported that AGEs generated under hyperglycemic conditions can specifically interact with CD36 on platelets. This interaction can trigger CD36-dependent JNK2 activation, enhance platelet aggregation, and accelerate thrombus formation. These findings represent new insights into the mechanisms underlying the increased risk of arterial thrombosis in diabetic patients (Zhu et al. 2012).

SR-BI has some structural homology to CD36, particularly at the transmembrane domains (Greenwalt et al. 1992). The first described function of SR-B1 was as a scavenger receptor able to bind and internalize acetyl-LDL and ox-LDL (Acton et al. 1994).

Some experimental data support the interference on SR-BI-mediated cholesterol transport that may be caused by AGE-modified proteins, and thus inhibiting the selective uptake of HDL-cholesteryl esters, as well as cholesterol efflux from peripheral cells to HDL, thereby accelerating diabetes-induced atherosclerosis (Ohgami et al. 2003). This interference is thought to occur by interference of the formation of a hydrophobic channel where the HDL-cholesteryl esters move between HDL particles and cell membrane instead of blocking the HDL binding to the receptor. Interestingly, both aminoguanidine and metformin prevent the reduced HDL-mediated cell cholesterol efflux induced by AGEs (Miyazaki et al. 2002; Machado et al. 2006).

3.3.1.3.2.2 SRE-1/Lox-1 The Class E, type 1 scavenger receptor, also known as lectin-like oxidase low-density lipoprotein receptor (LOX-1), was initially cloned in 1997 from bovine aortic endothelial cells and from human lung [21], as a novel receptor that mediates the endocytic uptake and subsequent degradation of ox-LDL (Sawamura et al. 1997). Briefly after, the expression of LOX-1 was reported in macrophages and was suggested as a scavenger receptor for ox-LDL (Yoshida et al. 1998).

The first mechanistic link between this receptor with the glycol-oxidative modification of lipoproteins was reported in a model of diabetic rats (Chen et al. 2001), and 1 year later, Jono et al. (2002) reported that LOX-1 functions as an endothelial receptor for AGE–BSA. Since then, a growing body of evidence has supported the role of LOX-1 as a receptor for AGEs. Interestingly, LOX-1 expression can be upregulated by AGE–BSA through a mechanism involving RAGE engagement and subsequent activation of the PI3K/PDK1/mTORC2 pathway. Additionally, metformin can reduce AGE-stimulated LOX-1 expression in endothelial cells *in vitro* (Shiu et al. 2012).

Finally, a soluble form of LOX-1 has been reported. In this context, increased levels of soluble LOX-1 are reported in type 2 diabetic patients, and the levels decreased after improvement of glycemic control, where the magnitude of reduction correlated with the reduction of AGEs (Tan et al. 2008).

3.3.1.3.2.3 FEEL-1/FEEL-2 Fascilin, EGF-like, lamin-type EGF-like, and link domain-containing scavenger receptor -1 (FEEL-1) and its paralogous protein FEEL-2 are multiligand receptors (also known as stabilin-1 and -2) able to endocyte not only AGEs but also modified LDL. FEEL-1 was initially cloned from human vein endothelial cells. Both receptors are quite structurally different when compared with other scavenger receptors, and the homology degree between both receptors is not higher than 40% (Tamura et al. 2003). FEEL-1 and -2 are highly expressed by the liver and vascular tissues, where they recognize AGEs, thereby contributing to the development of diabetic vascular complications and atherosclerosis. Additionally, stabilin-1 is also expressed in activated macrophages (Politz et al. 2002).

The binding and uptake of apoptotic bodies by FEEL-1 -2 (stabilin-1, -2) was reported to depend on the recognition of phosphatidylserine (PS). Of note, this binding specificity to PS has also been reported for RAGE, which actively participates in the clearance of apoptotic cells by the binding to PS (He et al. 2011).

Finally, a quite interesting hypothesis derived from the data obtained *in vitro* from choriocapillaris endothelial cells (CCEC) has been launched. Overload of the FEEL-1- and -2-mediated clearance system with AGEs in these cells (e.g., in diabetes) may hamper their ability to clear AGE, which could then ligate RAGE elsewhere in the retina and thus contributing to the development of diabetic retinopathy (McCourt et al. 2009).

3.3.2 Enzyme-Mediated Degradation

3.3.2.1 Glyoxalase System

In 1994, Professor Thornalley's group described for the first time the association of the detoxification of methylglyoxal by the glyoxalase system and its association with the development of diabetic complications (McLellan and Thornalley 1994).

The glyoxalase system is an enzymatic system located at the cytosolic compartment of all human cells and comprises two enzymes, glyoxalase-I (GLO-I) and glyoxalase-II (GLO-II). This enzymatic system mediates the conversion of methylglyoxal to D-lactate via the intermediate formation of S-D- lactoylglutathione. Further studies have revealed that reactive dicarbonyls, such as methylglyoxal, can react also with reduced glutathione thus forming hemithioacetal, which is then converted by GLO-I to s-2 hydroacetylglutathione, which under the action of GLO-II renders α-hydroxyacid and reduced glutathione (Thornalley 2003; Mannervik 2008).

GLO-I is the key enzyme in this antiglycation enzymatic defense mechanism because it is the rate-limiting step of this enzymatic pathway, which is now considered as the major detoxification system of reactive dicarbonyls (Fleming et al. 2011).

In 2001, a clinical observation on hemodialysis patients highlighted the role of the glyoxalase as a detoxification system of precursor reactive carbonyl compounds (RCOs) in the *in vivo* AGE formation (Miyata et al. 2001).

It is known that arginine residues have high-frequency occurrence in sites of protein–protein, enzyme substrate, and protein–nucleotide binding sites. Furthermore, a compelling body of evidence clearly shows that functionally important arginine residues in proteins undergo dicarbonyl glycation, thus leading to the functional impairment of several proteins linked to many physiopathological processes. Therefore, dicarbonyl glycation is a real threat to cellular proteome, and as such the term "dicarbonyl proteome" was coined in 2008 (Rabbani and Thornalley 2008).

It is known that cells respond to stress by several stress–response mechanisms as part of a general mechanism to maintain cellular homeostasis (Martindale and Holbrook 2002; Kourtis and Tavernarakis 2011). Of note, dicarbonyl stress has been reported to be countered by upregulation of GLO-I by the activation of the Nrf2-mediated anti-stress system, which coordinates the increased expression of several genes associated with protection against oxidative stress (Mingzhan et al. 2012).

Conversely, hyperglycemia, methylglyoxal, and AGEs are able to reduce GLO-I expression and activity in different cell types, while inhibition or *RAGE* gene ablation restores GLO-I (Bierhaus et al. 2005; Bierhaus and Nawroth 2009).

At present, it is well known that dysfunction of the glyoxalase system is linked to several age-related health problems, such as diabetes, cardiovascular disease, cancer, and disorders of the central nervous system (Maessen et al. 2015). Of note, the intake of dietary glycotoxins has been recently linked to a reduced activity in ovarian GLO-I activity in an androgenized prepubertal rat model (Kandaraki et al. 2012). Actually, reversal of suppressed GLO-1 mRNA has been demonstrated in MetSyn subjects on a low-AGE diet (Vlassara et al. 2016).

Finally, an interesting report highlighted the possibility of restoring glyoxalase-I function by pharmacological manipulation. In fact, candesartan, an angiotensin type 1 receptor blocker which is known to reduce the incidence of diabetic retinopathy and improve the regression of the retinal disease, is able to restore the GLO-I activity and expression in diabetics rats (Miller et al. 2010).

3.3.3 Conclusions

At present, compelling experimental and clinical data support the idea that accumulation of AGEs, either endogenously formed or derived from the diet, could be associated with diseases. During the last two decades, remarkable efforts have been made to unraveling how the body can manage carbonyl stress, being able to prevent AGEs from modifying key target proteins or activating proinflammatory pathways following engagement. However, it is very important to have in mind that RAGE also plays a key role in normal physiology. Therefore, it is imperative to develop more extensive research focused on clearly delineating the functional link between AGE-mediated receptor signaling and detoxification pathways not only in disease but also in the physiological context.

REFERENCES

Acton, S. L., P. E. Scherer, H. F Lodish, and M. Krieger. 1994. Expression cloning of SR-BI, a CD36-related class B scavenger receptor. *Journal of Biological Chemistry* 269 (33):21003–21009.

Araki, N., T. Higashi, T. Mori, R. Shibayama, Y. Kawabe, T. Kodama, K. Takahashi, M. Shichiri, and S. Horiuchi. 1995. Macrophage scavenger receptor mediates the endocytic uptake and degradation of advanced glycation end products of the Maillard reaction. *European Journal of Biochemistry* 230 (2):408–415.

Barondes, S. H., D.N. Cooper, M. A Gitt, and H. Leffler. 1994. Galectins. Structure and function of a large family of animal lectins. *Journal of Biological Chemistry* 269:20807–20807.

Bierhaus, A., P. Humpert, M. Morcos, T. Wendt, T. Chavakis, B. Arnold, D.M. Stern, and P.P Nawroth. 2005. Understanding RAGE, the receptor for advanced glycation end products. *Journal of Molecular Medicine* 83 (11):876–886. doi: 10.1007/s00109-005-0688-7.

Bierhaus, A., and P. P. Nawroth. 2009. Multiple levels of regulation determine the role of the receptor for AGE (RAGE) as common soil in inflammation, immune responses and diabetes mellitus and its complications. *Diabetologia* 52 (11):2251–2263. doi: 10.1007/s00125-009-1458-9.

Bowman, M. A. H., and A. M. Schmidt. 2013. The next generation of RAGE modulators: Implications for soluble RAGE therapies in vascular inflammation. *Journal of Molecular Medicine* 91 (12):1329–1331.

Brownlee, M., A. Cerami, and H. Vlassara. 1988. Advanced glycosylation end products in tissue and the biochemical basis of diabetic complications. *New England Journal of Medicine* 318 (20):1315–1321. doi: 10.1056/NEJM198805193182007.

Cai, W., J. C. He, L. Zhu, X. Chen, G. E Striker, and H. Vlassara. 2008. AGE-receptor-1 counteracts cellular oxidant stress induced by AGEs via negative regulation of p66shc-dependent FKHRL1 phosphorylation. *American Journal of Physiology-Cell Physiology* 294 (1):C145–C152.

Cai, W., J. C. He, L. Zhu, X. Chen, S. Wallenstein, G. E. Striker, and H. Vlassara. 2007. Reduced oxidant stress and extended lifespan in mice exposed to a low glycotoxin diet: Association with increased AGER1 expression. *The American Journal of Pathology* 170 (6):1893–1902.

Cai, W., J. C He, L. Zhu, C. Lu, and H. Vlassara. 2006. Advanced glycation end product (AGE) receptor 1 suppresses cell oxidant stress and activation signaling via EGF receptor. *Proceedings of the National Academy of Sciences* 103 (37):13801–13806.

Cai, W., M. Ramdas, L. Zhu, X. Chen, G. E. Striker, and H. Vlassara. 2012. Oral advanced glycation endproducts (AGEs) promote insulin resistance and diabetes by depleting the antioxidant defenses AGE receptor-1 and sirtuin 1. *Proceedings of the National Academy of Sciences* 109 (39):15888–15893.

Chen, M., M. Nagase, T. Fujita, S. Narumiya, T. Masaki, and T. Sawamura. 2001. Diabetes enhances lectin-like oxidized LDL receptor-1 (LOX-1) expression in the vascular endothelium: Possible role of LOX-1 ligand and AGE. *Biochemical and Biophysical Research Communications* 287 (4):962–968.

Febbraio, M., D. P Hajjar, and R. L. Silverstein. 2001. CD36: A class B scavenger receptor involved in angiogenesis, atherosclerosis, inflammation, and lipid metabolism. *Journal of Clinical Investigation* 108 (6):785.

Fleming, T. H, P. M. Humpert, P. P. Nawroth, and A. Bierhaus. 2011. Reactive metabolites and AGE/RAGE-mediated cellular dysfunction affect the aging process–a mini-review. *Gerontology* 57 (5):435–443.

Gkika, D., F. Mahieu, B. Nilius, J. G. J. Hoenderop, and R. J. M. Bindels. 2004. 80K-H as a new Ca2+ sensor regulating the activity of the epithelial Ca2+ channel transient receptor potential cation channel V5 (TRPV5). *Journal of Biological Chemistry* 279 (25):26351–26357.

Goldstein, J. L, Y. K. Ho, S. K. Basu, and M. S. Brown. 1979. Binding site on macrophages that mediates uptake and degradation of acetylated low density lipoprotein, producing massive cholesterol deposition. *Proceedings of the National Academy of Sciences* 76 (1):333–337.

González, I., J. Romero, B. L. Rodríguez, R. Pérez-Castro, and A. Rojas. 2013. The immunobiology of the receptor of advanced glycation end-products: Trends and challenges. *Immunobiology* 218 (5):790–797.

Greenwalt, D. E., R. H Lipsky, C. F. Ockenhouse, H. Ikeda, N. N. Tandon, and G. A. *Jamieson*. 1992. Membrane glycoprotein CD36: A review of its roles in adherence, signal transduction, and transfusion medicine. *Blood* 80 (5):1105–1115.

Gugliucci, A., and T. Menini. 2014. The axis AGE-RAGE-soluble RAGE and oxidative stress in chronic kidney disease. In *Oxidative Stress and Inflammation in Non-communicable Diseases-Molecular Mechanisms and Perspectives in Therapeutics*, Jordi Camps (Ed.), pp. 191–208. Springer, Heidelberg, Switzerland.

Haigis, M. C., and D. A. Sinclair. 2010. Mammalian sirtuins: Biological insights and disease relevance. *Annual Review of Pathology* 5:253.

He, C. J., T. Koschinsky, C. Buenting, and H. Vlassara. 2001. Presence of diabetic complications in type 1 diabetic patients correlates with low expression of mononuclear cell AGE-receptor-1 and elevated serum AGE. *Molecular Medicine* 7 (3):159.

He, M., H. Kubo, K. Morimoto, N. Fujino, T. Suzuki, T. Takahasi, M. Yamada, M. Yamaya, T. Maekawa, and Y. Yamamoto. 2011. Receptor for advanced glycation end products binds to phosphatidylserine and assists in the clearance of apoptotic cells. *EMBO Reports* 12 (4):358–364.

He, C-J., F. Zheng, A. Stitt, L. Striker, M. Hattori, and H. Vlassara. 2000. Differential expression of renal AGE-receptor genes in NOD mice: Possible role in nonobese diabetic renal disease. *Kidney International* 58 (5):1931–1940.

Henle, T., 2003. AGEs in foods: Do they play a role in uremia? *Kidney International* 63:S145–S147.

Hodgkinson, C., A. Mander, and G. Sale. 2005. Identification of 80K-H as a protein involved in GLUT4 vesicle trafficking. *Biochemistry Journal* 388:785–793.

Hofmann, M. A., S. Drury, C. Fu, W. Qu, A. Taguchi, Y. Lu, C. Avila, et al. 1999. RAGE mediates a novel proinflammatory axis: A central cell surface receptor for S100/calgranulin polypeptides. *Cell* 97:889–901.

Horiuchi, S., Y. Unno, H. Usui, K. Shikata, K. Takaki, W. Koito,Y. U. I. Sakamoto, R. Nagai, K. Makino, and A. Sasao. 2005. Pathological roles of advanced glycation end product Receptors SR-A and CD36. *Annals of the New York Academy of Sciences* 1043 (1):671–675.

Iacobini, C., S. Menini, G. Oddi, C. Ricci, L. Amadio, F. Pricci, A. Olivieri, M. Sorcini, U. D. Mario, and C. Pesce. 2004. Galectin-3/AGE-receptor 3 knockout mice show accelerated AGE-induced glomerular injury: Evidence for a protective role of galectin-3 as an AGE receptor. *The FASEB Journal* 18 (14):1773–1775.

Jono, T., A. Miyazaki, R. Nagai, T. Sawamura, T. Kitamura, and S. Horiuchi. 2002. Lectin-like oxidized low density lipoprotein receptor-1 (LOX-1) serves as an endothelial receptor for advanced glycation end products (AGE). *FEBS Letters* 511 (1):170–174.

Kandaraki, E., A. Chatzigeorgiou, C. Piperi, E. Palioura, S. Palimeri, P. Korkolopoulou, M. Koutsilieris, and A. G. Papavassiliou. 2012. Reduced ovarian glyoxalase-I activity by dietary glycotoxins and androgen excess: A causative link to polycystic ovarian syndrome. *Molecular Medicine* 18 (1):1183.

Kodama, T., M. Freeman, L. Rohrer, J. Zabrecky, P. Matsudaira, and M. Krieger. 1990. Type I macrophage scavenger receptor contains α-helical and collagen-like coiled coils. *Nature* 343 (6258):531–535.

Kourtis, N., and N. Tavernarakis. 2011. Cellular stress response pathways and ageing: Intricate molecular relationships. *The EMBO Journal* 30 (13):2520–2531.

Li, Y. M., T. Mitsuhashi, D. Wojciechowicz, N. Shimizu, J. Li, A. Stitt, C. He, D. Banerjee, and H. Vlassara. 1996. Molecular identity and cellular distribution of advanced glycation endproduct receptors: Relationship of p60 to OST-48 and p90 to 80K-H membrane proteins. *Proceedings of the National Academy of Sciences* 93 (20):11047–11052.

Lu, C., J. C. He, W. Cai, H. Liu, L. Zhu, and H. Vlassara. 2004. Advanced glycation endproduct (AGE) receptor 1 is a negative regulator of the inflammatory response to AGE in mesangial cells. *Proceedings of the National Academy of Sciences of the United States of America* 101 (32):11767–11772.

Ma, K., Y. Xu, C. Wang, N. Li, K. Li, Y. Zhang, X. Li, Q. Yang, H. Zhang, and X. Zhu. 2014. A cross talk between class a scavenger receptor and receptor for advanced glycation end-products contributes to diabetic retinopathy. *American Journal of Physiology-Endocrinology and Metabolism* 307 (12):E1153–E1165.

Machado, A. P., R. S. Pinto, Z. P Moysés, E. R Nakandakare, E. C. R. Quintão, and M. Passarelli. 2006. Aminoguanidine and metformin prevent the reduced rate of HDL-mediated cell cholesterol efflux induced by formation of advanced glycation end products. *The International Journal of Biochemistry & Cell Biology* 38 (3):392–403.

Maessen, D. E. M., C. D. A. Stehouwer, and C. G. Schalkwijk. 2015. The role of methylglyoxal and the glyoxalase system in diabetes and other age-related diseases. *Clinical Science* 128 (12):839–861.

Mannervik, B., 2008. Molecular enzymology of the glyoxalase system. *Drug Metabolism and Drug Interactions* 23 (1–2):13–28.

Martindale, J. L., and N. J. Holbrook. 2002. Cellular response to oxidative stress: Signaling for suicide and survival. *Journal of Cellular Physiology* 192 (1):1–15.

Martínez, V. G., S. K. Moestrup, U. Holmskov, J. Mollenhauer, and F. Lozano. 2011. The conserved scavenger receptor cysteine-rich superfamily in therapy and diagnosis. *Pharmacological Reviews* 63 (4):967–1000.

McCourt, P., K. Schledzewski, S. Goerdt, G. Moldenhauer, X. Liu, B. Smedsrød, and K. K. Sørensen. 2009. Endocytosis of advanced glycation end-products in Bovine Choriocapillaris Endothelial Cells. *Microcirculation* 16 (7):640–655.

McLellan, A. C., and J. Thornalley. 1994. Glyoxalase system in clinical diabetes mellitus and correlation with diabetic complications. *Clinical Science* 87:21–29.

Miller, A. G., G. Tan, K. J. Binger, R. J. Pickering, M. C. Thomas, R. H. Nagaraj, M. E. Cooper, and J. L. Wilkinson-Berka. 2010. Candesartan attenuates diabetic retinal vascular pathology by restoring glyoxalase-I function. *Diabetes* 59 (12):3208–3215.

Mingzhan, X., R. Naila, M. Hiroshi, I. Precious, K. Neil, S. Tomokazu, M. Takashi, Y. Masayuki, and J. T. Paul. 2012. Transcriptional control of glyoxalase 1 by Nrf2 provides a stress-responsive defence against dicarbonyl glycation. *Biochemical Journal* 443 (1):213–222.

Miyata, T., C. van Ypersele de Strihou, T. Imasawa, A. Yoshino, Y. Ueda, H. Ogura, K. Kominami, H. Onogi, R. Inagi, and M. Nangaku. 2001. Glyoxalase I deficiency is associated with an unusual level of advanced glycation end products in a hemodialysis patient. *Kidney International* 60 (6):2351–2359.

Miyazaki, A., H. Nakayama, and S. Horiuchi. 2002. Scavenger receptors that recognize advanced glycation end products. *Trends in Cardiovascular Medicine* 12 (6):258–262.

Miyazawa, T., K. Nakagawa, S. Shimasaki, and R. Nagai. 2012. Lipid glycation and protein glycation in diabetes and atherosclerosis. *Amino Acids* 42 (4):1163–1170.

Nieminen, J., A. Kuno, J. Hirabayashi, and S. Sato. 2007. Visualization of galectin-3 oligomerization on the surface of neutrophils and endothelial cells using fluorescence resonance energy transfer. *Journal of Biological Chemistry* 282 (2):1374–1383.

Ohgami, N., A. Miyazaki, M. Sakai, A. Kuniyasu, H. Nakayama, and S. Horiuchi. 2003. Advanced glycation end products (AGE) inhibit scavenger receptor class B type I-mediated reverse cholesterol transport: A new crossroad of AGE to cholesterol metabolism. *Journal of Atherosclerosis and Thrombosis* 10 (1):1–6.

Ohgami, N., R. Nagai, M. Ikemoto, H. Arai, A. Kuniyasu, S. Horiuchi, and H. Nakayamaa. 2001. CD36, a member of class B scavenger receptor family, is a receptor for advanced glycation end products. *Annals of the New York Academy of Sciences* 947 (1):350–355. doi: 10.1111/j.1749-6632.2001.tb03961.x.

Ohgami, N., R. Nagai, A. Miyazaki, M. Ikemoto, H. Arai, S. Horiuchi, and H. Nakayama. 2001. Scavenger receptor class B type I-mediated reverse cholesterol transport is inhibited by advanced glycation end products. *Journal of Biological Chemistry* 276 (16):13348–13355.

Ohgami, N., R. Nagai, H. Nakayama, M. Ikemoto, and S. Horiuchi. 2000. CD36, a member of class B scavenger receptor family, as a receptor for advanced glycation end products. Paper read at Diabetes. *J Biol Chem.* 276(5):3195–3202.

Park, H. J., and J. C. Boyington. 2010. The 1.5 A Crystal structure of human Receptor for Advanced Glycation Endproducts (RAGE) ectodomains reveals unique features determining ligand binding. *Journal of Biological Chemistry.* 285 (52):40762–40770.

Politz, O., A. Gratchev, P. McCourt, K. Schledzewski, P. Guillot, S. Johansson, G. Svineng, P. Franke, C. Kannicht, and J. Kszhyshkowska. 2002. Stabilin-1 and-2 constitute a novel family of fasciclin-like hyaluronan receptor homologues. *Biochemistry Journal* 362:155–164.

Poulsen, M. W, R. V. Hedegaard, J. M. Andersen, B. de Courten, S. Bügel, J. Nielsen, L. H. Skibsted, and L. O. Dragsted. 2013. Advanced glycation endproducts in food and their effects on health. *Food and Chemical Toxicology* 60:10–37.

Pugliese, G., C. Iacobini, C. M. Pesce, and S. Menini. 2015. Galectin-3: An emerging all-out player in metabolic disorders and their complications. *Glycobiology* 25:136–150.

Rabbani, N., and P. J. Thornalley. 2008. The dicarbonyl proteome. *Annals of the New York Academy of Sciences* 1126 (1):124–127.

Raucci, A., S. Cugusi, A. Antonelli, S. M. Barabino, L. Monti, A. Bierhaus, K. Reiss, P. Saftig, and M. E. Bianchi. 2008. A soluble form of the receptor for advanced glycation endproducts (RAGE) is produced by proteolytic cleavage of the membrane-bound form by the sheddase a disintegrin and metalloprotease 10 (ADAM10). *The FASEB Journal* 22 (10):3716–3727.

Rohrer, L., M. Freeman, T. Kodama, M. Penman, and M. Krieger. 1990. Coiled-coil fibrous domains mediate ligand binding by macrophage scavenger receptor type II. *Nature* 343(6258):570–572.

Rojas, A., F. Delgado-López, I. González, R. Pérez-Castro, J. Romero, and I. Rojas. 2013. The receptor for advanced glycation end-products: A complex signaling scenario for a promiscuous receptor. *Cellular Signalling* 25 (3):609–614.

Rojas, A., and M. A. Morales. 2004. Advanced glycation and endothelial functions: A link towards vascular complications in diabetes. *Life Sciences*, 76: 715–730.

Sawamura, T., N. Kume, T. Aoyama, H. Moriwaki, H. Hoshikawa, Y. Aiba, T. Tanaka, S. Miwa, Y. Katsura, and T. Kita. 1997. An endothelial receptor for oxidized low-density lipoprotein. *Nature* 386(6620):73–77.

Schmidt, A. M., 2015. Soluble RAGEs—Prospects for treating & tracking metabolic and inflammatory disease. *Vascular Pharmacology* 72:1–8.

Schmidt, A. M., S. D. Yan, J. L. Wautier, and D. Stern. 1999. Activation of receptor for advanced glycation end products: A mechanism for chronic vascular dysfunction in diabetic vasculopathy and atherosclerosis. *Circulation Research* 84 (5):489–497.

Schrijvers, B. F., A. S. D. Vriese, and A. Flyvbjerg. 2004. From hyperglycemia to diabetic kidney disease: The role of metabolic, hemodynamic, intracellular factors and growth factors/cytokines. *Endocrine Reviews* 25 (6):971–1010.

Shiu, S. W., Y. Wong, and K. C. Tan. 2012. Effect of advanced glycation end products on lectin-like oxidized low density lipoprotein receptor-1 expression in endothelial cells. *Journal of Atherosclerosis and Thrombosis* 19 (12):1083–1092.

Silberstein, S., D. J. Kelleher, and R. Gilmore. 1992. The 48-kDa subunit of the mammalian oligosaccharyltransferase complex is homologous to the essential yeast protein WBP1. *Journal of Biological Chemistry* 267 (33):23658–23663.

Suzuki, H., Y. Kurihara, M. Takeya, N. Kamada, M. Kataoka, K. Jishage, O. Ueda, et al. 1997. A role for macrophage scavenger receptors in atherosclerosis and susceptibility to infection. *Nature* 386 (6622):292–296.

Tamura, Y., H. Adachi, J-I. Osuga, K. Ohashi, N. Yahagi, M. Sekiya, H. Okazaki, S. Tomita, Y. Iizuka, and H. Shima. 2003. FEEL-1 and FEEL-2 are endocytic receptors for advanced glycation end products. *Journal of Biological Chemistry* 278 (15):12613–12617.

Tan, K. C., S. W. Shiu, Y. Wong, L. Leng, and R. Bucala. 2008. Soluble lectin-like oxidized low density lipoprotein receptor-1 in type 2 diabetes mellitus. *Journal of Lipid Research* 49 (7):1438–1444.

Thornalley, P. J., 2003. Glyoxalase I-structure, function and a critical role in the enzymatic defence against glycation. *Biochemical Society Transactions* 31 (6):1343–1348.

Turk, Z., 2010. Glycotoxines, carbonyl stress and relevance to diabetes and its complications. *Physiological Research* 59 (2):147–156.

Uribarri, J., W. Cai, M. Ramdas, S. Goodman, R. Pyzik, X. Chen, L. Zhu, G. E. Striker, and H. Vlassara. 2011. Restriction of advanced glycation end products improves insulin resistance in human type 2 diabetes potential role of AGER1 and SIRT1. *Diabetes Care* 34 (7):1610–1616.

Uribarri, J., M. D. del Castillo, M. P. de la Maza, R. Filip, A. Gugliucci, C. Luevano-Contreras, M. H. Macías-Cervantes, D. H Markowicz Bastos, A. Medrano, and T. Menini. 2015. Dietary advanced glycation end products and their role in health and disease. *Advances in Nutrition: An International Review Journal* 6 (4):461–473.

Virella, G., S. R. Thorpe, N. L. Alderson, M. B. Derrick, C. Chassereau, J. Matthew Rhett, and M. F. Lopes-Virella. 2004. Definition of the immunogenic forms of modified human LDL recognized by human autoantibodies and by rabbit hyperimmune antibodies. *Journal of Lipid Research* 45 (10):1859–1867.

Vistoli, G., D. De Maddis, A. Cipak, N. Zarkovic, M. Carini, and G. Aldini. 2013. Advanced glycoxidation and lipoxidation end products (AGEs and ALEs): An overview of their mechanisms of formation. *Free Radical Research* 47 (supl):3–27.

Vlassara, H., 1994. Recent progress on the biologic and clinical significance of advanced glycosylation end products. *The Journal of Laboratory and Clinical Medicine* 124 (1):19–30.

Vlassara, H., R. Bucala, and L. Striker. 1994. Pathogenic effects of advanced glycosylation: Biochemical, biologic, and clinical implications for diabetes and aging. *Laboratory Investigation; A Journal of Technical Methods and Pathology* 70 (2):138–151.

Vlassara, H., W. Cai, S. Goodman, R. Pyzik, A. Yong, X. Chen, L. Zhu, T. Neade, M. Beeri, and J. M. Silverman. 2009. Protection against loss of innate defenses in adulthood by low advanced glycation end products (AGE) intake: Role of the antiinflammatory AGE receptor-1. *The Journal of Clinical Endocrinology & Metabolism* 94 (11):4483–4491.

Vlassara, H., W. Cai, E. Tripp, R. Pyzik, K. Yee, L. Goldberg, L. Tansman, X. Chen, V. Mani, Z. A. Fayad, G. N. Nadkarni, G. E. Striker, J. C. He, J. Uribarri. 2016. AGE restriction ameliorates insulin resistance in obese individuals with the metabolic syndrome: A randomised controlled trial. *Diabetologia* 59(10):2181–2192.

Vlassara, H., Y. Ming Li, F. Imani, D. Wojciechowicz, Z. Yang, F. T. Liu, and A. Cerami. 1995. Identification of galectin-3 as a high-affinity binding protein for advanced glycation end products (AGE): A new member of the AGE-receptor complex. *Molecular Medicine* 1 (6):634.

Yan, S. F., R. Ramasamy, A. M. Schmidt. 2008. Mechanisms of disease: Advanced glycation end-products and their receptor in inflammation and diabetes complications. *Nature clinical practice. Endocrinology & Metabolism* 4:285–93.

Yang, Z., Z. Makita, Y. Horii, S. Brunelle, A. Cerami, P. Sehajpal, M. Suthanthiran, and H. Vlassara. 1991. Two novel rat liver membrane proteins that bind advanced glycosylation endproducts: Relationship to macrophage receptor for glucose-modified proteins. *The Journal of Experimental Medicine* 174 (3):515–524.

Yeh, C-H., L. Sturgis, J. Haidacher, X. N. Zhang, S. J. Sherwood, R. J. Bjercke, O. Juhasz, M. T. Crow, R. G. Tilton, L. Denner, 2001. Requirement for p38 and p44/p42 mitogen-activated protein kinases in RAGE-mediated nuclear factor-kappaB transcriptional activation and cytokine secretion. *Diabetes* 50: 1495–1504.

Yoshida, H., N. Kondratenko, S. Green, D. Steinberg, and O. Quehenberger. 1998. Identification of the lectin-like receptor for oxidized low-density lipoprotein in human macrophages and its potential role as a scavenger receptor. *Biochemistry Journal* 334:9–13.

Zhang, L., M. Bukulin, E. Kojro, A. Roth, V. V. Metz, F. Fahrenholz, P. P. Nawroth, A. Bierhaus, and R. Postina. 2008. Receptor for advanced glycation end products is subjected to protein ectodomain shedding by metalloproteinases. *Journal of Biological Chemistry* 283 (51):35507–35516.

Zhu, W., W. Li, and R. L. Silverstein. 2012. Advanced glycation end products induce a prothrombotic phenotype in mice via interaction with platelet CD36. *Blood* 119 (25):6136–6144.

Zong, H., A. Madden, M. Ward, M. H. Mooney, C. T. Elliott, and A. W. Stitt. 2010. Homodimerization is essential for the receptor for advanced glycation end products (RAGE)-mediated signal transduction. *Journal of Biological Chemistry* 285 (30), 23137–23146.

4

How Are AGEs Handled by the Kidney?

Alejandro Gugliucci
Touro University College of Osteopathic Medicine
Vallejo, CA

CONTENTS

KEY POINTS

- Advanced glycation end products (AGEs) are produced by the Maillard reaction between reactive dicarbonyls and amino groups, mainly in proteins, but also in lipids and nucleic acids. They have been associated with aging, diabetes, neurological disease, and kidney failure. AGEs have three main sources: intracellular, glycation occurring in plasma or in the extracellular matrix, and finally AGEs from food.
- Human serum contains partially hydrolyzed AGE-peptides and free AGE-adducts, stemming from incomplete cellular or macrophage catabolism. Final disposal of endogenous or exogenous AGEs is a key kidney function. AGE-peptides are filtered and then reabsorbed in the proximal tubules followed by excretion of free AGE.
- Chronic kidney disease (CKD) patients have the highest level of AGEs, AGE-peptides, and free adducts, due to impaired clearance coupled with increased production via oxidative stress. Exogenous glycotoxins derived from regular diets play an important role in producing high serum AGEs levels in renal failure.
- The proinflammatory self-perpetuating action of AGEs acting on their receptor (RAGE) perpetuates damage in renal failure.
- Dietary restriction of AGEs may be a sensible method to lessen the disproportionate burden of toxic AGES in tissues and seemingly the morbidity and mortality related to their accretion.

4.1 Background

Advanced glycation end products (AGEs) are produced in the classical Maillard reaction, discovered in 1913 and reviewed elsewhere in this book (Stevens et al. 1977; Cerami et al. 1979, 1985, 1986; Monnier and Cerami 1982; Brownlee et al. 1984, 1985).

4.2 Sources of AGEs

In healthy humans, AGEs have two sources, endogenous and exogenous.

4.2.1 Endogenous AGEs

AGEs are produced in cells or in long-lived extracellular protein by glycation. Protein glycation is an intricate series of consecutive reactions collectively called the Maillard reaction, present in all tissues and fluids where enough concentration of glucose or more reactive dicarbonyls react with proteins (Stevens et al. 1977; Sell et al. 1991; Monnier et al. 1992). In early stages, the glycation adduct fructosyl-lysine (FL) is formed, the reaction then proceeds to form AGEs. Degradation of glycated proteins, glycolytic intermediates, and lipid peroxidation gives rise to glyoxal (G), methylglyoxal (MG), and 3-deoxyglucosone (3-DG), which are much more potent glycating agents (Rabbani and Thornalley 2009). These compounds react with proteins (as well as phospholipids and DNA) to form more AGEs directly. Other significant sources of AGE-products are hydroimidazolones derived from arginine residues modified by glyoxal, MG, and 3-DG. Other key AGE compounds are N^{ε}-carboxymethyl-lysine (CML), N^{ε}-carboxyethyl-lysine (CEL), pentosidine, pyrraline, and glucosepane (Sell et al. 2005; Nemet et al. 2011; Sveen et al. 2015). Moreover, the catabolism of cell and tissue-bound AGEs leaks a new pool of second generation, highly reactive AGE intermediates (peptides and free adducts) in circulation, named glycotoxins by some authors (Koschinsky et al. 1997; He et al. 1999; Uribarri et al. 2003). Some of these serum AGE-peptide derivatives react with new proteins (e.g., LDL, collagen) perpetuating and propagating oxidative modifications and/or creating new AGES cross-links *in vitro* and *in vivo* (Vlassara et al. 1992; Bucala et al. 1994; Makita et al. 1994; Gugliucci and Bendayan 1996).

4.2.2 Exogenous AGEs

AGEs are also present in ingested food, indeed in huge amounts as compared to the endogenous source (Vlassara et al. 1992). The content of AGEs in food depends on the nutrient composition and on the way food is processed, with roasting, smoking, and baking producing the highest levels of AGEs (He et al. 1999; Uribarri et al. 2003). This exogenous source of AGEs seems to be significant since modulation of the intake has been shown to modify the circulating levels of AGEs. A pioneering work since then confirmed by other studies has shown increases in AGE concentration in serum and urine of normal individuals after ingesting an AGE-rich protein meal which confirmed that 30% of AGEs in foods survive digestion and absorption and appear in the circulation as low molecular weight adducts in a manner directly proportional to the amount ingested (Koschinsky et al. 1997). Likewise, 70% of the ingested AGEs escape absorption. Moreover, only one-third of the absorbed AGEs in the serum appear in urine, the rest probably binds covalently onto tissues and cells. In humans, the steady influx of food-derived AGEs may serve as a source of glycotoxins, which become very critical in renal failure as we will discuss later.

4.3 Deleterious Effects of AGEs

AGEs exert a direct effect on proteins and lipids as previously discussed as well as proinflammatory effects mediated by RAGE (the receptor for advanced glycation end-products), which is a multiligand protein first isolated from bovine lung. RAGE integrates the immunoglobulin superfamily of receptors, which has an extracellular region containing one "V"-type immunoglobulin domain and two "C"-type immunoglobulin domains (Schmidt et al. 1996; Ramasamy et al. 2012; Thallas-Bonke et al. 2013). The receptor has a hydrophobic transmembrane segment and a greatly charged cytoplasmic domain. The latter orchestrates intracellular RAGE signaling. RAGE recognizes a variety of ligands including high mobility group box 1 protein (HMGB1), the leukocyte integrin Mac-1, S100/calgranulins, modified LDL, DNA, RNA, and amyloid fibrils. When activated, RAGE leads to a sequence of signaling with activation of nuclear factor-κ B (NF-κB) and oxidative stress and inflammation. RAGE signals via phosphatidylinositol-3 kinase (PI-3K), Ki-Ras and the MAPKs, and Erk1 and Erk2 (Schmidt and Stern 2000; Rodriguez-Ayala et al. 2005). In a coordinated fashion, these pathways promote and sustain the translocation of NF-κB from the cytoplasm to the nucleus. This occurs in a variety of cell types: monocytes, endothelial cells, microglia, podocytes, etc. Activation promotes inflammation and tissue injury sustained by a RAGE-dependent expression of proinflammatory mediators such as monocyte chemoattractant protein-1 (MCP-1) and vascular cell adhesion molecule-1 (VCAM-1) (Schmidt and Stern 2000; Rodriguez-Ayala et al. 2005). In this way, RAGE activity is associated with diabetic microvascular complications including nephropathy, retinopathy, and neuropathy (Bowman and Schmidt 2013; Daffu et al. 2013; Manigrasso et al. 2013). In renal failure, given the fact that AGE levels are even higher than in diabetes, those events are magnified and compounded by an increase in oxidative stress from multiple sources associated with the impaired renal homeostatic function. In parallel with the aforementioned cascades leading to inflammation, in endothelial (glomerular) and mesangial cells, RAGE triggering spurs a surge of reactive oxygen species (ROS). Beyond the local renal level, whether RAGE is augmented in atherosclerotic lesions in CKD remains unclear for humans. CKD prominently hastens atherogenesis in apoE-deficient mice. Blocking RAGE decreases the proatherogenic effects of CKD, conceivably mediated by a reduction in oxidative stress (Thallas-Bonke et al. 2013).

4.4 Renal Handling of AGEs

AGEs from all sources described above circulate and are handled for the most part by the kidney as toxic waste products. More than two decades ago, it became apparent that human serum contains partially hydrolyzed AGE-peptides and free AGE-adducts (Makita et al. 1991).

4.4.1 Renal Failure as a Human Model to Understand AGE Catabolism

In a pioneering work by Vlassara's team, with the aid of a radioreceptor assay employing the recently discovered RAGE at the time, they measured AGE-modified collagen in vascular tissue and AGE-peptides and AGE-proteins in serum from normal subjects and diabetic and nondiabetic patients with various degrees of renal dysfunction (Makita et al. 1991). AGE-peptides accumulated in the serum of patients with diabetes as a function of progressive renal impairment. The concentrations dropped moderately after hemodialysis and markedly after kidney transplantation. Diabetic patients with ESRD had five times more circulating AGE-peptides than diabetic patients without clinical signs of renal disease. The amount of serum AGE-peptides was clearly related to the extent of remaining kidney function. AGE-peptides were progressively higher as renal deterioration increased and correlated with serum creatinine levels. These data, confirmed thereafter in several other papers (Sell et al. 1991; Makita et al. 1994; Vlassara 1994), suggested that circulating AGEs are efficiently cleared by the normal kidney. With kidney dysfunction, however, and particularly in association with diabetes, serum AGEs accumulate.

4.4.2 AGE-Peptides and Free Adducts as a "Second Glycation Hit"

These tissue-derived degradation products may be produced either by a specific macrophages AGE-receptor pathway or by extracellular proteolytic systems. AGE-peptides are extremely reactive substances capable of modifying circulating or tissue proteins. LDL, for instance, contains a fraction

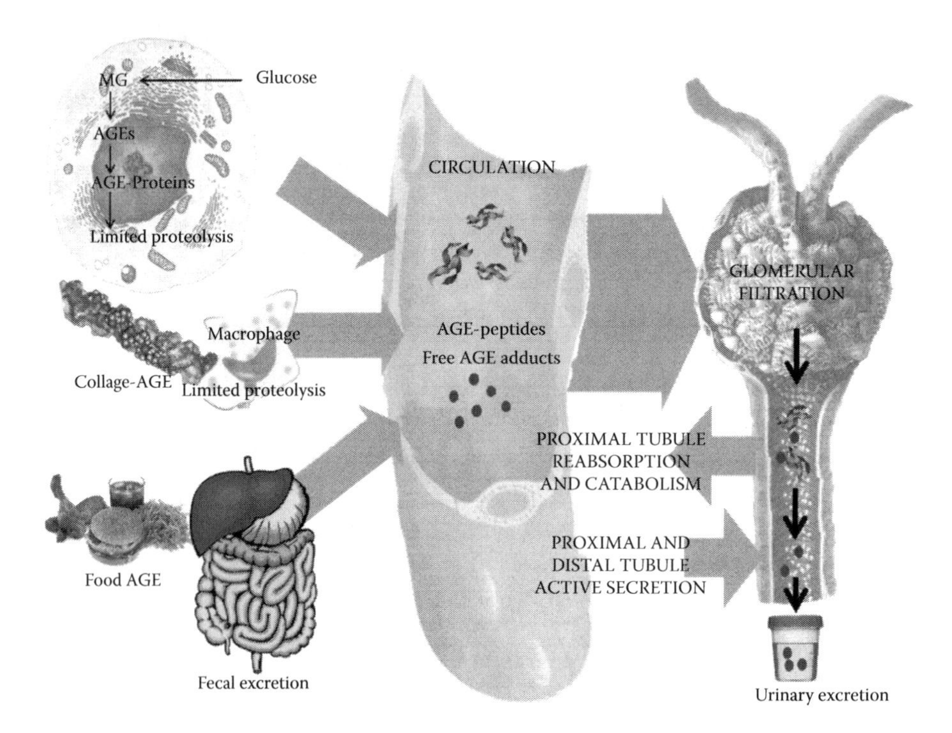

FIGURE 4.1 Role of the kidney in overall metabolism of AGEs. In the circulation and tissues, AGEs have three main sources, intracellular glycation, plasma and extracellular matrix glycation, as well as food-derived AGEs. Human serum contains partially hydrolyzed AGE-peptides and free AGE-adducts, stemming from incomplete cellular or macrophage catabolism. Endogenous AGE-peptides are filtered and then reabsorbed in the proximal tubules followed by excretion of free AGE. These processes, largely dependent on GFR and tubular function, are, by definition, severely impaired in CKD and ESRD. Therefore, as can be seen, CKD patients are prone to and certainly have the highest level of AGEs, AGE-peptides, and free adducts, due to increased production via oxidative stress and impaired clearance.

bearing AGE-adducts, AGE-LDL (Bucala et al. 1994). AGE-peptides, both synthetic and extracted from patients, readily bind to LDL altering its metabolism. Through this kind of evidence, it becomes clear that AGE-peptides are responsible for the modification of circulating and tissue resident proteins, leading to structural and functional changes, a damage added to that created by the original carbonyl (MG, glucose, etc.) attack on proteins. Evidently, partial cellular proteolysis of AGE-proteins as well as macrophage action on extracellular matrix generates a problem for the body to handle those partially degraded molecules, which still contain reactive groups (Figure 4.1).

4.4.3 Animal Mechanistic Studies Showing How the Kidneys Handle the "Second Hit" Problem: It Is Just Filtration?

As several lines of evidence suggested that AGE-peptides are eliminated by the kidney, early on we were the first to mechanistically show the renal fate of AGEs (Gugliucci and Bendayan 1995, 1996). AGE–BSA and AGE-peptides were injected and AGE-products in renal tissue of rats were monitored by colloidal gold post-embedding immunoelectron microscopy (Gugliucci and Bendayan 1995, 1996). When AGE-peptides were injected to normal rats, a short-term follow-up of their localization in the kidney showed they are easily filtered and actively reabsorbed by the proximal convoluted tubule. We showed that the endolysosomal apparatus of the proximal convoluted tubule plays a role in the disposal of AGE-peptides. The fact that AGE-peptide clearance in humans and rats is lower than the creatinine clearance indicates that not all of the circulating AGE-peptides are found in urine; some process of reabsorption occurs. The final fate of AGE-peptides also remains to be determined since no mammalian enzyme has been discovered that could mediate the catabolism of AGE moieties once the lysosomal hydrolysis of peptide bonds has taken place. We suggested the existence of a secretory process of resulting AGE-amino acids (free adducts) into urine that could also account for the presence of AGE-adducts such as pentosidine in the urine of diabetic patients. In the long run, the increased tubular charge of AGE-peptides due to diabetes may overwhelm the whole process and lead to tubular disorders (Gugliucci and Bendayan 1995, 1996). Another feature of AGE-peptides is the ability to bind covalently to phospholipids as described previously (Bucala et al. 1993). An accumulation of these adducts in tubular lysosomes as we have demonstrated might prove to be one further aggression to membranes and yet another process contributing to the overall toxicity.

4.4.4 Renal Handling of AGEs in Humans Confirms Animal Studies

With the advent of sensitive and sophisticated LCMS MS techniques to measure adducts, a more complete picture of the role of the kidney in AGEs handling emerged, including not only the fate of small peptides but also that of circulating free adducts (Agalou et al. 2005; Thornalley 2005; Rabbani et al. 2007; Rabbani and Thornalley 2009; Thornalley and Rabbani 2009). Glycation, oxidation, and nitration of endogenous proteins occur spontaneously and these modifications are also present in foods. Quantitatively important AGEs are hydro-imidazolones derived from arginine residues modified by glyoxal, methylglyoxal, and 3-DG: N_δ-(5-hydro-4-imidazolon-2-yl)ornithine, N_δ-(5-hydro-5-methyl-4-imidazolon-2-yl)-ornithine (MG-H1), N_δ-(5-hydro-5-(2,3,4-trihydroxybutyl)-4-imidazolon-2-yl)ornithine, and related structural isomers (3DG-H). Other key AGEs are N_ε-carboxymethyllysine (CML) and N_ε-carboxyethyllysine (CEL) and the protein cross-links pentosidine and glucosepane (Thornalley 2006). Further AGEs and related derivatives of emerging importance are N_ε-carboxymethylcysteine and N_ω-carboxymethylarginine.

4.4.5 Further Proof from Intervention Studies Causing Acute Renal Failure in Animals

Increased levels of these chemical changes were shown in chronic renal failure as well as acute renal failure. In rats, following bilateral nephrectomy and bilateral ureteral obstruction AGES residues of plasma protein were increased 3 h post-surgery, and afterward decreased in all groups (Rabbani et al. 2007). There were also marked increases in AGEs, dityrosine, or 3-nitrotyrosine free adducts in both nephrectomized and ureter-ligated rats compared to controls. There were lower modified adduct concentrations in the ureter-ligated rats compared to the nephrectomized rats, reflecting residual glomerular filtration and tubular removal and confirming our previous results (Gugliucci and Bendayan 1996; Rabbani et al. 2007).

4.4.6 Renal Failure Causes Dangerous Accumulation of AGEs: Middle Toxins

AGE-peptides are filtered and then reabsorbed in the proximal tubules followed by excretion of free AGE-adducts. These processes, largely dependent on GFR and tubular function are, by definition, severely impaired in CKD and ESRD. Therefore, as can be seen, CKD patients are prone to and certainly have the highest level of AGEs, AGEs-peptides, and free adducts, due to increased production via oxidative stress and impaired clearance (Miyata et al. 1996). In that sense, AGEs qualify as one of the classical "middle toxins" typical of uremia (Vlassara 1994). Unlike creatinine, which is reduced by three-fourths, AGE-peptides are only reduced by one-third in a typical hemodialysis (HD) session since AGE-peptides do not pass as efficiently through the dialyzer membrane. The pathological role of various low- to middle-molecular-weight compounds, termed "middle molecules" or "uremic toxins," that are not removed effectively by hemodialysis has always been a concern for nephrologists. They may have a significant etiologic role in the progress of several complications related to dialysis, including peripheral neuropathy, microangiopathy and macroangiopathy. The fast progression of these complications in diabetic patients on HD is surprising; half the patients with diabetes that start HD die within 2 years (Vlassara 1994). The higher levels of AGE-peptides in diabetic patients with ESRD might explain, for instance, the increased amounts of AGEs in their vessel-wall tissues. Circulating AGEs, with their innate chemical and biologic activities, could contribute to further organ damage via oxidative stress and actual protein modification. The role of both filtration and tubular processes in renal handling of AGEs is clear: a functioning kidney appears to be outstandingly effective and far better than hemodialysis: in ESRD patients, kidney transplantation reduced levels of circulating AGES-peptides to the normal range within days (Vlassara 1994).

4.4.7 Hemodialysis Lowers AGE-Peptides that Modify HDL Function

ESRD patients have increased oxidative stress, dyslipoproteinemia, and accelerated atherosclerosis. AGEs may play a role and certainly modify LDL (Bucala et al. 1993, 1994; Makita et al. 1994). We conducted a study to explore a putative role of LMW AGE-peptides accumulating in ESRD on HDL dysfunction, which may precipitate atherogenesis in this patient population (Gugliucci et al. 2007). Our ESRD patients had a 3-fold increase in serum AGEs and a striking 10-fold increase in low molecular weight AGEs, again showing the key role of the kidneys in the appropriate disposal of these molecules. We were the first to show that PON-1 activity actually changes favorably as a result of dialysis. One of the PON-1 physiological functions is to protect LDL from oxidative changes and ESRD is an oxidative stress disorder (Gugliucci et al. 2013; Gugliucci and Menini 2015; Mackness and Mackness 2013, 2015). We showed that the changes in PON-1 activity cannot be easily explained by changes in HDL-C nor subclasses per se (Gugliucci et al. 2007, 2013). Since we showed that increases in PON-1 are well predicted by changes in serum creatinine and urea, we suspected a role for dialyzable solutes and middle molecules. Low molecular weight AGEs decreased 3–4 times (on average) after dialysis. This rate of change correlated well with the changes in serum creatinine, pointing to low molecular weight species on the1 kDa range. Clearance of low molecular weight AGEs after hemodialysis correlated even better and predicted 79% of the changes in PON-1 activity. Although this correlation does not prove causation, it suggests this could be the case, especially when we consider the high reactivity of AGE-adducts. The effect of low molecular weight molecules retained in renal failure on PON-1 was replicated *in vitro*, showing time and dose dependency. These data serve as proof of principle that modulating AGEs can have a quick translation on changes in protein function, reversing deleterious effects. In renal failure patients, one means to achieve that is dialysis and another powerful one is to curtail exogenous AGEs.

4.5 Exogenous AGEs and Renal Failure: Benefits of Modulating Exogenous AGEs

CKD patients display increased concentrations of many α-oxoaldehydes, particularly glyoxal, MG, and 3-DG (Thornalley 2006). The key role of the kidney in handling the AGEs load is shown by the dramatic effect on AGEs and oxidative stress produced when they fail as described above. Interventions to curtail exogenous AGEs load are particularly illustrative as further proof, as decreasing endogenous sources have proven to be difficult. Pioneering work by Uribarri and Vlassara et al. has defined the relationship between dietary AGE content and serum AGEs levels. In a study that included 139 hemodialysis and 50 peritoneal dialysis patients, serum CML level correlated significantly with dietary AGEs intake (Uribarri et al. 2003). Dietary AGEs content, regardless of other diet components, is a significant contributor to high serum AGE levels in patients with renal failure. In a prospective and randomized 4-week study, the same group showed that a short-term low-AGE diet can significantly modify circulating AGE levels in renal failure patients on maintenance peritoneal dialysis (Uribarri et al. 2003). These findings support the hypothesis that exogenous glycotoxins derived from regular diets, comprising those suggested for dialysis patients, play an important role in producing high serum AGE levels in renal failure. Circulating AGE levels also decreased after dietary AGEs restriction in other conditions (Mallipattu and Uribarri 2014; Macias-Cervantes et al. 2015). Finally, proof of the proinflammatory self-perpetuating action of AGEs comes from several publications (Uribarri et al. 2005; Bengmark 2007; Cottone et al. 2008; Vlassara et al. 2012). Dietary restriction of AGEs may be a sensible method to lessen the disproportionate burden of toxic AGEs in tissues and seemingly the morbidity and mortality related to their accretion.

REFERENCES

Agalou, S., N. Ahmed, R. Babaei-Jadidi, A. Dawnay, and P. J. Thornalley. 2005. Profound mishandling of protein glycation degradation products in uremia and dialysis. *J Am Soc Nephrol* 16 (5):1471–85. doi: 10.1681/ASN.2004080635.

Bengmark, S. 2007. Advanced glycation and lipoxidation end products—Amplifiers of inflammation: The role of food. *JPEN J Parenter Enteral Nutr* 31 (5):430–40.

Bowman, M. A., and A. M. Schmidt. 2013. The next generation of RAGE modulators: Implications for soluble RAGE therapies in vascular inflammation. *J Mol Med (Berl)* 91 (12):1329–31. doi: 10.1007/s00109-013-1097-y.

Brownlee, M., H. Vlassara, and A. Cerami. 1984. Nonenzymatic glycosylation and the pathogenesis of diabetic complications. *Ann Intern Med* 101 (4):527–37.

Brownlee, M., H. Vlassara, and A. Cerami. 1985. Nonenzymatic glycosylation products on collagen covalently trap low-density lipoprotein. *Diabetes* 34 (9):938–41.

Bucala, R., Z. Makita, T. Koschinsky, A. Cerami, and H. Vlassara. 1993. Lipid advanced glycosylation: Pathway for lipid oxidation *in vivo*. *Proc Natl Acad Sci U S A* 90 (14):6434–8.

Bucala, R., Z. Makita, G. Vega, S. Grundy, T. Koschinsky, A. Cerami, and H. Vlassara.1994. Modification of low density lipoprotein by advanced glycation end products contributes to the dyslipidemia of diabetes and renal insufficiency. *Proc Natl Acad Sci U S A* 91 (20):9441–5.

Cerami, A., V. J. Stevens, and V. M. Monnier. 1979. Role of nonenzymatic glycosylation in the development of the sequelae of diabetes mellitus. *Metabolism* 28 (4 Suppl 1):431–7.

Cerami, A., H. Vlassara, and M. Brownlee. 1985. Protein glycosylation and the pathogenesis of atherosclerosis. *Metabolism* 34 (12 Suppl 1):37–42.

Cerami, A., H. Vlassara, and M. Brownlee. 1986. Role of nonenzymatic glycosylation in atherogenesis. *J Cell Biochem* 30 (2):111–20. doi: 10.1002/jcb.240300203.

Cottone, S., M. C. Lorito, R. Riccobene, E. Nardi, G. Mule, S. Buscemi, C. Geraci, M. Guarneri, R. Arsena, and G. Cerasola. 2008. Oxidative stress, inflammation and cardiovascular disease in chronic renal failure. *J Nephrol* 21 (2):175–9.

Daffu, G., C. H. del Pozo, K. M. O'Shea, R. Ananthakrishnan, R. Ramasamy, and A. M. Schmidt. 2013. Radical roles for RAGE in the pathogenesis of oxidative stress in cardiovascular diseases and beyond. *Int J Mol Sci* 14 (10):19891–910. doi: 10.3390/ijms141019891.

Gugliucci, A., and M. Bendayan. 1995. Reaction of advanced glycation endproducts with renal tissue from normal and streptozotocin-induced diabetic rats: An ultrastructural study using colloidal gold cytochemistry. *J Histochem Cytochem* 43 (6):591–600.

Gugliucci, A., and M. Bendayan. 1996. Renal fate of circulating advanced glycated end products (AGE): Evidence for reabsorption and catabolism of AGE-peptides by renal proximal tubular cells. *Diabetologia* 39 (2):149–60.

Gugliucci, A., E. Kinugasa, H. Ogata, R. Caccavello, and S. Kimura. 2014. Activation of paraoxonase 1 after hemodialysis is associated with HDL remodeling and its increase in the HDL fraction and VLDL. *Clin Chim Acta* 430:9–14.

Gugliucci, A., K. Mehlhaff, E. Kinugasa, H. Ogata, R. Hermo, J. Schulze, and S. Kimura. 2007. Paraoxonase-1 concentrations in end-stage renal disease patients increase after hemodialysis: Correlation with low molecular AGE adduct clearance. *Clin Chim Acta* 377 (1–2):213–20. doi: 10.1016/j.cca.2006.09.028.

Gugliucci, A., and T. Menini. 2015. Paraoxonase 1 and HDL maturation. *Clin Chim Acta* 439:5–13. doi: 10.1016/j.cca.2014.09.016.

He, C., J. Sabol, T. Mitsuhashi, and H. Vlassara. 1999. Dietary glycotoxins: Inhibition of reactive products by aminoguanidine facilitates renal clearance and reduces tissue sequestration. *Diabetes* 48 (6):1308–15.

Koschinsky, T., C. J. He, T. Mitsuhashi, R. Bucala, C. Liu, C. Buenting, K. Heitmann, and H. Vlassara. 1997. Orally absorbed reactive glycation products (glycotoxins): An environmental risk factor in diabetic nephropathy. *Proc Natl Acad Sci U S A* 94 (12):6474–9.

Macias-Cervantes, M. H., J. M. Rodriguez-Soto, J. Uribarri, F. J. Diaz-Cisneros, W. Cai, and M. E. Garay-Sevilla. 2015. Effect of an advanced glycation end product-restricted diet and exercise on metabolic parameters in adult overweight men. *Nutrition* 31 (3):446–51. doi: 10.1016/j.nut.2014.10.004.

Mackness, M., and B. Mackness. 2013. Targeting paraoxonase-1 in atherosclerosis. *Expert Opin Ther Targets* 17 (7):829–37. doi: 10.1517/14728222.2013.790367.

Mackness, M., and B. Mackness. 2015. Human paraoxonase-1 (PON1): Gene structure and expression, promiscuous activities and multiple physiological roles. *Gene* 567 (1):12–21. doi: 10.1016/j.gene.2015.04.088.

Makita, Z., R. Bucala, E. J. Rayfield, E. A. Friedman, A. M. Kaufman, S. M. Korbet, R. H. Barth, J. A. Winston, H. Fuh, K. R. Manogue, et al. 1994. Reactive glycosylation endproducts in diabetic uraemia and treatment of renal failure. *Lancet* 343 (8912):1519–22.

Makita, Z., S. Radoff, E. J. Rayfield, Z. Yang, E. Skolnik, V. Delaney, E. A. Friedman, A. Cerami, and H. Vlassara. 1991. Advanced glycosylation end products in patients with diabetic nephropathy. *N Engl J Med* 325 (12):836–42. doi: 10.1056/NEJM199109193251202.

Mallipattu, S. K., and J. Uribarri. 2014. Advanced glycation end product accumulation: A new enemy to target in chronic kidney disease? *Curr Opin Nephrol Hypertens* 23 (6):547–54. doi: 10.1097/MNH.0000000000000062.

Manigrasso, M. B., J. Juranek, R. Ramasamy, and A. M. Schmidt. 2014. Unlocking the biology of RAGE in diabetic microvascular complications. *Trends Endocrinol Metab* 25(1):15–22.

Miyata, T., Y. Iida, K. Horie, Z. Cai, S. Sugiyama, and K. Maeda. 1996. Pathophysiology of advanced glycation end-products in renal failure. *Nephrol Dial Transplant* 11 Suppl 5:27–30.

Monnier, V. M., and A. Cerami. 1982. Non-enzymatic glycosylation and browning of proteins in diabetes. *Clin Endocrinol Metab* 11 (2):431–52.

Monnier, V. M., D. R. Sell, R. H. Nagaraj, S. Miyata, S. Grandhee, P. Odetti, and S. A. Ibrahim. 1992. Maillard reaction-mediated molecular damage to extracellular matrix and other tissue proteins in diabetes, aging, and uremia. *Diabetes* 41 Suppl 2:36–41.

Nemet, I., C. M. Strauch, and V. M. Monnier. 2011. Favored and disfavored pathways of protein crosslinking by glucose: Glucose lysine dimer (GLUCOLD) and crossline versus glucosepane. *Amino Acids* 40 (1):167–81. doi: 10.1007/s00726-010-0631-2.

Rabbani, N., K. Sebekova, K. Sebekova, Jr., A. Heidland, and P. J. Thornalley. 2007. Accumulation of free adduct glycation, oxidation, and nitration products follows acute loss of renal function. *Kidney Int* 72 (9):1113–21. doi: 10.1038/sj.ki.5002513.

Rabbani, N., and P. J. Thornalley. 2009. Quantitation of markers of protein damage by glycation, oxidation, and nitration in peritoneal dialysis. *Perit Dial Int* 29 Suppl 2:S51–6.

Ramasamy, R., S. F. Yan, and A. M. Schmidt. 2012. Advanced glycation endproducts: From precursors to RAGE: Round and round we go. *Amino Acids* 42 (4):1151–61. doi: 10.1007/s00726-010-0773-2.

Rodriguez-Ayala, E., B. Anderstam, M. E. Suliman, A. Seeberger, O. Heimburger, B. Lindholm, and P. Stenvinkel. 2005. Enhanced RAGE-mediated NFkappaB stimulation in inflamed hemodialysis patients. *Atherosclerosis* 180 (2):333–40. doi: 10.1016/j.atherosclerosis.2004.12.007.

Schmidt, A. M., O. Hori, R. Cao, S. D. Yan, J. Brett, J. L. Wautier, S. Ogawa, K. Kuwabara, M. Matsumoto, and D. Stern. 1996. RAGE: A novel cellular receptor for advanced glycation end products. *Diabetes* 45 Suppl 3:S77–80.

Schmidt, A. M., and D. Stern. 2000. Atherosclerosis and diabetes: The RAGE connection. *Curr Atheroscler Rep* 2 (5):430–6.

Sell, D. R., K. M. Biemel, O. Reihl, M. O. Lederer, C. M. Strauch, and V. M. Monnier. 2005. Glucosepane is a major protein cross-link of the senescent human extracellular matrix. Relationship with diabetes. *J Biol Chem* 280 (13):12310–5. doi: 10.1074/jbc.M500733200.

Sell, D. R., R. H. Nagaraj, S. K. Grandhee, P. Odetti, A. Lapolla, J. Fogarty, and V. M. Monnier. 1991. Pentosidine: A molecular marker for the cumulative damage to proteins in diabetes, aging, and uremia. *Diabetes Metab Rev* 7 (4):239–51.

Stevens, V. J., H. Vlassara, A. Abati, and A. Cerami. 1977. Nonenzymatic glycosylation of hemoglobin. *J Biol Chem* 252 (9):2998–3002.

Sveen, K. A., K. Dahl-Jorgensen, K. H. Stensaeth, K. Angel, I. Seljeflot, D. R. Sell, V. M. Monnier, and K. F. Hanssen. 2015. Glucosepane and oxidative markers in skin collagen correlate with intima media thickness and arterial stiffness in long-term type 1 diabetes. *J Diabetes Complications* 29 (3):407–12. doi: 10.1016/j.jdiacomp.2014.12.011.

Thallas-Bonke, V., M. T. Coughlan, A. L. Tan, B. E. Harcourt, P. E. Morgan, M. J. Davies, L. A. Bach, M. E. Cooper, and J. M. Forbes. 2013. Targeting the AGE-RAGE axis improves renal function in the context of a healthy diet low in advanced glycation end-product content. *Nephrology* (Carlton) 18 (1):47–56. doi: 10.1111/j.1440-1797.2012.01665.x.

Thornalley, P. J. 2005. Glycation free adduct accumulation in renal disease: The new AGE. *Pediatr Nephrol* 20 (11):1515–22. doi: 10.1007/s00467-005-2011-9.

Thornalley, P. J. 2006. Advanced glycation end products in renal failure. *J Ren Nutr* 16 (3):178–84. doi: 10.1053/j.jrn.2006.04.012.

Thornalley, P. J., and N. Rabbani. 2009. Highlights and hotspots of protein glycation in end-stage renal disease. *Semin Dial* 22 (4):400–4. doi: 10.1111/j.1525-139X.2009.00589.x.

Uribarri, J., W. Cai, O. Sandu, M. Peppa, T. Goldberg, and H. Vlassara. 2005. Diet-derived advanced glycation end products are major contributors to the body's AGE pool and induce inflammation in healthy subjects. *Ann N Y Acad Sci* 1043:461–6. doi: 10.1196/annals.1333.052.

Uribarri, J., M. Peppa, W. Cai, T. Goldberg, M. Lu, S. Baliga, J. A. Vassalotti, and H. Vlassara. 2003. Dietary glycotoxins correlate with circulating advanced glycation end product levels in renal failure patients. *Am J Kidney Dis* 42 (3):532–8.

Uribarri, J., M. Peppa, W. Cai, T. Goldberg, M. Lu, C. He, and H. Vlassara. 2003. Restriction of dietary glycotoxins reduces excessive advanced glycation end products in renal failure patients. *J Am Soc Nephrol* 14 (3):728–31.

Vlassara, H. 1994. Serum advanced glycosylation end products: A new class of uremic toxins? *Blood Purif* 12 (1):54–9.

Vlassara, H., H. Fuh, Z. Makita, S. Krungkrai, A. Cerami, and R. Bucala. 1992. Exogenous advanced glycosylation end products induce complex vascular dysfunction in normal animals: A model for diabetic and aging complications. *Proc Natl Acad Sci U S A* 89 (24):12043–7.

Vlassara, H., J. Uribarri, W. Cai, S. Goodman, R. Pyzik, J. Post, F. Grosjean, M. Woodward, and G. E. Striker. 2012. Effects of sevelamer on HbA1c, inflammation, and advanced glycation end products in diabetic kidney disease. *Clin J Am Soc Nephrol* 7 (6):934–42. doi: 10.2215/CJN.12891211.

Section II

The Modern Diet & AGEs: How Do Exogenous AGEs Become Incorporated into Our Body?

5

Dietary Advanced Glycation End Products: Animal Studies

Melpomeni Peppa
Attikon University Hospital
Athens, Greece

CONTENTS

KEY POINTS

- The current epidemics of obesity, diabetes mellitus, and aging-related diseases indicate the interplay between heritable aberrations and environmental influences.
- Various environmental factors have been identified to be strongly associated with the pathogenesis of obesity, aging, diabetes, and their complications, including several dietary factors.
- Advanced glycation end products (AGEs) which are generated throughout the preparation or processing of food are absorbed in the gastrointestinal system and partially excreted in the urine.
- Animal studies in wild-type and experimental models of diabetes, obesity, and aging have shown that diet-derived AGEs exert deleterious effects in the body, including induction of oxidative stress, insulin resistance, β-cell dysfunction and apoptosis, and inflammation and altered immune function, in a similar way to the endogenously formed counterparts.
- Dietary AGE restriction prevents or delays the progression of obesity, diabetes, aging, and their complications, in various animal experimental models.
- The beneficial results from the dietary AGE restriction can be extrapolated in humans and the modification of these products in the diet is emerging as a promising, cost-effective, and applicable therapeutic intervention.

5.1 Introduction

The current epidemics of diabetes mellitus and aging-related diseases may largely be due to environmental factors. In addition to the existing knowledge that advanced glycation end products (AGEs) contribute to the pathogenesis of those diseases and their complications, a large body of evidence supports the fact that diet-derived AGEs (dAGE) play an important role as well. Methods of food preparation and processing have a significant effect in the generation of diverse unstable carbonyl derivatives of glycoxidation and lipoxidation reactions, which can be partly absorbed in the gastrointestinal system, contributing to the total AGE body burden. Industrial and societal changes have led to the production and consumption of foods rich in AGE.

The sustained influx of AGEs leads to suppression of host defenses and induction of intracellular reactive oxygen species, which can shift basal oxidative stress and lead to inflammation, insulin resistance, obesity, β-cell dysfunction, impaired insulin secretion, and insulin resistance, leading to diabetes, aging as well as their complications. *In vivo* studies using wild-type but also experimental animal models of obesity, insulin resistance, and diabetes, fed with a defined oral test prepared with or without carbohydrate, or a single rodent diet prepared under different temperatures, are important to clarify the role of dAGE in various pathologies. These studies emphasize that dAGE restriction reduces basal oxidative stress and inflammation; restores host defenses and increases life span; prevents or improves dementia, type 1 and type 2 diabetes mellitus, renal disease, and their complications.

In this chapter, we will review data emerging from studies in experimental animal models, which greatly support the important role of dAGE in various pathologies and suggest that dAGE could be a promising, cost-effective, and broadly applicable intervention in humans.

5.2 Dietary AGE Homeostasis—Animal Studies

The presence of toxic dAGEs in modern foodstuffs has resulted from vast socioeconomic changes in the past 50 years and new technologies employed in the mass production of food, including heat, dehydration, ionization, irradiation, and the desirable effect of dAGEs on food flavor [1–4].

Kinetic studies in normal rats, using orally administered double-labeled AGE tracers (121I–14Cglucose-derived AGE–ovalbumin) and an AGE inhibitor, aminoguanidine, showed that the main "entry" for dAGEs is the gastrointestinal tract. About 10% of a single AGE-rich protein preparation is absorbed, mostly as a single peptide, dipeptides, or tripeptides, and approximately two-thirds remained in contact with tissues for >72h, whereas the rest was rapidly excreted by the kidneys. Based on these kinetic studies, the rate of tissue AGE accumulation due to dAGEs was estimated to be with the exogenously derived dAGEs compared to the endogenously formed AGEs [5,6].

In addition, animal studies showed that the main "exit" of the dAGEs is the kidney, which seems to be a key component of host defenses, by filtration or by active uptake and secretion, two processes that result in the net excretion of AGEs in urine [5,6]. Any increase in the ingestion of dAGEs or reduction in renal AGE clearance may potentially cause a generation of prerenal AGEs and an increase in the formation of new AGEs and oxidant stress within both renal and extrarenal tissues, suppression of AGER1 levels, and augmentation of oxidant stress and inflammation. Although functional renal end points are not yet available in humans, a common thread across animal and human studies is emerging: a pre-existing oxidant overload may reduce host defenses before the onset of a pathology, for example, diabetes mellitus and set the stage for diabetic renal disease.

5.3 Dietary AGE Effects on Different Pathologies—Animal Studies

The actual effect of sustained exposure to dAGEs was evaluated in a series of studies in mice. As described later, several animal studies provide a new framework and an experimental setting from which to revisit the pathogenesis and treatment of various pathologies.

5.3.1 Prevention Studies

Intraperitoneal injections of AGEs in healthy male Sprague-Dawley rats for 16 weeks resulted in impaired insulin secretion, decreased islet preproinsulin gene expression, and a characteristic decline in first-phase insulin secretion in response to glucose. These changes were attributed to the stimulation of the superoxide production within mitochondria and the interruption of a number of critical sequential steps, including changes in cellular glucose uptake, alteration of cellular calcium flux, and loss of mitochondrial ATP content, prevented by alagebrium [7,8]. In addition, parenteral or oral administration of AGEs in healthy mice leads to a cycle of increased cell and tissue AGEs, oxidative stress, and inflammation and tissue injury similar to the diabetic vascular or renal complications, without hyperglycemia, reversed by anti-AGE agents (9–14). These studies indicate that the dAGEs contribute significantly to the total body AGEs and induce oxidant stress, impaired insulin secretion, insulin resistance, and inflammation in healthy mice. They also demonstrate that these changes can be diminished and further pathology can be prevented in several mouse models by restricting the intake of dAGEs without reducing energy intake (15–22).

5.3.2 Type 1 Diabetes Mellitus

A large body of evidence in experimental animals suggests that AGEs are implicated in the pathogenesis of type 1 diabetes mellitus (T1D) by affecting directly the β-cell causing defective insulin secretion and cell apoptosis or indirectly through the induction of systemic inflammation and oxidative stress, through the AGE–RAGE interaction, as well as altered immune cell activation [7,8,23–26].

Diet-derived AGEs seem to affect the various pathways linked to the pathogenesis of T1D, in a similar way to the endogenously formed counterparts. Peppa et al. showed that early exposure to AGEs taken in with regular nutrients had a role in the pathogenesis of T1D, in an experimental animal of T1D, the NOD mice. The mice were exposed to a high-AGE diet (H-AGE) and to a nutritionally similar diet with approximately 5-fold lower levels of N^{ε}-carboxymethyllysine (CML) and methylglyoxal-derivatives (MG) (L-AGE), due to the shorter heat exposure during processing. Diabetes suppressive effects under L-AGE feeding were significant across three generations in founder mice, initiated at 3 or 6 weeks of age, and were extended throughout two generations of offspring, F1 and F2, if kept on the L-AGE maternal regimen. L-AGE mice exhibited a diabetes-free rate of 86%, greatly increased survival rates by 76% for up to 56 weeks of age, and a delay in disease onset (4-month lag). Survival for L-AGE mice was 76% versus 0% for H-AGE mice after 44 weeks. T1D reduction (33% to 14%) coincided with initiation to the L-AGE diet during the perinatal period. The greatest disease prevention (14%) was associated with exposure to a low AGE maternal environment, suggesting that toxic AGEs are transportable via the placenta (Figure 5.1).

However, the protective maternal effect of the L-AGE diet was reversed after crossing over to the H-AGE diet, as readily as the normally H-AGE maternal effect was reversed by the L-AGE diet, when applied at weaning (3 or 6 weeks). These data confirmed the plasticity inherent in this period and reinforced the importance of "dose," "time," and "duration" of exposure to toxic factor(s). The majority of mice exposed to L-AGE environment maternally or at weaning displayed modest insulitis and no diabetes for 1 year. A milder insulitis and a milder diabetes characterized L-AGE mice that did become diabetic, as compared with those with severely damaged islets and overt diabetes seen in H-AGE–fed mice by 25 weeks [21]. Furthermore, the 16-week-old prediabetic L-AGE NOD mice exhibited near-normal glucose and insulin responses to glucose challenge compared with the typically dysfunctional pattern of age-matched H-AGE–fed mice (Figure 5.2). Reduced insulitis in L-AGE versus H-AGE mice was marked by GAD- and insulin-unresponsive pancreatic interleukin (IL)-4–positive $CD4^+$ cells compared with the GAD and insulin-responsive interferon (IFN)-γ positive T-cells from H-AGE mice. Splenocytes from L-AGE mice consisted of GAD- and insulin-responsive IL-10–positive $CD4^+$ cells compared with the IFN-γ positive T-cells from H-AGE mice [21] (Figure 5.3).

Therefore, high-AGE intake may provide excess antigenic stimulus for T-cell–mediated diabetes or direct β-cell injury in NOD mice being ameliorated by maternal or neonatal exposure to L-AGE nutrition. A marked suppression of total pancreatic lymphocytes was observed in the L-AGE–fed mice (15-fold) compared with the H-AGE NOD group fed a regular diet. In addition, the L-AGE–fed mice displayed a pattern of predominantly IL-4–positive $CD4^+$ cells. There were virtually no infiltrates in

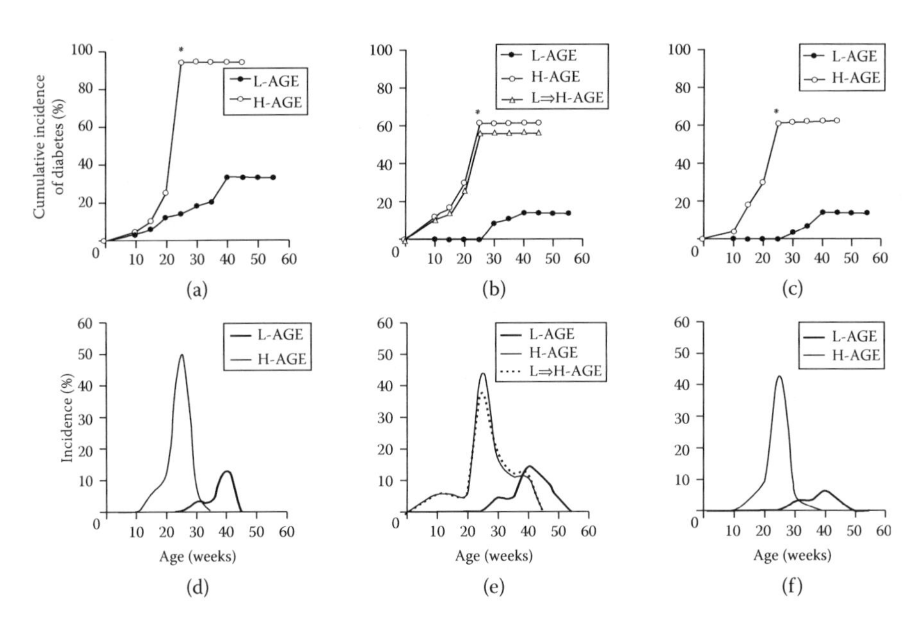

FIGURE 5.1 Incidence of type 1 diabetes in F0, F1, and F2 generations of female NOD mice exposed to LAGE or H-AGE diet. (a) By 6 weeks of age, F0 mice were placed on H-AGE (n = 16) or L-AGE diet (n = 30). (b) After weaning (3 weeks), F1 offspring were placed on H-AGE (n = 18) or L-AGE diet (n = 21). Also, a subgroup of F1 mice (n = 16) from L-age–fed mothers was switched to H-AGE diet (L- to H-AGE). (c) After weaning (3 weeks), F2 offspring were placed on an H-AGE (n = 21) or L-AGE diet (n = 30). (a–c) Cumulative incidence of type 1 diabetes. (d–f) Incidence of type 1 diabetes in F0, F1, and F2 mice on H-AGE diet (e) on H-AGE diet from LAGE mothers (L- to H-AGE) and L-AGE diet (f). Diabetes incidence was monitored for 56 weeks. *P = 0.000 (a), *P = 0.006 (b), *P = 0.000 (c) for H-AGE or L3HAGE (L- to H-AGE diet) versus L-AGE groups.

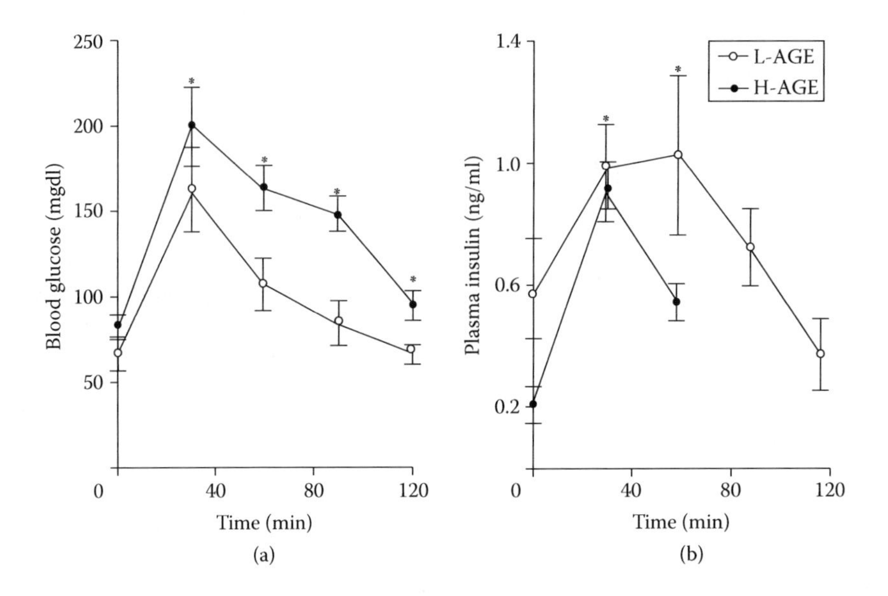

FIGURE 5.2 Cell function of NOD mice exposed to L-AGE or H-AGE diet. After glucose challenge (IGTT, 5% dextrose solution, 2 mg/g body wt i.p.) in 16-week-old nondiabetic female F1 mice from H-AGE–fed (F) and L-AGE–fed groups (E) (n = 12/group). Glucose (a) and insulin (b) responses were estimated at half-hour intervals up to 120 minutes. Data are the mean = SE of 12 measurements per time point per group. (a) *Glucose in H-AGE versus L-AGE at 0 minute, P = 0.021; at 30 minutes, P = 0.036; at 60 minutes, P = 0.009; at 90 minutes, P = 0.009; and at 120 minutes, P = 0.009. (b) *Insulin in H-AGE versus L-AGE at 0 minute, P = 0.009; at 30 minutes, P = 0.009; and at 60 minutes, P = 0.009.

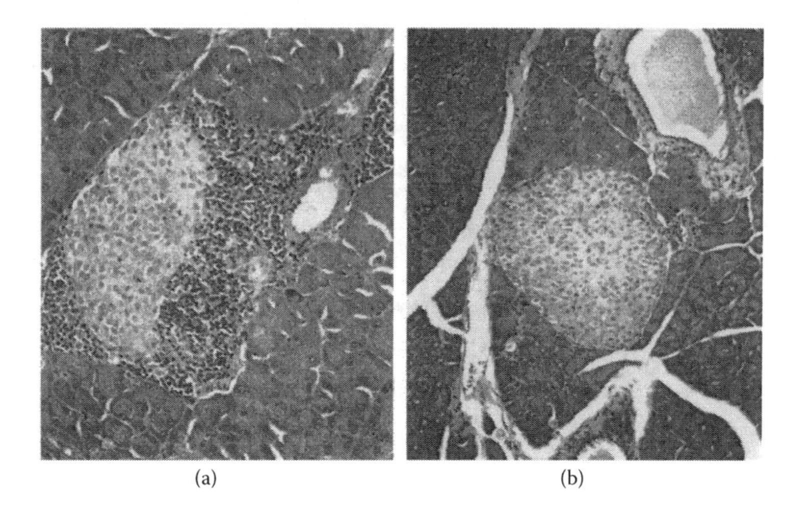

FIGURE 5.3 Islet morphology in nondiabetic F1 NOD mice exposed to L-AGE or H-AGE diet. (a) Pancreatic tissues retrieved from 9-week-old F1 H-AGE–fed mice, stained by H&E, showed severe mononuclear cell infiltration and disruption of pancreatic islet architecture. (b) Islets of age-matched F1 NOD mice from the L-AGE–fed group did not exhibit these changes. Magnification x400.

islets from two generations of mice exposed to L-AGE nutrients during the fetal stage or early in life. In these mice, there was also a marked unresponsiveness of pancreatic T-cells to β-cell antigens, insulin, and GAD. This might indicate blocked autoreactive T-cell recruitment due to low local expression of these antigens under a "safer" AGE-poor diet [21].

While these effects were readily attributable to the food, they were not due to differences in nutrient composition, as the diets used were of a single origin, with equivalent energy profiles. A prominent feature, however, was their distinctly different glycotoxin content. A large proportion of CML or MG derivatives found in the regular or H-AGE diet did not develop in the L-AGE preparation, which resulted from the shorter heat exposure during processing.

The above data indicate that the AGEs components of the diets enriched in AGE products are involved in the pathogenesis of T1D. It is plausible that early exposure of gut lympoid tissue to excess diet-derived AGE-peptides (e.g., AGEGAD peptides) results in a population of nondeleted autoreactive T-cells, which in a predisposed setting, as in the NOD mouse, offsets the balance in favor of tissue-specific GAD-cytotoxic T-cell clones and β-cell damage. It can be thus speculated that the L-AGE diet provided the young lymphoid tissue system with a low dose of certain AGE-related antigen(s), which enabled Th2 cells to actively suppress nondeleted autoreactive T-cells [21]. These findings have been confirmed *in vitro* and in rodents parenterally administered AGE and anti-AGE agents or an AGE-restricted diet (J. M. Forbes, personal communication)

These data support the notion that dietary AGE restriction results in suppression of islet infiltration by β-cell cytotoxic T-cells and islet toxicity; significantly delayed onset, reduced severity of disease, and marked increase in overall survival occurred [15,21]. However, future studies are required to define how exposure to excess AGEs specifically contributes to T1D development and autoimmunity and whether this is via direct or indirect pathways. Taken together, the existing data suggest dAGE as a modifiable risk factor and therapeutic target for the prevention of T1D.

5.3.3 Type 2 Diabetes

AGEs have been involved in the pathogenesis of insulin resistance (IR), which is the main underlying mechanism of type 2 diabetes (T2D) [27].

AGEs contribute to IR by a variety of mechanisms, including a direct modification of the insulin molecule, thereby leading to its impaired action, generation of oxidative stress, and impairment of mitochondrial function or an indirect action through AGE receptors mainly RAGE. These processes are ameliorated by anti-AGE agents [28].

Hofmann et al. investigated the effect of dAGEs on the progression of IR resistance in C57/BL/KsJ *db/db* mice, a well-established animal model for obesity and T2D. The mice were fed with two different diets similar to all the nutrients differing in the AGE content, low in AGE (LAD) and high in AGE (HAD) [20].

A significant relationship between dAGEs, circulating AGEs, and insulin sensitivity was observed. Despite equal food intake in the two groups, LAD mice, already obese and diabetic, ceased to gain weight within 10 weeks of study, and, by 20 weeks, they exhibited a significant weight loss which was consistent with a shift in endogenous glucose metabolism, resulting in a more efficient glucose disposal rate. Throughout this period, fasting serum insulin levels, a well-established indicator for the progression of IR, were significantly lower in LAD than in HAD mice, without the characteristic rise and fall typically seen in the strain and in the HAD mice. In addition, LAD mice exhibited a nearly complete restoration of glycemic response to intravenous glucose and insulin tolerance tests. The insulin kinetics seen in the LAD mice were consistent with the well-preserved pancreatic islet morphology and function demonstrated in this group at the end of the study in contrast with the HAD mice which displayed the expected hypertrophy coupled with a loss of insulin-producing cells and the normal islet architecture [20].

Glucose uptake in abdominal adipose tissue revealed that LAD improved IR by partially restoring the severely impaired insulin-stimulated glucose uptake by adipocytes. There were significantly higher total serum cholesterol levels in the LAD mice, attributable almost exclusively to a marked increase in HDL cholesterol concentrations [20].

This study provides further support that dAGEs may be important contributors to the circulating AGEs and influence the progression of IR in an experimental model of T2D. Furthermore, this study suggests that dAGE restriction might prevent the development of IR and T2D [20].

Similar findings were found by Sandu et al. in a study performed in normal C57/BL6 mice which were randomly assigned to high-fat diets (35% g fat), either high (HAGE-HF group; 995.4 units/mg AGE) or low (by 2.4-fold LAGE-HF group; 329.6 units/mg AGE) in AGE content [22]. After 6 months, 75% of HAGE-HF mice were diabetic and exhibited higher body weight, fasting glucose, insulin and serum AGE than control mice, while none of the LAGE-HF mice were diabetic despite a similar rise in body weight and plasma lipids. The HAGE-HF group displayed markedly impaired glucose and insulin responses during glucose tolerance tests, euglycemic and hyperglycemic clamps, altered pancreatic islet structure and function, higher plasma 8-isoprostane and lower adiponectin levels, compared with those of LAGE-HF mice, in which findings resembled those of control mice. The HAGE-HF group had more visceral fat (by 2- and 4-fold) and more AGE-modified fat (by 2- and 5-fold) than LAGE-HF and control mice, respectively, despite similar dietary fat intake and body weight gain by both groups. These findings strongly suggest a protective role for a low-AGE diet, even if the fat content is elevated [22].

Cai et al. performed a study in four generations of F3/MG+ mice which manifested increased adiposity and premature IR, marked by severe deficiency of anti-AGE advanced glycation receptor 1 (AGER1) and of survival factor sirtuin 1 (SIRT1) in white adipose tissue (WAT), skeletal muscle, and liver. The mice fed isocaloric diets with or without AGEs [synthetic methyl-glyoxal-derivatives (MG+)] [29].

Increased adiposity, glucose intolerance, hyperinsulinemia, elevated leptin, and decreased adiponectin levels appeared prematurely in F3/MG+ mice, namely 6 months before its onset in Reg-fed mice and 12 mo before that in F3/MG− mice. The expanded WAT in MG+ or Reg mice was also rich in AGE lipids (by ~ 3- to 4-fold above MG−). In MG+ mice, there was a marked increase in NF-κB acetylated-p65 in WAT adipocytes, high TNF-α, and CD11c in peritoneal macrophages and suppressed AGER1, SIRT1, PPARγ, IL-10, and CD206 mRNA levels, compared with the MG⁻ mice. These data demonstrate that MG-derived AGE, present in thermally treated food, can profoundly alter the inflammation/insulin axis, in the absence of excess intake of nutrients or genetic susceptibility [29].

5.4 Vascular Disease

Several studies in experimental animals demonstrate that AGEs play an important role in the pathogenesis of microangiopathy and macroangiopathy, and animal studies support a similar role for dAGEs.

Atherosclerosis-prone mice are useful models for assessing the role of various determinants of atherosclerotic lesions at the site of vascular injury. Lin et al. investigated the effect of dAGEs on arterial stenosis in genetically hypercholesterolemic apolipoprotein E–deficient (apoE/), streptozotocin-induced diabetic mice. Diabetic and nondiabetic apoE/mice (6–8 weeks old) were randomized into either a standard AIN-93G chow (AGE 12 500/700 U/mg, termed high-AGE diet, H-AGE) or the same chow having four to 5-fold lower AGE level (L-AGE: 27009/830 U/mg). The L-AGE mice exhibited lower AGE levels, 50% smaller lesions at the aortic root, markedly suppressed tissue AGEs, AGE-Receptor-1, AGE-Receptor-2 and RAGE expression, reduced numbers of inflammatory cells, tissue factor, vascular cell adhesion molecule-1, and MCP-1 levels. These findings suggested an important link between dAGEs, tissue-incorporated AGEs, and diabetes-accelerated arterial stenosis, expressing an antiatherogenic profile [30].

In another study, Lin et al. evaluated the association between dAGE content and neointimal formation after arterial injury in genetically hypercholesterolemic mice. Male, 12-week-old, apolipoprotein E–deficient ($apoE^{-/-}$) mice were randomly assigned to receive either a high-AGE diet (HAD; AGE/15,000 U/mg), or a similar diet with 10-fold lower AGE (LAD; AGE/1,500 U/mg). These mice underwent femoral artery injury 1 week later and were maintained on their diets. At 4 weeks after injury, a significant decrease in circulating AGE levels, intimal formation, neointimal area, intima/media ratio, and stenotic luminal area was noted in LAD mice in association with a marked reduction (56%) of macrophages in the neointimal lesions, as well as an obvious reduction of smooth muscle cell content, and a reduced deposition of AGE in the endothelia, SMC, and macrophages in neointimal lesions. These results support the causal relationship between dAGE and the vessel wall response to acute injury, suggesting a significant potential for dAGE restriction in the prevention of restenosis after angioplasty [31].

Peppa et al. investigated the effects of dAGEs on wound healing in female db/db mice, an experimental model of T2D. The mice were randomly assigned on two diets that differed only in AGE content (high [H-AGE] versus low [L-AGE] ratio, 5:1) for 3 months. L-AGE–fed mice displayed lower circulating and skin AGE deposits, increased epithelialization, angiogenesis, inflammation, granulation tissue deposition, enhanced collagen organization, and more rapid wound closure time, compared with H-AGE mice. These results support the notion that dAGE restriction may improve impaired diabetic wound healing [32,33] (Figure 5.4).

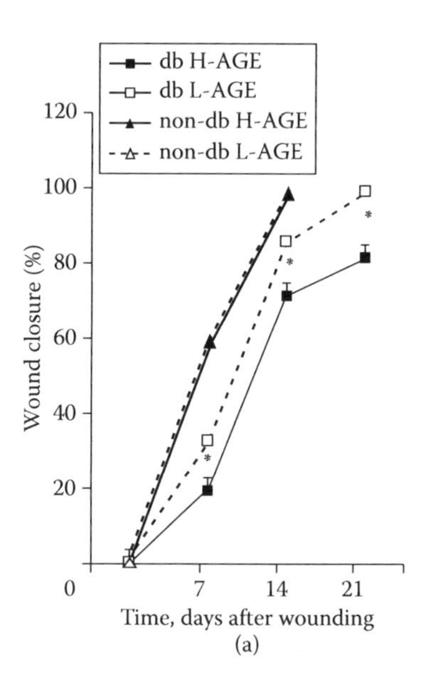

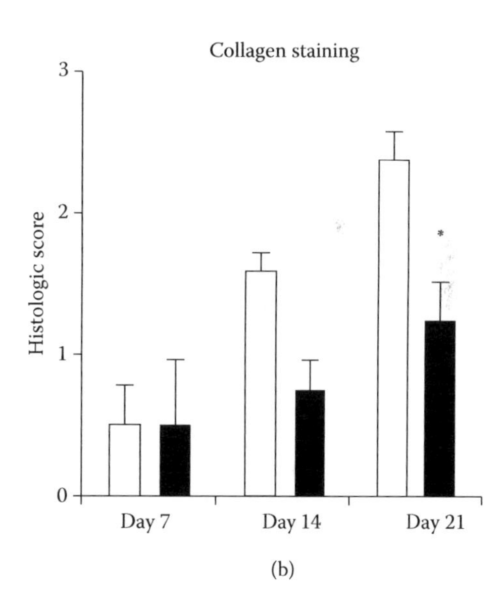

FIGURE 5.4 Time to closure and histologic changes of diabetic wounds correlate with dietary AGE intake. (a) After 12 weeks' exposure to either L-AGE or H-AGE diets, full excisional wounds (1 cm) were created at the back of the mice and the time to closure was evaluated at days 7, 14, and 21 after wounding (data shown as percentage of change from baseline). (b) Sections were stained with Sirius red, and collagen deposition was scored according to the intensity of the staining (score 1–3). Data are expressed as mean = SE. $^*P < 0.05$ between diet groups at the end of the study.

5.5 Aging-Life Span

Senescence and aging seems to share genetic and environmental factors including elevated oxidant stress, cumulative DNA damage, altered gene expression, telomere shortening, energy utilization, and caloric consumption [34,35].

Cai et al. showed that C57BL6 male mice with a lifelong exposure to a low-AGE diet (LAD) had higher than baseline levels of tissue AGER1 and glutathione/oxidized glutathione, and reduced plasma 8-isoprostanes, tissue RAGE, and p66shc levels, compared with mice pair- fed the regular diet. This was associated with a reduction in systemic AGE accumulation, amelioration of IR, albuminuria, glomerulosclerosis, and extended lifespan. These results support the notion that oxidant stress metabolic and end organ dysfunction of aging may result from lifelong exposure to high levels of glycoxidants that exceed AGER1 and antioxidant reserve capacity, suggesting that dAGE restriction may preserve these innate defenses, resulting in decreased tissue damage and a longer lifespan [18].

Although caloric restriction constitutes an effective way to extend lifespan, Cai et al. examined whether the beneficial effects of caloric restriction are related to the restriction of oxidants or energy. Pair-fed mice were provided either a caloric restricted (CR) diet or a CR diet in which AGEs were elevated by brief heat treatment (CR-HAD). In contrast with CR mice, old CR-HAD mice developed high levels of 8-isoprostanes, AGE, RAGE, and p66*shc*, coupled with low AGER1 and GSH/GSSG levels, IR, marked myocardial and renal fibrosis, and shortened lifespan. In the current study, high levels of oxidants in the CR-HAD diet may have competed against the benefits of CR by mechanisms that remain to be identified. Therefore, the beneficial effects of a CR diet may be partly related to reduced oxidant intake, and partially mediated by reduced dAGE. The findings support evidence that oxidant stress can be reduced, and health span increased, in mice fed a diet that is restricted in the content of AGEs [19].

5.6 Dementia

Dementia, the most frequent form of which is Alzheimer's disease (AD), has been associated with the metabolic syndrome (MS), (T2D) all of them linked to environmental factors and oxidative stress [36,37].

Higher histochemical levels of AGEs have been found in the brain of AD patients than in normal controls, constituting components of senile plaques and neurofibrillary tangles [38]. In addition, AGE receptors are expressed in brain neurons, microglia, and endothelium [39]. Due to their chemical structure, AGEs may take part in the transformation of soluble into insoluble β amyloid and the aggregation of microtubule associated tau protein and amplify the proinflammatory properties of amyloid β1–42 (Aβ) or tau protein as well [40,41].

The role of dAGEs on dementia was investigated by Cai et al. in an animal study using the MG+/MG− mouse model which provides an opportunity to explore the link of oral AGE to these chronic conditions, free of either genetic or caloric manipulations. WT mice pair-fed three diets throughout life: low-AGE (MG−), MG-supplemented low-AGE (MG+), and regular (Reg) chow. In contrast with MG- and regular mice, older MG+ mice, similar to old Reg controls, developed MS, increased brain amyloid-β42 and deposits of AGEs, gliosis, cognitive deficits, accompanied by suppressed SIRT1, nicotinamide phosphoribosyltransferase, AGE-receptor-1, and PPARγ [42]. The data from neocortical neurons of MG+ mice suggest a placental mode of transfer of excessive AGEs to the fetal brain, which might render the brain more susceptible to oxidant stress injury. Importantly, this injurious process appears to be preventable in brains of MG− mice, a finding of significant therapeutic importance. These changes were not due to aging or caloric intake, as neither these changes nor the MS were present in age-matched, pair-fed MG− mice. Whether the effects in MG+ mice are a reflection of altered blood–brain barrier, high intracerebral oxidant stress, or both, remains to be established. However, the fact is that restriction of dAGEs seems to be a promising therapeutic strategy to combat the epidemics of AD and MS.

5.7 Conclusions

Animal studies using experimental models of various pathologies clearly show the important role of dAGEs in several metabolic diseases. Given the marked expansion of processed foods and the close relationship of AGEs to food preparation and processing, these data may have direct relevance to humans. The net result of those studies is that dAGE restriction may be a modifiable factor for the prevention or delayed progression of various metabolic diseases and their complications.

REFERENCES

1. O'Brien, J. & Morrissey, P. A. Nutritional and toxicological aspects of the Maillard browning reaction in foods. *Crit. Rev. Food Sci. Nutr.* 1989; 28: 211–248.
2. van Boekel, M. A. Formation of flavour compounds in the Maillard reaction. *Biotechnol. Adv.* 2006; 24: 230–233.
3. Zamora, R. & Hidalgo, F. J. Coordinate contribution of lipid oxidation and maillard reaction to the nonenzymatic food browning. *Crit. Rev. Food Sci. Nutr.* 2005; 45: 49–59.
4. Tessier, F. J. & Niquet, C. The metabolic, nutritional and toxicological consequences of ingested dietary Maillard reaction products: A literature review [French]. *J. Soc. Biol.* 2007; 201:199–207.
5. He, C., Sabol, J., Mitsuhashi, T., Vlassara, H. Dietary glycotoxins: Inhibition of reactive products by aminoguanidine facilitates renal clearance and reduces tissue sequestration. *Diabetes.* 1999; 48: 1308–1315.
6. Koschinsky, T., He, C.J., Mitsuhashi, T., Bucala, R., Liu, C., Buenting, C., Heitmann, K. & Vlassara, H. Orally absorbed reactive glycation products (glycotoxins): An environmental risk factor in diabetic nephropathy. *Proc. Natl Acad. Sci. U. S. A.* 1997; 94: 6474–6479.
7. Coughlan, M.T., Yap, F., Tong, D., Andrikopoulos, S., Gasser, A., Thallas-Bonke, V., Webster, D., et al. Advanced glycation end products are direct modulators of b-Cell function. *Diabetes.* 2011; 60: 2523–2532.
8. Kano, Y., Kanatsuna, T., Nakamura, N., Kitagawa, Y., Mori, H., Kajiyama, S., Nakano, K., Kondo, M. Defect of the first-phase insulin secretion to glucose stimulation in the perfused pancreas of the non-obese diabetic (NOD) mouse. *Diabetes.* 1986; 35: 486–490.
9. Vlassara, H., Striker, L.J., Teichberg, S., Fuh, H., Li, Y. M. & Steffes, M. Advanced glycation end products induce glomerular sclerosis and albuminuria in normal rats. *Proc. Natl Acad. Sci. U. S. A.* 1994; 91: 11704–11708.
10. Vlassara, H., Fuh, H., Makita, Z., Krungkrai, S., Cerami, A. & Bucala, R. Exogenous advanced glycosylation end products induce complex vascular dysfunction in normal animals: A model for diabetic and aging complications. *Proc. Natl Acad. Sci. U. S. A.* 1992; 89: 12043–12047.
11. Onorato, J. M., Jenkins, A. J., Thorpe, S. R., Baynes, J. W. Pyridoxamine, an inhibitor of advanced glycation reactions, also inhibits advanced lipoxidation reactions. Mechanism of action of pyridoxamine. *J. Biol. Chem.* 2000; 275: 21177–21184.
12. Metz, T. O., Alderson, N. L., Chahich, M. E., Thorpe, S. R., Baynes, J. W. Pyridoxamine traps intermediates in lipid peroxidation reactions in vivo: Evidence on the role of lipids in chemical modification of protein and development of diabetic complications. *J. Biol. Chem.* 2003; 278: 42012–42019.
13. Wolffenbuttel, B. H., Boulanger, C. M., Crijns, Huijberts, M. S., Poitevin, P., Swennen, G. N. & Vasan, S., Breakers of advanced glycation end products restore large artery properties in experimental diabetes. *Proc. Natl Acad. Sci. U. S. A.* 1998; 95: 4630–4634.
14. Degenhardt, T. P., Alderson, N. L., Arrington, D. D., Beattie, R. J., Basgen, J. M., Steffes, M. W., Thorpe, S. R., et al. Pyridoxamine inhibits early renal disease and dyslipidemia in the streptozotocin-diabetic rat. *Kidney Int.* 2002; 61: 939–950.
15. Zheng, F., He, C., Cai, W., Hattori, M., Steffes, M. & Vlassara, H. Prevention of diabetic nephropathy in mice by a diet low in glycoxidation products. *Diabetes. Metab. Res. Rev.* 2002; 18: 224–237.
16. Uribarri, J., Cai, W., Peppa, M., Goodman, S., Ferrucci, L., Striker, G. & Vlassara, H., Circulating glycotoxins and dietary advanced glycation endproducts: Two links to inflammatory response, oxidative stress, and aging. *J. Gerontol. A Biol. Sci. Med. Sci.* 2007; 62: 427–433.
17. Vlassara, H., Cai, W., Goodman, S., Pyzik, R., Yong, A., Chen, X., Zhu, L., et al. Protection against loss of innate defenses in adulthood by low advanced glycation end products (AGE) intake: Role of the antiinflammatory AGE receptor-1. *J. Clin. Endocrinol. Metab.* 2009; 94: 4483–4491.

18. Cai, W., He, J.C., Zhu, L., Chen, X., Wallenstein, S., Striker, G.E. & Vlassara, H. Reduced oxidant stress and extended lifespan in mice exposed to a low glycotoxin diet: Association with increased AGER1 expression. *Am. J. Pathol.* 2007; 170: 1893–1902.
19. Cai, W., He, J.C., Zhu, L., Chen, X., Zheng, F., Striker, G.E. & Vlassara, H. Oral glycotoxins determine the effects of calorie restriction on oxidant stress, age-related diseases, and lifespan. *Am. J. Pathol.* 2008; 173: 327–336.
20. Hofmann, S.M., Dong, H.J., Li, Z., Cai, W., Altomonte, J., Thung, S.N., Zeng, F., Fisher, E.A. & Vlassara, H. Improved insulin sensitivity is associated with restricted intake of dietary glycoxidation products in the db/db mouse. *Diabetes.* 2002; 51: 2082–2089.
21. Peppa, M., He, C., Hattori, M., McEvoy, R., Zheng, F. & Vlassara, H. Fetal or neonatal low-glycotoxin environment prevents autoimmune diabetes in NOD mice. *Diabetes.* 2003; 52: 1441–1448.
22. Sandu, O., Song, K., Cai, W., Zheng, F., Uribarri, J. & Vlassara, H. Insulin resistance and type 2 diabetes in high-fat-fed mice are linked to high glycotoxin intake. *Diabetes.* 2005; 54: 2314–2319.
23. Kaneto, H., Fujii, J., Myint, T., Miyazawa, N., Islam, K.N., Kawasaki, Y., Suzuki, K., Nakamura, M., Tatsumi, H., Yamasaki, Y. & Taniguchi, N. Reducing sugars trigger oxidative modification and apoptosis in pancreatic β-cells by provoking oxidative stress through the glycation reaction. *Biochem. J.* 1996; 320: 855–863.
24. Kapurniotu, A., Bernhagen, J., Greenfield, N., Al-Abed, Y., Teichberg, S., Frank, R.W., Voelter, W. & Bucala, R. Contribution of advanced glycosylation to the amyloidogenicity of islet amyloid polypeptide. *Eur. J. Biochem.* 1998; 251: 208–216.
25. Ivanov, G.I., Chaushev, T.A., Dakovska, L.N. & Kyurkchiev, S.D., Increased adhesion of lymphoid cells to glycated proteins. *Int. J. Biochem. Cell. Biol.* 1999; 31: 797–804.
26. Imani, F., Horii, Y., Suthanthiran, M., Skolnik, E.Y., Makita, Z., Sharma, V., Sehajpal, P. & Vlassara, H. Advanced glycosylation endproduct-specific receptors on human and rat T-lymphocytes mediate synthesis of interferon gamma: Role in tissue remodeling. *J. Exp. Med.* 1993; 178(6): 2165–2172.
27. Singh, R., Barden, A., Mori, T. & Beilin, L. Advanced glycation end-products: A review. *Diabetologia.* 2001; 44: 129–146.
28. Song, F. & Schmidt, A.M., Glycation & insulin resistance: Novel mechanisms and unique targets? *Arterioscler. Thromb. Vasc. Biol.* 2012; 32(8): 1760–1765.
29. Cai, W., Ramdas, M., Zhu, L., Chen, X., Striker, G.E. & Vlassara, H. Oral advanced glycation end-products (AGEs) promote insulin resistance and diabetes by depleting the antioxidant defenses AGE receptor-1 and sirtuin 1. *Proc. Natl. Acad. Sci. U. S. A.* 2012; 109(39): 15888–15893.
30. Lin, R.Y., Choudhury, R.P., Cai, W., Lu, M., Fallon, J.T., Fisher, E.A. & Vlassara, H. Dietary glycotoxins promote diabetic atherosclerosis in apolipoprotein E-deficient mice. *Atherosclerosis.* 2003; 168(2): 213–220.
31. Lin, R.Y., Reis, E.D., Dore, A.T., Lu, M., Ghodsi, N., Fallon, J.T., Fisher, E.A. & Vlassara, H. Lowering of dietary advanced glycation endproducts (AGE) reduces neointimal formation after arterial injury in genetically hypercholesterolemic mice. *Atherosclerosis.* 2002; 163(2): 303–11.
32. Peppa, M., Brem, H., Ehrlich, P., Zhang, J.G., Cai, W., Li, Z., Croitoru, A., Thung, S. & Vlassara, H. Adverse effects of dietary glycotoxins on wound healing in genetically diabetic mice. *Diabetes.* 2003; 52(11): 2805–2813.
33. Peppa, M., Stavroulakis, P. & Raptis, S.A. Advanced glycoxidation products and impaired diabetic wound healing. *Wound Repair Regen.* 2009; 17(4): 461–472.
34. Masoro, E,J., Overview of caloric restriction and ageing. *Mech. Ageing Dev.* 2005; 126: 913–922.
35. Madsen, M.A., Hsieh, C.C., Boylston, W.H., Flurkey, K., Harrison, D. & Papaconstantinou, J. Altered oxidative stress response of the long-lived Snell dwarf mouse. *Biochem. Biophys. Res. Commun.* 2004; 318: 998–1005.
36. Janson, J., Laedtke, T., Parisi, J.E., O'Brien, P., Petersen, R.C. & Butler, P.C. Increased risk of type 2 diabetes in Alzheimer disease. *Diabetes.* 2004; 53(2): 474–481.
37. Talbot, K., Wang. H.Y., Kazi, H., Han, L.Y., Bakshi, K.P., Stucky, A., Fuino, R.L., et al. Demonstrated brain insulin resistance in Alzheimer's disease patients is associated with IGF-1 resistance, IRS-1 dysregulation, and cognitive decline. *J. Clin. Invest.* 2012;122(4):1316–1338.
38. Vitek, M.P., Bhattacharya, K., Glendening, J.M., Stopa, E., Vlassara, H., Bucala, R., Manogue, K. & Cerami, A. Advanced glycation end products contribute to amyloidosis in Alzheimer disease. *Proc. Natl. Acad. Sci. U. S. A.* 1994; 91: 4766–4770.

39. Li, J.J., Dickson, D., Hof, P.R. & Vlassara, H. Receptors for advanced glycosylation endproducts in human brain: Role in brain homeostasis. *Mol. Med.* 1998; 4(1): 46–60.
40. Li, X.H., Xie, J.Z., Jiang, X., Lv, B.L., Cheng, X.S., Du, L.L., Zhang, J.Y., Wang, J.Z. & Zhou, X.W. Methylglyoxal induces tau hyperphosphorylation via promoting AGEs formation. *Neuromolecular. Med.* 2012; 4(4): 338–348.
41. Malherbe, P., Richards, J.G., Gaillard, H., Thompson, A., Diener, C., Schuler, A., Huber, G. & Yan, S.D. RAGE and amyloid-beta peptide neurotoxicity in Alzheimer's disease. *Nature.* 1996; 382: 685–691.
42. Cai, W., Uribarri, J., Zhu, L., Chen, X., Swamy, S., Zhao, Z., Grosjean, F., et al. Oral glycotoxins are a modifiable cause of dementia and the metabolic syndrome in mice and humans. *Proc. Natl. Acad. Sci. U. S. A.* 2014; 111(13): 4940–4945.

6

AGEs in Infant Formulas: Chemical and Physiological Aspects

Latifa Abdennebi-Najar
Société Francophone pour la recherche et l'éducation sur les origines développementales, environnementales et épigénétiques de la santé et des maladies (SF-DOHaD)
Viry Chatillon, France

Ghada Elmhiri
PRP-HOM/SRBE/LRTOX, Laboratoire de Radiotoxicologie Expérimentale
Fontenay-aux-Roses, France

CONTENTS

KEY POINTS

- Infant formula is a complex pre-substitute human milk matrix predetermined to ensure appropriate infant growth and development.
- Processing and storage of infant formula affect its composition and nutritional quality, in part due to the production of glycation end products (AGEs).
- AGEs absorbed from the infant formula become part of the body AGE pool.
- AGEs may potentially affect infant health through several mechanisms.
- It remains to be elucidated whether the high load of AGEs in the infant diet during the early 1,000 days of life, the critical period of child development and health, could exert long-term negative effects.

6.1 Introduction

Mother's milk is the first known human food for as long as the human race has existed. Mother's milk supplies all the energy and nutrients needed to ensure infant growth and development in the postnatal period. Infants who cannot be fed at the breast or for whom breast milk is not available need infant formula milk. These formulas are designed to provide infants with optimum nutrition for normal growth and development and are available in either powdered or liquid forms. Infant formula (IF) is intended to mimic the nutritional composition of breast milk. Its composition is therefore scrupulously adapted to the nutritional needs of the newborn.

Infant formula is a product based on milk from cows or other animals or a mixture of these and/or other ingredients, which were proven to be suitable for infant feeding (Stan 2007). During the standard production of IF, the raw material mix is blended, pasteurized, homogenized, condensed, and spray-dried or sterilized to obtain powdered formulas (Figure 6.1). To ensure appropriate microbial quality, rigorous heating processes are applied. Such processes induce major undesirable changes in the initial composition and the nutritional value of IF (Birlouez-Aragon et al. 2004). The main degradation reactions causing these nutritional changes and damages to the products are linked to protein glycation, which occurs during the Maillard reaction (Boekel and Van 1998).

6.2 Description of the Chemistry Behind the Maillard Reaction in Milk

The Maillard reaction (nonenzymatic glycation) is a chemical reaction between an amino group and a carbonyl group that usually takes place during food processing or storage. The Maillard reaction can be decomposed into three stages (Figure 6.2). First, a reducing sugar, lactose, a disaccharide of glucose and

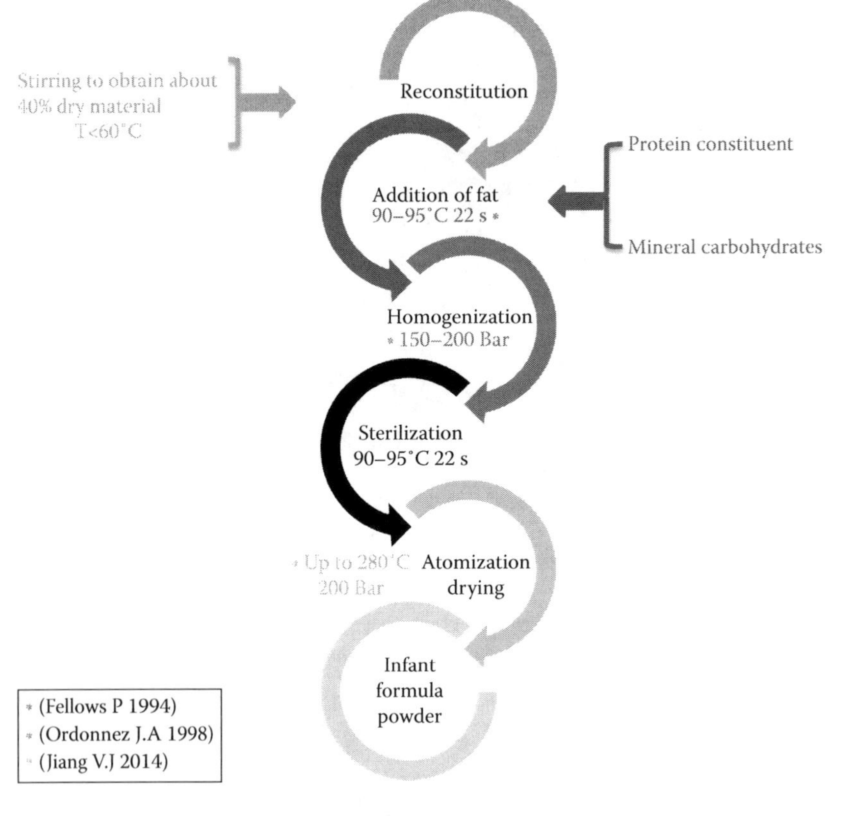

FIGURE 6.1 The different steps for elaboration of infant formula powder.

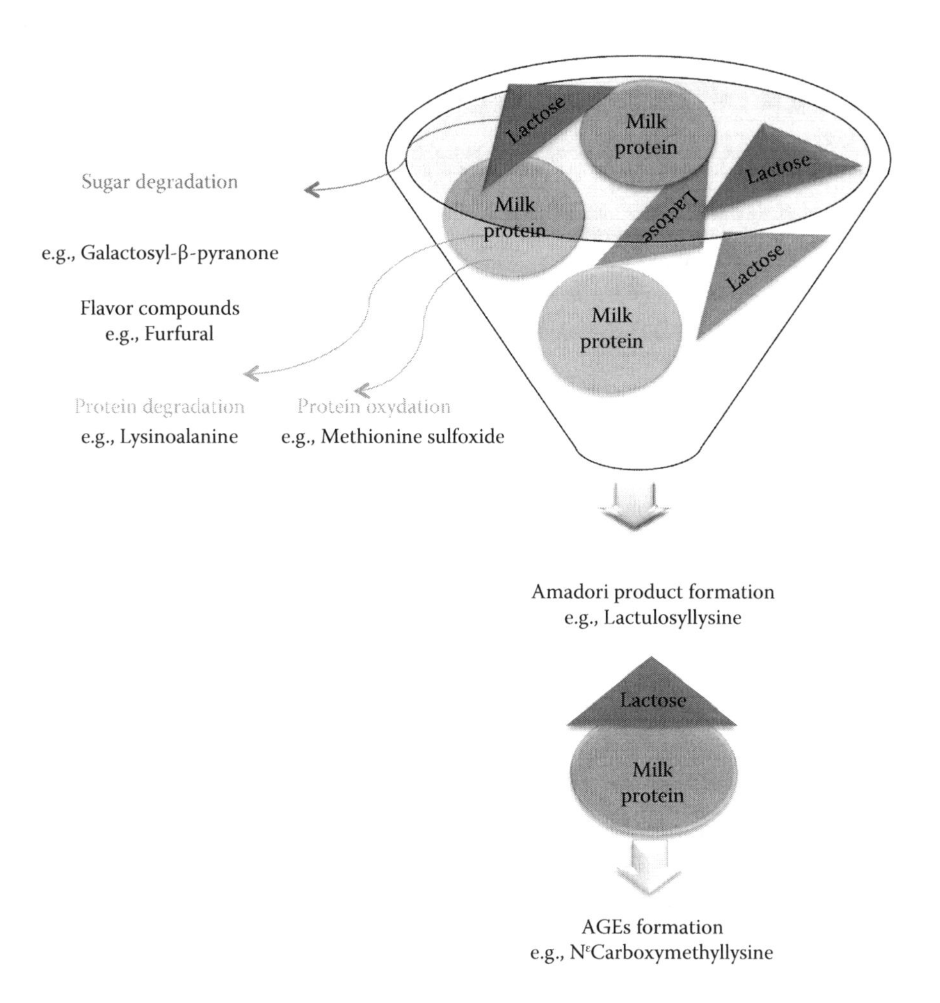

FIGURE 6.2 Maillard reaction in milk.

galactose (the monosaccharides glucose and galactose are found in raw milk only in very low concentrations) condenses with the free amino acid side chains of milk proteins (mainly ε-amino group of lysine residue), via formation of a Schiff base giving rise to stable Amadori compounds. Lactosyllysine is the Amadori product in milk (bound to the protein). In some milk products, such as skimmed milk powder, up to 50% of the lysine residues are converted to lactulosyllysine (Finot et al. 1981; Henle et al. 1991). Lactulosyllysine compound can be measured after conversion into furosine, which is the result of its acid hydrolysis. Second, Amadori products turn into advanced glycation end products (AGEs). The best characterized example is the oxidative degradation of lactulosyllysine yielding N^{ε}-carboxymethyllysine (CML) (Büser et al. 1987). AGEs can also be generated by the reaction of glucose degradation products, such as methylglyoxal, with the amino acid side chains of proteins (Henle et al. 1994). More AGEs have been identified in processed milk such as N^{ε}-carboxyethyllysine (CEL), pentosidine, oxalic acid monolysinylamide (OMA) (Hasenkopf et al. 2001), and pyrraline (Henle and Miyata 2003). Furfurals are both the result of Amadori compounds from the Maillard reaction and of lactose isomerization, also known as the Lobry De Bruyn–Alberda van Ekenstein transformation (Boekel and Van 1998; Morales and Jimenez-Perez 1998; Chavez-Servin et al. 2005). The main furfurals reported in milk are 5-hydroxymethyl-2-furaldehyde. Third, the final steps of the Maillard reaction consists of the condensation of amino compounds and sugar fragments into polymerized protein and brown pigments, called the melanoidins. Fluorescence and browning development in the Maillard reaction are generally used as indicators of the reaction rate and formation of MRP (Yeboah et al. 1999).

6.3 Major Glycation Products in Infant Formula during Heat Process and Storage

6.3.1 IF Composition and Type

Bovine milk is the basis for most infant formulas. It contains higher levels of fat, minerals, and protein compared to human milk (Table 6.1), so it is skimmed and diluted to be as close as possible to breast milk composition (Stan 2007). High standards of hygiene are maintained throughout the production process of IF. Powdered infant formula is not a sterile product. It has, however, a longer shelf life than the liquid forms of IF and is cheaper.

IFs are usually supplemented with lactose and whey protein (Nasirpour et al. 2006) to reflect the higher concentration of lactose found in human milk (7.1%) and the lower casein to whey ratio of human milk compared to cow's milk (40:60 vs. 82:18, respectively). Proteins present in milk are recognized as the main cause of allergic reactions. Specific hypoallergenic infant formulas are generated via enzymatic hydrolysis and heat-denaturation of the intact proteins for infants who have milk proteins hypersensitivity (Ragno et al. 1993; Chung et al. 2012). In addition, for infants developing lactose intolerance symptoms, specific IFs without lactose are also developed (Table 6.1).

Although the fat content of human milk is very similar to cow's milk, there are major differences in the fatty acid composition. IFs are therefore modified or supplemented. IF supplementation with long-chain polyunsaturated fatty acids docosahexaenoic acid (DHA) and arachidonic acid (AA) has beneficial effects for infant brain development and vision (Fleith and Clandinin 2005).

6.3.2 Glycation Products in IF during Heat Process

Due to their specific composition with high lactose and protein and the application of drastic heat processing, IFs show higher levels of glycation markers than cow milk products (Birlouez-Aragon et al. 2004) denoting a lower quality of the formula compared to regular milk. Importantly, the increased levels of lysine loss, lactulosyllysine, and AGEs are observed in IFs. Moreover, (Albalá-Hurtado et al. 1997) found an increased level of hydroxymethylfurfural (HMF) indicating lower milk quality. The Maillard reaction has been thought to be responsible for the solubility loss of protein in powder IF (Le et al. 2011).

It is, however, relatively difficult to precisely evaluate the effect of Maillard reaction on IFs due to the different existing types and the variability of glycation molecules among the different samples of the same group of IF. In Table 6.2, we report the potential degree of glycation in IFs according to some of their components and type. In hypoallergenic formula (HA), protein hydrolysis activates the Maillard reaction (Birlouez-Aragon et al. 2004) due to the proteolysis reaction that releases N-terminal ε-amino groups, which are targeted by glycation (Penndorf et al. 2007). HA formulas contain higher CML levels than regular formulas of the same consistency (liquid or powdered, respectively) (Dittrich et al. 2006; Delatour et al. 2009). In contrast, the lactulosyllysine content in powdered HA formulas was even lower than in regular powdered formulas. The type of sugar present (Fenaille et al. 2006) in IF is also an

TABLE 6.1

Cow's Milk, Breast Milk, and Infant Formula Composition[a]

	Human Milk	Infant Formula	Cow's Milk
Proteins Range (g)	1.2–1.5	1.2–1.9	3.5
Casein (%)	40	–	80
Whey (%)	60	–	20
Carbohydrates (g)	6–7	7.2–8.9	5
Lactose (g)	6	4.7–7.4	5
Oligosaccharides (g)	1	–	0
Lipids (g)	3.6	3.6	3.6
Linoleic acid (%)	10–15	–	3

[a] composition per 100 mL.

TABLE 6.2
Glycation Markers Level According to the Type of Infant Formula (++: reactive; +++: highly reactive)

Specific Formula Type	To Whom	Glycation Reactivity	References
Standard milk-based formulas: • Casein • Whey	All infants	++	Fenaille et al. 2006; Naranjo et al. 1998; Pereyra Gonzales et al. 2003
Hypoallergenic formulas	Allergy to milk proteins	+++	Dittrich et al. 2006; Delatour et al. 2009; Birlouez-Aragon 2004
Soy-based formulas (free of animal proteins)	Galactosemia	++	Bhatia and Greer 2008
Lactose-free formulas	Congenital lactase deficiency Galactosemia	++	Oh et al. 2014
Special formulas Formula for premature and low birth weight	Extra calories Minerals Protein fortification	+++	Leclère et al. 2002
Supplemented formulas Long-chain polyunsaturated fatty acids Prebiotics and probiotics	• Arachidonic acid and Docosahexaenoic acid • Nucleotides, Prebiotics and Probiotics	+++	Nielsen et al. 1985

important determinant of glycation formation. Glucose seems to be more reactive than complex sugars like lactose (Naranjo et al. 1998; Pereyra Gonzales et al. 2003). Furthermore, the high content of polyunsaturated fatty acids also plays a major role in Maillard reaction (Nielsen et al. 1985a, 1985b). Indeed, long-chain polyunsaturated fatty acids are easily oxidized during the production of IF and induce glycation precursors, such as glyoxal (Lima et al. 2010). Regarding minerals and vitamins, supplementation of iron and ascorbic acid is known to enhance protein damage from a Fenton-type reaction (Leclère et al. 2002) and an increase of the hydroxyl radical formation (Almaas et al. 1997) the lysine glycation and the tryptophan oxidation (Leclère et al. 2002). Finally, volatile Maillard reaction products are shown to be present in low quantities in IF (Colahan-Sederstrom and Peterson 2005).

6.3.3 Effect of Heat Process on Protein Bioavailability in IFs

As mentioned previously, heat process induces formation of several glycation markers that reduce the quality of an infant formula. Protein quality is mainly evaluated by the amino acid proportionality pattern, protein digestibility, and amino acid bioavailability of the protein used in the preparation of IF. It is suggested that infant formula consistency (powder, ready-to-use, and liquid concentrate) may influence amino acid availability as previously shown. The availability of lysine is most marked in spray-dried and ultra-high temperature treated formulas (Sarwar et al. 1989). Heating in liquid concentrate causes more loss of lysine by Maillard reactions and sulfur amino acids by oxidation reactions than in powder form. In fact, liquid concentrates have lower protein, lysine, methionine, and cystine digestibilities, and protein quality than powders prepared by the same manufacturer (Sarwar et al. 1988).

Strong protein–protein and protein–lipid interactions are more actively generated after heat process in sterilized than in spray-dried and UHT-treated products demonstrating that these protein modifications are dependent on the applied temperature (Salamon et al. 2009). The total protein turnover of whey-predominant and casein-predominant formulas was compared in term and low-birth-weight infants (Jarvenpaa et al. 1982a). No difference was observed in growth or nitrogen retention or protein synthesis or urinary 3-methylhistidine excretion in preterm infants fed with the two types of formulas (Pencharz et al. 1983). However, it is worth taking into account that the concentration of some amino acids like taurine in the plasma and urine was significantly higher in low-birth-weight infants fed with whey-predominant as compared to those fed with casein-predominant formulas (Jarvenpaa et al. 1982a, 1982b; Kashyap et al. 1987).

It has been demonstrated that the elimination pattern of α-amino nitrogen from an infant that was fed a spray-dried formula was closest to that resulting from human milk, whereas the sterilized product seemed to be less digestible (Boehm and Raiha 1994). This is particularly important for preterm infants that are commonly fed with sterilized liquid products or hydrolyzed formula.

6.3.4 Impact of Storage on the Shelf Life of IF

The detection of Maillard reaction products is important for the quality control of milk during storage. In most cases, the industrial sterilization thermal treatments are designed to avoid reaching the coloring step although it is likely to develop during storage (Ferrer et al. 2005; Bosch et al. 2007). So far, several heat-induced markers have been proposed to evaluate the quality of IFs such as furosine, HMF, and lactulose concentrations. These have been recognized as useful indicators to control the extent of browning reactions during storage. However, these indicators do not show the same trend according to the type of formula and the duration time. Ferrer demonstrated that for an adapted infant formula, over a period of 24 months, the lysine decreased from 9.78 to 7.85 and 7.45 g/kg^{-1} at 20°C and 37 °C, respectively (Ferrer et al. 2003). Conversely, furosine increased correspondingly from 187 to 750 and 1,001 g/ kg^{-1}, respectively. It appeared that the furosine increase correlated well with the lysine loss over the first 12 months of storage, but less well thereafter. Recently, Chavez-Servin et al. (2015) showed that the range of potential HMF consumed for an infant about 6 months old feeding only on formula was estimated between 0.63 mg and 3.25 mg per day.

The impact of storage on vitamins is less studied. Certain pre-melanoidins could react with vitamins and destroy them. Storage at 60°C caused rapid destruction of folic acid (53% loss at 4 weeks) and slower loss of thiamin, vitamin B6, and pantothenic acid (18% at 8 weeks). At 70°C, the rate of destruction is much higher and occurs in parallel to the destruction of lactosyllysine and to the apparition of other Maillard products. For the four aforementioned labile vitamins, 18% or less survived at 4 weeks (Ford et al. 1983).

6.4 Implication of the High Load of AGEs in IFs on Health and Diseases Outcomes

6.4.1 Diabetes and Kidney Failure

The composition of IFs differs remarkably from breast milk with higher protein content, lower concentration of long-chain polyunsaturated fatty acids, and a lack of hormones such as insulin, leptin, IGF, as well as numerous other biological substances. These differences between IFs and breast milk have been assumed to be the cause of the decrease of insulin sensitivity and the development of diabetes and obesity in bottle fed infants (Das 2002; Kerkhof et al. 2012). Formula-derived-AGEs might in certain cases exceed up to 670-fold the level of breast milk (Sebekova et al. 2008). This fact represents a potential supplementary risk factor of developing insulin resistance and obesity (Mericq et al. 2010). Studies in humans and animals have shown that IF AGEs are absorbed and excreted in the urine (Dittrich et al. 2006; Sebekova et al. 2008; Elmhiri et al. 2015). Compared with breast-fed infants, 3- to 6-month-old and 7- to 10-month-old formula-fed infants displayed higher plasma total CML concentrations than breast-fed ones (Mericq et al. 2010). However, no direct evidence of high load, formula-derived-AGEs effect on insulin resistance, inflammation, or oxidative stress in young infants was found (Klenovics et al. 2013).

Numerous babies such as low-birth-weight babies who suffered from intrauterine growth restriction (IUGR) are fed with a high-protein formula to ensure a rapid postnatal catch up growth (Embleton and Cooke 2005). However a high protein intake in the first 2 years of life has been related to negative effects such as a risk for obesity and metabolic programming. Whether these negative outcomes are associated to the high load of AGEs in formula is unknown. However, we should consider that the protein content must be handled with care especially for those infants born with IUGR.

Several studies suggested that milk AGEs are involved in renal defects (Henle 2003). Precisely, AGEs and also lysinoalanine that are largely formed in IF were reported to induce histological changes in the

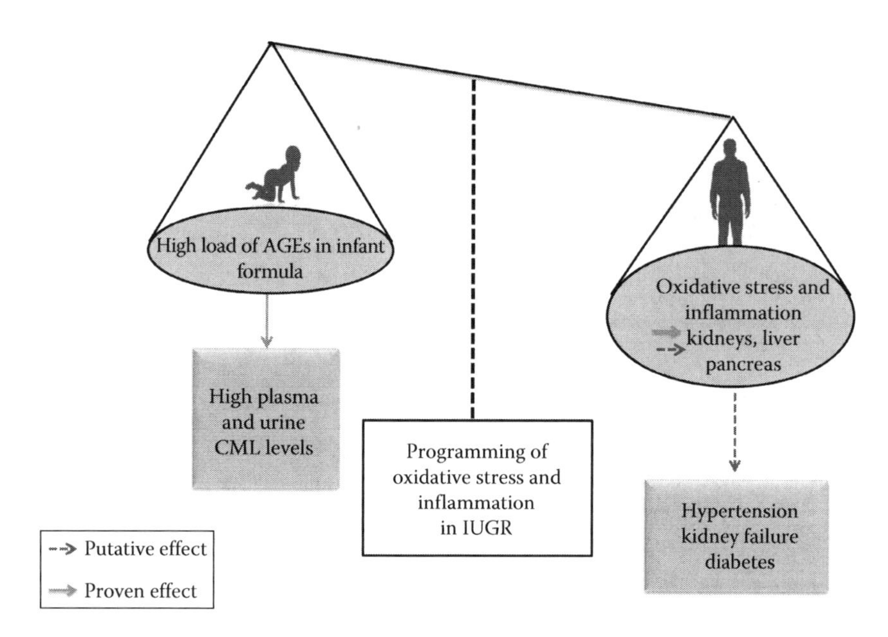

FIGURE 6.3 AGEs derived from formulas and their long-term health outcomes.

straight part of the proximal tubule in rat kidney (Gould and MacGregor 1977). In a pilot study, however, Langhendries showed that short-term feeding of different types of infant formulas in preterm infants did not induce changes in the kidney function but observed an increase in urinary micro-protein levels compared to infants fed with breast milk (Langhendries et al. 1992). Whether AGEs and lysinoalanine in early childhood affects postnatal programming of kidney function and hypertension remains to be elucidated (Figure 6.3).

Among the different species, the piglet is the best for assessing the effect of infant formulas because of the close anatomical and physiological similarities between neonatal piglets and human neonates (Attig et al. 2008). We used piglets to evaluate the effect of glycation end products in IF on long-term oxidative stress and inflammation in the kidney (Elmhiri et al. 2015). Our results indicated that a high level of postnatal AGEs exposed IUGR piglets to an elevated oxidative stress in both kidney and liver during the juvenile stage. Moreover, a concomitant expression of proapoptotic genes, target renin–angiotensin system genes, the expression and activation of the proinflammatory factor NF-κB, and the secretion of IL-18 were also observed. In agreement with others (Cai et al. 2002), the observed effects of AGEs in kidney seem to be mediated through the synthesis and activation of RAGE. Findings in human and rodents suggest that a high level of RAGE and AGEs correlates with a high risk for several diseases, including diabetes and chronic kidney disease (Sebekova and Somoza 2007; Birlouez-Aragon et al. 2010; Mericq et al. 2010).

6.4.2 Potential Effects of Glycation Products in IF on Microbiota

The metabolic output of the human colonic microbiota is increasingly understood to play a central role in modulating human health. The microbiota acts in concert with the host to transform a range of dietary compounds that drives the metabolism. Melanoidins and some AGE-modified proteins are partially digestible and reach the colon. However, little is known about their consequent degradation and/or transformation by the gut microbiota.

In vivo studies on the effect of AGEs in IF on microbial structure and composition are scarce. It can be postulated that a number of potential mechanisms by which AGEs derived formula colonic degradation may contribute to inflammatory and/or oxidative processes (O'Brien and Morrissey 1989). Ames showed that the number of anaerobic species including lactobacilli increased following fermentation of Maillard reaction products prepared from glucose and lysine (Ames et al. 1999). In a recent study, it was reported that the Maillard reaction products generated from milk proteins (cMRP) and MRP fermented by *Lactobacillus gasseri* H10 or by *Lactobacillus fermentum* H9 (F-cMRP) have an important anti-cardiovascular activity (Oh et al. 2014). Rats receiving a high cholesterol diet showed that F-cMRP and cMRP have the potential to play preventive and therapeutic roles in the management of cardiovascular disease. This is achieved by activating an antioxidative defense mechanism that regulates cholesterol synthesis and metabolism. Based on these results, the physiological and biological functions of milk protein could be improved by the Maillard reaction (Oh et al. 2015).

Following the same thought, our recent *in vivo* study on a piglet demonstrated that consumption of a high load of IF-derived-AGEs postnatally induced an enhancement of antioxidant enzyme expression including superoxide dismutase (SOD), catalase (CAT), and glutathione peroxidase (GSH-Px). It also increased the activity of GSH-Px in the colon of IUGR piglets 3 months after milk feeding (Elmhiri et al. 2016). The primary antioxidant enzymes SOD, CAT, and GSH-Px protect against molecular and cellular damage caused by reactive oxygen species. Wang et al. reported that the antioxidative defense mechanism protects against the development of atherosclerosis (Wang et al. 2004). A transient postnatal increase of the total count of lactobacilli and bifidobacteria was associated with the enhancement of the antioxidant status in juvenile animals. Bifidobacteria in the infant gut are important for inhibiting the growth of pathogenic organisms, modulating mucosal barrier function, and promoting immunological and inflammatory responses (Sudo et al. 1997; Coppa et al. 2004; Bode 2009; Barile and Rastall 2013). Whether IF melanoidins or fermented MRP are involved in such modification of the microbiota composition and the antioxidant status remains unknown. Further studies on IF-derived-AGEs are needed to determine the nature of these components and the extent of their effects over age on gut microbiota.

6.5 Conclusions

Infant formula is a complex pre-substitute human milk matrix predetermined to ensure appropriate infant growth and development. Industrial processing and long-term storage of IF induce a higher degree of damage to its composition and nutritional quality, largely due to the production of glycation end products, the so-called Maillard reaction products or AGEs. High dietary intake of AGE induces a rise in circulating AGEs in formula-consuming infants and is associated with the development of transient insulin resistance. The kidney has been shown to be the major target of AGEs. AGEs absorbed from infant formula may disturb the kidney function by inducing early oxidative stress and micro-inflammation and also a lipoxidative state in the liver. These physiological dysregulations of AGEs in IF could threaten the equilibrium of the redox balance leading to low run of the defense system of the infant over time. However, the potential beneficial effects of fermented AGEs to counteract harmful AGEs' side effects remains to be determined. It remains to be elucidated whether the high load of AGEs in the infant diet during the early 1,000 days of life, the critical period of child development and health, could exert long-term negative effects in vulnerable children such as premature, IUGR, or diseased ones, or predispose them to more serious manifestation of chronic diseases later in life.

ACKNOWLEDGEMENTS

The authors thank Dr. Monia BOUKTHIR (Children's Hospital, Department of Pediatrics, Tunisia), Dr Mustapha ROUIS (8256 UPMC Université Paris 6, CNRS INSERM, Adaptations biologiques et Vieillissement 8256/ERL 1164, Paris), Dr Stéphane FIRMIN (LaSalle Institute) for their comments. Thanks to Mous Ismael and Mariem for their support.

REFERENCES

Albalá-Hurtado, S., M. T. Veciana-Nogués, M. Izquierdo-Pulido, and M. C. Vidal-Carou. 1997. Determination of free and total furfural compounds in infant milk formulas by high-performance liquid chromatography. *J Agric Food Chem* 45 (6):2128–2133.

Almaas, R., T. Rootwelt, S. Oyasaeter, and O. D. Saugstad. 1997. Ascorbic acid enhances hydroxyl radical formation in iron-fortified infant cereals and infant formulas. *Eur J Pediatr* 156 (6):488–92.

Ames, J. M., A. Wynne, A. Hofmann, S. Plos, and G. R. Gibson. 1999. The effect of a model melanoidin mixture on faecal bacterial populations in vitro. *Br J Nutr* 82 (6):489–95.

Attig, L., J. Djiane, A. Gertler, O. Rampin, T. Larcher, S. Boukthir, P. M. Anton, J. Y. Madec, I. Gourdou, and L. Abdennebi-Najar. 2008. Study of hypothalamic leptin receptor expression in low-birth-weight piglets and effects of leptin supplementation on neonatal growth and development. *Am J Physiol Endocrinol Metab* 295 (5):E1117–25. doi: 10.1152/ajpendo.90542.2008.

Barile, D., and R. A. Rastall. 2013. Human milk and related oligosaccharides as prebiotics. *Curr Opin Biotechnol* 24 (2):214–9. doi: 10.1016/j.copbio.2013.01.008.

Bhatia, J., and F. Greer. 2008. Use of soy protein-based formulas in infant feeding. *Pediatrics* 121 (5):1062–8. doi: 10.1542/peds.2008-0564.

Birlouez-Aragon, I., E. De St Louvent, P. Stahl, and L. Eveleigh. 2004. O0102 Protein hydrolysis of infant formulas strongly activates the maillard reaction. *J Pediatr Gastroenterol Nutr* 39:S47.

Birlouez-Aragon, I., G. Saavedra, F. J. Tessier, A. Galinier, L. Ait-Ameur, F. Lacoste, C. N. Niamba, N. Alt, V. Somoza, and J. M. Lecerf. 2010. A diet based on high-heat-treated foods promotes risk factors for diabetes mellitus and cardiovascular diseases. *Am J Clin Nutr* 91 (5):1220–6. doi: 10.3945/ajcn.2009.28737.

Bode, L. 2009. Human milk oligosaccharides: Prebiotics and beyond. *Nutr Rev* 67 Suppl 2:S183–91. doi: 10.1111/j.1753-4887.2009.00239.x.

Boehm, G., and N. C. Raiha. 1994. Heat treatment of infant formula: Effect on postprandial serum alpha-amino-nitrogen concentrations in very-low-birth-weight infants. *J Pediatr Gastroenterol Nutr* 18 (3):371–4.

Boekel, M. A., and J. S. Van. 1998. Effect of heating on Maillard reactions in milk. *Food Chem* 62 (4):403–414.

Bosch, L., Alegria, A., Farré, R., and Clemente, G. 2007. Fluorescence and color as markers for the Maillard reaction in milk–cereal based infant foods during storage. *Food Chem* 105 (3): 1135–1143.

Büser, W., H. F. Erbersdobler, and R. Liardon. 1987. Identification and determination of N-ε-carboxymethyllysine by gas-liquid chromatography. *J Chrom A* 387:515–519.

Cai, W., Q. D. Gao, L. Zhu, M. Peppa, C. He, and H. Vlassara. 2002. Oxidative stress-inducing carbonyl compounds from common foods: Novel mediators of cellular dysfunction. *Mol Med* 8 (7):337–46.

Chavez-Servin, J. L., A. I. Castellote, and M. C. Lopez-Sabater. 2005. Analysis of potential and free furfural compounds in milk-based formulae by high-performance liquid chromatography. Evolution during storage. *J Chromatogr A* 1076 (1–2):133–40.

Chavez-Servin, J. L., K. de la Torre Carbot, T. Garcia-Gasca, A. I. Castellote, and M. C. Lopez-Sabater. 2015. Content and evolution of potential furfural compounds in commercial milk-based infant formula powder after opening the packet. *Food Chem* 166:486–91. doi: 10.1016/j.foodchem.2014.06.050.

Chung, C. S., S. Yamini, and P. R. Trumbo. 2012. FDA's health claim review: Whey-protein partially hydrolyzed infant formula and atopic dermatitis. *Pediatrics* 130 (2):e408–14. doi: 10.1542/peds.2012-0333.

Colahan-Sederstrom, P. M., and D. G. Peterson. 2005. Inhibition of key aroma compound generated during ultrahigh-temperature processing of bovine milk via epicatechin addition. *J Agric Food Chem* 53 (2):398–402. doi: 10.1021/jf0487248.

Coppa, G. V., S. Bruni, L. Morelli, S. Soldi, and O. Gabrielli. 2004. The first prebiotics in humans: Human milk oligosaccharides. *J Clin Gastroenterol* 38 (6 Suppl):S80–3.

Das, U. N. 2002. The lipids that matter from infant nutrition to insulin resistance. *Prostag Leukot Essent Fatty Acids* 67 (1):1–12.

Delatour, T., J. Hegele, V. Parisod, J. Richoz, S. Maurer, M. Steven, and T. Buetler. 2009. Analysis of advanced glycation endproducts in dairy products by isotope dilution liquid chromatography-electrospray tandem mass spectrometry. The particular case of carboxymethyllysine. *J Chromatogr A* 1216 (12):2371–81.

Dittrich, R., I. Hoffmann, P. Stahl, A. Muller, M. W. Beckmann, and M. Pischetsrieder. 2006. Concentrations of Nepsilon-carboxymethyllysine in human breast milk, infant formulas, and urine of infants. *J Agric Food Chem* 54 (18):6924–8.

Elmhiri, G., D. Hamoudi, S. Dou, N. Bahi-jaber, J. Reygnier, T. Larcher, S. Firmin, and L. Abdennebi-Najar. 2016. Antioxydant properties of formula derived Maillard reaction products in colon of intrauterine growth restricted pigs. *Food Funct* 7 (6):2582–90.

Elmhiri, G., D. F. Mahmood, C. Niquet-Leridon, P. Jacolot, S. Firmin, L. Guigand, F. J. Tessier, T. Larcher, and L. Abdennebi-Najar. 2015. Formula-derived advanced glycation end products are involved in the development of long-term inflammation and oxidative stress in kidney of IUGR piglets. *Mol Nutr Food Res* 59 (5):939–47. doi: 10.1002/mnfr.201400722.

Embleton, N. D., and R. J. Cooke. 2005. Protein requirements in preterm infants: Effect of different levels of protein intake on growth and body composition. *Pediatr Res* 58 (5):855–60. doi: 10.1203/01.pdr.0000182586.46532.7c.

Fenaille, F., V. Parisod, P. Visani, S. Populaire, J. C. Tabet, and P. A. Guy. 2006. Modifications of milk constituents during processing: A preliminary benchmarking study. *Int Dairy J* 16 (7):728–739.

Ferrer, E., A. Alegria, R. Farre, P. Abellan, F. Romero, and G. Clemente. 2003. Evolution of available lysine and furosine contents in milk-based infant formulas throughout the shelf-life storage period. *J Sci Food Agric* 83:465–472.

Ferrer, E., A. Alegria, R. Farre, G. Clemente, and C. Calvo. 2005. Fluorescence, browning index, and color in infant formulas during storage. *J Agric Food Chem* 53 (12):4911–7. doi: 10.1021/jf0403585.

Finot, P. A., R. Deutsch, and E. Bujard. 1981. The extent of the Maillard reaction during the processing of milk. *Prog Food Nutr Sci* 5:345–355.

Fleith, M., and M. T. Clandinin. 2005. Dietary PUFA for preterm and term infants: Review of clinical studies. *Crit Rev Food Sci Nutr* 45 (3):205–29.

Ford, J. E., R. F. Hurrell, and P. A. Finot. 1983. Storage of milk powders under adverse conditions. 2. Influence on the content of water-soluble vitamins. *Br J Nutr* 49 (3):355–64.

Gould, D. H., and J. T. MacGregor. 1977. Biological effects of alkali-treated protein and lysinoalanine: An overview. *Adv Exp Med Biol* 86B:29–48.

Hasenkopf, K., B. Ubel, T. Bordiehn, and M. Pischetsrieder. 2001. Determination of the Maillard product oxalic acidmonolysinylamide (OMA) in heated milk products by ELISA. *Nahrung* 45 (3):206–9.

Henle, T., 2003. AGEs in foods: Do they play a role in uremia? *Kidney Int Suppl* (84):S145–7. doi: 10.1046/j.1523-1755.63.s84.16.x.

Henle, T., and T. Miyata, 2003. Advanced glycation end products in uremia. *Adv Ren Repl Ther* 10:321–331.

Henle, T., A. W. Walter, R. Haeßner, and H. Klostermeyer. 1994. Detection and identification of a protein-bound imidazolone resulting from the reaction of arginine residues and methylglyoxal. *Zeitschrift für Lebensmittel-Untersuchung und Forschung* 199 (1):55–58.

Henle, T., H. Walter, and H. Klostermeyer. 1991. Evaluation of the extent of the early Maillard-reaction in milk products by direct measurement of the Amadori-product lactuloselysine. *Z Lebensm Unters Forsch* 193 (2):119–22.

Jarvenpaa, A. L., N. C. Raiha, D. K. Rassin, and G. E. Gaull. 1982a. Milk protein quantity and quality in the term infant. I. Metabolic responses and effects on growth. *Pediatrics* 70 (2):214–20.

Jarvenpaa, A. L., D. K. Rassin, N. C. Raiha, and G. E. Gaull. 1982b. Milk protein quantity and quality in the term infant. II. Effects on acidic and neutral amino acids. *Pediatrics* 70 (2):221–30.

Kashyap, S., E. Okamoto, S. Kanaya, C. Zucker, K. Abildskov, R. B. Dell, and W. C. Heird. 1987. Protein quality in feeding low birth weight infants: A comparison of whey-predominant versus casein-predominant formulas. *Pediatrics* 79 (5):748–55.

Kerkhof, G. F., R. W. Leunissen, and A. C. Hokken-Koelega. 2012. Early origins of the metabolic syndrome: Role of small size at birth, early postnatal weight gain, and adult IGF-I. *J Clin Endocrinol Metab* 97 (8):2637–43. doi: 10.1210/jc.2012-1426.

Klenovics, K. S., P. Boor, V. Somoza, P. Celec, V. Fogliano, and K. Sebekova. 2013. Advanced glycation end products in infant formulas do not contribute to insulin resistance associated with their consumption. *PLoS One* 8 (1):e53056. doi: 10.1371/journal.pone.0053056.

Langhendries, J. P., R. F. Hurrell, D. E. Furniss, C. Hischenhuber, P. A. Finot, A. Bernard, O. Battisti, J. M. Bertrand, and J. Senterre. 1992. Maillard reaction products and lysinoalanine: Urinary excretion and the effects on kidney function of preterm infants fed heat-processed milk formula. *J Pediatr Gastroenterol Nutr* 14 (1):62–70.

Le, T. T., B. Bhandari, and H. C. Deeth. 2011. Chemical and physical changes in milk protein concentrate (MPC80) powder during storage. *J Agric Food Chem* 59 (10):5465–73. doi: 10.1021/jf2003464.

Leclère, J., I. Birlouez-Aragon, and M. Meli. 2002. Fortification of milk with iron-ascorbate promotes lysine glycation and tryptophan oxidation. *Food Chem* 76 (4):491–499.

Lima, M., S. H. Assar, and J. M. Ames. 2010. Formation of N(epsilon)-(carboxymethyl)lysine and loss of lysine in casein glucose-fatty acid model systems. *J Agric Food Chem* 58 (3):1954–8. doi: 10.1021/jf903562c.

Mericq, V., C. Piccardo, W. Cai, X. Chen, L. Zhu, G. E. Striker, H. Vlassara, and J. Uribarri. 2010. Maternally transmitted and food-derived glycotoxins: A factor preconditioning the young to diabetes? *Diabetes Care* 33 (10):2232–7. doi: 10.2337/dc10-1058.

Morales, F. J., and S. Jimenez-Perez. 1998. Study of hydroxymethylfurfural formation from acid degradation of the amadori product in milk-resembling systems. *J Agric Food Chem* 46 (10):3885–3890.

Naranjo, G. B., L. S. Malec, and M. S. Vigo. 1998. Reducing sugars effect on available lysine loss of casein by moderate heat treatment. *Food Chem* 62 (3):309–313.

Nasirpour, A., J. Scher, M. Linder, and S. Desobry. 2006. Modeling of lactose crystallization and color changes in model infant foods. *J Dairy Sci* 89 (7):2365–73. doi: 10.3168/jds.S0022-0302(06)72309-8.

Nielsen, H. K., P. A. Finot, and R. F. Hurrell. 1985a. Reactions of proteins with oxidizing lipids. 2. Influence on protein quality and on the bioavailability of lysine, methionine, cyst(e)ine and tryptophan as measured in rat assays. *Br J Nutr* 53 (1):75–86.

Nielsen, H. K., J. Loliger, and R. F. Hurrell. 1985b. Reactions of proteins with oxidizing lipids. 1. Analytical measurements of lipid oxidation and of amino acid losses in a whey protein-methyl linolenate model system. *Br J Nutr* 53 (1):61–73.

O'Brien, J., and P. A. Morrissey. 1989. Nutritional and toxicological aspects of the Maillard browning reaction in foods. *Crit Rev Food Sci Nutr* 28 (3):211–48.

Oh, N. S., H. S. Kwon, H. A. Lee, J. Y. Joung, J. Y. Lee, K. B. Lee, Y. K. Shin, et al. 2014. Preventive effect of fermented Maillard reaction products from milk proteins in cardiovascular health. *J Dairy Sci* 97 (6):3300–13. doi: 10.3168/jds.2013-7728.

Oh, N. S., M. R. Park, K. W. Lee, S. H. Kim, and Y. Kim. 2015. Dietary Maillard reaction products and their fermented products reduce cardiovascular risk in an animal model. *J Dairy Sci* 98 (8):5102–12. doi: 10.3168/jds.2015-9308.

Pencharz, P. B., L. Farri, and A. Papageorgiou. 1983. The effects of human milk and low-protein formulae on the rates of total body protein turnover and urinary 3-methyl-histidine excretion of preterm infants. *Clin Sci (Lond)* 64 (6):611–16.

Penndorf, I., D. Biedermann, S. V. Maurer, and T. Henle. 2007. Studies on N-terminal glycation of peptides in hypoallergenic infant formulas: Quantification of alpha-N-(2-furoylmethyl) amino acids. *J Agric Food Chem* 55 (3):723–7. doi: 10.1021/jf061821b.

Pereyra Gonzales, A. S., G. B. Naranjo, L. S. Malec, and M. S. Vigo. 2003. Available lysine, protein digestibility and lactulose in commercial infant formulas. *Int Dairy J* 13 (2–3):95–99.

Ragno, V., P. G. Giampietro, G. Bruno, and L. Businco. 1993. Allergenicity of milk protein hydrolysate formulae in children with cow's milk allergy. *Eur J Pediatr* 152 (9):760–2.

Salamon, R. V., Z. màndoki, Z. Csapó-Kiss, A. Győri, Z. Gyrői, and J. Csapó. 2009. Changes in fatty acid composition of diferent milk products caused by diferent technology. *Acta Univ Sapientiae Alimentaria* 2 (1):101–109.

Sarwar, G., R. W. Peace, and H. G. Bouing. 1988. Bioavailability of lysine in milk-based infant formulas as determined by rat growth response method. *Nutr Res* 8:47–55.

Sarwar, G., R. W. Peace, and H. G. Botting. 1989. Differences in protein digestibility and quality of liquid concentrate and powder forms of milk-based infant formulas fed to rats. *Am J Clin Nutr* 49 (5):806–13.

Sebekova, K., G. Saavedra, C. Zumpe, V. Somoza, K. Klenovicsova, and I. Birlouez-Aragon. 2008. Plasma concentration and urinary excretion of N epsilon-(carboxymethyl)lysine in breast milk- and formula-fed infants. *Ann N Y Acad Sci* 1126:177–80.

Sebekova, K., and V. Somoza. 2007. Dietary advanced glycation endproducts (AGEs) and their health effects—PRO. *Mol Nutr Food Res* 51 (9):1079–84. doi: 10.1002/mnfr.200700035.

Stan, C., 2007. *FAO/WHO Food Standards Programme*. Food and Agriculture Organization of the United Nations, Rome, Italy, pp. 72–108.

Sudo, N., S. Sawamura, K. Tanaka, Y. Aiba, C. Kubo, and Y. Koga. 1997. The requirement of intestinal bacterial flora for the development of an IgE production system fully susceptible to oral tolerance induction. *J Immunol* 159 (4):1739–45.

Wang, H. H., T. M. Hung, J. Wei, and A. N. Chiang. 2004. Fish oil increases antioxidant enzyme activities in macrophages and reduces atherosclerotic lesions in apoE-knockout mice. *Cardiovasc Res* 61 (1):169–76.

Yeboah, F. K., I. Alli, and V. A. Yaylayan. 1999. Reactivities of D-glucose and D-fructose during glycation of bovine serum albumin. *J Agric Food Chem* 47 (8):3164–72.

7

Potentially Toxic Food Components Formed by Excessive Heat Processing

Franco Pedreschi
Pontificia Universidad de Católica de Chile
Santiago de Chile, Chile

Michael Murkovic
Graz University of Technology
Graz, Austria

CONTENTS

KEY POINTS

- Neoformed contaminants generated during processing of food have become an area of contention because of the potential toxic health effects of these compounds.
- Specific neoformed contaminants formed depends not only on the high processing temperature but also on the original chemical composition of the foods to be cooked.
- Neoformed contaminants in foods processed in high temperature are related to Maillard reaction and other reaction mechanisms according to the chemical composition of the raw materials.
- Mitigation formation of neoformed contaminants could be achieved by diminishing the food precursors in the raw food and inhibiting the processing conditions which favored the reactions that led to the formation of neoformed contaminants.
- It is not only important to mitigate formation of neoformed contaminants in foods processed in high temperature but also to select the proper mitigation conditions in order to affect negatively the attractive sensorial properties of the cooked products.

7.1 Introduction

Household and industrial heat treatments induce a number of important functions in food preparation, improving its digestibility, ensuring microbiological safety, and developing flavor and taste to name just three (Pedreschi et al. 2014). While these kinds of processes are an integral part of food production, recent research on neoformed contaminants (NFCs), a range of compounds produced during heat treatment, paints a worrying picture of their wider health effects. In the Maillard Reaction (MR)—the chemical processes that cause food to brown as it cooks—sugars including glucose, fructose, and lactose react with free amino acids in foods. These MR products (MRPs) give food its appetizing color, aroma, and flavor. Other well-known heat-generated food toxicants include nitrosamines, carcinogens that form in meats and cheeses preserved with nitrites and increased by frying; heterocyclic amines (HA), carcinogens that form in meat well-done, fried, or barbecued; and furan (Jaeger et al. 2010).

NFCs are compounds formed during heating processes that exhibit potential harmful effects to humans. Among the several NFCs described in literature, acrylamide (AA) and furan are mainly formed through the MR in potatoes and cereal products. These can be regarded as some of the most important heat-induced contaminants occurring in potato, bread, and other bakery products (Birlouez-Aragon et al. 2010). High levels of AA—an NFC present in staple foods like potatoes, breakfast cereals, and even infant formulas—have been linked to a potential increased risk of cancer, while research on HAs suggests that high doses from heated meats may have a carcinogenic impact, as well. These compounds are not external to the process but are formed naturally during thermal processing of foods through the complex set of chemical reactions taking place (Gerrard 2006). For instance, AA is known as a neurotoxin in humans which is classified as a probable human carcinogen by the International Agency of Research on Cancer (IARC). Similarly, furan is considered a potential carcinogen to humans by the IARC. Furthermore, HAs formed in cooked protein-rich foods such as meat and fish are carcinogenic in animal models and form DNA adducts in human beings. HAs are readily produced by cooking of meat in the household and most people are exposed to appreciable, although very small, amounts of these unequivocal carcinogens. HAs are formed from amino acids, creatine or creatinine, and sugar during cooking at temperatures higher than 150°C, and were initially found in the charred parts of meat and fish. HAs are formed during heating of food (meat, fish) that contains creatine, free amino acids, and carbohydrates as the result of very complex reactions (Zöchling and Murkovic 2002). Besides creatinine and amino acids, monosaccharides are involved in the MR. Finally, meats cooked well-done by high-temperature techniques contain also mutagenic compounds such as HAs, but the amounts of these compounds vary by cooking techniques, temperature, time, and type of meat. The amounts of the HAs are in the low ng/g range but can reach high levels on excessive heating (Sugimura et al. 2004).

Since NFC formation reactions are usually also responsible for the attractive color, flavor, and texture of the final products, the challenge is how to mitigate the formation of these compounds without affecting negatively the attractive sensory attributes of the foods and thus the consumer acceptance. NFC formation could be mitigated by removing NFC precursors (free asparagine, ascorbic acid, reducing sugars, creatinine, free amino acids, etc.) present in raw materials or by favoring conditions under which critical NFC formation reactions are inhibited (thermal load reduction, formulation change, addition of amino acids, addition of antioxidants, etc.) (Mariotti et al. 2012, 2013; Pedreschi et al. 2014).

7.2 Excessive Heat Application in Food Processing

Modern science has shown that heating of meat and other protein-rich foods can generate various kinds of potentially hazardous compounds, some of which are genotoxic and carcinogenic. In the last years, heat treated carbohydrate-rich foods where substantial amounts of AA and similar compounds can be formed were put into focus as a hot topic. However, other toxic compounds formed during cooking of food such as furan, and a variety of MRPs and lipid oxidation products may also constitute an increased risk of cancer for consumers (Birlouez-Aragon et al. 2010; Morales et al. 2008).

Heating of food gives many advantages in processing: it adds taste, color, and texture, and minimizes harmful bacteria. However, modern science has shown that heating of foods also can generate potentially hazardous compounds. Cooking tends to destroy nutrients as well as microbes; nutritionists often advocate eating raw food. However, another aspect, and one which less people are aware of, is the presence of toxins (including carcinogens) that exist when food is heated past a certain temperature over time (Birlouez-Aragon et al. 2010). Some of the toxic substances are as follows: (1) AA—a carcinogen found in cigarettes, coffee, baked and fried potato, bread products, among others; (2) nitrates, nitrites, and HAs; (3) advanced glycation end products (AGEs); and (4) oxidized unsaturated oils.

NFCs are contaminants supposed to be essentially formed at high temperatures during the MR from reactive amino groups of proteins or free amino acids and carbonylated derivatives of sugars (O'Brien and Morrisey 1989). Additionally, a wide range of food ingredients (lipids and vitamin C) may be degraded upon heating, especially in the presence of iron and carbonyl compounds which are highly reactive in the MR. From these carcinogenic compounds, furan can be formed easily (Birlouez_aragon et al 2010; Yaylayan et al 2000). In the case of lipids, besides the carbonyl compounds entering the MR, a number of thermoxidized products with possible adverse health effects are formed during frying. Amino acids can also be degraded via the Strecker reaction in particular conditions (low water activity and basic pH). The Strecker aldehydes react further with MR products and creatinine in meat/fish to form HA (Cheng et al. 2006). In this network of reactions, asparagine can react to form AA (Mottram et al. 2002). The high level of free asparagine in potatoes, cereal grains, and coffee, in combination with severe heat treatment applied during frying, cooking, and roasting explains why such processed food products contain the highest levels of AA (Pedreschi et al. 2014).

The main variables affecting the extent of the MR are temperature and time which depend on processing conditions as well as pH, water activity, and type and availability of the reactants which are based on food matrix properties but may be changed as a result of the processing of food and raw materials (Rufián-Henares et al. 2009). Since the MR requires reducing sugars and amino compounds as reactants, the successful post-harvest removal of these compounds from the food raw material is a promising possibility to reduce the formation of MRPs during subsequent heat processing (Pedreschi et al. 2014). Additionally, the reduction of the thermal load to which a food is exposed during heat processing is a key factor to control the extent of the MR. Unit operations such as frying, baking, roasting, or extrusion rely on favorable effects of the MR such as color and flavor formation. On the contrary, nutritional losses of essential amino acids occur during the MR as well as the formation of some undesired reaction products (Gerrard 2006).

7.3 Potential Toxic Compounds Induced in Foods by Excessive Heating

The MR can be considered as one of the most important chemical reactions taking place during food processing. A series of chemical reactions between reducing sugars and amino compounds occurring during food production can be summarized as the MR (Jaeger et al. 2010). Desired consequences like the formation of flavor and brown color of some cooked foods and also the destruction of essential amino acids and the production of antinutritive compounds require the consideration of the MR and relevant mechanisms for its control. A multitude of reaction products can be formed from the MR which have been attributed to display characteristics such as antioxidative, antimicrobial, mutagenic, or carcinogenic (Brands et al. 2000; Rufián-Henares and Morales 2007). 5-Hydroxymethylfurfural (=5-(hydroxymethyl) furan-2-carbaldehyde), 5-HMF, is a furan derivative which forms in the MR (Ames 1992) when carbohydrates are heated in the presence of amino acids or proteins (Mauron 1981) or, alternatively, by thermal dehydration of a sugar under acidic conditions (Kroh 1994). Interestingly, according to the current state of scientific knowledge, 5-HMF concentrations occurring in foods do not give rise to safety concerns (BfR 2011).

7.3.1 Acrylamide

AA (2-propenamide, CAS No. 79-06-01) is a colorless and odorless crystalline solid. AA was propelled into the spotlight in 2002 when the Swedish National Food Administration and the University of Stockholm reported considerable high levels of this probably carcinogenic compound in commonly consumed foods such as bread, coffee, potato crisps, French fries, and many others (Rosén and Hellenäs 2002). AA is known as a neurotoxin in humans, and it is classified as a probable human carcinogen by the IARC). As a genotoxic carcinogen, AA is considered to have no threshold limit of exposure, for example, a single exposure to one molecule of carcinogen can trigger the biological process leading to cancer (Felsot 2002). Current policy in Europe is that practical measures should be taken voluntarily to reduce AA formation in vulnerable foods since AA is considered a health risk at the concentrations found in foods (Capuano and Fogliano 2011; Pedreschi et al. 2014). As a guide for the food industry to reduce the levels of AA in processed food, Food Drink Europe has developed a "Toolbox." With the tools published in this document, the levels of AA should be reduced. With more and more knowledge available, the toolbox is updated regularly (http://www.fooddrinkeurope.eu).

AA is produced as a by-product of the MR in starchy foods processed at high temperatures (>120°C). Reducing sugars such as glucose and fructose are the major contributors to AA in potato-based products. On the contrary, the limiting substrate of AA formation in cereals and coffee is the free amino acid asparagine (Brathen et al. 2005). It is evident that the main sources of human dietary exposure to AA are those of fried potatoes (272–570 μg kg^{-1}), bakery products (75–1044 μg kg^{-1}), breakfast cereals (149 μg kg^{-1}), and coffee (229–890 μg kg^{-1}) (EFSA 2012). AA mitigation techniques are based principally on removing AA precursors from raw materials and/or diminishing the intensity of the factors which favor MR (Pedreschi et al. 2014).

The MR, in the presence of asparagine, has been shown to be the main pathway for AA formation in a wide range of foods processed at high temperatures (Yaylayan et al. 2003a; Zyzak et al. 2003). The key intermediate is an oxazolidin-5-one which is rearranged, decarboxylated, and the amino group eliminated forming the AA (Yaylayan et al. 2003b). Propionamide is another possible precursor which gives AA in high yields after the elimination of an amino group but with low relevance in foods (Granvogl and Schieberle 2006) (Figure 7.1). AA is mainly formed during heat processing (>120°C) of foods—primarily those derived from plant origin such as potato and cereal products (Mottram et al. 2002; Stadler et al. 2002; Zyzak et al. 2003). Stable isotope-labeled experiments have shown that the backbone of the AA molecule originates from the amino acid asparagine (Stadler et al. 2002; Zyzak et al. 2003). Asparagine alone could in principle form AA by direct decarboxylation and deamination, but the reaction is inefficient, with extremely low yields (Granvogl and Schieberle 2006). However, asparagine in the presence of reducing sugars (a hydroxycarbonyl moiety) or reactive dicarbonyls furnishes AA in the range up to 1 mol percent in model systems (Stadler et al. 2002).

AA induces tumors in several organs in mice and rats (Friedman et al. 1995; Johnson et al. 1986) and exerts reproductive (Chapin et al. 1995; Tyl et al. 2000) and neurotoxic damage (LoPachin 2004). After dietary consumption, AA is rapidly absorbed from the gastrointestinal tract and widely distributed to the tissues (Fennell et al. 2005). In the liver, AA is metabolized to glycidamide (GA), which is more reactive toward DNA and proteins.

Since 2007, the European Commission has recommended monitoring and investigating of the levels of AA in food (EU 2007, 2011). As AA is a genotoxic compound, no threshold level exists below which food safety concerns can be disregarded. For that reason the ALARA ("as low as reasonably achievable") principle should be followed with regard to levels of AA in food (Tardiff et al. 2010). In their latest recommendation, the European Commission recommends investigations into the production and processing methods for products exceeding the indicative values, which are set for most food categories except products for home cooking and other products (EU 2011).

7.3.2 Heterocyclic Amines

HAs are well known for their mutagenicity and for the carcinogenicity in laboratory rodents. Although the results from the animal and tissue culture studies are unambiguous, it is difficult to derive these results from epidemiological studies. The epidemiological evidence suggests that consumption of well-done or grilled meat may be associated with increased cancer risk in humans. However, the presence of an individual HA in cooked meat is highly correlated with the presence of other HAs and with many other constituents, including protein, animal fat, nitrosamines, and substances other than HAs formed during cooking, such as polycyclic aromatic hydrocarbons. Furthermore, the carcinogenic effects of these HAs may be

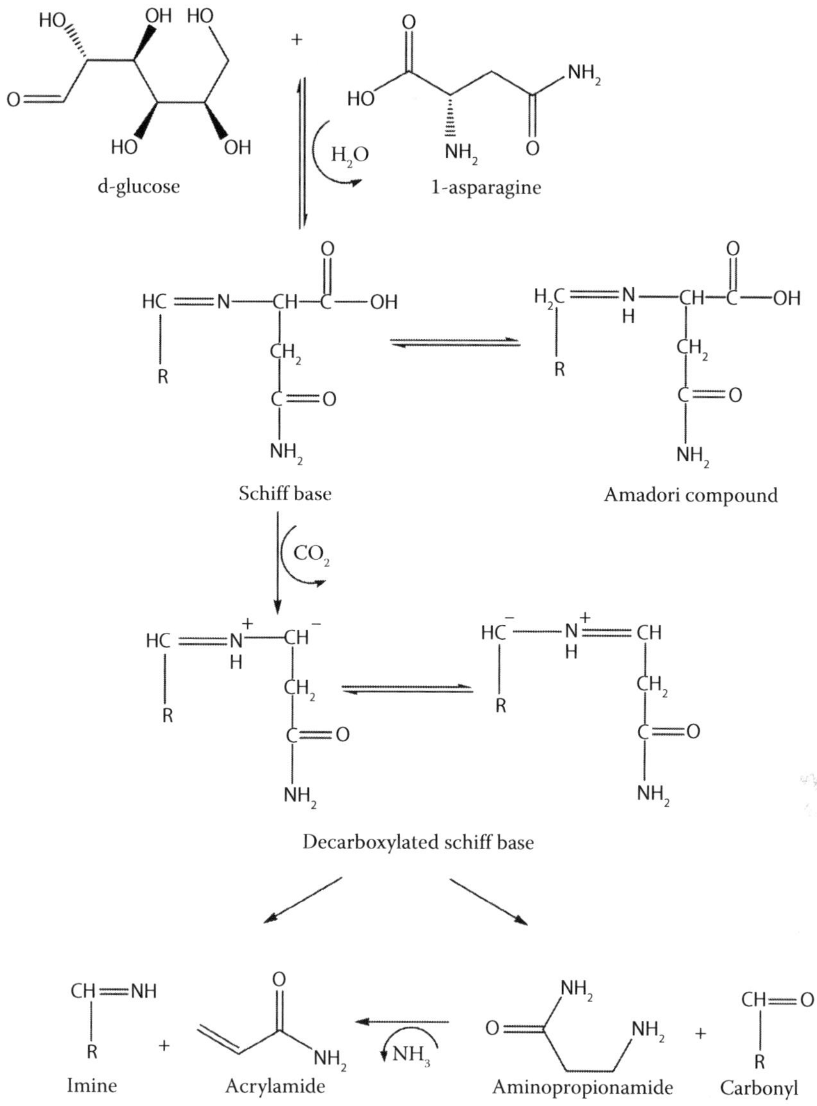

FIGURE 7.1 Acrylamide formation by Maillard reaction in heated foods. (Adapted from Hedegaard et al. *Food Chemistry* 108:917–925, 2008.)

inhibited or enhanced by many factors, including interactions of HA mixtures. It is therefore difficult for human epidemiological studies to establish associations between cancer risk and specific HAs (NTP 2014). A comprehensive overview of the literature revealed that four of these substances (MeIQ, MeIQx, IQ, PhIP) (Table 7.1) are reasonably anticipated to be human carcinogens based on sufficient evidence of carcinogenicity from studies in experimental animals and supporting genotoxicity data (NTP 2014). The outcome of this report is similar to an evaluation by the IARC which was published earlier (IARC 1993).

This group of compounds is formed during cooking of specific foods. For the formation some precursors are necessary. These comprise mainly carbohydrates, amino acids, and in some cases creatine such as shown in Figure 7.2. Complex and to a great extent not yet characterized reaction pathways result in the formation of HAs. Some of the compounds contain an imidazole group, which is derived from creatine directly. The other parts of the molecules are formed from the carbohydrates and amino acids. The complex reaction pathways need high temperatures (above 150°C) to proceed significantly.

TABLE 7.1

Typical Content of Polar and Nonpolar Heterocyclic Aromatic Amines in Meat and Fish Products (ng/g)

	MeIQx	IQ	4,8-DiMeIQx	PhIP	AαC	Trp-P-1	Trp-P-2	Norharman	Harman
Red meat	0–10	0–2	0–5	0–35	0–20	0–1	0–2	0–30	0–20
Poultry	0–3	0–1	0–3	0–10	0–1	0–2	0–1		
Fish	0–2	0–1	0–1	0–10	0–10	0–1	ND	0–200	0–130
Meat extract, gravy	0–80	0–15	0–9	0–10	0–3	0–5	ND	0–100	0–120

Source: Jägerstad, M, et al., *Eur. Food Res. Technol. A*, 207, 419–427, 1998.
ND, not determined.

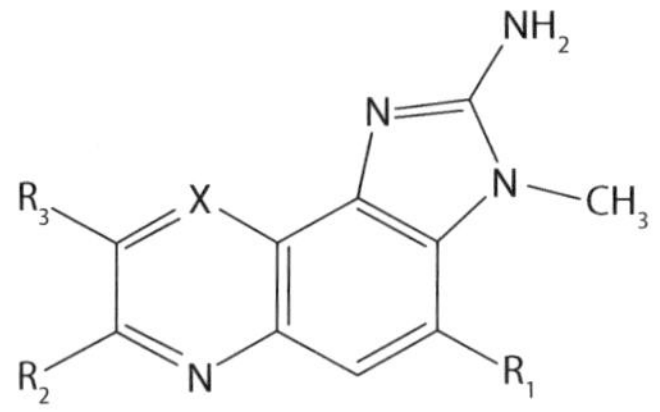

	R_1	R_2	R_3	X
IQ	H	H	H	C
MeIQ	CH_3	H	H	C
IQx	H	H	H	N
MeIQx	H	H	CH_3	N
4,8-DiMeIQx	CH_3	H	CH_3	N
7,8-DiMeIQx	H	CH_3	CH_3	N
4,7,8-TriMeIQx	CH_3	CH_3	CH_3	N

PhIP
4'-OH-PhIP

FIGURE 7.2 Structures of polar heterocyclic aromatic amines, which are derived from amino acids, carbohydrates, and creatine.

Therefore, during boiling negligible amounts are formed. Typical cooking procedures, which tend to produce heterocyclic aromatic amines, comprise frying, grilling, and roasting. Depending on the duration of cooking, temperature, water activity, and precursor concentrations, these substances can be formed at concentrations which can increase the risk of cancer (Jägerstad et al. 1983). A detailed pathway of formation of PhIP was published by Murkovic et al. (1999).

Figure 7.3 gives an example of fried meat with low (normal) concentrations of HAs formed at normal cooking procedures. However, it can be seen that when the meat is fried for a prolonged time and the temperature increases, the concentrations can be extremely high. Especially, the consumption of well-done and over-done meat results in high exposure. Over-done and burnt parts of the grilled meat should be removed before eating or the grilling procedure has to be adapted accordingly.

This group comprises ca. 20 compounds, of which 10 have been demonstrated to be carcinogenic. The IQ-type substances can be methylated at the positions 4, 7, and 8 and they could be derived from quinoxaline (Qx) which contains a nitrogen atom at position 1 or from quinolone (Q) which contains a carbon atom at the respective position. Different substances are the imidazo-pyridines (PhIP, 4'-OH-PhIP) which are derived from the amino acid phenylalanine or tyrosine. The "nonpolar" HAs are formed from direct degradation of amino acids. These substances do not contain the imidazole moiety. Depending on the type, composition, and concentration of the precursors tested, different mixtures of HAs are formed.

7.3.2.1 Occurrence in Foods

Normally, the concentrations are in the low ng/g range (or even lower) (Tables 7.1 and 7.2) and the substances are formed at the high-temperature zones, which means that they are occurring mainly in the surface or crust of the cooked product. During cooking, the aqueous phase including the dissolved

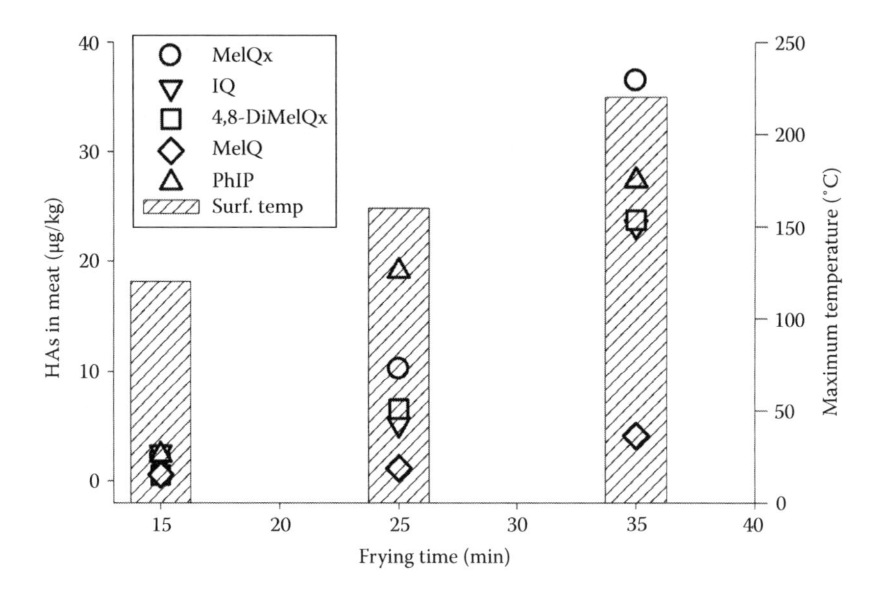

FIGURE 7.3 Concentrations of HAs in pan fried meat related to the maximum surface temperature of the pan. (Murkovic, unpublished data)

TABLE 7.2

Systematic Names of the Heterocyclic Aromatic Amines that Have Been Identified in Heated Foods or Model Systems (Mixture of the Precursors Dissolved in, for example, Diethylene Glycol)

Quinolines	
IQ	2-Amino-3-methylimidazo[4,5-f]quinoline
MeIQ	2-Amino-3,4-dimethylimidazo[4,5-f]quinoline
Quinoxalines	
IQx	2-Amino-3-methylimidazo[4,5-f]quinoxaline
MeIQx	2-Amino-3,8-dimethylimidazo[4,5-f]quinoxaline
4,8-DiMeIQx	2-Amino-3,4,8-trimethylimidazo[4,5-f]quinoxaline
7,8-DiMeIQx	2-Amino-3,7,8-trimethylimidazo[4,5-f]quinoxaline
4,7,8-TriMeIQx	2-Amino-3,4,7,8-tetramethylimidazo[4,5-f]quinoxaline
4-CH_2OH-8-MeIQx	2-Amino-4-hydroxymethyl-3,8-dimethylimidazo[4,5-f]quinoxaline
7,9-DiMeI*g*Qx	2-Amino-1,7,9-trimethylimidazo[4,5-g]quinoxaline
Pyridines	
PhIP	2-Amino-1-methyl-6-phenylimidazo[4,5-b]pyridine
4'-OH-PhIP	2-Amino-1-methyl-6-(4-hydroxyphenyl)imidazo[4,5-b]pyridine
DMIP	Dimethylimidazopyridine
TMIP	Trimethylimidazopyridine
Pyridoimidazoles and Indoles	
Trp-P-1	3-Amino-1,4-dimethyl-5H-pyrido[4,3-b]indole
Trp-P-2	3-Amino-1-methyl-5H-pyrido[4,3-b]indole
Glu-P-1	2-Amino-6-methyl-dipyrido[1,2-a:3',2'-d]imidazole
Glu-P-2	2-Amino-dipyrido[1,2-a:3',2'-d]imidazole
AαC	2-Amino-9H-dipyrido[2,3-b]indole
MeAαC	2-Amino-3-methyl-9H-dipyrido[2,3-b]indole

(Continued)

TABLE 7.2 *(Continued)*

Systematic Names of the Heterocyclic Aromatic Amines that Have Been Identified in Heated Foods or Model Systems (Mixture of the Precursors Dissolved in, for example, Diethylene Glycol)

Furopyridine	
MeIFP	2-Amino-(1 or 3),6-dimethylfuro-[2,3(or 3,2)-e]imidazo[4,5-b]pyridine
Benzoxazines	
	2-Amino-3-methylimidazo[4,5-f]-4H-1,4-benzoxazine
	2-Amino-3,4-dimethylimidazo[4,5-f]-4H-1,4-benzoxazine
Other Structures	
Lys-P-1	3,4-Cyclopentenopyrido-[3,2-a]carbazole
Orn-P-1	4-Amino-6-methyl-1H-2,5,10,10b-tetraaza-fluoranthene
Phe-P-1	2-Amino-5-phenylpyridine

Source: Sugimura, T., *Heterocyclic Amines in Cooked Foods: Possible Human Carcinogens*, Princeton Scientific, Princeton, NJ, pp. 214–231, 1995.

precursors from the cells is transported to the surface of the meat. Therefore, in the contact zones with the pan, these spots are significantly hotter (temperature close to the surface temperature of the pan) and the browning reaction is much stronger, resulting not only in a nice color, aroma, and texture but also in high concentrations of the heterocyclic aromatic amines.

7.3.2.2 Analysis of HAs

Originally a method for liquid chromatography was developed by Groß and Grüter which has been modified many times but is still in use by many groups (Gross and Grüter 1992). As the analysis is difficult due to the low concentrations and the complex matrix, a one- or two-step solid phase extraction (SPE) has to be done of the ethyl acetate extract which is obtained from the saponified samples. A very selective SPE material is "blue cotton" which was first used by Hayatsu et al. (1983). This material—containing a copper phthalocyanine complex as interacting ligand—was also used to enrich the HAs from environmental samples (e.g., river water). A huge number of publications are available which show the development of new—small scale—extractions using membrane technologies or different SPE materials (Busquets et al. 2009).

Chromatography is normally done on reversed phase columns with gradient elution. When selecting the column, whether the highly polar and basic amino-imidazole group can interact with the stationary phase resulting in significant tailing has to be considered. This can be reduced by adding, for example, triethylamine to the eluent or carrying out the chromatography on pH stable phases at pH values of above 9.

Detection is normally done by MS and recently more and more MS/MS methods have been published. Mass spectrometry is useful due to its high selectivity and sufficient sensitivity. UV detection is only partially useful since the complex matrix—even after clean-up—reduces the sensitivity. Some of the HAs have an excellent fluorescence (e.g., PhIP, λ_{ex} = 316 nm, λ_{em} = 370 nm) which can be used for detection. Under reversed phase conditions, the quinolines and quinoxalines show no fluorescence. Using fluorescence detection, very decent chromatograms can be obtained from meat. However, when analyzing coffee, the fluorescence detection is of limited use. Electrochemical detection can also be used due to a selective redox potential (500–600 mV). Both amperometric and coulometric detection can be applied. The advantage of coulometric detection is that there is an additional useful feature which can show hydrodynamic voltammograms. These can be used for identification of the substances (Gerbl et al. 2004). A comprehensive overview on liquid and gas chromatographic methods as well as electrophoretic and immunological techniques was given by Katoka (1997).

7.3.2.3 Possibilities to Reduce the Exposure

There are several ways to reduce the exposure to HAs. The simplest way is to reduce the consumption of red meat, especially when it is over-done. During cooking, too high temperatures for much time should be avoided. The selection of specific varieties of pigs (with optimal glycogen content) can also be advantageous (Olsson et al. 2002). Many controversial results have been obtained for the use of, for example, antioxidant spices or a variety of other food additives or ingredients. It is not clear whether antioxidants can reduce the formation of HAs by a simple mechanism removing activated electrons from the formation pathway. On the contrary, reduced temperature cooking (e.g., boiling or sous vide) eliminates the formation of the HAs completely. When using microwaves for heating, it has to be considered that not only water but also fat absorbs the radiation, resulting in significantly higher temperatures of up to 300°C in high-fat foods.

7.3.3 Furan

Furan (C_4H_4O) is a small organic compound (Mw: 68 g mol^{-1}) with high volatility (boiling point: 31°C) and lipophilicity (Crews et al. 2007; IARC 1995). The presence of furan in a broad range of heat-processed foods (0–6000 μg kg^{-1}) has received considerable attention due to the fact that this heat-induced contaminant is considered as a "possible carcinogenic compound to humans" (Mariotti et al. 2013). In the mid-nineties, this contaminant was considered as a possible carcinogen to humans (2B) by the IARC based on research done in laboratories with animals exposed to high furan doses (IARC 1995). Currently, there are still no reports about epidemiological studies that show possible associations between furan exposure and human cancer (Mariotti et al. 2013).

Carbohydrates, amino acids, carbohydrate-amino acid mixtures, vitamins, polyunsaturated fatty acids (PUFAs), and carotenoids have been reported as precursors for furan formation. The broad number of foods that has been shown to contain furan suggests that multiple pathways might be involved in its formation in foods (Fan 2005). An in-depth description of precursors and mechanisms of furan accumulation in food has been published by Maga (1979), Yaylayan et al. (2000), and Crews and Castle (2007). Thermal degradation and rearrangement of sugars was suggested as the primary source of furan in food; more recently, amino acids, PUFAs, and ascorbic acid have also been implicated (Crews and Castle 2007; Fan 2005; Hasnip et al. 2006; Vranová and Ciesarova 2009; Zoller et al. 2007). Due to its low boiling point, furan generated during thermal processes is easily vaporized, accumulating in the headspace of canned or jarred foods (Goldmann et al. 2005; Hasnip et al. 2006). However, despite its high volatility, furan has also been found in low-moisture foods processed in open containers, such as potato chips, crackers, crisp breads, and toasted breads (Anese and Suman 2013; Crews and Castle 2007; Guenther et al. 2010; Mariotti et al. 2013a).

Since current human exposure levels to dietary intake indicate a risk to human health and the necessity for its mitigation, it is a main issue to develop potential methodologies for furan mitigation in a wide range of heated foods (Anese and Suman 2013; Mariotti et al. 2012, 2013). Our research group has estimated the dietary exposure to furan in Chile (Mariotti et al. 2013b). Of the food surveyed, "American"-type coffee (espresso coffee plus hot water) obtained from automatic coffee machine (936 ng g^{-1}) and low-moisture starchy products like potato chips showed the highest furan concentrations (259 ng g^{-1}). Furthermore, furan was also found in samples of breakfast cereals (approximately 20 ng g^{-1}), jarred fruit baby foods (8.5 ng g^{-1}), and orange juice (7.0 ng g^{-1}). School children (aged 9–13 years) represented the highest intake of furan (about 500 ng kg^{-1} body weight day^{-1}).

The primary source of furan in food was thought to be from thermal degradation and rearrangement of organic compounds, particularly carbohydrates (Maga 1979). Furan and its derivatives have been associated with the flavor of many foods and some studies have shown that there are several distinct pathways responsible for its formation (Morehouse et al. 2008; Zoller et al. 2007). Data from the literature suggest multiple sources of furan formation originating from (1) thermal degradation/MR of reducing sugars, alone or in the presence of amino acids, (2) thermal degradation of certain amino acids, and thermal oxidation of (3) ascorbic acid, (4) polyunsaturated fatty acids, and (5) carotenoids (Becalski and Seaman 2005; Perez-Locas and Yaylayan 2004). A variety of carbohydrate–amino acid mixtures or protein model systems (e.g., alanine, cysteine, and casein) and vitamins (ascorbic acid,

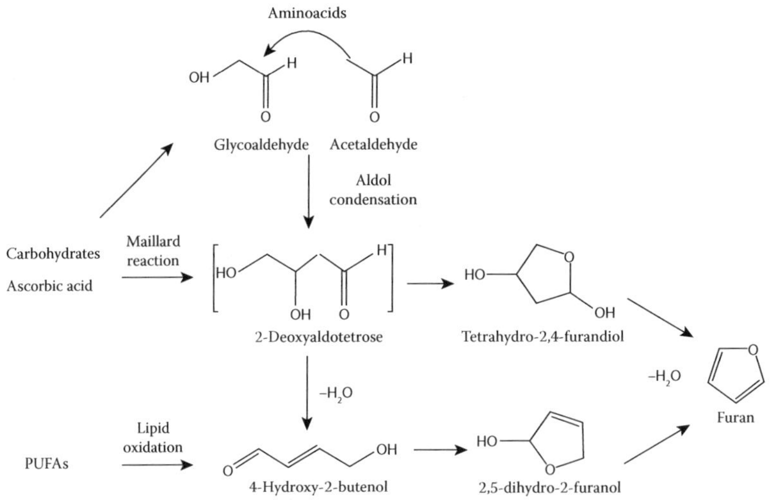

FIGURE 7.4 Different origins of furan formation. (Adapted from Crews, L., and Castle, L., *Trends Food Sci. Technol.*, 18, 365–372, 2007; Perez–Locas, C., and Yaylayan, V. A., *J. Agric. Food Chem.*, 52, 6830–6836, 2004; Vranová, J., and Ciesarova, Z., *Czech J. Food Sci.*, 27, 1–10, 2009; Mariotti, M., et al., *J. Agric. Food Chem.*, 60, 10162–10169, 2013a.)

dehydroascorbic acid, and thiamin) have been used to generate furan in food. In this respect, some factors such as the heating temperature, pH, and moisture content have been shown to have a considerable effect on furan generation, since most of the mechanistic insights into the formation of furan depend on them (Fan et al. 2008; Owczarek-Fendor et al. 2010). Figure 7.4 summarizes the general pathways leading to the formation of furan from these sources.

The presence of furan in a broad range of heat-processed foods (0–6,000 μg kg^{-1}) has received considerable attention due to the fact that this heat-induced contaminant is considered as a "possible carcinogenic compound to humans." Since a genotoxic mode of action could be associated with furan-induced tumor formation, current human exposure levels to this contaminant may indicate a risk to human health and the necessity for its mitigation (Mariotti et al. 2013). Toxicology and carcinogenesis studies of furan indicated that it is clearly carcinogenic to rats and mice, showing a dose-dependent increase in hepatocellular adenomas and carcinomas in both sexes (EFSA 2004). Several studies have been conducted on furan toxicity; however, the mechanism(s) of tumor induction by furan induction in laboratory animals have not been elucidated.

7.4 AGEs in Heat-Processed Foods

AGEs are formed when protein is cooked in the presence of sugars. AGEs are created through a nonenzymatic reaction between reducing sugars and free amino groups of proteins, lipids, or nucleic acids (Zhang et al. 2008). This reaction is also known as the MR or browning reaction (O'Brien and Morrissey 1989; Uribarri et al. 2010). The formation of AGEs is part of normal metabolism, but if excessively high levels of AGEs reach the tissues, the circulation pathogenic mechanism can predominate (Ulrich and Cerami 2001). The pathological effects of AGEs are related to their ability to promote oxidative stress and inflammation by binding to cell surface receptors or by cross-linking of body proteins, altering their structure and function (Eble et al. 1983; Schmidt et al. 2000). Among the better-studied AGEs are the stable and relatively inert N^{ε}-carboxymethyl-lysine (CML) and the highly reactive glyoxal (GO) and methylglyoxal (MGO). Both of these AGEs can be derived from protein and lipid glycoxidation (Abordo et al. 1999; Fu et al. 1996).

In addition to AGEs that are formed within the body, AGEs also exist in foods. AGEs are naturally present in uncooked animal-derived foods, and cooking results in the formation of new AGEs within these foods (Uribarri et al. 2010). In particular, grilling, broiling, roasting, searing, and frying propagate and accelerate new AGE formation (Goldberg et al. 2004; O'Brien and Morrissey 1989). A wide variety of foods in modern diets are exposed to cooking or thermal processing for reasons of safety and convenience as well as to enhance flavor, color, and appearance. The fact that the modern diet is a large source of AGEs is now well documented (Goldberg et al. 2004; O'Brien and Morrissey 1989; Vlassara and Uribarri 2004). Because it had previously been assumed that dietary AGEs are poorly absorbed, their potential role in human health and disease was largely ignored. However, recent studies with the oral administration of a single AGE-rich meal to human beings as well as labeled single protein-AGEs or diets enriched with specific AGEs such as MG to mice clearly show that dietary AGEs are absorbed and contribute significantly to the body's AGEs pool (Cai et al. 2008; Koschinsky et al. 1997).

Interestingly, modern diets are largely heat processed and as a result contain high levels of AGEs. Dry heat promotes new dietary AGEs formation by10- to 100-fold compared to the uncooked state across all food categories. Animal-derived foods that are high in fat and protein are generally AGE rich and prone to new AGE formation during cooking. In contrast, carbohydrate-rich foods such as vegetables, fruits, whole grains, and milk contain relatively few AGEs, even after cooking. The formation of new dietary AGEs during cooking was prevented by the AGEs inhibitory compound amino guanidine and significantly reduced by cooking with moist heat, using shorter cooking times, cooking at lower temperatures, and by the use of acidic ingredients such as lemon juice or vinegar. A new dietary AGEs database provides a valuable instrument for estimating dietary AGEs intake and for guiding food choices to reduce dietary AGE intake (Uribarri et al. 2010).

7.5 Conclusions

Heating of foods is primarily necessary for improving the digestibility and increasing the safety by eliminating pathogenic microorganisms. During heating, significant chemical changes are induced that improve the sensory quality of the foods; either by changing the aroma and color or by changing the texture. In addition to the improved quality, chemical changes can occur, resulting in a formation of toxicologically relevant substances that could also be carcinogenic. During recent decades several different contaminants with mutagenic properties were identified; that is, HAs, AA, and furan derivatives. For the formation of these compounds, heat-intensive cooking procedures are necessary. All the precursors necessary for the formation of these contaminants have nutritional properties.

Excessive heating results in high concentrations of all of these compounds, resulting in a higher health risk the more intensive the heat treatment is. For the formation of relevant amounts of HAs as well as AA, temperatures of more than 150°C are necessary. These high temperatures are relevant at frying, grilling, or broiling. To reduce the exposure, lower cooking temperatures should be used as is common during boiling or steaming. However, this change would also change the texture and the aroma of the foods. In the case of the furan derivatives, the situation is different as these can be formed at lower temperatures and even during storage. In all cases, reduction of the uptake of typically "highly contaminated" foods (e.g., well-done grilled or fried meat, typical AA- rich products) or reduction of the concentration of furan by evaporating it should be considered.

All these compounds discussed here are naturally occurring constituents of our daily diet. Avoiding them will be a difficult task but reducing the uptake will be possible by responsible cooking and change in the eating habits.

ACKNOWLEDGMENTS

Authors acknowledge financial support from FONDECYT Project No. 1150146.

REFERENCES

Abordo, E., Minhas, H. & Thornalley, P. (1999). Accumulation of alpha-oxoaldehydes during oxidative stress: A role in cytotoxicity. *Biochemistry and Pharmacology* **58**:641–648.

Ames, J. (1992). The Maillard reaction, in *Biochemistry of Food Proteins*. Hudson, B.J.F., Ed., Elsevier, London, pp. 99–153.

Anese, M. & Suman, M. (2013). Mitigation strategies of furan and 5-hydroxymethylfurfural in food. *Food Research International* **51**:1257–264.

Becalski, A. & Seaman, S. (2005). Furan precursors in food: A model study and development of a simple headspace method for determination of furan. *Journal of AOAC International* **88:**102–106.

BfR (2011). *Opinion Nr. 030. According to the current state of scientific knowledge 5-HMF concentrations occurring in foods do not give rise to safety concerns.* Available at: http://www.bfr.bund.de/cm/349/according-to-the-current-state-of-scientific-knowledge-5-hmf concentrations-occuring-in-foods-do-not-give-rise-to-safety.pdf. (Accessed December 13, 2015).

Birlouez-Aragon, I., Morales, F., Fogliano, V. & Pain J-P. (2010). The health and technological implications of a better control of neoformed contaminants by the food industry. *Pathologie Biologie* **58**:232–238.

Brands, C., Alink, G., van Boekel, M. & Jongen, W. (2000). Mutagenicity of heated sugar-casein systems: Effect of the Maillard reaction. *Journal of Agricultural and Food Chemistry* **48:**2271–2275.

Bråthen, E., Kita, A., Knutsen, S. & Wicklund, T. (2005). Addition of glycine reduces the content of acrylamide in cereal and potato products. *Journal of Agricultural and Food Chemistry* **53**:3259–3264.

Busquets, R., Jönsson, J.A., Frandsen, H., Puignou, L., Galceran, M.T. & Skog, K. (2009). Hollow fibre-supported liquid membrane extraction and LC-MS/MS detection for the analysis of heterocyclic amines in urine samples. *Molecular Nutrition and Food Research* **53**:1496–1504.

Cai, W., He, J. Zhu, L., Lu, C. & Vlassara, H. (2006). Advanced glycation end product (AGE) receptor 1 suppresses cell oxidant stress and activation signaling via EGF receptor. *Proceedings of the National Academy of Sciences United States America* **103:**13801–13806.

Capuano, E., & Fogliano, V. (2011). Acrylamide and 5-hydroxymethylfurfural (HMF): A review on metabolism, toxicity, occurrence in food and mitigation strategies. *LWT—Food Science and Technology* **44:**793–810.

Chapin, R., Fail, P., George, J., Grizzle, T., Heindel, J., Harry, G., Collins, B. & Teague, J. (1995). The reproductive and neural toxicities of acrylamide and three analogues in Swiss mice, evaluated using the continuous breeding protocol. *Fundamentals in Applied Toxicology* **27:**9–24.

Cheng, X., Graham, D., Castner, D. & Ratner, B. (2006). Temperature dependent activity and structure of adsorbed proteins on plasma polymerized N-isopropyl acrylamide. *Biointerphases* **1:**61–72.

Crews, C. & Castle, L. (2007). A review of the occurrence, formation and analysis of furan in heat-processed foods. *Trends in Food Science and Technology* **18**:365–372.

Eble, A., Thorpe, S. & Baynes, J. (1983). Non-enzymatic glycosylation and glucose-dependent cross-linking of proteins. *Journal of Biological Chemistry* **258:**9406–9412.

EFSA (European Food Safety Authority). (2004). Report of the scientific panel on contaminants in the food chain in furan in food. *EFSA Journal* **137**:1–20.

EFSA (European Food Safety Authority). (2012). Update on acrylamide levels in food from monitoring years 2007 to 2010. *EFSA Journal* **10**:2938–2976.

EU (European Commission). (2007). Commission recommendations of 3 May 2007 on the monitoring of acrylamide levels in food. *Official Journal of the EU* **L137**:33–39.

EU (European Commission). (2011). *Commission recommendation of 11 January 2011 on investigations into the levels of acrylamide in food.* Available at: http://ec.europa.eu/food/food/chemicalsafety/contaminants/recommendation_10012011_acrylamide_food_en.pdf. (Accessed October 10, 2015).

Fan, X. (2005). Formation of furan from carbohydrates and ascorbic acid following exposure to ionizing radiation and thermal processing. *Journal of Agricultural and Food Chemistry* **53:**7826–7831.

Fan, X., Huang, L. & Sokorai, K. (2008). Factors affecting thermally induced furan formation. *Journal of Agricultural and Food Chemistry* **56**:9490–9494.

Felsot, A. (2002). *Acrylamide angst: Another annoying distraction about food safety agrichemical and environmental news: A monthly report on environmental and pesticide related issues.* Washington State University, Washington, DC.

Fennell, T., Sumner, S., Snyder, R., Burgess, J., Spicer, R., Bridson, W. & Friedman, M. (2005). Metabolism and hemoglobin adduct formation of acrylamide in humans. *Toxicological Sciences* **85**:447–459.

Friedman, M., Dulak, L. & Stedham, M. (1995). A lifetime oncogenicity study in rats with acrylamide. *Toxicological Sciences* **27:**95–105.

Fu, M., Requena, J., Jenkins, A., Lyons, T., Baynes, J. & Thorpe, S. (1996). The advanced glycation end product, N^{ε}-carboxymethyl-lysine, is a product of both lipid peroxidation and glycoxidation reactions. *The Journal of Biological Chemistry* **271:**9982–9986.

Gerbl, U., Cichna, M., Zsivkovits, M., Knasmüller, S. & Sontag, G. (2004). Determination of heterocyclic aromatic amines in beef extract, cooked meat and rat urine by liquid chromatography with coulometric electrode array detection. *Journal of Chromatography B* **802**:107–113.

Gerrard, J. (2006). The Maillard reaction in food: Progress made, challenges ahead – Conference Report from the Eighth International Symposium on the Maillard Reaction. *Trends in Food Science & Technology* **17**:324–330.

Goldberg, T., Cai, W., Peppa, M., Dardaine, V., Baliga, B., Uribarri, J. & Vlassara, H. (2004). Advanced glycoxidation end products in commonly consumed foods. *Journal of the American Dietetic Association* **104:**1287–1291.

Goldmann, T., Perisset, A., Scanlan, F. & Stadler, R. (2005). Rapid determination of furan in heated foodstuffs by isotope dilution solid phase micro-extraction-gas chromatography-mass spectrometry (SPME-GC-MS). *The Analyst* **130:**878–883.

Granvogl, M. & Schieberle, P. (2006). Thermally generated 3-aminopropionamide as a transient intermediate in the formation of acrylamide. *Journal of Agricultural and Food Chemistry* **9:**5933–5938.

Gross, G. & Grüter, A. (1992). Quantitation of mutagenic/carcinogenic heterocyclic aromatic amines in food products. *Journal of Chromatography A* **592**:271–278.

Guenther, H., Hoenicke, K., Biesterveld, S., Gerhard-Rieben, E. & Lantz, I. (2010). Furan in coffee: Pilot studies on formation during roasting and losses during production steps and consumer handling. *Food Additives and Contaminants* **27:**283–290.

Hasnip, S., Crews, C. & Castle, L. (2006). Some factors affecting the formation of furan in heated foods. *Food Additives and Contaminants* **23:**219–227.

Hayatsu, H., Matsui, Y., Ohara, Y., Oka, T. & Hayatsu, T. (1983). Characterization of mutagenic fractions in beef extract and in cooked ground beef. Use of blue-cotton for efficient extraction. *Gann* **74**:472–482.

IARC. (1993). Heterocyclic aromatic amines. In Some Naturally Occurring Substances: Food Items and Constituents, Heterocyclic Aromatic Amines, and Mycotoxins. IARC Monographs on the Evaluation of Carcinogenic Risk of Chemicals to Humans, vol. **56**., International Agency for Research on Cancer, Lyon, France, pp. 165–242.

IARC. (1995). *Cancer, Dry cleaning, some chlorinated solvents and other industrial chemicals, Monographs on the evaluation of carcinogenic risks to humans*, Lyon, France, ch. 63, pp. 394–407.

Jaeger, H., Janositz, A. & Knorr, D. (2010).The Maillard Reaction and its control during food processing. The potential of emerging technologies. *Pathologie Biologie* **58:**207–213.

Jägerstad, M., Laser Reutersward, A., Olsson, R., Grivas, S., Nyhammar, T., Olsson, K. & Dahlqvist, A. (1983). Creatin(in)e and Maillard reaction products as precursors of mutagenic compounds: Effects of various amino acids. *Food Chemistry* **12**:255–264.

Jägerstad, M., Skog, K., Arvidsson, P. & Solyakov, A. (1998). Chemistry, formation and occurrence of genotoxic heterocyclic amines identified in model systems and cooked foods. *European Food Research and Technology A* **207**:419–427.

Johnson, K.A., Gorzinski, S.J., Bodner, K.M., Campbell, R.A., Wolf, C.H., Friedman, M.A. & Mast, R.W. (1986). Chronic toxicity and oncogenicity study on acrylamide incorporated in the drinking water of Fischer 344 rats. *Toxicology and Applied Pharmacology* **85:**154–168.

Koschinsky, T., He, C. & Mitsuhashi, T. (1997). Orally absorbed reactive glycation products (glycotoxins): An environmental risk factor in diabetic nephropathy. *Proceedings of the National Academy of Sciences United States of America* **94**:6474–6479.

Katoka, H. (1997). Methods for the determination of mutagenic heterocyclic amines and their applications in environmental analysis. *Journal of Chromatography A* **774**:121–142.

Kroh, L. (1994). Caramelisation in food and beverages. *Food Chemistry* **51:**373–379.

LoPachin R. (2004). The changing view of acrylamide neurotoxicity. *NeuroToxicology* **25**, 617–630.

Maga, J. (1979). Furans in foods. *CRC Critical Reviews in Food Science and Nutrition* **11:**355–400.

Mariotti, M., Granby, K., Fromberg, A., Risum, J., Agosin, E. & Pedreschi, F. (2012). Furan occurrence in starchy food model systems processed at high temperatures: Effect of ascorbic acid and heating conditions. *Journal of Agricultural and Food Chemistry* **60**:10162–10169.

Mariotti, M., Granby, K., Rozowski, J. & Pedreschi, F. (2013a). Furan: A critical heat induced dietary contaminant. *Food & Function* **4**:1001–1015.

Mariotti, M., Toledo, C., Hevia, K., Gómez, J.P., Fromberg, A., Granby, K., Rosowski, J., Castillo, O. & Pedreschi, F. (2013b). Are Chileans exposed to dietary furan? *Food Additives and Contaminants Part A-Chemistry Analysis Control Exposure & Risk Assessment* **10:**1715–1721.

Mauron, J. (1981). The Maillard reaction in food: A critical review from the nutritional standpoint. *Progress in Food Nutrition Sciences* **5**:5–35.

Morales, F., Capuano, E. & Fogliano, V. (2008). Mitigation strategies to reduce acrylamide formation in fried potato products. *Annals of the New York Academy of Sciences* **1126:**89–100.

Morehouse, K., Nyman, P., McNeal, T., DiNovi, M. & Perfetti, G. (2008). Survey of furan in heat processed foods by headspace gas chromatography/mass spectrometry and estimated adult exposure. *Food Additives & Contaminants: Part A* **253:**259–264.

Mottram, D., Wedzicha, A. & Dodson, A. (2002). Acrylamide is formed in the Maillard reaction. *Nature* **419**:448–449.

Murkovic, M., Weber, H.-J., Geiszler, S., Fröhlich, K. & Pfannhauser, W. (1999). Formation of the food associated carcinogen 2-amino-1-methyl-6-phenylimidazo[4,5-b]pyridine (PhIP) in model systems. *Food Chemistry* **65**:233–237.

NTP (National Toxicology Program). (2014). *Report on Carcinogens*, 13th ed. U.S. Department of Health and Human Services, Public Health Service, Research Triangle Park, NC.

O'Brien, J. & Morrissey, P. (1989). Nutritional and toxicological aspects of the Maillard browning reaction in foods. *Critical Reviews in Food Science and Nutrition* **28:**211–248.

Olsson, V., Solyakov, A., Skog, K., Lundström, K. & Jägerstad, M. (2002). Natural variations of precursors in pig meat affect the yield of heterocyclic amines—Effects of RN genotype, feeding regime, and sex. *Journal of Agricultural and Food Chemistry* **50**:2962–2969.

Owczarek-Fendor, A., De Meulenaer, B., Scholl, G., Adams, A., Van Lancker, F., Yogendrarajah, P., Uytterhoeven, V., Eppe, G., De Pauw, E. & Scippo, M. (2010). Importance of fat oxidation in starch-based emulsions in the generation of the process contaminant furan. *Journal of Agricultural and Food Chemistry* **58**:9579–9586.

Pedreschi, F., Mariotti, M. & Granby, K. (2014). Current issues in dietary acrylamide: Formation, mitigation and risk assessment. *Journal of the Science of Food and Agriculture* **94:**9–20.

Perez-Locas, C. & Yaylayan, V.A. (2004). Origin and mechanistic pathways of formation of the parent furan. A food toxicant. *Journal of Agricultural and Food Chemistry* **52**:6830–6836.

Rikke V. Hegegaard, Henrik Frandsen, Leif H. & Skibsted. (2008). Kinetics of formation of acrylamide and Schiff base intermediates from asparagine and glucose. *Food Chemistry* 108:917–925.

Rosén, J. & Hellenäs, K. (2002). Analysis of acrylamide in cooked foods by liquid chromatography tandem mass spectrometry. *The Analyst* **127**:880–882.

Rufián-Henares, J., Delgado-Andrade, C. & Morales, F. (2009). Non-enzymatic browning: The case of the Maillard reaction. In *Assessing the generation and bioactivity of neo-formed compounds in thermally treated foods*, Cristina Delgado-Andrade and Jose Angel Rufian-Henares (Eds.), Editorial Atrio, Granada, Spain, pp. 4–9.

Rufián-Henares, J. & Morales, F. (2007). Angiotensin-I converting enzyme inhibitory activity of coffee melanoidins. *Journal of Agricultural and Food Chemistry* **21**:1480–1485.

Schmidt, A., Hofmann, M., Taguchi, A., Yan, S. & Stern, D. (2000). RAGE: A multiligand receptor contributing to the cellular response in diabetic vasculopathy and inflammation. *Seminars in Thrombosis and Hemostasis* **26**:485–493.

Stadler, R., Blank, I., Varga, N., Robert, F., Hau, J. & Guy, P. (2002). Acrylamide from Maillard reaction products. *Nature* **419**:449–450.

Sugimura, T. (1995). History, present and future of heterocyclic amines, cooked food mutagens. In: *Heterocyclic amines in cooked foods: Possible human carcinogens*, R. Adamson, R., Gustafsson, J., Ito, N., Nagao, M., Sugimura, T., Wakabayashi, K. & Yamazoe, Y., (Eds.), pp. 214–231, Princeton Scientific, Princeton, NJ.

Sugimura, T., Wakabayashi, K., Nakagama, W. & Nagao, M. (2004). Heterocyclic amines: Mutagens/carcinogens produced during cooking of meat and fish. *Cancer Science* **95**:290–299.

Tardiff, R., Gargas, M., Kirman, C., Carson, L. & Sweeney, L. (2010). Estimation of safe dietary intake levels of acrylamide for humans. *Food and Chemical Toxicology* **48**:658–667.

Tyl, R., Marra, M., Myersa, C., Rossa, W. & Friedman, M. (2000). Relationship between acrylamide reproductive and neurotoxicity in male rats. *Reproductive Toxicology* **14**:147–157.

Ulrich, P. & Cerami, A. (2001). Protein glycation, diabetes, and aging. *Recent Progress in Hormone Research* **56**:1–21.

Uribarri, J., Woodruff, S., Cai, W., Chen, X., Pyzik, R., Striker, G. & Vlassara, H. (2010). Advanced glycation end products in foods and a practical guide to their reduction in the diet. *Journal of the American Dietic Association* **110**:911–918.

Vlassara, H. & Uribarri, J. (2004). Glycoxidation and diabetic complications: Modern lessons and a warning? *Reviews in Endocrinology & Metabolic Disease* **5**:181–188.

Vranová, J. & Ciesarova, Z. (2009). Furan in food—A review. *Czech Journal of Food Sciences* **27**:1–10.

Yaylayan, V., Keyhani, A. & Wnorowsski, A. (2000). Formation of sugar-specific reactive intermediates from C-13-labeled L-serines. *Journal of Agricultural and Food Chemistry* **48**:636–641.

Yaylayan, V., Machiels, D. & Istasse, L. (2003a). Thermal decomposition of specifically phosphorylated D-glucoses and their role in the control of the Maillard reaction. *Journal of Agricultural and Food Chemistry* **51**:3358–3366.

Yaylayan, V., Wnorowski, A. & Perez Locas, C. (2003b). Why asparagine needs carbohydrates to generate acrylamide. *Journal of Agricultural and Food Chemistry* **51**:1753–1757.

Zhang, L., Bukulin, M. & Kojro, E. (2008). Receptor for advanced glycation end products is subjected to protein ectodomain shedding by metalloproteinases. *Journal of Biological Chemistry* **283**:35507–35516.

Zöchling, S. & Murkovic, M. (2002). Formation of the heterocyclic aromatic amine PhIP: Identification of precursors and intermediates. *Food Chemistry* **79**:125–134.

Zoller, O., Sager, F. & Reinhard, H. (2007). Furan in food: Headspace method and product survey. *Food Additives and Contaminants* **24**:91–107.

Zyzak, D., Sanders, R., Stojanovic, M., Tallmadge, D. & Eberhart, H. (2003). Acrylamide formation mechanism in heated foods. *Journal of Agricultural and Food Chemistry* **51**:4782–4787.

8

Is Part of the Fructose Effects on Health Related to Increased AGE Formation?

Halyna Semchyshyn
Vasyl Stefanyk Precarpathian National University
Ivano-Frankivsk, Ukraine

CONTENTS

KEY POINTS

- There is a compelling evidence that long-term intake of excessive fructose can have deleterious side effects, while acute temporary application of fructose has defensive effects under pathophysiological conditions associated with oxidative stress.
- Fructation (nonenzymatic glycosylation involving fructose), a source of reactive metabolites, is suggested as an important mechanism underlying either beneficial or harmful effects of fructose.
- Detrimental impact of fructose is assumed to be mediated and amplified by AGEs that are produced in the late stages of fructation and are able to generate additional reactive species forming a vicious cycle of chronic/severe carbonyl/oxidative stress.
- Short-term consumption of low doses of fructose seems to induce temporary/mild carbonyl/oxidative stress stimulating defensive mechanisms; therefore, the levels of AGEs are rather negligible and insufficient for pathological changes in the organism.
- At normal consumption levels, fructose is a healthy and valuable nutrient, which does not cause discernible biological effects substantially different from other dietary carbohydrates.

8.1 Introduction

Over recent decades, the effect of fructose on human health has attracted growing attention not only from the scientific community. The "fructose hypothesis," based on numerous publications, alleges that dietary fructose plays a unique and causative role at the root of modern health problems with a detrimental impact on humans (>1,100 publications in Pubmed). On the contrary, some authors state that fructose is a valuable, healthy and safe nutrient at normal intake levels (>210 publications in Pubmed). The hot debate continues, since both controversy and confusion exist concerning fructose, its metabolism and health effects. In this chapter, we invite you to listen to the arguments on both sides before declaration of the "guilty" or "not guilty" verdict.

8.2 Detrimental Impact—"Guilty"

The increased fructose intake (quadrupled since the early 1900s) parallels the epidemic of obesity, and as a consequence, diabetes and its complications, cardiovascular and neurodegenerative disorders, gout, liver, and kidney diseases (Gaby 2005; Johnson et al. 2007; Stanhope et al. 2009; Tappy and Lê 2010; Tappy et al. 2010; Rebollo et al. 2012; Bray 2013; Stanhope et al. 2013; Sloboda et al. 2014). This correlation is evidence in favor of harmful effect of fructose on humans. Although a lot of truly constructive criticism exists (White 2013; Chiavaroli et al. 2014; Laughlin et al. 2014), experimental studies on animals also show that chronic intake of excessive fructose can induce most features of the metabolic syndrome (Rebollo et al. 2012; Sloboda et al. 2014). An obvious question arises: What mechanism(s) is (are) responsible for the detrimental effect of fructose?

Glycation (Figure 8.1), a nonenzymatic glycosylation involving reducing carbohydrates (e.g., glucose and fructose), is suggested to be a potential mechanism underlying the adverse metabolic changes in humans and animals. In general, unlike enzymatic reactions, nonenzymatic processes are not under tight control in the organism, and therefore can be harmful under certain conditions. The chemical reaction between a free carbonyl group of reducing monosaccharide and an amino group of amino acid was first described by Louis Camille Maillard in 1912 (1912a, 1912b). Several decades later, the Maillard reaction was recognized as one of the main reasons for the occurrence of the nonenzymatic food browning demonstrating an importance in food science (Hodge 1953; Tessier 2010). In the late 1960s, the products of nonenzymatic glycosylation similar to those of food browning were identified in the human body (Rahbar 1968; Rahbar et al. 1969). Thus, it took a lot of time to realize the physiological significance of the reaction described by Maillard, which received renewed attention in biochemistry and medicine. In the early 1980s, it was postulated that glycation had a causative role in aging and age-related pathologies (Monnier and Cerami 1981). Nowadays, the theory originally called "the glycation hypothesis of aging" is at the origin of the growing interest in the field of *in vivo* glycation, aging, and age-related diseases (Yin and Chen 2005; Semchyshyn and Lushchak 2012).

The majority of studies in the field of glycation are focused on glucose ("glycation") as the most abundant intra- and extracellular monosaccharide in living organisms (Tessier 2010; Robert et al. 2010, 2011),

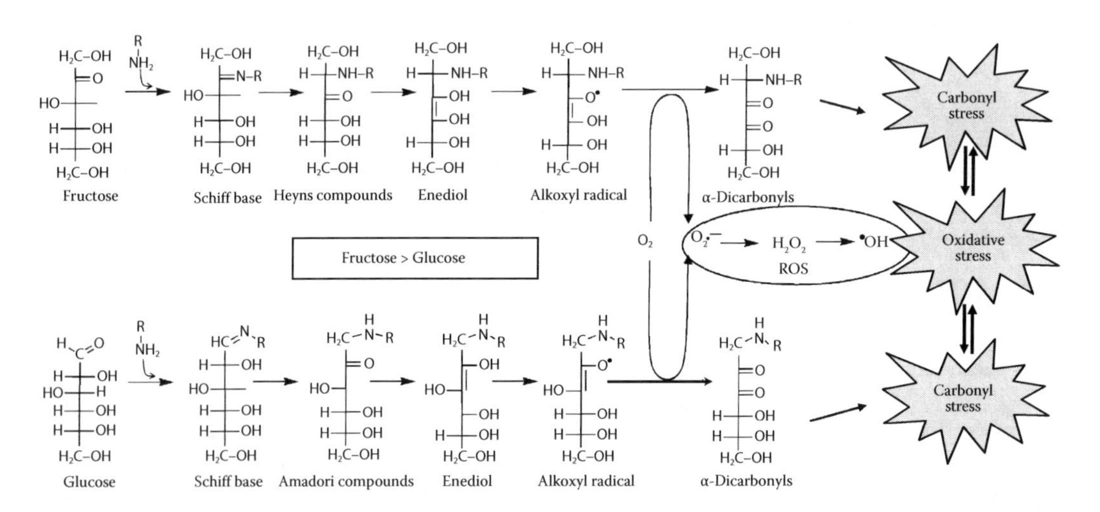

FIGURE 8.1 Involvement of fructose and glucose in the glycation, resulting in RCS/ROS generation and induction of carbonyl/oxidative stress.

and therefore thought to play a primary biological role in the *in vivo* Maillard chemistry, whereas glycation by fructose ("fructation") has not been as thoroughly investigated as that of glucose. To clarify a potential role of fructose in the Maillard reaction, some studies compare glucose and fructose involvement in the generation of glycation products. Although there is a little information regarding higher reactivity of glucose versus fructose in nonenzymatic processes *in vitro* (Wijewickreme et al. 1997; Yeboah et al. 1999; Rangsansarid et al. 2008), the opposite is reported in numerous *in vitro* and *in vivo* studies, demonstrating that fructose compared with glucose is a more potent glycoxidation agent (Suárez et al. 1991; Sakai et al. 2002; Lawrence et al. 2008; Robert et al. 2010; Semchyshyn et al. 2011, 2014). From a theoretical point of view, the latter may seem somewhat confusing. Due to a higher electrophilicity and accessibility of the carbonyl group of an aldose (e.g., glucose), its reactivity should be greater than that of the respective ketose (e.g., fructose). As an explanation, glucose is less reactive due to the formation of very stable ring structures in aqueous solutions (glucopyranose and glucofuranose) that retard its reactivity. Fructose also forms both pyranose and furanose structures but exists to a greater extent in the open-chain active form than glucose does. The proportion of reactive acyclic forms of glucose and fructose in aqueous solution accounts for 0.001–0.002% and 0.7%, respectively (Hayward and Angyal 1977; Turk 2010). This seems to be the most appropriate reason for higher *vitro* and *in vivo* reactivity of fructose versus glucose in aqueous solutions.

The initial step of fructation is the covalent interaction between free carbonyl group of open-chain fructose and amino group of any biomolecule, resulting in the Schiff base formation (Figure 8.1). The latter is an unstable compound that can be subjected to further isomerization (Heyns rearrangement) and formation of more stable Heyns adducts. The Heyns compounds as well as Amadori products (the later one derived from glucation) are so-called "early glycation products." The fructose moiety of the Heyns products can undergo enolization followed by dehydration, oxidation, and/or fragmentation reactions, consequently producing a variety of highly reactive carbonyl species (RCS) and reactive oxygen species (ROS) (Dyer et al. 1991; Thornalley 2005; Tessier 2010). The most common reactive species produced by fructose *in vivo* are presented in Table 8.1. Besides fructation, such nonenzymatic reactions as autoxidation of fructose (Wolff pathway) or Heyns compounds (Hodge pathway), and oxidative fragmentation of the Schiff base (Namiki pathway) result in RCS and ROS generation (Namiki and Hayashi 1983; Peng et al. 2011; Semchyshyn and Lushchak 2012; Semchyshyn et al. 2014). It should be noted that reactive species can also be formed due to enzymatic reactions of fructose (Table 8.1), for example, polyol pathway and glycolysis (Semchyshyn 2014; Takeuchi et al. 2015).

Most of the biological damage caused by RCS is related to dicarbonyls—compounds with two reactive carbonyl groups (glyoxal, methylglyoxal, glucosone, 3-deoxyglucosone, 3-deoxyfructose, etc.). In the advanced stages of glycation, dicarbonyls interact with free amino, sulfhydryl, and guanidine functional groups of intracellular or extracellular biomolecules like proteins, nucleic acids, and aminophospholipids, resulting in their nonenzymatic, irreversible modification, and formation of a variety of adducts and cross-links collectively named AGEs (Tessier 2010; Peng et al. 2011; Robert et al. 2011; Voziyan et al. 2014; Uribarri et al. 2015).

Extensive study of AGEs has revealed many stable, end-stage adducts resulted from the interactions between fructation-derived RCS/ROS and biomolecules (Table 8.1). The accumulation of poorly degraded AGEs increases with age and progression of age-related disorders (Gaby 2005; Tessier 2010; Robert and Labat-Robert 2014; Uribarri et al. 2015). These adducts have been detected in various tissues and peripheral blood and are considered to be pathogenic. AGEs as well as RCS/ROS are found to induce most features of the metabolic syndrome, including glucose intolerance, hyperglycemia, hyperlipidemia, hyperuricemia, and lactacidemia (Gaby 2005; Tessier 2010; Voziyan et al. 2014; Mallipattu and Uribarri 2014). It is important to note that AGEs may continue covalent interactions with biomolecules giving more complex cross-links. In addition, AGEs are efficient sources of RCS and ROS *in vivo* (Yim et al. 2001; Thornalley 2005; Shumaev et al. 2009; Peng et al. 2011). This next round of increases in RCS/ROS concentration may result in a chronic carbonyl/oxidative stress and further increase in the level of AGEs—generally, this is a way to form a vicious cycle (Figure 8.2). Being a more potent glycation agent than glucose, fructose produces higher level of reactive species and AGEs, and its long-term excessive consumption might lead to AGEs-mediated adverse effects on human health.

TABLE 8.1

Reactive Intermediate Species and End Products Generated by Fructose and Its Derivatives *in vivo*

Nonenzymatic Reactions				Enzymatic Reactions		
Fructation		Autoxidation and Fragmentation		Polyol Pathway		Glycolysis
Reactive Intermediate Products						
RCS	ROS	RCS	ROS	RCS	ROS	RCS
Glyoxal Methylglyoxal	Superoxide anion radical	Glyoxal Methylglyoxal	Superoxide anion radical	3-Deoxyfructose	Superoxide anion radical	Acetaldehyde
Glucosone	Hydrogen peroxide	Glycolaldehyde	Hydrogen peroxide	3-Deoxyglucosone	Hydrogen peroxide	Glyceraldehyde
3-Deoxyglucosone	Hydroxyl radical	3-Deoxyglucosone	Hydroxyl radical	Fructose-3-phosphate	Hydroxyl radical	Glyceraldehyde-3-phosphate
Acrolein	Alkoxyl radicals			2-keto-3-Deoxygluconic acid		Dioxyacetone phosphate
						Methylglyoxal
Fructose-Derived AGEs						
GOLD		GOLD		DOLD		GLAP
MOLD		MOLD		Pyrraline		MOLD
DOLD		CEL				
CMC		CML				
CMG		GA-pyridine				
CMPE		Pyrraline				
Pyrraline		Pentosidine				
		Argpyrimidine				
		Imidazolone				
		DOLD				
		Glucosepane				

AGEs, advanced glycation end products; CEL, carboxyethyllysine; CMC, carboxymethylcysteine; CMG, carboxymethylguanosine; CML, carboxymethyllysine; CMPE, carboxymethylphosphatidylethanolamine; DOLD, 3-deoxyglucosone-lysine dimer; GA-pyridine, glycolaldehyde-pyridine; GLAP, glyceraldehyde-derived pyridinium compound; GOLD, glyoxal-lysine dimmer; MOLD, methylglyoxal-lysine dimmer; RCS, reactive carbonyl species; ROS, reactive oxygen species.

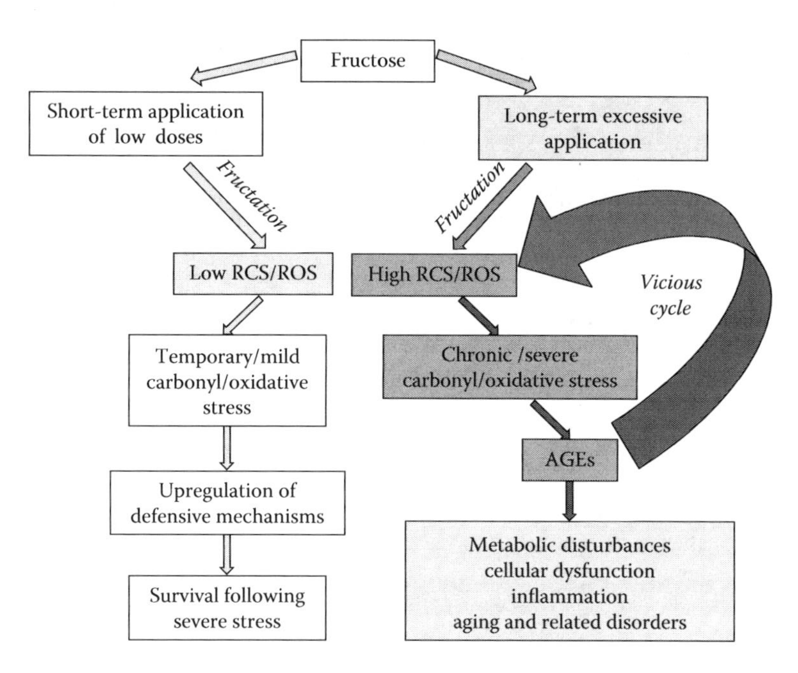

FIGURE 8.2 Involvement of reactive oxygen and carbonyl species in cytotoxic and defensive effects of fructose.

8.3 Beneficial Impact—"Not Guilty"

Besides the above mentioned detrimental impact of fructose and its reactive metabolites, beneficial effects of the monosaccharide are also known. Short-term application of fructose or its phosphorylated derivatives has been found to protect different cultured cell lines against exogenous stresses and demonstrate the defensive effect under pathophysiological conditions related to oxidative stress. It has been demonstrated that fructose and fructose-1,6-bisphosphate had significantly higher antioxidant capacities against hydroxyl radical than other carbohydrates (Spasojević et al. 2009a). Fructose has been shown to defend rat hepatocytes against oxidative stress (Valeri et al. 1996; MacAllister et al. 2011). In contrast to glucose, fructose inhibited apoptosis in rat hepatocytes by decreasing the level of ROS (Frenzel et al. 2002) and protected astroglial C6 cells exposed to exogenous hydrogen peroxide (Spasojević et al. 2009b). These data prompted some authors to suggest that acute supplementation of fructose and its phosphorylated forms in the diet or infusion could be of benefit in cytoprotective therapy of pathologies related to uncontrolled nonenzymatic oxidation (Spasojević et al. 2009b).

Based on the aforementioned *in vitro* experiments, several mechanisms responsible for the defensive effect of fructose can be postulated: (1) protection of the cell against oxidative damage by iron binding (Valeri et al. 1996), (2) stabilization of the pool of reduced glutathione, an important part of antiglycation/antioxidant system in the cell (Frenzel et al. 2002; Semchyshyn et al. 2014; Townsend et al. 2014), and (3) upregulation of the pentose phosphate pathway producing the reduced equivalents NADPH (Spasojević et al. 2009a).

Recently, our *in vivo* experiment with intact *Saccharomyces cerevisiae* cells has shown that fructose-grown yeast at exponential phase (short-term model) exposed to H_2O_2 demonstrated higher survival compared to glucose-grown yeast (Semchyshyn and Lozinska 2012). It is important to note that, in contrast to the short-term model, the higher level of carbonyl/oxidative stress markers, which were correlated with a higher aging and mortality rate of fructose- than glucose-grown yeast, have been previously detected at stationary phase (long-term model) (Semchyshyn et al. 2011). Acute application of fructose seemed to induce temporary, defensive mechanisms, stimulated by mild carbonyl/oxidative stress, responsible for cell survival under lethal H_2O_2-stress; reduced level of ROS in fructose-grown cells after exposure to H_2O_2 was consistent with a broad peak of superoxide dismutase and catalase activation by hydrogen peroxide. At the same time, cells grown on glucose demonstrated an increase in the level of ROS and a sharp rise in the antioxidant enzyme activities followed by their rapid inactivation (Semchyshyn and Lozinska 2012).

Thus, we suggested the involvement of RCS/ROS in both the cytotoxic and defensive effects of fructose (Semchyshyn 2013). However, the level of AGEs which mediate and amplify detrimental effect of long-term intake of excessive fructose is rather negligible at short-term consumption of low concentrations of fructose.

8.4 Conclusions and Perspectives

The current debate and controversy regarding the biological role of fructose and its impact on human health is an area of growing interest among researchers. Many scientists and nutritionists believe that fructose is safer and healthier than glucose; therefore, fructose has been promoted as a dietary sweetener with unique properties. At the same time, numerous epidemiological, clinical, and experimental studies demonstrate strong positive correlation between the increased intake of dietary fructose and the progression of metabolic disturbances. We suppose that nonenzymatic glycosylation involved fructose is an important mechanism underlying both the beneficial and detrimental effects of fructose.

Despite the fact that biochemistry has evolved from organic chemistry, the problem of modern concepts of metabolism is that they ignore nonenzymatic processes, and there is no place in basic biochemistry for any reaction other than those catalyzed by enzymes. However, nonenzymatic processes, such as glycation, free radical chain reactions, that are not tightly controlled by the organism-like enzymatic reactions have to be incorporated in the concepts of modern biochemistry in order to understand how they affect metabolism and human health (Yin and Chen 2005; Robert et al. 2010; Robert and Labat-Robert 2014).

Although reactive species can be formed due to enzymatic reactions of fructose (Table 8.1), we believe that it is mostly the nonenzymatically produced reactive species by fructose, as the most potent glycation agent among reducing monosaccharides, which are responsible for its biological effects (Figure 8.2). Fructose-generated reactive metabolites can modulate homeostasis at various levels by both participating in signaling/transcription regulation and damaging biological molecules. Intracellular formation of AGEs initiated by reactive species is considered a marker of chronic/severe carbonyl/oxidative stress,

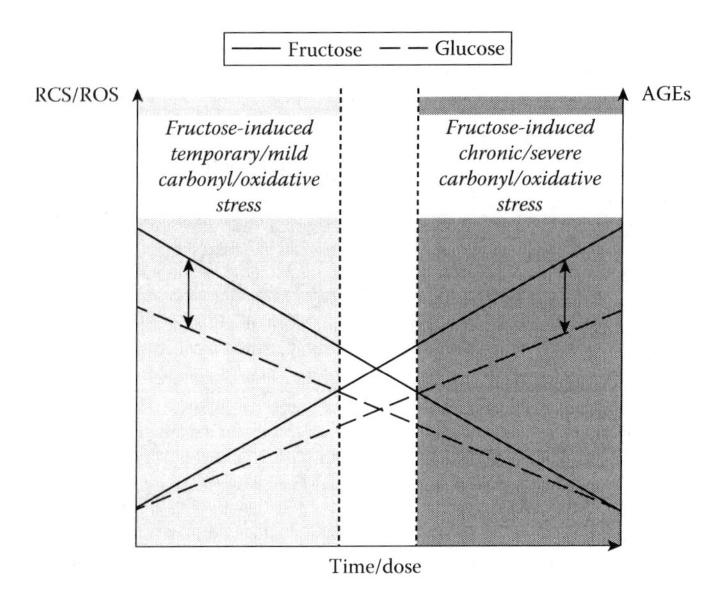

FIGURE 8.3 Time- and dose-dependent induction of temporary/mild or chronic/severe stresses by fructose that generates higher level of RCS/ROS and AGEs than glucose.

leading to metabolic disorders and aging. Since AGEs efficiently produce RCS and ROS, a vicious cycle is formed, and therefore fructose adverse effect seems to be AGE-amplified.

Being a more potent glycation agent than glucose, fructose nonenzymatically produces a higher level of reactive species, which during long-term excessive fructose consumption leads to chronic/severe carbonyl/oxidative stress and AGEs-mediated adverse effects on human health. In contrast, acute intake of low doses of fructose induces temporary/mild stress stimulating defensive mechanisms against stressful conditions (Figure 8.3). It is important that increased AGE formation seems to be related to harmful but not beneficial effects of fructose on health. We also believe that fructose intake at normal levels does not have discernible biological effects substantially different from other dietary carbohydrates.

REFERENCES

Bray, G. A. 2013. Energy and fructose from beverages sweetened with sugar or high-fructose corn syrup pose a health risk for some people. *Adv Nutr* 4:220–5.

Chiavaroli, L., Ha, V., de Souza, R. J., Kendall, C. W., and Sievenpiper, J. L. 2014. Fructose in obesity and cognitive decline: Is it the fructose or the excess energy? *Nutr J* 13:27.

Dyer, D. G., Blackledge, J. A., Katz, B. M. et al. 1991. The Maillard reaction *in vivo*. *Z Ernahrungswiss* 30:29–45.

Frenzel, J., Richter, J., and Eschrich, K. 2002. Fructose inhibits apoptosis induced by reoxygenation in rat hepatocytes by decreasing reactive oxygen species via stabilization of the glutathione pool. *Biochim Biophys Acta* 1542:82–94.

Gaby, A. R. 2005. Adverse effects of dietary fructose. *Altern Med Rev* 10:294–306.

Hayward, L. D., and Angyal, S. J. 1977. A symmetry rule for the circular dichroism of reducing sugars, and the proportion of carbonyl forms in aqueous solutions thereof. *Carbohydr Res* 53:13–20.

Hodge, J. E. 1953. Chemistry of browning reactions in model systems. *J Agric Food Chem* 1:928–43.

Johnson, R. J., Segal, M. S., Sautin, Y. et al. 2007. Potential role of sugar (fructose) in the epidemic of hypertension, obesity and the metabolic syndrome, diabetes, kidney disease, and cardiovascular disease. *Am J Clin Nutr* 86:899–906.

Laughlin, M. R., Bantle, J. P., Havel, P. J. et al. 2014. Clinical research strategies for fructose metabolism. *Adv Nutr* 5:248–59.

Lawrence, G. D. Mavi, A., and Meral, K. 2008. Promotion by phosphate of Fe(III)- and Cu(II)-catalyzed autoxidation of fructose. *Carbohydr Res* 343:626–35.

MacAllister, S. L., Choi, J., Dedina, L., and O'Brien P. J. 2011. Metabolic mechanisms of methanol/formaldehyde in isolated rat hepatocytes: Carbonyl-metabolizing enzymes versus oxidative stress. *Chem Biol Interact* 191:308–14.

Maillard, L. C. 1912a. Action des acides aminés sur les sucres: Formation des mélanoïdines par voie méthodique. *C R Acad Sci* 154:66–8.

Maillard, L. C. 1912b. Formation d'humus et de combustibles mineraux sans intervention de l'oxygene atmospherique des microorganismes, des hautes temperatures, ou des fortes pressions. *C R Acad Sci* 155:1554–6.

Mallipattu, S. K., and Uribarri, J. 2014. Advanced glycation end product accumulation: A new enemy to target in chronic kidney disease? *Curr Opin Nephrol Hypertens* 23:547–54.

Monnier, V. M., and Cerami, A. 1981. Nonenzymatic browning *in vivo*: Possible process for aging of long-lived proteins. *Science* 211:491–3.

Namiki, M., and Hayashi, T. 1983. A new mechanism of the Maillard reaction involving sugar fragmentation and free radical formation. In *The Maillard reaction in foods and nutrition*, ed. G. R. Waller, and M. S. Feather, pp. 21–46. ACS Symposium, Series 215. Washington DC: American Chemical Society.

Peng, X., Ma, J., Chen, F., and Wang, M. 2011. Naturally occurring inhibitors against the formation of advanced glycation end-products. *Food Funct* 2:289–301.

Rahbar, S. 1968. Hemoglobin H disease in two Iranian families. *Clin Chim Acta* 20:381–5.

Rahbar, S., Blumenfeld, O., and Ranney, H. M. 1969. Studies of an unusual hemoglobin in patients with diabetes mellitus. *Biochem Biophys Res Commun* 36:838–43.

Rangsansarid, J., Cheetangdee, N., Kinoshita, N., and Fukuda, K. 2008. Bovine serum albumin-sugar conjugates through the Maillard reaction: Effects on interfacial behavior and emulsifying ability. *J Oleo Sci* 57:539–47.

Rebollo, A., Roglans, N., Alegret, M., and Laguna, J. C. 2012. Way back for fructose and liver metabolism: Bench side to molecular insights. *World J Gastroenterol* 45:6552–9.

Robert, L., and Labat-Robert, J. 2014. Role of the Maillard reaction in aging and age-related diseases. Studies at the cellular-molecular level. *Clin Chem Lab Med* 52:5–10.

Robert, L., Labat-Robert, J., and Robert, A. M. 2010. The Maillard reaction. From nutritional problems to preventive medicine. *Pathol Biol (Paris)* 58:200–6.

Robert, L., Robert, A. M., and Labat-Robert, J. 2011. The Maillard reaction—Illicite (bio)chemistry in tissues and food. *Pathol Biol (Paris)* 59:321–8.

Sakai, M., Oimomi, M., and Kasuga, M. 2002. Experimental studies on the role of fructose in the development of diabetic complications. *Kobe J Med Sci* 48:125–36.

Semchyshyn, H. M. 2013. Fructation *in vivo*: Detrimental and protective effects of fructose. *BioMed Res Int* 2013:343914.

Semchyshyn, H. M. 2014. Reactive carbonyl species *in vivo*: Generation and dual biological effects. *Scientific World J* 2014:417842.

Semchyshyn, H. M., and Lozinska, L. M. 2012. Fructose protects baker's yeast against peroxide stress: Potential role of catalase and superoxide dismutase. *FEMS Yeast Res* 12:761–73.

Semchyshyn, H. M., Lozinska, L. M., Miedzobrodzki, J., and Lushchak, V. I. 2011. Fructose and glucose differentially affect aging and carbonyl/oxidative stress parameters in *Saccharomyces cerevisiae* cells. *Carbohydr Res* 346:933–8.

Semchyshyn, H. M., and Lushchak, V. I. 2012. Interplay between oxidative and carbonyl stresses: Molecular mechanisms, biological effects and therapeutic strategies of protection. In *Oxidative Stress—Molecular Mechanisms and Biological Effects*, V. I. Lushchak and H. M. Semchyshyn, (Eds.), pp. 15–46, InTech, Rijeka, Croatia.

Semchyshyn, H., Miedzobrodzki, J., Bayliak, M., Lozinska, L., and Homza, B. 2014. Fructose compared with glucose is more a potent glycoxidation agent *in vitro*, but not under carbohydrate-induced stress *in vivo*: Potential role of antioxidant and antiglycation enzymes. *Carbohydr Res* 384:61–9.

Shumaev, K. B., Gubkina, S. A., Kumskova, E. M., Shepelkova, G. S., Ruuge, E. K., and Lankin, V. Z. 2009. Superoxide formation as a result of interaction of L-lysine with dicarbonyl compounds and its possible mechanism. *Biochemistry (Mosc.)* 74:461–6.

Sloboda, D. M., Li, M., Patel, R., Clayton, Z. E., Yap, C., and Vickers, M. H. 2014. Early life exposure to fructose and offspring phenotype: Implications for long term metabolic homeostasis. *J Obes* 2014:203474.

Spasojević, I., Bajić, A., Jovanović, K., Spasić, M., and Andjus P. 2009b. Protective role of fructose in the metabolism of astroglial C6 cells exposed to hydrogen peroxide. *Carbohydr Res* 344:1676–81.

Spasojević, I., Mojović, M., Blagojević, D. et al. 2009a. Relevance of the capacity of phosphorylated fructose to scavenge the hydroxyl radical. *Carbohydr Res* 344:80–4.

Stanhope, K. L. Schwarz, J. M., and Havel, P. J. 2013. Adverse metabolic effects of dietary fructose: Results from the recent epidemiological, clinical, and mechanistic studies. *Curr Opin Lipidol* 24:198–206.

Stanhope, K. L., Schwarz, J. M., Keim N. L. et al. 2009. Consuming fructose-sweetened, not glucose-sweetened, beverages increases visceral adiposity and lipids and decreases insulin sensitivity in overweight/obese humans. *J Clin Invest* 119:1322–34.

Suárez, G., Maturana, J., Oronsky, A. L., and Raventos-Suárez, C. 1991. Fructose-induced fluorescence generation of reductively methylated glycated bovine serum albumin: Evidence for nonenzymatic glycation of Amadori adducts. *Biochim Biophys Acta* 1075:12–9.

Takeuchi, M., Takino, J., Furuno, S. et al. 2015. Assessment of the concentrations of various advanced glycation end-products in beverages and foods that are commonly consumed in Japan. *PLoS One* 10:e0118652.

Tappy, L., and Lê, K. A. 2010. Metabolic effects of fructose and the worldwide increase in obesity. *Physiol Rev* 90:23–46.

Tappy, L., Lê, K. A., Tran, C., and Paquot, N. 2010. Fructose and metabolic diseases: New findings, new questions. *Nutrition* 26:1044–9.

Tessier, F. J. 2010. The Maillard reaction in the human body. The main discoveries and factors that affect glycation. *Pathol. Biol. (Paris)* 58:214–9.

Thornalley, P. J. 2005. Dicarbonyl intermediates in the Maillard reaction. *Ann N Y Acad Sci* 1043:111–17.

Townsend, D. M., Lushchak, V. I., and Cooper, A. J. 2014. A comparison of reversible versus irreversible protein glutathionylation. *Adv Cancer Res* 122:177–198.

Turk, Z., 2010. Glycotoxines, carbonyl stress and relevance to diabetes and its complications. *Physiol Res* 59:147–56.

Uribarri, J., Del Castillo, M. D., de la Maza, M. P. et al. 2015. Dietary advanced glycation end products and their role in health and disease. *Adv Nutr* 6:461–73.

Valeri, F., Boess, F., Wolf, A., Göldlin, C., and Boelsterli U. A. 1996. Fructose and tagatose protect against oxidative cell injury by iron chelation. *Free Radic Biol Med* 22:257–68.

Voziyan, P., Brown, K. L., Chetyrkin, S., and Hudson, B. 2014. Site-specific AGE modifications in the extracellular matrix: A role for glyoxal in protein damage in diabetes. *Clin Chem Lab Med* 52:39–45.

White, J. S. 2013. Challenging the fructose hypothesis: New perspectives on fructose consumption and metabolism. *Adv Nutr* 4:246–56.

Wijewickreme, A. N., Kitts, D. D., and Durance, T. D. 1997. Reaction conditions influence the elementary composition and metal chelating affinity of nondialyzable model Maillard reaction products. *J. Agric Food Chem* 45:4577–83.

Yeboah, F. K., Alli, I., and Yaylayan, V. A. 1999. Reactivities of D-glucose and D-fructose during glycation of bovine serum albumin. *J Agric Food Chem* 47:3164–72.

Yim, M. B., Yim, H. S., Lee, C., Kang, S. O., and Chock, P. B. 2001. Protein glycation: Creation of catalytic sites for free radical generation. *Ann N Y Acad Sci* 928:48–53.

Yin, D., and Chen, K. 2005. The essential mechanisms of aging: Irreparable damage accumulation of biochemical side-reactions. *Exp Gerontol* 40:455–65.

Section III

Role of AGEs in the Pathogenesis of Chronic Diseases

9

Role of Advanced Glycation Products in Health and Disease in Children

Anshu Gupta and Tasnim Rahman
Virginia Commonwealth University
Richmond, VA

CONTENTS

KEY POINTS

- Obesity and diabetes in children have risen to epidemic proportions.
- Caloric excess and increasing consumption of processed foods play a major role in the pathogenesis of obesity and diabetes in children.
- Advanced glycation end products (AGEs) derived from diet are implicated in the pathogenesis of both type 1 and type 2 diabetes as well as in complications resulting from long-standing hyperglycemia.
- Dietary AGEs are suggested to play a role in adipogenesis and insulin resistance as early as infancy.
- Future studies are needed to clarify the interactions between genetic polymorphisms and secretory isoforms, protective and pathogenic, and the AGE-rich environment.

9.1 Introduction

The ever decreasing age at onset of obesity and diabetes in the modern world predicts shortened life expectancy for mankind if not deterred with urgent measures. While the role of genetic predisposition in these rapidly spreading modern epidemics is generally recognized, it has also brought the issue of food environment, both in terms of food quantity and quality, to the forefront of scientific debate. Most of the scientific community now agrees that we need to address not only the caloric content of a food but also the quality in terms of macronutrient composition as well as presence of prooxidative compounds; viz. agents used to add flavor and increase palatability, but that might be deleterious to an individual's health in the long term. One such category of products is a heterogeneous group of compounds, collectively known as advanced glycation end products (AGEs). The role played by AGEs generated from chronic hyperglycemia in long-standing type 1 diabetes mellitus (T1DM) in children in the pathogenesis of microvascular and macrovascular complications has been studied extensively. Recent studies have added further evidence in support of adverse effects of AGEs derived exogenously from diet in obesity and its comorbidities as well as in destruction of β-cells that produce insulin, thus highlighting their hitherto unrecognized contribution in the pathogenesis of diabetes. Also, the role of AGEs in renal injury in children in the absence of diabetes is under active investigation. In this chapter, we will focus on studies pertaining to AGEs in healthy infants and children, those with obesity, prediabetes as well as in newly diagnosed and long-standing diabetes with complications such as atherosclerosis, nephropathy, neuropathy, and retinopathy. Further, we will briefly review evidence supporting a role of AGEs and their receptor in children with renal disease without pre-existing diabetes.

9.2 Healthy Infants and Children

In other chapters of this book, it has been shown that exogenous AGEs derived from diet and tobacco exposure can be at least partially absorbed into the circulation and that the dietary AGE intake correlates with blood levels of AGEs as well as markers of inflammation and insulin resistance in adults. This has implications for women during pregnancy since these prooxidants in the maternal circulation can create an adverse intrauterine environment for the fetus; this can bear a negative impact on fetal development as well as enhance risk of future adulthood cardiovascular diseases and type 2 diabetes mellitus (T2DM) as suggested by Barker [1]. In support of this hypothesis, animal studies demonstrated an earlier onset of adiposity and increased insulin resistance in neonatal mice (third-generation offspring) when first-generation dams were fed a diet high in methylglyoxal (MG), an intermediate reactive glycation product, generated by exposure of food to high heat and dry conditions [2]. In order to examine this further in humans, investigators studied mother–infant pairs at birth, as well as at 6 and 12 months of age after infant foods (a source of AGEs) were introduced [3]. They noted a strong correlation of maternal serum AGE levels (represented by N-ε carboxy methyllysine [CML] and MG) with those of neonates, suggesting that AGEs can be transferred across the placenta from the mother to the fetus and contribute to an adverse intrauterine environment. Further, as expected, with introduction of processed infant foods, there was a parallel rise in both dietary AGE consumption and serum AGE level in infants at 6 and 12 months. This positive relationship was also not only demonstrated with isoprostane-8, a circulating oxidative stress marker, but notably a negative correlation of serum AGEs was found with adiponectin, an anti-inflammatory adipokine in the infants. These findings suggest a potential role of AGEs in pathogenesis of future obesity in these children. In fact, a study by Monden et al. [4] in mice showed a central role of the receptor for AGEs (RAGE) in adipocyte hypertrophy and differentiation and that RAGE deficiency ameliorated the adverse effect of a high-fat diet replete with AGEs. Similarly, Klenovics et al. independently confirmed higher serum CML levels and lower insulin sensitivity in formula-fed infants at age 3–6 months compared with breastfed infants, although these differences did not persist at follow-up at age 12–14 months [5]. In another study of infants, while dietary AGEs were not measured, Boor et al. compared insulin sensitivity and soluble cell adhesion molecule (siCAM-1), an inflammatory marker, in formula-fed and breastfed infants and its interaction with RAGE gene polymorphisms [6]. The authors observed that minor allele of 374A/T RAGE gene polymorphism was associated with increased siCAM-1 level and decreased insulin sensitivity in mothers; similar results were noted in older children as well as in infants who were formula-fed compared with those who were breastfed. Additionally, children who carried the major allele were noted be more insulin-sensitive if breastfed compared with those who were formula-fed. Interestingly, those who carried the major allele had improved insulin resistance measure at follow-up; this suggests an interaction of diet and RAGE polymorphism and warrants further investigation. In summary, the above studies suggest a possible relationship of dietary AGEs, adipogenesis, and insulin sensitivity in infancy, likely moderated by genetic makeup.

Given the implications of intrauterine and early neonatal environments on the long-term health of an individual, it is imperative to answer the important questions raised by the aforementioned studies in relation to the perinatal and postnatal programming effects of AGEs. Also, the interaction of genetic factors such as RAGE polymorphism with dietary AGEs should be assessed in studies designed to investigate these interactions.

9.3 Children with Obesity and Prediabetes (at Risk of Diabetes)

While studies in healthy adults and those without diabetes [7] have shown a positive correlation of dietary AGEs with circulating levels of CML and MG as well as with inflammatory markers and indices of insulin resistance, data are limited in children. Investigators are now beginning to examine the role of AGEs in younger cohorts and its impact on obesity, inflammatory markers, indices of insulin secretion, and sensitivity.

In a study of middle school children, when comparing lean children and those with obesity, AGE levels in blood (represented by CML) were noted to be 10%–15% lower in the group with obesity; this finding was intriguing since children with obesity showed higher levels of C-reactive protein (CRP) and IL-6 and comparable renal function. These results are in contrast with those observed in adults. The authors noted that children with obesity manifested higher renal creatinine clearance and suggested renal hyperfiltration of AGEs as a compensatory mechanism that might explain the paradoxical results in children [8]. Similarly, another group demonstrated a negative correlation of CML with adiposity and inflammatory markers in a cross-sectional study of obese middle school children [9]. The investigators posited that AGEs might be trapped in adipose tissue macrophages as an initial protective response that becomes maladaptive in the presence of a chronic AGE overload and leads to inflammation. The notion is supported by studies of Monden et al., as previously discussed, which showed a prominent role of RAGE in adipose tissue hypertrophy and differentiation. Taken together, these studies support an active role of AGE–RAGE axis in adipose tissue inflammation, which might affect systemic AGE levels in an age-dependent manner. Future investigations that assess the role of adipose tissue macrophages and RAGE, in those who develop obesity and diabetes in the context of a high-AGE diet, could provide further insight; studies that assess the role of polymorphisms of RAGE as well as enzymes that detoxify AGEs such as glyoxalases and studies to demonstrate whether there is an age-dependent expression of these genes and proteins will expand our understanding of these interactions further.

9.4 Children with Newly Diagnosed Type 1 Diabetes

According to the American Diabetes Association, T1DM is an autoimmune disease characterized by cell-mediated destruction of pancreatic β-cells over a period of time, progressing to absolute insulin deficiency when approximately only 20% cell mass is remaining [10]. This is followed by clinical symptoms of excessive urination, thirst, nighttime voiding, and ultimately diabetic coma if not evaluated in a timely manner. Three-quarters of all T1DM are diagnosed in patients <18 years of age [11]. In children, progression of disease is relatively rapid compared to adults. T1DM accounts for 5%–10% of all diabetes diagnosis (http://www.diabetes.org/diabetes-basics/type-1/) and correlates with genetic predispositions; however, it is also related to environmental factors that are relatively poorly defined. Several hypotheses have been proposed in the past such as viral triggers, exposure to cow's milk, egg allergy, vitamin D deficiency, and vaccinations but none have proved to be definitive [12].

In vitro studies of pancreatic islets incubated with AGEs demonstrated enhanced cell apoptosis and decreased insulin secretion [13,14] mediated by RAGE-dependent and RAGE-independent pathways. It was also suggested that AGEs might bind to insulin and decrease its biological activity. Further, apoptosis and impaired glucose-stimulated insulin secretion in the islets reversed in response to incubation with glucagon-like peptide-1 (GLP-1), suggesting it has a protective action against AGEs. Whether GLP-1 action is at pre-receptor or post-receptor level remains to be established. In summary, AGEs potentially act via different receptors to exert their actions on insulin secretion as well as apoptosis.

Interestingly, there is an animal model of nonobese diabetic mice (NOD) that develops diabetes spontaneously at a very young age resembling T1DM in humans. In a dietary approach to assess the response to dietary AGE reduction [15], two groups of NOD mice were fed different levels of AGEs in their diet in the neonatal period equivalent of childhood in human beings. Mice fed low-AGE diet had a lower occurrence, delayed onset, and reduced severity of autoimmune diabetes compared with the animal group that was fed a diet with high levels of AGEs. Animals in low-AGE diet group also survived significantly longer (76% low-AGE-fed mice survived up to 56 weeks, whereas none of the high-AGE-fed mice lived past 44 weeks) and manifested significantly lower inflammatory damage in islet cells than their high-AGE diet counterparts. These effects were maintained in the progeny of low-AGE diet dams as long as the dams were maintained on the low-AGE diet during pregnancy and to weaning. The study is yet to be replicated in humans but to support the theory, a study of population-based and twin cohorts of T1DM children showed elevated serum CML levels to be a strong predictor of T1DM. Genetic model fitting showed CML levels to be an environmentally acquired risk factor for T1DM [16]. Dietary AGEs are absorbed when consuming foods that are processed using dry heat and dehydration, both methods prevalent in highly industrialized food environment of Western diets and, therefore, are a major candidate in this scenario as a source of AGEs in the circulation. Thus, there is compelling evidence suggesting that elevated levels of AGEs are involved in the pathogenesis of T1DM and modifying these levels could be a noninvasive way to modify the T-cell autoimmune response, the hallmark feature of T1DM.

Role for receptor of advanced glycation product (RAGE): According to Yap et al. [17], there may be an interaction between dietary AGEs and RAGE or they may operate independently and cause activation of the immune-mediated T-cell response that leads to insulitis, which is a central feature of T1DM. Another approach to assess the AGE–RAGE axis has involved studying the modified RAGE subtypes produced as a result of differential transcription (endogenous secretory RAGE [esRAGE] and proteolytic cleavage (soluble RAGE [sRAGE]); these variants are hypothesized to play a cytoprotective role in the pathogenesis of diabetes. In a study by Chen et al., when NOD mice were treated with sRAGE, the rate of transfer of diabetes was significantly reduced even when diabetogenic splenocytes were introduced. Compared to control animals, islets of sRAGE-treated mice manifested significantly lower inflammation [18]. This suggests that RAGE is centrally involved in the inflammatory responses in diabetic animal models; blockade of RAGE may represent a putative approach to prevent the immune response seen in preclinical stages of T1DM.

Additionally, polymorphisms of RAGE, which is encoded by the *AGER* gene, have been associated with HLA-DQ/DR haplotypes, which predict increased or decreased risk of T1DM. Further, Salonen et al. [19] showed that concentrations of sRAGE correlated with AGER polymorphisms, which have been independently associated with HLA-DQ/DR haplotypes that predict risk for T1DM. This was also confirmed in a study performed on Finnish children with T1DM; among the three polymorphisms of AGER, two were highly associated with sRAGE concentrations (rs2070600 being predictive of higher risk and rs9469089 being protective) and the third was not (rs17493811). As discussed previously, Chen et al. have shown that administration of sRAGE blocks RAGE binding and prevents adoptive transfer of autoimmune diabetes in an animal model. RAGE was found to be expressed on both immune and non-immune cells, and the AGE–RAGE axis was clearly involved in differentiation of T-cells into pathogenic cells that led to insulitis and development of diabetes. Therefore, RAGE blockade may be an innovative option to treat individuals at risk of T1DM with high cellular RAGE levels.

Furthermore, Salonen studied sRAGE levels among very young children with newly diagnosed T1DM who are considered to have an aggressive form of the disease and healthy controls in Finland. Children who were diagnosed at a young age of less than 2 years had the lowest sRAGE concentrations as opposed to the healthy controls who had the highest sRAGE concentrations. This suggests that lower sRAGE concentrations may be associated with accelerated progression of T1DM. Thus, sRAGE levels may also serve as a prognostic indicator for more aggressive disease once it is validated in additional studies.

Taken together, results from animal models and clinical observational studies suggest an important role of AGEs in autoimmune diabetes that needs to be further investigated.

Going beyond T1DM, it has been noted that children and adolescents with T2DM [20] lose their β-cells at a faster pace compared with adults [21] for reasons that are not yet clear. In light of the impact of AGEs on insulin secretion, independent of immune-mediated response of T1DM discussed above, an important consequence to consider is the adverse impact of AGEs on glucose metabolism in children with obesity predisposed to develop T2DM. Dietary AGEs could provide a further hit to the already stressed β-cell burdened to produce extra insulin in order to compensate for the obesity-associated insulin resistance. Therefore, it would be important to study the effect of a low-AGE dietary intervention in this population as a potential approach to mitigate the epidemic of T2DM that threatens future generations.

9.5 Children with Long-Standing DM and Its Complications

Patients with long-standing DM are at an increased risk for developing atherosclerosis, retinopathy, nephropathy, neuropathy, and cardiovascular disease [22]. AGEs have been long known to be elevated at an earlier age in the presence of DM and are also involved in the pathogenesis of diabetic atherosclerosis. Increased production of AGEs induces oxidative stress and chronic inflammation (as discussed in earlier chapters), both via receptor and nonreceptor mediator mechanisms, and has been identified as an initiating factor for the development of diabetic complications. MG is a highly reactive α-oxoaldehyde and an intermediate reactive AGE produced in glycolysis. MG reacts with arginine residue of a protein, forming methylglyoxal-derived hydroimidazolone (MG-H1, an AGE) and is found in abundance in serum and tissue in long-standing diabetes [23]. Recently, Heier and his colleagues assessed the role of MG in the pathogenesis of atherosclerosis and inflammation, as assessed by ultrasound of carotid intima-media thickness and CRP, respectively, in children with T1DM [24]. Patients in the study were in intensive insulin treatment and were between the ages of 8 and 18 years. Levels of MG-H1 were significantly higher in the diabetic (DM) group compared to controls. MG-H1 levels correlated positively with HbA1c (glycated hemoglobin) as well as CRP. However, no significant relationship was noted between MG-H1 and arterial stiffness. Studies in adults have demonstrated relationship between dietary AGEs, serum AGE levels, and endothelial function as well as arterial stiffness [25]; lack of this relationship in children could be related to the study population being young with an average age of 13.2 years and a relatively shorter mean duration of disease of 5.5 years. Similarly, a study by Han et al. [26] also showed increased levels of MG-H1 AGEs in young patients with short duration of disease. Additionally, another study of children with T1DM of a mean duration of 4 years noted increased levels and accumulation of other AGEs like pentosidine and CML [27]. These studies underscore the presence of elevated AGEs prior to clinical evidence of atherosclerosis, presenting a window for timely intervention to reduce AGEs, before the complications have set in.

Since the most effective preventative measure against diabetic complications is adequate control of hyperglycemia, monitoring, detection, and early management of signs of diabetic sequelae, availability of markers that signal their onset can be valuable in mitigating the progression of complications of DM. Kostolanska et al. studied children with long-standing T1DM to check for the possibility of using serum/plasma AGE as an indicator of potential diabetic complications [28]. A total of 50 patients with T1DM between ages of 7 and 19 years and 5 years duration of disease as well as healthy controls were assessed. Patients with T1DM were classified based on the presence (DC+)/absence of (DC–) diabetic complications. Hb1Ac, serum AGEs, and lipid peroxidation were significantly higher in DC+ group and DC– group compared to controls. Difference in serum AGE levels between the diabetic groups and controls was also significant. Overall, AGEs were concluded to be reliable markers of diabetic complications and were suggested as a potential marker to follow for the detection of complications of long-standing DM. More recently, a novel tool used to measure skin fluorescence of AGEs has been strongly positively correlated with HbA1c in children with T1DM [29], this might emerge as a noninvasive tool to measure diabetes control/monitor for complications once validated in prospective studies.

As an alternative approach in the search of protective mechanism(s) against oxidative stress and angiopathy in young diabetic patients, Koutroumani et al. [30] studied levels of putative inhibitors of AGEs formed by enzymatic catalysis (sRAGE) and alternative splicing (endogenous sRAGE [esRAGE]) in the blood of children with T1DM. Patients with T1DM duration greater than 5 years, with moderately controlled Hb1Ac (8.0% ± 1.8%), demonstrated higher levels of sRAGE in plasma compared with healthy adolescents, which tended to increase further with higher levels of HbA1c. Also, esRAGE levels were increased with longer duration of diabetes. RAGE mRNA expression was noticeably higher only in "older" T1DM patients (>13 years of age) with longer duration of disease (>5 years). On the contrary, the study found increased plasma levels of AGEs (CML), particularly in younger patients (≤13 years), only with shorter duration of diabetes (≤5 years) compared to controls. The difference persisted in older patients but was not statistically significant. Based on their observations, authors posited that sRAGE and esRAGE may play a protective role by binding to AGEs and decreasing RAGE receptor activation. Early experimental studies using sRAGE to prevent atherosclerosis in diabetic murine models have produced encouraging results but need to be validated in clinical studies. The exact role of sRAGE and esRAGE as biomarkers versus being protective in patients with long-standing diabetes remains to be established.

Whether changes in dietary AGEs can modify the course of T1DM in children has not been studied. Improved inflammation and decreased insulin resistance from studies in adults with diabetes involving dietary AGE reduction [31], however, support the view that it would be beneficial. Therefore, dietary AGE reduction counseling should be a consistent feature of current medical nutrition therapy for diabetes.

9.6 AGEs and Childhood Renal Disease

Studies in children with diabetic kidney disease as well as chronic renal insufficiency clearly point to an increasing accumulation of AGEs. In a case–control study of children with average age 12 years [32], those with chronic kidney disease (CKD) were noted to manifest twice the level of fluorescent AGEs compared to healthy controls, which were even higher in those undergoing dialysis. Subsequent to renal transplantation, fluorescent AGEs were reduced but did not normalize, while AGEs such as CML and products of lipid peroxidation did not manifest any significant decrease from pretransplant levels. Authors concluded that ongoing renal impairment with oxidative stress as well as the immunosuppressive therapy was likely factor contributing to persistently elevated AGE levels despite transplant. In a similar study by Misselwitz et al. [27], a 10-fold elevation was noted in levels of another AGE, namely pentosidine, in those with end stage renal disease, which correlated significantly with renal function as represented by creatinine clearance. Free pentosidine levels declined markedly, while total pentosidine and CML levels did not decrease significantly after a single round of hemodialysis. However, pentosidine and CML did decrease significantly after renal transplant, although not normalized. These observations support the view that high-molecular-weight AGEs persist in tissues for longer duration. Studies in adults have shown that low-AGE diets can be effective in decreasing CML levels in patients with ESRD; whether it is feasible in adolescents with CKD is yet to be studied.

9.7 Conclusions

In summary, we believe that there is enough evidence that the AGE–RAGE axis is involved in the modern day epidemics of obesity and diabetes and its influence starts early in childhood. However, there appears to be a complex interaction of the genetic polymorphisms of RAGE, dietary AGEs, and the proinflammatory AGE and RAGE action which needs to be addressed in future studies by systematically measuring dietary AGEs and assessing effectiveness and feasibility of manipulating dietary AGE intake to prevent these chronic diseases in the younger population.

REFERENCES

1. Barker DJ, Winter PD, Osmond C, Margetts B, Simmonds SJ. Weight in infancy and death from ischaemic heart disease. *Lancet.* 1989; 2(8663): 577–80.
2. Cai WJ, Ramdas M, Zhu Li, Chen X, Striker GE, Vlassara H. Oral advanced glycation endproducts (AGEs) promote insulin resistance and diabetes by depleting the antioxidant defenses AGE receptor-1 and sirtuin-1. *Proc Natl Acad Sci USA.* 2012; 109(39): 15888–93.
3. Mericq V, Piccardo C, Cai W, Chen X, Zhu L, Striker GE, Vlassara H, Uribarri J. Maternally transmitted and food-derived glycotoxins: A factor preconditioning the young to diabetes? *Diabetes Care.* 2010; 33(10): 2232–7.
4. Monden M, Koyama H, Otsuka Y, Morioka T, Mori K, Shoji T, Mima Y, et al. Receptor for advanced glycation end products regulates adipocyte hypertrophy and insulin sensitivity in mice: Involvement of Toll-like receptor 2. *Diabetes.* 2013; 62(2): 478–89.
5. Klenovics KS, Boor P, Somoza V, Celec P, Fogliano V, Sebekova K. Advanced glycation end products in infant formulas do not contribute to insulin resistance associated with their consumption. *PLoS One.* 2013; 8(1): e53056.

6. Boor P, Celec P, Klenovicsová K, Vlková B, Szemes T, Minárik G, Turna J, Sebeková K. Association of biochemical parameters and RAGE gene polymorphisms in healthy infants and their mothers. *Clin Chim Acta.* 2010; 411(15–16): 1034–40.
7. Vlassara H, Cai W, Goodman S, Pyzik R, Yong A, Chen X, Zhu L, et al. Protection against loss of innate defenses in adulthood by low advanced glycation end products (AGE) intake: Role of the antiinflammatory AGE receptor-1. *J Clin Endocrinol Metab.* 2009; 94: 4483–91.
8. Sebekova K, Somoza V, Jarcuskova M, Heidland A, Podracka L. Plasma advanced glycation end products are decreased in obese children compared with lean controls. *Int J Pediatr Obes.* 2009; 4: 112–18.
9. Accacha S, Rosenfeld W, Jacobson A, Michel L, Schnurr FJ, Shelov S, Ten S, et al. Plasma advanced glycation end products (AGEs), receptors for AGEs and their correlation with inflammatory markers in middle school-age children. *Horm Res Paediatr.* 2013; 80(5): 318–27.
10. Klöppel G, Löhr M, Habich K, Oberholzer M, Heitz PU. Islet pathology and the pathogenesis of type 1 and type 2 diabetes mellitus revisited. *Surv Synth Pathol Res.* 1985; 4: 110–25.
11. American Diabetes Association. Standards of Medical Care in Diabetes. *Diabetes Care* 2015; 38: S1, S70–S76.
12. Knip M, Veijola R, Virtanen SM, Hyöty H, Vaarala O, Åkerblom HK. Environmental triggers and determinants of type 1 diabetes. *Diabetes.* 2005; 54(Suppl. 2): S125–36.
13. Luciano Viviani G, Puddu A, Sacchi G, Garuti A, Storace D, Durante A, Monacelli F, Odetti P. Glycated fetal calf serum affects the viability of an insulin-secreting cell line in vitro. *Metabolism.* 2008; 57(2): 163–9.
14. Lin N, Zhang H, Su Q. Advanced glycation end-products induce injury to pancreatic beta cells through oxidative stress. *Diabetes Metab.* 2012; 38(3): 250–7.
15. Peppa M, He C, Hattori M, McEvoy R, Zheng F, Vlassara H. Fetal or neonatal low-glycotoxin environment prevents autoimmune diabetes in NOD mice. *Diabetes.* 2003; 52: 1441–8.
16. Beyan H, Riese H, Hawa MI, Beretta G, Davidson HW, Hutton JC, Burger H, et al. Glycotoxin and autoantibodies are additive environmentally determined predictors of type 1 diabetes: A twin and population study. *Diabetes.* 2012; 61(5): 1192–8.
17. Yap FY, Kantharidis P, Coughlan MT, Slattery R, Forbes JM. Advanced glycation end products as environmental risk factors for the development of type 1 diabetes. *Curr Drug Targets.* 2012; 13(4): 526–40.
18. Chen Y, Yan SS, Colgan J, Zhang HP, Luban J, Schmidt AM, Stern D, Herold KC. Blockade of late stages of autoimmune diabetes by inhibition of the receptor for advanced glycation end products. *J Immunol (Baltimore, Md.: 1950).* 2004; 173(2): 1399–405.
19. Salonen KM, Ryhanen SJ, Forbes JM, Borg DJ, Harkonen T, Ilonen J, Simell O, Veijola R, Groop PH, Knip M. Decrease in circulating concentrations of soluble receptors for advanced glycation end products at the time of seroconversion to autoantibody positivity in children with prediabetes. *Diabetes Care.* 2015; 38(4): 665–70.
20. TODAY Study Group. Effects of metformin, metformin plus rosiglitazone, and metformin plus lifestyle on insulin sensitivity and β-cell function in TODAY. *Diabetes Care.* 2013; 36(6): 1749–57.
21. UK Prospective Diabetes Study (UKPDS) Group. Intensive blood- glucose control with sulphonylureas or insulin compared with conventional treatment and risk of complications in patients with type 2 diabetes (UKPDS 33). *Lancet* 1998; 352: 837–53.
22. American Diabetes Association. Standards of Medical Care in Diabetes. *Diabetes Care* 2015; 38:S1, S49–66.
23. Thornalley PJ. Pharmacology of methylglyoxal: Formation,modification of proteins and nucleic acids, and enzymatic detoxification—A role in pathogenesis and antiproliferative chemotherapy. *Gen Pharmacol.* 1996; 27: 565–73.
24. Heier M, Margeirsdottir HD, Torjesen PA, Seljeflot I, Stensaeth KH, Gaarder M, Brunborg C, Hanssen KF, Dahl-Jørgensen K. The advanced glycation end product methylglyoxal-derived hydroimidazolone-1 and early signs of atherosclerosis in childhood diabetes. *Diabetes Vasc Dis Res.* 2015; 12(2): 139–45.
25. Negrean M, Stirban A, Stratmann B, Gawlowski T, Horstmann T, Götting C, Kleesiek K, et al. Effects of low- and high-advanced glycation endproduct meals on macro- and microvascular endothelial function and oxidative stress in patients with type 2 diabetes mellitus. *Am J Clin Nutr.* 2007; 85: 1236–43.
26. Han Y, Randell E, Vasdev S, Gill V, Curran M, Newhook LA, Grant M, Hagerty D, Schneider C. Plasma advanced glycation endproduct, methylglyoxal-derived hydroimidazolone is elevated in young, complication-free patients with type 1 diabetes. *Clin Biochem.* 2009; 42(7–8): 562–9.

27. Misselwitz J, Franke S, Kauf E, John U, Stein G. Advanced glycation end products in children with chronic renal failure and type 1 diabetes. *Pediatr Nephrol.* 2002; 17(5): 316–21.
28. Kostolanska J, Jakus V, Barak, L. Glycation and lipid peroxidation in children and adolescents with type 1 diabetes mellitus with and without diabetic complications. *J Pediatr Endocrinol Metab.* 2009; 22(7): 635–43.
29. Banser A, Naafs JC, Hoorweg-Nijman JJ, van de Garde EM, van der Vorst MM. Advanced glycation end products, measured in skin, vs. HbA1c in children with type 1 diabetes mellitus. *Pediatr Diabetes.* 2016; 17:426–432. doi: 10.1111/pedi.12311.
30. Koutroumani N, Partsalaki I, Lamari F, Dettoraki A, Gil, A. P., Karvela, A., Kostopoulou E, Spiliotis BE. Protective mechanisms against oxidative stress and angiopathy in young patients with diabetes type 1 (DM1). *J Pediatr Endocrinol Metab.* 2013; 26(3–4): 309–17.
31. Uribarri J, Cai W, Peppa M, Goodman S, Ferrucci L, Striker G, Vlassara H. Circulating glycotoxins and dietary advanced glycation endproducts: Two links to inflammatory response, oxidative stress, and aging. *J Gerontol A Biol Sci Med Sci.* 2007; 62(4): 427–33.
32. Sebeková K, Podracká L, Blazícek P, Syrová D, Heidland A, Schinzel R. Plasma levels of advanced glycation end products in children with renal disease. *Pediatr Nephrol.* 2001; 16(12): 1105–12.

10

The Role of Advanced Glycation End Products in Cognitive Decline and Dementia

Roni Lotan
The Joseph Sagol Neuroscience Center Tel Hashomer
Ramat Gan, Israel

Aron M. Troen
The Hebrew University of Jerusalem
Rehovot Israel

Michal Schnaider Beeri
Interdisciplinary Center (IDC) Herzliya
Herzliya, Israel

CONTENTS

KEY POINTS

- Dementia and Alzheimer's disease (AD) pose one of the greatest social and economic burdens to public health.
- AD has currently no cure, thus lifestyle interventions to prevent the disease are crucial.
- Advanced glycation end products (AGEs) are a heterogeneous group of compounds also present in foods that are linked to several chronic diseases of aging.
- Recent evidence supports the hypothesis that AGEs are involved in the pathology of AD and in cognitive decline.
- Intervening to reduce AGEs is feasible and thus offers a potential new therapy to prevent or slow AD and cognitive decline.

10.1 Advanced Glycation End Products

Advanced glycation end products (AGEs) are a class of chemical compounds that are formed by the non-enzymatic reaction between reducing sugars and free amino groups. This reaction occurs endogenously in the course of normal cellular metabolism. AGEs tend to be more abundant in the tissues of older than in younger animals, and under conditions where the precursors for the reaction, such as glucose, are in excess (Poulsen et al. 2013).

In addition to the endogenous creation of AGEs, exogenous sources such as tobacco smoking and preformed AGEs from food also contribute significantly to the body's pool of AGEs. AGEs exist in most foods, but they are particularly abundant in animal-derived foods and fats. Cooking and exposure to high temperatures (i.e., grilling, broiling, roasting, searing, and frying) and long cooking times can greatly increase the amount of AGEs in food (Goldberg et al. 2004; Uribarri et al. 2010). Because dietary AGEs are absorbed in the gut (Koschinsky et al. 1997), choice of food and cooking patterns can greatly influence their accumulation in the body.

Among the most studied AGEs are pentosidine and carboxymethyllysine (CML) and their precursor methylglyoxal (MG), which are considered indicative of the body's overall AGE burden, although many other types of AGEs exist (Goldin et al. 2006; Poulsen et al. 2013; Salahuddin et al. 2014; Stirban et al. 2014).

AGEs can affect cellular functions by acting as ligands for several receptors. The AGE receptor, receptor for AGEs (RAGE), is a member of the immunoglobulin family, and its cellular signaling activates transcription factors such as NF-κB, AP-1, and FOXO that regulate inflammation and oxidative stress by inducing the expression of cytokines, adhesion molecules, and prothrombotic and vasoconstrictive products. In parallel, a second receptor, AGER1 facilitates AGE breakdown and can downregulate the proinflammatory signals induced by the binding of AGEs to RAGE. While RAGE expression seems to be upregulated by chronic exposure to high levels of AGEs, AGER1 expression is downregulated. Thus, under some conditions, AGE accumulation might create a persistent or self-amplifying signal by limiting AGE clearance. In addition to these membrane-bound receptors, sRAGE—a soluble RAGE isoform consisting of the RAGE extracellular domain—can act as a decoy to RAGE and thereby may contribute to the removal or detoxification of AGEs and the downregulation of their signaling cascades (Bierhaus et al. 2005; Toth et al. 2008; Srikanth et al. 2011; Poulsen et al. 2013).

In addition to their harmful capacity to overactivate receptor-mediated, proinflammatory signaling, AGEs can also inflict cellular damage by directly modifying the structure and function of cellular proteins and other macromolecules (Giardino et al. 1994; Khechai et al. 1997; Rondeau and Bourdon 2011). The indirect effects of AGE-induced changes in cellular signaling and their direct toxicity may explain the observed association between elevated concentrations of circulating AGEs with a wide range of chronic diseases including diabetes, atherosclerosis, cancer, and kidney disease. The growing evidence for a causal link between AGEs and neurodegenerative disorders, especially Alzheimer's disease (AD) (Sttit 2001; Ahmed 2005; Van Heijst et al. 2005; Hartog et al. 2007; Salahuddin et al. 2014), is the focus of this short review.

10.2 Cognitive Impairment, Dementia, and Alzheimer's Disease

Dementia is a clinical syndrome characterized by the development of multiple cognitive deficits including memory, orientation in space and time, attention, and executive functions, leading to a substantial decline from previous functioning levels and causing significant loss in social and/or occupational functioning (American Psychiatric Association 1994). Mild cognitive impairment (MCI) is an intermediate stage of decline between normal aging and dementia (Petersen et al. 2001) during which the incipient pathology first becomes symptomatic. A diagnosis of MCI therefore increases the likelihood of progression to clinical dementia although it does not always progress (Tschanz et al. 2006; Lee et al. 2014). The cognitive symptoms of dementia may arise due to different underlying pathologies, alone or in combination. AD pathology is the most frequent finding upon postmortem examination of clinical dementia cases accounting for approximately 70% of cases, with the remainder typically attributed to vascular dementia, or other neurodegenerative pathologies such as Parkinson's disease. Although these diseases are considered to be clinically distinct, the majority of dementia patients display mixed vascular and neurodegenerative pathologies upon postmortem examination.

AD prevalence increases exponentially with age, affecting 5% of people aged 65–75 years and almost 50% of elderly above the age of 85. As the elderly are the fastest growing segment of the Western population, the prevalence and incidence of AD are growing and they are expected to quadruple by the year 2050. This poses a profound social and economic challenge not only to patients and their families but also to societies' capacity to meet the resulting public health crisis (Brookmeyer et al. 2007; Prince et al. 2013).

The neuropathological hallmarks of AD are extracellular amyloid plaques, which are comprised primarily of aggregates of the amyloid β (Aβ) peptide, and intracellular neurofibrillary tangles, which are aggregations of abnormally phosphorylated tau proteins. Both plaques and tangles result in the degradation, dysfunction, and death of neurons and synapses (Swerdlow 2007; Kumar et al. 2015).

Five approved medications are currently in use for AD; however, none of them cure the disease, but rather treat the symptoms and somewhat slow down its progression (Kumar et al. 2015). The failure of numerous clinical trials, with candidate drugs targeting the hallmark pathology, has refocused attention on the potential benefit of lifestyle interventions (e.g., on physical inactivity, diet) that aim to reduce the risk of disease that is associated with those factors that can be effectively modified. Analysis of attributable risk predicts that reduction of exposure to modifiable factors such as smoking, diabetes, and obesity (which are also associated with AGEs) could prevent a substantial proportion of cases (Barnes and Yaffe 2011).

Here, we briefly review recent evidence from animal and human studies that underpins the hypothesis that AGEs are causally involved in age-associated neurodegenerative disease and cognitive impairment, which, if true, would suggest that dietary AGE reduction may prevent or slow down the progression of these conditions.

10.3 AGEs and Their Association with Cognition and Neuropathology

10.3.1 Observational and Postmortem Studies in Humans

Over the past decade, a growing number of epidemiological and neuropathological studies have yielded evidence of significant associations between exposures to high levels of dietary, circulating, or brain AGEs and cognitive or clinical outcomes in both nondemented older adults and in patients with dementia (Table 10.1).

Several cross-sectional studies have documented the association between AGE accumulation and cognition in nondemented individuals. A recent cross-sectional study in 764 cognitively nondemented older adults determined the association of cognitive function with a noninvasive marker for AGEs, skin autofluorescence (SAF—which indicates the level of AGE accumulation in the skin) (Spauwen et al. 2015). Higher SAF was associated with poorer cognitive function in all cognitive domains (verbal memory, response inhibition, information processing speed, and global functioning) when adjusted for age. Verbal memory and response inhibition were still significant after further adjustment for sex, diabetes, educational level, smoking, alcohol consumption, waist circumference, total cholesterol/high-density lipoprotein (HDL) cholesterol ratio, triglycerides, and lipid-lowering medication use. However, significance was lost when the model was adjusted for systolic blood pressure, cardiovascular disease, depression, and estimated glomerular filtration rate (eGFR), suggesting that these covariates might mediate this association. In the same study, of the three AGEs that were measured in blood (CML, carboxyethyllysine, and pentosidine), pentosidine alone was associated with cognitive impairment as assessed by the mini-mental state examination (MMSE) (Spauwen et al. 2015). A similar cross-sectional study (Moran et al. 2015) of patients with and without type 2 diabetes found that higher SAF was significantly associated with increased risk of cognitive impairment, where impairment was defined as a score that was less than 1.5 standard deviations below

TABLE 10.1

Characteristics of the Observational Studies of AGEs and Cognitive Decline

Study	Design	Sample Size	Population (Mean Age)	AGEs Assessments	Cognitive Assessments	Other Assessments	Adjustments	Main Outcomes
Spauwen et al. 2015	Cross-sectional	764	Nondemented (59.6)	SAF and plasma AGEs	Global cognitive functioning, speed, immediate, and delayed memory		• Age, sex, diabetes, educational level, smoking, alcohol consumption, waist circumference, cholesterol, triglycerides, lipid-lowering medication use • Further adjustment for systolic blood pressure, cardiovascular disease, depression, eGFR	• Response inhibition and delayed word recall were significantly associated with SAF. • Delayed word recall was significantly associated with plasma Pentosidine. • Global cognitive functioning was significantly associated with plasma Pentosidine
Moran et al. 2015	Cross-sectional	486	Nondemented (69.9)	SAF	Neuropsychological battery including memory, speed, and executive and visuospatial functions	brain MRI	Age, sex, smoking, serum creatinine, total intracranial volume, BMI, HbA1c, duration of T2DM	greater levels of SAF were significantly associated with the risk of any cognitive impairment and with lower GMV
Srikanth et al. 2013	Cross-sectional	378	Nondemented (72.1)	MG in serum	Neuropsychological battery including verbal memory, visual memory, working memory, speed, attention, and spatial ability	Brain MRI	Age, sex, education, HOMA_IR, stroke	Greater MG in serum was associated independently with poorer memory and lower gray matter
Shuvaev et al. 2001	Cross-sectional	99	AD patients ($n = 20$) and nondemented controls ($n = 79$)	Amadori products in CSF	MMSE test to assess the severity of probable AD		Age, glucose level	AD group was characterized by a significantly higher glycation level in CSF

(Continued)

TABLE 10.1 *(Continued)*

Characteristics of the Observational Studies of AGEs and Cognitive Decline

Study	Design	Sample Size	Population (Mean Age)	AGEs Assessments	Cognitive Assessments	Other Assessments	Adjustments	Main Outcomes
Ahmed et al. 2005	Cross-sectional	50	AD patients ($n = 32$, mean age 71) and nondemented age-matched controls ($n = 18$, mean age 69)	Glycation adducts in CSF	MMSE			Level of some of the glycation adducts was significantly higher in AD patients compared with controls. MMSE was correlated negatively with some of the glycation adducts
Bär et al. 2003	Cross-sectional	66	AD patients ($n = 15$, mean age 69.1), vascular dementia patients ($n = 20$, mean age 70.6), age-matched controls ($n = 14$, mean age 66.8), younger controls ($n = 17$, mean age 32.3)	CML and pentosidine in serum and CSF	MMSE, Wechlser Memory Scale	Brain MRI		• In AD patients, CML levels were significantly higher in CSF but lower in serum compared to age-matched controls. No difference was observed for Pentosidine. • In vascular dementia patients, Pentosidine levels were significantly higher in serum and CSF compared to aged matched controls. No difference was observed for CML.
Kuhla et al. 2005	Cross-sectional	12	AD patients ($n = 6$, mean age 74) and health controls ($n = 6$, mean age 54)	MG and glyoxal in CSF, GLO-1 (detoxification system of MG in brain (AD patients $n = 5$ and controls $n = 5$)				• No statistical difference in MG and glyoxal in CSF between health and AD. • GLO-1 was significantly increased in AD brains compared to healthy controls.

(Continued)

TABLE 10.1 ***(Continued)***

Characteristics of the Observational Studies of AGEs and Cognitive Decline

Study	Design	Sample Size	Population (Mean Age)	AGEs Assessments	Cognitive Assessments	Other Assessments	Adjustments	Main Outcomes
Ge et al. 2013	Cross-sectional	443	Patients with cognitive impairment (n = 377, mean age 63.10) and controls (n = 66, mean age 55.09)	RAGE in serum	MMSE and MoCA	STEAM 1H-MRS of the left hippocampus and thalamus (to assess metabolic changes)		• Serum RAGE was significantly negatively correlated with MMSE and MoCA scores • No difference between serum RAGE and metabolic changes as assessed by MRS
Ghidoni et al. 2008	Cross-sectional	327	AD patients (n = 100, mean age 76.88), MCI patients (n = 66, mean age 72.43), controls (n = 161, mean age 72.28),	sRAGE in plasma	MMSE			Levels of sRAGE were significantly different among the study groups, the highest sRAGE levels were detected in healthy controls and the lowest in the AD group, with intermediate concentrations in the MCI group
Emanuele et al. 2005	Cross-sectional	404	AD patients (n = 152, mean age 73.11), vascular dementia (n = 91, mean age 80.10), and healthy controls (n = 161, mean age 72.28)	sRAGE in plasma	MMSE			Concentrations of sRAGE had significantly decreased in patients with AD and in patients with VaD compared with cognitively healthy controls
Yaffe et al. 2011	Prospective cohort	920	Nondemented (74)	Pentosidine in urine	Modified mini-mental state examination (3MS), DSST		Age, sex, race, education, HT, cardiovascular disease, eGFR, DM	Incident cognitive decline was significantly greater in high or mild pentosidine level in baseline. Results remain significant only for DSST in the adjusted model, but the trend for 3MS remained.

(Continued)

TABLE 10.1 ***(Continued)***

Characteristics of the Observational Studies of AGEs and Cognitive Decline

Study	Design	Sample Size	Population (Mean Age)	AGEs Assessments	Cognitive Assessments	Other Assessments	Adjustments	Main Outcomes
Beeri et al. 2011	Prospective cohort	267	Nondemented (83.5)	MG in serum	MMSE		Age, sex, and years of education, diabetes and presence of an APOE4 allele and kidney function	Baseline serum MG was significantly associated with annual decline in MMSE
West et al. 2014	Prospective cohort	49	Nondemented (71)	Dietary AGEs and MG in serum	Neuropsychological battery assessing 4 domains: attention, executive, memory, language		Month of follow-up, baseline cognitive outcome, age, education, sex, DM, blood pressure, APOE4 genotype, BMI	Baseline dietary AGEs was significantly associated with greater memory decline. Baseline serum MG was significantly associated with greater decline in attention
Cai et al. 2014	Prospective cohort	93	Nondemented	MG in serum	MMSE		Age, sex, education, and baseline MMSE	High baseline sMG levels are significantly associated with cognitive decline over time

Note: AGE, advanced glycation end product; AD, Alzheimer's disease; BMI, body mass index; CML, carboxymethyllysine; CSF, cerebrospinal fluid; DM, diabetes mellitus; DSST, digit symbol substitution test; eGFR, estimated glomerular filtration rate; MG, methylglyoxal; MMSE, mini-mental state examination; MoCA, Montreal Cognitive Assessment; MRI, magnetic resonance imaging; SAF, skin autofluorescence; sRAGE, soluble RAGE; T2DM, type 2 diabetes mellitus.

age, sex, and education-matched population norms for one or more cognitive domains (memory, processing speed, and executive and visuospatial functions). Higher SAF was also associated with brain atrophy as indicated by lower gray matter volume (GMV) measured by magnetic resonance imaging, as well as with age and diabetes. Diabetes was also associated with GMV, but the association was attenuated by 20% when adding SAF to a multivariable model, rendering it nonsignificant. The authors interpreted these findings as suggesting that AGE accumulation in tissue (as reflected in SAF) partially mediates the association between diabetes and lower GMV (Moran et al. 2015). These findings in diabetics were consistent with an association between higher serum MG, lower GMV, and poorer cognition in another cross-sectional study of nondemented older adults (Srikanth et al. 2013).

Although an observation of correlation cannot prove causation, prospective cohort studies support a stronger inference of causation than that offered by cross-sectional studies.

We found five such prospective studies of longitudinal change in cognition in nondemented elderly adults, two of which estimated dietary intake of AGEs and three of which measured circulating AGEs, but all of which found more rapid cognitive decline in subjects with higher levels of AGEs at baseline. In very elderly adults, higher serum MG was associated with a faster rate of cognitive decline measured by change in MMSE (Beeri et al. 2011). In a second study, dietary AGEs intake was positively associated with a faster rate of memory decline (as assessed by a composite of memory tests) and serum MG concentration was associated with decline in attention (West et al. 2014). Similarly, in a study by Cai and colleagues, baseline levels of sMG in adults that were cognitively normal at the beginning of the study correlated significantly with cognitive decline assessed by the MMSE 9 months later. In the same study, baseline dietary AGEs consumption and serum MG were also associated with RAGE mRNA levels, serum CML, plasma 8-isoprostanes, leptin, and mononuclear cell TNFα protein, and inversely correlated with SIRT1 mRNA and adiponectin levels (Cai et al. 2014). These results underscore the close association of AGEs with inflammation, another pivotal process in AD (Wyss-Coray and Rogers 2012). In another prospective study of nondemented elderly adults with and without diabetes, higher levels of urine pentosidine were associated with more rapid cognitive decline as measured by a modified MMSE, the 3MS, and the digit symbol substitution test (DSST). After adjustment for age, sex, education, hypertension, cardiovascular disease, and eGFR, odds of decline on the DSST remained significantly greater for higher level of urine pentosidine (Yaffe et al. 2011). Finally, a study using cohort and ecological data reported a temporal association between higher estimated levels of dietary AGE consumption and higher incidence of AD in different countries up to 20 years later (Perrone and Grant 2015).

As with studies of nondemented individuals, studies of postmortem brain tissue, blood, and cerebrospinal fluid (CSF) from AD patients tend to show similar associations between AGEs accumulation and clinical, cognitive, and pathological outcomes. For example, in a postmortem case–control brain study by Lüth and colleagues, the percentage of AGE-positive neurons increased with both age and advancing stage of the disease (Lüth et al. 2005). Furthermore, AGEs co-localized with hyperphosphorylated tau protein, nNOS (a marker for nitroxidative stress), and caspase-3 (a marker of apoptotic cell death), all of which are features of neurodegeneration (Lüth et al. 2005). Additional studies by Cruz-Sánchez et al. (2010), Lue et al. (2001), and Vitek et al. (1994) consistently found higher AGEs and RAGE expression in AD brain compared to controls.

Elevated AGE concentrations have also been demonstrated in CSF of patients with AD. Amadori products, precursors of AGE formation, were found to be significantly higher in CSF of AD patients than that of controls. However, CSF and plasma glucose did not differ between the groups, suggesting that the increase in Amadori products is not due to higher glucose levels. In addition, the levels of Amadori products were nominally higher in more severe patients but the difference between sub-groups of patients did not reach statistical significance (Shuvaev et al. 2001). Similarly, in a study by Ahmed and colleagues, levels of the glycated proteins CML and 3-DG-H (3-deoxyglucosone-derived hydroimidazolone) in CSF were significantly higher in AD patients compared with controls. Also, higher levels of fructosyl-lysine (a marker for early-stage reactions of glycation) were significantly associated with poorer cognitive function assessed by MMSE (Ahmed et al. 2005).

Cross-sectional findings with respect to serum AGE biomarkers are somewhat less consistent. In a study by Bär and colleagues (2003), CML concentrations were significantly higher in CSF of AD patients compared to age-matched controls; however, they were significantly decreased in serum. As for pentosidine concentrations, no significant change was observed between AD patients and controls in either serum or CSF. Interestingly, in one study that failed to show significant differences in CSF AGEs of AD patients and controls, the levels of glyoxalase 1 (GLO-1), which converts MG by to D-lactoylglutathione, were significantly higher in AD brains, suggesting that in some cases, it may act to detoxify MG and limit its accumulation in the central nervous system (Kuhla et al. 2005).

Data on the association between RAGE receptors and cognition lend further support to the hypothesized role of AGEs in cognitive impairment and dementia. Serum RAGE concentrations (as distinct from sRAGE) have been found to be significantly higher among AD cases in a cross-sectional case–control study, where cognition was assessed by MMSE and the Montreal Cognitive Assessment (MoCA) (Ge et al. 2013). Similarly, other studies have reported that concentrations of the circulating soluble sRAGE receptor (which acts as a decoy to AGE substrates and downregulates the RAGE pathway) were significantly lower in AD patients compared to controls and vascular dementia patients (Emanuele et al. 2005) and in MCI patients compared to controls (Ghidoni et al. 2008), pointing to the involvement of RAGE ligands in the early stage of the disease. Since RAGE is a multiligand receptor, its association with neurodegenerative and other chronic diseases is not attributed solely to its interaction with AGEs, and the extent to which AGEs exposure activates the RAGE pathway in AD is less clear. The involvement of RAGE signaling in AD is discussed broadly elsewhere and is beyond the scope of this review (Cai et al. 2015).

In addition to their involvement in AD pathology, or in parallel to them, AGEs may also be specifically related to cerebrovascular diseases (Emanuele et al. 2005; Southern et al. 2007; Honjo et al. 2012). For example, CML expression in brain sections of patients with cerebrovascular disease was higher in cases with worse cognition as assessed by Camcog (Southern et al. 2007), and CSF pentosidine concentrations were higher in vascular dementia patients compared to controls (Bär et al. 2003). Additional supporting evidence is that compared to controls, sRAGE levels are significantly lower in patients with vascular dementia and lowest in AD patients (Emanuele et al. 2005).

It is interesting that associations between AGEs and cognitive outcomes are similar in both diabetic and nondiabetic populations, suggesting that the association may reflect a general mechanism and not one dependent on abnormal glucose metabolism. The associations described above are also consistent with the suggestion that AGEs mediate the relation between diabetes and cognitive decline (Ravona-Springer and Schnaider Beeri 2011). Indeed, a postmortem study comparing nondiabetic and nondemented controls with diabetics, AD patients, and patients with both AD and diabetes found that the brain levels of AGEs, RAGE, and β plaques were higher in patients with combined AD and diabetes compared to patients with AD alone, suggesting pathological synergism of these two diseases (Valente et al. 2010). This possibility is reinforced by data from mouse studies, where RAGE-null diabetic mice had significantly less neurodegenerative changes compared to wild-type diabetic mice (Toth et al. 2006).

10.3.2 Studies in Animal Models

Several animal studies have examined the biological mechanism underlying the association of AGEs with cognition. In a recent study, wild-type mice fed a high-MG diet showed higher levels of brain Aβ and brain and serum AGEs, upregulation of RAGE, and downregulation of AGER-1, compared with those fed with low-MG diet or regular chow (Cai et al. 2014). Levels of plasma 8-isoprostane and leptin were increased, while adiponectin decreased in the group fed with high-MG diet compared to low-MG diet, suggesting elevated oxidative stress and inflammation as potential mediators of the higher Aβ levels. The MG diet also resulted in poor behavioral outcomes; mice in the high-MG group were slower, travelled for a shorter distance, and fell faster than those in the low-MG group on the accelerating rotarod test. They also had worse cognitive performance in the novel object recognition and replacement test, suggesting a memory deficit. Similarly, AD-model mice fed a high-AGE diet had significantly poorer memory, higher hippocampal levels of insoluble Aβ, higher expression of RAGE receptors, and higher levels of vascular oxidative stress compared with littermates fed an isocaloric, low-AGE diet (Lubitz et al. 2016).

Diabetic mice also have significantly higher levels of MG in plasma compared with wild-type mice and they perform poorly on the Morris water maze test of spatial learning and memory. Apoptotic regulators in the hippocampus are upregulated in diabetic mice, suggesting that MG may be neurotoxic.

To test this possibility, Huang and colleagues cultured hippocampal neurons with MG. This caused a significant increase in the percentage of apoptotic cells along with an increase in the expression of apoptotic regulators (e.g., Bax, Caspase 3), and a decrease in the expression of the antiapoptotic protein Bcl-2 (Huang et al. 2012).

Finally, a study by Liu and colleagues in diabetic rats (2013) showed that the antioxidant compound mangiferin reduced hippocampal AGE and RAGE concentrations, as well as oxidative stress and inflammatory markers, and improved cognitive performance on the Morris water maze. Mangiferin also increased hippocampal levels of GLO-1, which may help clear brain MG (Liu et al. 2013).

Although this study could not determine whether the reductions in AGE and RAGE preceded or followed the reduction in inflammation and oxidative stress, the latter are consistently associated with AGE accumulation (Nitti et al. 2007; Uribarri et al. 2007; Bigl et al. 2008) and implicated in the pathogenesis and progression of AD (Sastre 2011; Torres 2011). Thus, these experimental results highlight the close connection between AGEs, neurodegenerative processes, and cognition, and underscore the potential to intervene on AGE-associated pathophysiology.

10.3.3 Interaction of AGEs with AD Pathology

In addition to activating RAGE-mediated pathways, the accumulation of AGEs in the brain could directly cause or exacerbate cerebrovascular and AD pathology. Theoretically, AGE accumulation might alter the transport and clearance of soluble Aβ peptides across the blood–brain barrier via a RAGE-mediated process. In AD, there may be an imbalance between overexpression of RAGE, which transports Aβ into the brain, and the LRP-1 receptor, which mediates transport of Aβ out of the brain (Donahue et al. 2006).

Because Aβ are long-lived proteins, they are more liable to undergo extensive glycation and cross-linking, which can accelerate plaque formation (Vitek et al. 1994; Münch et al. 1997; Loske et al. 2000). Glycated Aβ is also prone to be more toxic. Hippocampal neurons that were cultured with glycated Aβ compared to Aβ alone showed decreased cell viability, increase in cell apoptosis, tau hyperphosphorylation, and activity of glycogen synthase kinase-3 (GSK-3), which phosphorylates tau protein. In addition, glycated Aβ is more suitable ligand for RAGE than Aβ alone and contributes to the upregulation of RAGE (Li et al. 2013). In mice, glycated Aβ has been shown to impair cognitive function on the Morris water maze test, together with significantly increasing RAGE mRNA expression, GSK-3 phosphorylation, and NF-κB and p-38 expression (Chen et al. 2014). In rats, AGEs also appear to enhance the expression of the amyloid precursor protein (APP), the precursor of Aβ (Ko et al. 2010). In addition to their effects on amyloid pathology, AGEs are also able to increase the phosphorylation of tau proteins both *in vitro* (Li et al. 2012a) and *in vivo*, through GSK-3-related mechanisms (Li et al. 2012b).

Lastly, AGE formation in AD may lead to a vicious cycle. AD neuropathology, inflammation, and oxidative stressors can each cause intracellular AGEs precursors to accumulate along with metals that promote oxidation and glycation of proteins and further AGE formation (Srikanth et al. 2011).

10.4 Conclusions

Collectively, the data presented above strongly support the tenable hypothesis that AGEs are causally involved in age-associated neurodegenerative diseases, and particularly in AD and cerebrovascular disease (Table 10.2). However, despite compelling mechanistic evidence from animal studies, the observational human studies cannot establish whether the observed associations are causal. Research is needed to clarify several open questions. First, if the causal hypothesis is correct, then interventions that target the AGEs pathway should yield cognitive benefit, but human randomized clinical trials are needed to test this. As mentioned above, in some cases, reducing modifiable risk factors for AD might prevent some disease (Barnes 2011); this potential for prevention might also pertain to AGE reduction, since exposure to circulating AGEs can be reduced significantly by dietary interventions (Kellow and Savige 2013). Thus, in addition to pharmacological approaches, testing the efficacy of dietary reduction

TABLE 10.2

Possible Mechanisms between AGEs and Cognitive Decline

Direct effects of AGEs

- Receptor for AGEs transfers Aß through the BBB.
- Aggregation of Aß is increasing due to glycation.
- Glycated Aß are more toxic.
- APP is higher due to AGEs.
- AGEs promote phosphorylation of tau proteins.
- Promoting apoptosis in neuron cells.

Mediating effects of AGEs on dementia

- AGEs increase oxidative stress.
- AGEs promote inflammation.
- AGEs promote diabetes and its complications.
- AGEs promote cardiovascular and cerebrovascular diseases.

of AGEs intake in populations with high habitual AGEs consumption would be of considerable interest. It will also be important to identify high-risk populations that may benefit from such interventions, such as diabetics. Second, clarifying whether there is any specific cognitive vulnerability to high AGEs exposure may help to better understand the mechanisms of putative AGE toxicity. From the available data, it seems that memory, which is processed in the hippocampus, is sensitive but AGE levels also appear related to differences in processing speed, suggesting prefrontal damage. Third, the biological mechanisms underlying the AGE–dementia link remain to be fully elucidated: Do AGEs directly cause pathology, or do they reflect oxidative stress and inflammation? If they directly cause pathology, what are the distinct neurodegenerative and cerebrovascular mechanisms? Do different AGEs have specific neuropathologic toxicities? Ultimately, evidence must be obtained to determine whether AGEs reduction is a viable and effective approach to prevention of age-related cognitive decline in diabetics and in the general aging population.

REFERENCES

Ahmed N. 2005. Advanced glycation endproducts—Role in pathology of diabetic complications. *Diabetes Res Clin Pract.* 67(1):3–21.

Ahmed N, Ahmed U, Thornalley PJ, Hager K, Fleischer G, Münch G. 2005. Protein glycation, oxidation and nitration adduct residues and free adducts of cerebrospinal fluid in Alzheimer's disease and link to cognitive impairment. *J Neurochem.* 92(2):255–63.

American Psychiatric Association. 1994. *Diagnostic and Statistical Manual of Mental Disorders*, 4th ed. Washington, DC: American Psychiatric Association.

Bär KJ, Franke S, Wenda B, Müller S, Kientsch-Engel R, Stein G, Sauer H. 2003. Pentosidine and N(epsilon)-(carboxymethyl)-lysine in Alzheimer's disease and vascular dementia. *Neurobiol Aging* 24(2):333–8.

Barnes DE, Yaffe K. 2011.The projected effect of risk factor reduction on Alzheimer's disease prevalence. *Lancet Neurol.* 10(9):819–28.

Beeri MS, Moshier E, Schmeidler J, Godbold J, Uribarri J, Reddy S, Sano M, Grossman HT, Cai W, Vlassara H, Silverman JM. 2011. Serum concentration of an inflammatory glycotoxin, methylglyoxal, is associated with increased cognitive decline in elderly individuals. *Mech Ageing Dev.* 132(11–12):583–7.

Bierhaus A, Humpert PM, Morcos M, Wendt T, Chavakis T, Arnold B, Stern DM, Nawroth PP. 2005. Understanding RAGE, the receptor for advanced glycation end products. *J Mol Med* (Berl) 83(11):876–86.

Bigl K, Gaunitz F, Schmitt A, Rothemund S, Schliebs R, Münch G, Arendt T. 2008. cytotoxicity of AGEs in human micro and astroglial cell lines depends on the degree of protein glycation. *J Neural Transm.* 115(11):1545–56.

Brookmeyer R, Johnson E, Ziegler-Graham K, Arrighi HM. 2007. Forecasting the global burden of Alzheimer's disease. *Alzheimers Dement.* 3:186–191.

Cai Z, Liu N, Wang C, Qin B, Zhou Y, Xiao M, Chang L, Yan LJ, Zhao B. 2015. Role of RAGE in Alzheimer's Disease. *Cell Mol Neurobiol.* 36:483–95.

Cai W, Uribarri J, Zhu L, Chen X, Swamy S, Zhao Z, Grosjean F, et al. 2014. Oral glycotoxins are a modifiable cause of dementia and the metabolic syndrome in mice and humans. *Proc Natl Acad Sci U. S. A.* 111(13):4940–5.

Chen C, Li XH, Tu Y, Sun HT, Liang HQ, Cheng SX, Zhang S. 2014. Aβ-AGE aggravates cognitive deficit in rats via RAGE. *Neuroscience.* 257:1–10.

Cruz-Sánchez FF, Gironès X, Ortega A, Alameda F, Lafuente JV. 2010. Oxidative stress in Alzheimer's disease hippocampus: A topographical study. *J Neurol Sci.* 299(1–2):163–7.

Donahue JE, Flaherty SL, Johanson CE, Duncan JA 3rd, Silverberg GD, Miller MC, Tavares R, Yang W, Wu Q, Sabo E, Hovanesian V, Stopa EG. 2006. RAGE, LRP-1, and amyloid-beta protein in Alzheimer's disease. *Acta Neuropathol.* 112:405–15.

Emanuele E, D'Angelo A, Tomaino C, Binetti G, Ghidoni R, Politi P, Bernardi L, Maletta R, Bruni AC, Geroldi D. 2005. Circulating levels of soluble receptor for advanced glycation end products in Alzheimer disease and vascular dementia. *Arch Neurol.* 62(11):1734–6.

Ge X, Xu X, Feng C, Wang Y, Li Y, Fen B. 2013. Relationships among serum C-reactive protein, receptor for advanced glycation products, metabolic dysfunction, and cognitive impairments. *BMC Neurol.* 2013, 13:110.

Ghidoni R, Benussi L, Glionna M, Franzoni M, Geroldi D, Emanuele E, Binetti G. 2008. Decreased plasma levels of soluble receptor for advanced glycation end products in mild cognitive impairment. *J Neural Transm.* 115(7):1047–50.

Giardino I, Edelstein D, Brownlee M. 1994. Nonenzymaic glycosylation in vitro and in bovine endothelial cells alters basic fibroblast growth factor activity. *J Clin Invest.* 94(1):110–17.

Goldberg T, Cai W, Peppa M, Dardaine V, Baliga BS, Uribarri J, Vlassara, H. 2004. Advanced glycoxidation end products in commonly consumed foods. *J Am Diet Assoc.* 104:1287–91.

Goldin A, Beckman JA, Schmidt AM, Creager MA. 2006. Advanced glycation end products sparking the development of diabetic vascular injury. *Circulation.* 114(6):597–605.

Hartog J, Voors AA, Bakker S, Smit A, Veldhuisen D. 2007. Advanced glycation end-products (AGEs) and heart failure: Pathophysiology and clinical implications. *Eur J Heart Failure.* 9:1146–1155.

Honjo K, Black SE, Verhoeff NP. 2012. Alzheimer's disease, cerebrovascular disease, and the β-amyloid cascade. *Can J Neurol Sci.* 39:712–28.

Huang X, Wang F, Chen W, Chen Y, Wang N, Von Maltan K. 2012. Possible link between the cognitive dysfunction associated with diabetes mellitus and the neurotoxicity of methylglyoxal. *Brain Res.* 1469:82–91.

Kellow NJ, Savige GS. 2013. Dietary advanced glycation end-product restriction for the attenuation of insulin resistance, oxidative stress and endothelial dysfunction: A systematic review. *Eur J Clin Nutr.* 67:239–48.

Khechai F, Ollivier V, Bridey F, Amar M, Hakim J, Prost D. 1997. Effect of advanced glycation end product-modified albumin on tissue factor expression by monocytes. Role of oxidant stress and protein tyrosine kinase activation. *Arterioscler Thromb Vasc Biol.* 17(11):2885–90.

Ko SY, Lin YP, Lin YS, Chang SS. 2010. Advanced glycation end products enhance amyloid precursor protein expression by inducing reactive oxygen species. *Free Radic Biol Med.* 49(3):474–80.

Koschinsky T, He C-J, Mitsuhashi T, Bucala R, Liu C, Buenting C, Heitmann K, Vlassara H. 1997. Orally absorbed reactive glycation products (glycotoxins): An environmental risk factor in diabetic nephropathy. *Proc Natl Acad Sci U S A.* 94:6474–9.

Kuhla B, Lüth HJ, Haferburg D, Boeck K, Arendt T, Münch G. 2005. Methylglyoxal, glyoxal, and their detoxification in Alzheimer's disease. *Ann N Y Acad Sci.* 1043:211–16.

Kumar A, Singh A, Ekavali. 2015. A review on Alzheimers disease pathophysiology and its management: An update. *Pharmacolog Rep.* 67:195–203.

Lee SJ, Ritchie CS, Yaffe K, Stijacic Cenzer I, Barnes DE. 2014. A clinical index to predict progression from mild cognitive impairment to dementia due to Alzheimer's disease. *PLoS One.* 9(12):e113535.

Li XH, Xie JZ, Jiang X, Lv BL, Cheng XS, Du LL, Zhang JY, Wang JZ, Zhou XW. 2012a. Methylglyoxal induces tau hyperphosphorylation via promoting AGEs formation. *Neuromolecular Med.* 14(4):338–48.

Li XH, Lv BL, Xie JZ, Liu J, Zhou XW, Wang JZ. 2012b. AGEs induce Alzheimer-like tau pathology and memory deficit via RAGE-mediated GSK-3 activation. *Neurobiol Aging.* 33(7):1400–10.

Li XH, Du LL, Cheng XS, Jiang X, Zhang Y, Lv BL, Liu R, Wang JZ, Zhou XW. 2013. Glycation exacerbates the neuronal toxicity of β-amyloid. *Cell Death Dis.* 4:e673

Liu YW, Zhu X, Yang QQ, Lu Q, Wang JY, Li HP, Wei YQ, Yin JL, Yin XX. 2013. Suppression of methylglyoxal hyperactivity by mangiferin can prevent diabetes-associated cognitive decline in rats. *Psychopharmacology (Berl)*. 2013;228:585–94.

Loske C, Gerdemann A, Schepl W, Wycislo M, Schinzel R, Palm D, Riederer P, Münch G. 2000. Transition metal-mediated glycoxidation accelerates cross linking of beta amyloid peptide. *Eur J Biochem*. 267(13):4171–8.

Lubitz I, Ricny J, Atrakchi-Baranes D, Shemesh C, Kravitz E, Liraz-Zaltsman S, Maksin-Matveev A, Cooper I, Leibowitz A, Uribarri J, Schmeidler J, Cai W, Kristofikova Z, Ripova D, LeRoith D, Schnaider-Beeri M. 2016. High dietary advanced glycation end products are associated with poorer spatial learning and accelerated Aβ deposition in an Alzheimer mouse model. *Aging Cell* 15:309–16

Lue LF, Walker DG, Brachova L, Beach TG, Rogers J, Schmidt AM, Stern DM, Yan SD 2001. Involvement of microglial receptor for advanced glycation endproducts (RAGE) in Alzheimer's disease: Identification of a cellular activation mechanism. *Exp Neurol*. 171:29–45.

Lüth HJ, Ogunlade V, Kuhla B, Kientsch-Engel R, Stahl P, Webster J, Arendt T, Münch G. 2005. Age- and stage-dependent accumulation of advanced glycation end products in intracellular deposits in normal and Alzheimer's disease brains. *Cereb Cortex*.15(2):211–20.

Moran C, Münch G, Forbes JM, Beare R, Blizzard L, Venn AJ, Phan TG, Chen J, Srikanth V 2015. Type 2 diabetes, skin autofluorescence, and brain atrophy. *Diabetes* 64(1):279–83.

Münch G, Mayer S, Michaelis J, Hipkiss AR, Riederer P, Müller R, Neumann A, Schinzel R, Cunningham AM. 1997. Influence of advanced glycation end-products and AGE-inhibitors on nucleation-dependent polymerization of beta-amyloid peptide. *Biochim Biophys Acta*. 1360(1):17–29.

Nitti M, Furfaro AL, Traverso N, Odetti P, Storace D, Cottalasso D, Pronzato MA, Marinari UM, Domenicotti C. 2007. PKC delta and NADPH oxidase in AGE- induced neuronal death. *Neurosci Lett*. 416(3):261–5.

Perrone L, Grant WB, 2015. Observational and ecological studies of dietary advanced glycation end products in national diets and Alzheimer's disease incidence and prevalence. *J Alzheimer's Dis*. 45(3):679–688.

Petersen RC, Doody R, Kurz A, Mohs RC, Morris JC, Rabins PV, Ritchie K, Rossor M, Thal L, Winblad B. 2001. Current concepts in mild cognitive impairment. *Arch Neurol*. 58(12):1985–92.

Poulsen MW, Hedegaard RV, Andersen JM, Courten BD, Bugel S, Nielsen J, Skibsted LH, Dragsted LO. 2013. Advanced glycation end products in food and their effects on health. *Food Chem Toxicol*. 60:10–37.

Prince M, Bryce R, Albanese E, Wimo A, Ribeiro W, Ferri CP. 2013. The global prevalence of dementia: A systematic review and metaanalysis. *Alzheimers Dement*. 9(1):63–75.

Ravona-Springer R, Schnaider-Beeri M. 2011.The association of diabetes and dementia and possible implications for nondiabetic populations. *Expert Rev Neurother*. 11(11):1609–1.

Rondeau P, Bourdon E, 2011. The glycation of albumin: Structural and functional impacts. *Biochimie*. 93(4):645–58.

Salahuddin P, Rabbani G, Khan R, 2014.The role of advanced glycation end products in various types of neurodegenerative diseases: A therapeutic approach. *Cell Mol Biol Lett*. 19:407–37.

Sastre M, Richardson JC, Gentleman SM, Brooks DJ. 2011 Inflammatory risk factors and pathologies associated with Alzheimer's disease. *Curr Alzheimer Res*. 8(2):132–41.

Shuvaev VV, Laffont I, Serot JM, Fujii J, Taniguchi N, Siest G. 2001. Increased protein glycation in cerebrospinal fluid of Alzheimer's disease. *Neurobiol Aging*. 22(3):397–402.

Southern L, Williams J, Esiri MM, 2007. immuouhistochmical study of N-epsilon-carboxymethyl lysine (CML) in human brain: Relation to vascular dementia. *BMC Neurol*. 7:35–42.

Spauwen PJ, van Eupen MG, Köhler S, Stehouwer CD, Verhey FR, van der Kallen CJ, Sep SJ, et al. 2015. Associations of advanced glycation end-products with cognitive functions in individuals with and without type 2 diabetes: The maastricht study. *J Clin Endocrinol Metab*. 100(3):951–60.

Srikanth V, Maczurek A, Phan T, Steele M, Westcott B, Juskiw D, Münch G. 2011. Advanced glycation endproducts and their receptor RAGE in Alzheimer's disease. *Neurobiol Aging*. 32(5):763–77.

Srikanth V, Westcott B, Forbes J, Phan TG, Beare R, Venn A, Pearson S, Greenaway T, Parameswaran V, Münch G.2013. Methylglyoxal, cognitive function and cerebral atrophy in older people. *J Gerontol A Biol Sci Med Sci*. 68(1):68–73.

Stirban A, Gawlowski T, Roden M, 2014.Vascular effects of advanced glycation end products: Clinical effects and molecular mechanisms. *Mol Metab*. 3(2):94–108.

Sttit A. 2001. Advanced glycation: An important pathological event in diabetic and age related ocular disease. *Br J Ophthalmol*. 85(6):746–53.

Swerdlow RH. 2007. Pathogenesis of Alzheimer's disease. *Clinical Intervention Aging.* 2(3):347–59.

Torres LL, Quaglio NB, de Souza GT, Garcia RT, Dati LM, Moreira WL, Loureiro AP, et al. 2011. Peripheral oxidative stress biomarkers in mild cognitive impairment and Alzheimer's disease. *J Alzheimers Dis.* 26(1):59–68.

Toth C, Rong LL, Yang C, Martinez J, Song F, Ramji N, Brussee V, et al. 2008. Receptor for Advanced Glycation End Products (RAGEs) and experimental diabetic neuropathy. *Diabetes.* 57(4):1002–17.

Toth C, Schmidt AM, Tuor UI, Francis G, Foniok T, Brussee V, Kaur J, et al. 2006. Diabetes, leukoencephalopathy and rage. *Neurobiol Dis.* 23(2):445–61.

Tschanz JT, Welsh-Bohmer KA, Lyketsos CG, Corcoran C, Green RC, Hayden K, Norton MC, et al. 2006. Conversion to dementia from mild cognitive disorder: The Cache County Study. *Neurology.* 67(2):229–234.

Uribarri J, Cai W, Peppa M, Goodman S, Ferrucci L, Striker G, Vlassara H. 2007. Circulating glycotoxins and dietary advanced glycation endproducts: Two links to inflammatory response, oxidative stress, and aging. *J Gerontol A Biol Sci Med Sci.* 62:427–33.

Uribarri J, Woodruff S, Goodman S, Cai W, Chen X, Pyzik R, Yong A, Striker G E, Vlassara H. 2010. Advanced glycation end products in foods and a practical guide to their reduction in diet. *J Am Diet Assoc.* 110(6):911–16.

Valente T, Gella A, Fernàndez-Busquets X, Unzeta M, Durany N. 2010. Immunohistochemical analysis of human brain suggests pathological synergism of Alzheimer's disease and diabetes mellitus. *Neurobiol Dis.* 37(1):67–76.

Van Heijst J, Nieseen H, Hoekman K, Schalkwijk CG. 2005. Advanced glycation end products in human cancer tissues: Detection of Nepsilon-(carboxymethyl)lysine and argpyrimidine. *Ann N Y Acad Sci.* 1043:725–33.

Vitek MP, Bhattacharya K, Glendening JM, Stopa E, Vlassara H, Bucala R, Manogue K, Cerami A. 1994. Advanced glycation end products contribute to amyloidosis in Alzheimer disease. *Proc Natl Acad Sci U S A.* 91:4766–70.

West RK, Moshier E, Lubitz I, Schmeidler J, Godbold J, Cai W, Uribarri J, Vlassara H, Silverman JM, Beeri MS. 2014. Dietary advanced glycation end products are associated with decline in memory in young elderly. *Mech Ageing Dev.* 140:10–12.

Wyss-Coray T, Rogers J. 2012. Inflammation in Alzheimer Disease—A brief review of the basic science and clinical literature. *Cold Spring Harb Perspect Med.* 2:a006346.

Yaffe K, Lindquist K, Schwartz AV, Vitartas C, Vittinghoff E, Satterfield S, Simonsick EM, et al. 2011. Advanced glycation end product level, diabetes, and accelerated cognitive aging. *Neurology.* 77(14):1351–6.

11

Advanced Glycation End Products and Polycystic Ovarian Syndrome

Eleni A. Kandaraki
Medical School of Athens University
Athens, Greece

Evanthia Diamanti-Kandarakis
Hygiea Hospital
Athens, Greece

CONTENTS

KEY POINTS

- Advanced glycation end products (AGEs) represent a complex group of compounds derived from endogenous as well as exogenous sources.
- Women with polycystic ovarian syndrome (PCOS) have elevated serum AGEs compared to age and BMI-matched women.
- Ovarian tissue from women with PCOS has increased AGEs deposition, detected by immunostaining, compared to ovarian tissue from non-PCOS women.
- This excess deposition is due to the impairment of the AGE clearance system, either via decreased enzymatic activity of glyoxalase-1 or via decreased function of scavenger receptors.
- Lifestyle modifications constitute the cornerstone of PCOS management. A combination of high-protein and low-glycemic food diet, with low concentrations of AGEs and rich in fruits and vegetables, improves metabolic and reproductive dysfunction in women with the syndrome either obese or lean.

11.1 Introduction

The exact impact of environmental compounds and specifically the role of dietary factors on female reproductive system function and regulation remains to date a challenging field. A great spectrum of dietary components, in the Westernized types of diets, seems to interfere in several intracellular pathways and has negative functional and structural consequences in different tissues of the body. Recent data reveal that plenty of harmful molecules ingested from the food on a daily basis are absorbed through the intestine via mechanisms that are not well defined and are deposited on tissues where different scavenger receptor systems are responsible for their clearance. Among the known target tissues, such as liver and kidney, recently the ovarian tissue has been included. In experimental models, *in vivo* and *in vitro* studies support the systematic effect of dietary glycotoxins (advanced glycation end products, AGEs) on the female reproductive system and particularly on the ovarian tissue (1–4). Nevertheless, the increased endogenous accumulation of these molecules has been already associated with chronic conditions, such as diabetes mellitus, cardiovascular diseases, Alzheimer's disease, and the aging process [5]. The endogenous production of these deleterious compounds, their exogenous absorption, their accumulation on body tissues, in particular the ovarian tissue, as well as their clearing mechanisms are some of the most promising and challenging research fields, since they seem to influence various molecular pathways, including metabolic, inflammatory, and reproductive parameters.

11.2 Endogenous AGEs (Nonenzymatic Glycation Products)

AGEs or glycotoxins are a heterogeneous group of compounds formed through the Maillard reaction (Figure 11.1). This is a multistep chemical reaction, where sugars react in a nonenzymatic way with amino acids, lipids, or nucleic acids and have a final irreversible step with the production of AGEs.

The Maillard reaction has been used for years in the food industry, in order to obtain the desired taste and color of ingredients.

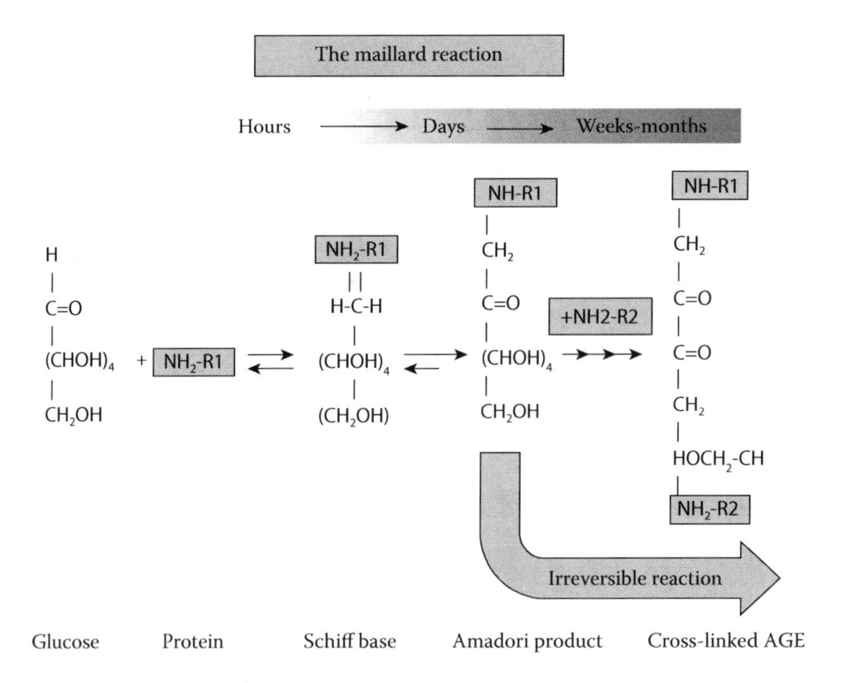

FIGURE 11.1 The Maillard reaction.

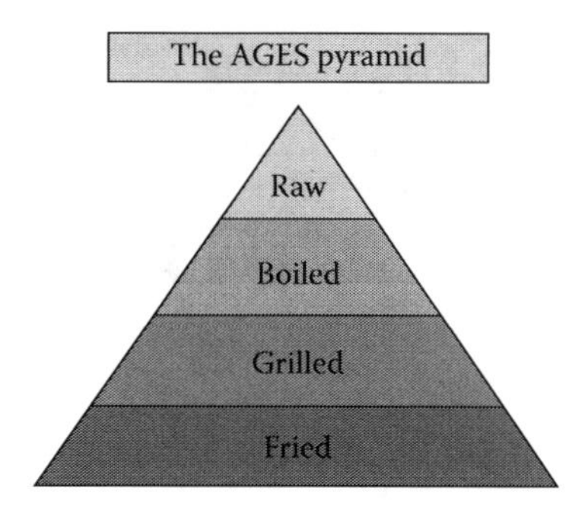

FIGURE 11.2 The AGE pyramid. The more the food processing during preparation, the higher the AGE concentration in food.

11.3 Exogenous AGEs (Dietary Glycotoxins)

Other than the endogenous AGEs, nonenzymatic glycation end products have been found to accumulate on tissues via exogenous sources, such as diet and cigarette smoke. Tobacco leaves have been suggested as a source of compounds that can rapidly increase AGEs. Cerami et al. showed that glycotoxins are inhaled through cigarette smoking into lung alveoli and subsequently are transported into the blood circulation or lung cells, where they interact with other glycated products contributing to their accumulation [6]. In addition, tobacco components have been blamed to disrupt mechanisms of intraovulatory maturation [7]. In the food industry, heating is widely used in order to improve safety, bioavailability, and taste of ingredients.

However, other than the positive effects, food heating can cause degradation of proteins and other catabolic reactions [8]. Cooking at high temperatures promotes the Maillard reaction, which provides the desired color, taste, and aroma. This process is used in the coffee production, coffee aroma, and pastries. Some of the Maillard reaction products are also used as preservatives in beverages and juices [9]. Thus, the Western-type diet is a rich source of exogenous AGEs. Food concentration in AGEs depends not only on the ingredients but also on the method of preparation [3,10]. Although foods rich in proteins and fat have higher concentration of AGEs, increasing the time and temperature of cooking can also achieve high AGE concentration. The more the food processing during their preparation (boiling, grilling, frying), the higher the AGE concentration in the food (Figure 11.2). As a result, these toxic products can easily enter the body via ingestion of highly processed food items [3,8,10]. Moreover, data show that the 10% of these exogenous AGEs enter the blood circulation, two-thirds of them get accumulated in the various body tissues, and the rest are excreted through the renal tract [11].

11.4 The Impact of Endogenous AGEs on the Female Reproductive System

The ovarian function declines as the age advances with reduced follicular reservoir and decreased fertility rate of the remaining follicles [12]. The ovarian microenvironment is vulnerable to exposure to several factors, which may accumulate and interfere with the ovulatory process [13]. One of the most widely recognized biological mechanisms, which leads to ovarian impairment, is the oxidative stress [14]. Increased production of carbonyl molecules from the intermediate products of glycation via nonenzymatic pathways, leading to the accumulation of AGEs, is one of the mechanisms via which oxidative stress has been shown to interfere with different tissue functions, including the ovary [15,16]. Increased levels of methylglyoxal, a precursor of AGEs, have been retrieved in ovarian cell cultures of Chinese hamsters [17]. Ovarian cell exposure to carbonyl overload promoted by high concentration of methylglyoxal has a catastrophic impact on cellular DNA, delays cell proliferation, and leads to a decreased ability of fertilization and follicle maturation, facts similar to the aging process [18]. This is in agreement with the results of Jinno et al., where the high serum and follicular fluid levels of AGEs were associated with decreased follicular and fetal development, as well as a decreased fertility rate via *in vitro* fertilization method [19]. Increased concentrations of AGEs and sRAGE (the soluble isoform of the AGE receptor) have been found in serum and follicular fluid of women older than 35 years when compared with women of younger reproductive age [20], which may be responsible for the chronic inflammatory effect of these toxic molecules on the ovulation process [21]. The production of follicles adequate for ovulation depends on the preservation of homeostatic mechanisms in the ovarian and follicular environment, which means that follicles age as the ovary ages. The female reproductive system ages much more rapidly compared to other organs, as it is shown by the reduced number of follicles and their reduced ability for fertilization [21]. In conclusion, current data demonstrate that the sustained accumulation of endogenous AGEs, either due to aging or other chronic pathological conditions, interferes in signaling and activation of inflammatory pathways, promotes the oxidative overload, and deranges the energy availability and reproductive function of the female reproductive system [22].

11.5 The Impact of Exogenous AGEs (Dietary Glycotoxins) on Female Reproductive System

Other than the endogenous production and accumulation of AGEs, ingestion of AGEs through exogenous sources like food or cigarette smoking seems to lead to similar results of AGEs accumulation in tissues with their catastrophic consequences. In the modern world, the Western-type of diet is increasingly adapted because of people's daily living needs resulting in various metabolic changes, regardless of their genetic background. More specifically, the impact of Western dietary habits on the female reproductive system has been attracting a growing research interest during the last years. Recent studies confirm the absorption and accumulation of exogenous AGEs on body tissues and report a positive correlation with AGE serum levels, overcoming their endogenous production [23]. Data in human and animal models support that dietary glycotoxins promote the accumulation of their toxic metabolites in blood and tissues [24,25]. In particular, with regard to the ovarian tissue, it showed an increased accumulation of glycotoxins and their receptor RAGE on ovarian layers of female rats fed with high concentration of AGEs in their diet for 6 months, compared to female rats fed with low concentration of dietary AGEs. In the high AGEs group, measurements of increased insulin, glucose, and testosterone levels confirm the impact of glycotoxins on the reproductive and metabolic profiles of these animal models [26]. Further supporting data have come from the study of Chang and Chan, where adding methylglyoxal in the drinking water of female rats was associated with decreased follicular maturation rate, fertilization, and *in vitro* fetal development [27].

11.6 The Impact of Endogenous and Exogenous AGEs on Polycystic Ovarian Syndrome

Since 2005, a clear association has been demonstrated between AGEs and polycystic ovarian syndrome (PCOS). Increased levels of serum AGEs and increased expression of their receptor RAGE were found in women with PCOS compared to control women without the syndrome [28]. In the same study, a linear positive correlation was shown between serum androgens and serum AGEs in polycystic women. Additionally, the several different phenotypes of the syndrome were studied and serum AGEs were found to be higher in those women diagnosed with PCOS compared to those having isolated characteristic of the syndrome, whereas no differences were found with regard to serum AGEs in the various different phenotypes of the syndrome. Bearing in mind that chronic inflammation and oxidative stress are parts of the pathophysiology of the syndrome, AGEs seem to play a connecting role between the metabolic and reproductive derangements of the syndrome [1]. A study of 151 pairs of mother–neonates showed that the oxidative stress of neonates from mothers with PCOS was comparable to those with gestational diabetes mellitus, and there was a strong correlation between the oxidative stress of neonates and the oxidative stress of their mothers [29]. Furthermore, achievement of ovulation in women with PCOS has repeatedly attracted research interest. In fact, a positive correlation of increased serum AGEs was found in women without ovulation compared to those who have the syndrome but yet achieve ovulation. In the same study, in ovulating women serum, AGEs had a positive correlation with the increased levels of anti-Mullerian hormone, a hormone with inhibitory effect on the follicle-stimulating hormone, produced by the granulosa cells of primary follicle and used as a marker of increased immature oocytes which do not get promoted to maturation and ovulation [30]. Other than the serum AGEs, the immunohistochemical expression of these molecules and their receptor RAGE on polycystic ovaries were also studied. Biopsies from ovarian tissue of normal and PCOS women showed increased AGE expression on endothelial, theca, and granulosa cells of PCOS women compared to normal controls. The immunohistochemical expression of RAGE was also found to be stronger on granulosa layer, whereas the inflammatory factor NF-κB 55 p65 was found only in the nucleus of granulosa cells retrieved from polycystic ovaries [2].

Normal function of ovary and follicles requires a normal structure and elasticity of contouring connective tissue, the principal component of ovarian stroma. PCOS is characterized by derangement in collagen synthesis, volume, and density of stroma. It has been shown that AGE accumulation promotes overproduction of extracellular matrix and abnormal collagen cross-links formation, leading to disruption of the required environment for follicular maturation [31]. Apart from the surrounding connective tissue, intact ovarian blood supply is of major importance for normal ovarian function. The catastrophic impact of AGEs on blood vessels is well known due to stimulation of inflammatory factors. In particular, a strong positive correlation was seen between serum AGEs and levels of endothelin-1, a peptide causing endothelial damage in both normal and PCOS women [32]. In fact, increased cardiovascular risk has been found in patients with PCOS, due to endothelial damage caused by these toxic molecules [33].

Recently, Tatone et al. demonstrated the important role of increased endogenous AGE accumulation in the process of ovarian aging. It was found that aged rat ovaries had a 30-fold increase in endogenous AGE accumulation compared to the ovaries of younger rats. It seems there is an association between elevated AGE concentration and ovarian function decline, either due to aging or other pathological conditions with similar pathophysiology to the aging process, such as diabetes and PCOS. The new data that came out from this study were decreased enzymatic activity of glyoxalase-1 (GLO-1). GLO-1 has a key role in the glyoxalase enzymatic process, which contributes to AGE clearing (Figure 11.3). It is unclear if the decreased activity of this enzyme is the cause of an augmented accumulation of AGEs, or, more interestingly, there could be a negative feedback mechanism inhibiting the enzymatic activity of GLO-1 in high AGE concentrations, leading to further AGE accumulation [34].

The glyoxalase enzymatic system is located in the cytoplasm of all cells of mammals and takes part in the clearing process of glycated molecules. The enzymatic defense against glycation limits the structural damage and functional impairment caused by glycated products. However, it consists of an incomplete mechanism. These products are constantly produced and accumulated in low concentrations under normal circumstances. The greatest part of the glycated proteins, nucleic acids, and lipids are either catabolized or excreted via the renal tract. In conditions of overproduction of AGEs, such as renal failure, diabetes mellitus, or aging, the system is unable to achieve a complete clearance of these toxic molecules,

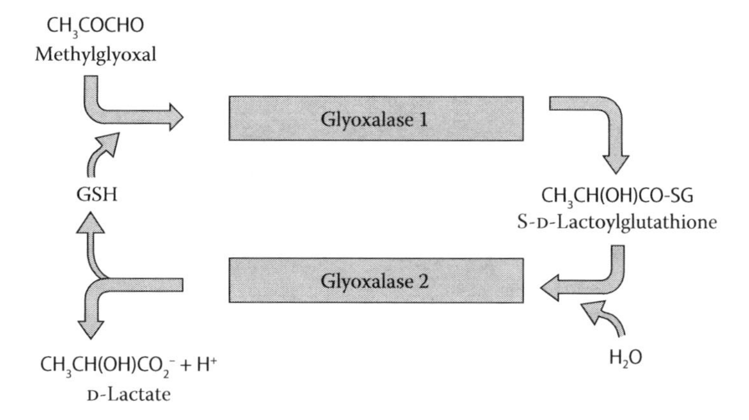

FIGURE 11.3 The glyoxalase system. Glyoxalase-1 (GLO-1) catalyzes the formation of S-D-lactoylglutathione from methylglyoxal via reduction of glutathione (GSH). Glyoxalase 2 (GLO-2) catalyzes the hydrolysis of S-D-lactoylglutathione to D-lactate and regenerates GSH.

leading to their accumulation [41]. In addition, in these conditions of AGE overload and consequently of high oxidative stress, there is a great consumption of glutathione (GSH) and NADPH, leading to in situ reduction of GLO-1 enzymatic efficacy [35], contributing even further to the accumulation of glyoxal, methylglyoxal, and other glycation products. The above observations are in agreement with the results of our study [36] on androgenized female rats compared to nonandrogenized controls, both fed with high- and low-AGE diets. More specifically, the rats of the androgenized group underwent subcutaneous implantation of dihydrotestosterone pellets, aiming to resemble the metabolic and reproductive characteristics of PCOS-like animal models. Both androgenized and nonandrogenized rats were divided in two subgroups, where diet of high- and low-AGE concentrations was randomly assigned. In the ovarian tissue extracts retrieved from rats fed high-AGE diet for 3 months, the GLO-1 activity was found to be reduced compared to the extracts from rats fed with low-AGE diet (p = 0.006). Moreover, the enzymatic activity was further reduced in the androgenized group of rats compared with the nonandrogenized

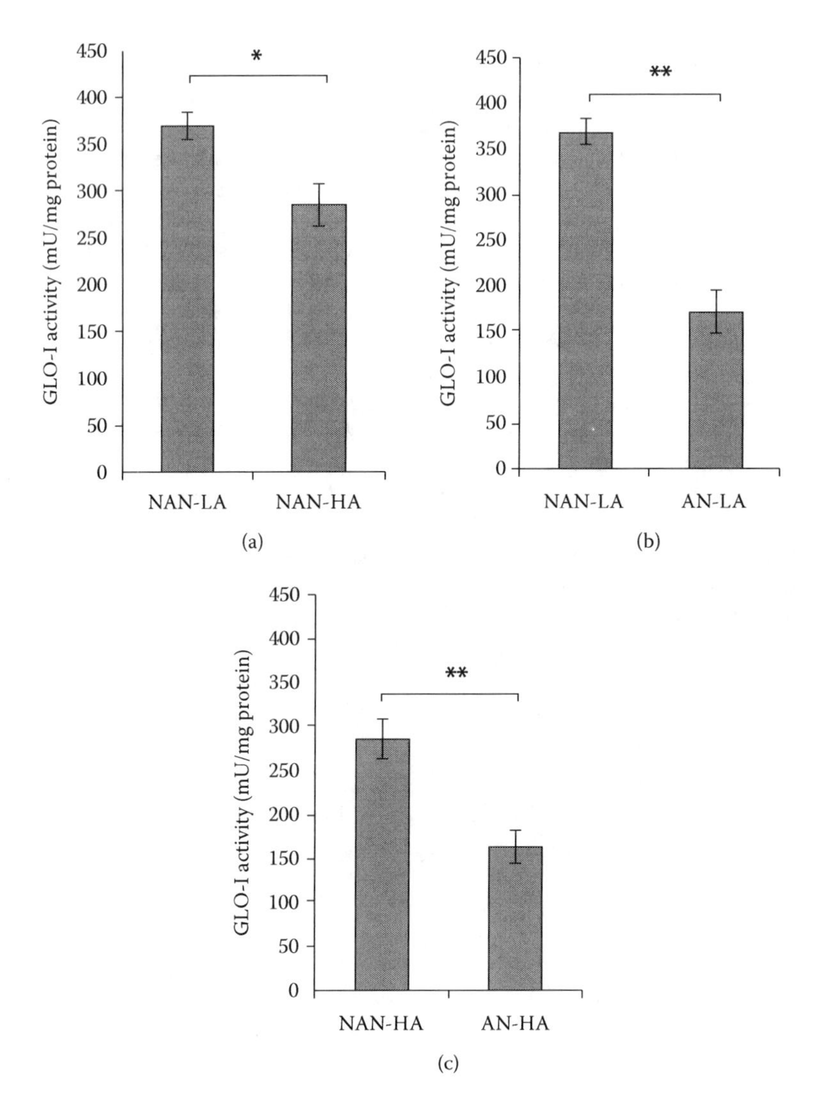

FIGURE 11.4 The impact of androgens excess and high AGEs diet on GLO-1 activity. (a) Reduced GLO-I activity is observed in NAN-HA-fed rats compared to NAN-LA. (b) GLO-I activity is remarkably reduced in AN-LA compared to NAN-LA. (c) GLO-I activity is decreased in AN-HA compared to NAN-HA-fed rats. NAN-LA, nonandrogenized low-AGEs-fed rats; NAN-HA, nonandrogenized high-AGEs-fed rats; AN-LA, androgenized low-AGEs-fed rats; AN-HA, androgenized high-AGEs-fed rats. $*p < 0.05$; $**p < 0.001$. (From Kandaraki, E., et al., *Mol. Med.*, 18, 1183–1189, 2012.)

group fed with the same diet, high or low AGEs, respectively ($p \leq 0.001$) (Figure 11.4). In conclusion, it seems that the enzymatic activity of GLO-1 is reduced in the presence of dietary AGE overconsumption and tissue accumulation, but also in the presence of hyperandrogenemia as it occurs in PCOS, another high-AGE state.

11.7 Management

Lifestyle modifications constitute the cornerstone of PCOS management although the optimal dietary management remains unknown. A combination of high-protein and low-glycemic food diet, with low concentrations of AGEs and rich in fruits, vegetables, whole grains, and low-fat dairy products improves metabolic and reproductive dysfunction in women with the syndrome either obese or lean. The impact of AGE accumulation on the metabolic and reproductive profiles of PCOS women has been identified as one of the targets for therapeutic strategies. More specifically, changes in dietary AGEs seem to be linked to changes in insulin sensitivity, oxidative stress, and hormonal status; it should be noticed that these findings are novel and have never been reported before in women with PCOS [37]. Additionally to dietary modifications, pharmaceutical interventions have also a place in lowering serum AGEs in women affected by the PCOS syndrome. Metformin administration for 6 months in 22 PCOS women has shown a decrease in serum AGEs and a subsequent improvement of metabolic parameters [38]. Similar results were seen in patients' hormonal and metabolic profiles after orlistat administration for 6 months, regardless of body weight variations [39]. Apart from endogenous AGEs, orlistat administration seems to play a beneficial role in decreasing absorption of exogenously ingested AGEs. A study in 36 women, 21 with PCOS and 15 normal controls, measured serum AGE levels before and after a high-AGE meal. Serum levels were found to be increased in both PCOS and control women after the meal administration, whereas a significant decrease of these levels was found when the high-AGE meal was combined with orlistat administration in both patient groups [40].

Since the high dietary intake of AGEs has an impact on the hormonal and metabolic profiles of women with PCOS, lowering dietary AGE intake could be a novel treatment strategy in women with the syndrome.

11.8 Conclusions

AGEs seem to interfere in the intraovarian pathophysiology, either by increased dietary consumption, absorption, and tissue accumulation, or by increased endogenous overproduction in pathological conditions, such as PCOS. It has been shown that there is not only a positive correlation between serum AGEs and androgen levels in women with PCOS, but also an increased accumulation of AGEs and their receptor RAGE on their ovarian layers. Interestingly, it seems that both high-AGE diets and hyperandrogenemic states promote an overproduction and accumulation of AGEs, possibly due to a defective clearing mechanism represented by the reduced activity of GLO-1, which again may be triggered by the AGE overload, leading to a vicious circle of reduced clearance and over-accumulation of AGEs. As a result, a low-AGE diet along with therapeutic agents, which improve androgen excess and/or reduce AGE accumulation, could point to new optimistic targets in the treatment of PCOS.

REFERENCES

1. Diamanti-Kandarakis E, Katsikis I, Piperi C, Kandaraki E, Piouka A, Papavassiliou AG, Panidis D. Increased serum advanced glycation end-products is a distinct finding in lean women with polycystic ovary syndrome (PCOS). *Clinical Endocrinology*. 2008; **69**(4): 634–41.
2. Diamanti-Kandarakis E, Piperi C, Patsouris E, Korkolopoulou P, Panidis D, Pawelczyk L, Papavassiliou AG, Duleba AJ. Immunohistochemical localization of advanced glycation end-products (AGEs) and their receptor (RAGE) in polycystic and normal ovaries. *Histochemistry and Cell Biology*. 2007; **127**(6): 581–9.

3. Goldberg T, Cai W, Peppa M, Dardaine V, Baliga BS, Uribarri J, Vlassara H. Advanced glycoxidation end products in commonly consumed foods. *Journal of the American Dietetic Association*. 2004; **104**(8): 1287–91.
4. Vlassara H. Advanced glycation in health and disease: Role of the modern environment. *Annals of the New York Academy of Sciences*. 2005; **1043**: 452–60.
5. Luevano-Contreras C, Chapman-Novakofski K. Dietary advanced glycation end products and aging. *Nutrients*. 2010; **2**(12): 1247–65.
6. Cerami C, Founds H, Nicholl I, Mitsuhashi T, Giordano D, Vanpatten S, Lee A, et al. Tobacco smoke is a source of toxic reactive glycation products. *Proceedings of the National Academy of Sciences of the United States of America*. 1997; **94**(25): 13915–20.
7. Mlynarcikova A, Fickova M, Scsukova S. Ovarian intrafollicular processes as a target for cigarette smoke components and selected environmental reproductive disruptors. *Endocrine Regulations*. 2005; **39**(1): 21–32.
8. Faist V, Erbersdobler HF. Metabolic transit and in vivo effects of melanoidins and precursor compounds deriving from the Maillard reaction. *Annals of Nutrition & Metabolism*. 2001; **45**(1): 1–12.
9. O'Brien J, Morrissey PA. Nutritional and toxicological aspects of the Maillard browning reaction in foods. *Critical Reviews in Food Science and Nutrition*. 1989; **28**(3): 211–48.
10. Uribarri J, Woodruff S, Goodman S, Cai W, Chen X, Pyzik R, Yong A, Striker GE, Vlassara H. Advanced glycation end products in foods and a practical guide to their reduction in the diet. *Journal of the American Dietetic Association*. 2010; **110**(6): 911–16 e12.
11. Koschinsky T, He CJ, Mitsuhashi T, Bucala R, Liu C, Buenting C, Heitmann K, Vlassara H. Orally absorbed reactive glycation products (glycotoxins): An environmental risk factor in diabetic nephropathy. *Proceedings of the National Academy of Sciences of the United States of America*. 1997; **94**(12): 6474–9.
12. Tatone C, Amicarelli F, Carbone MC, Monteleone P, Caserta D, Marci R, Artini PG, Piomboni P, Focarelli R. Cellular and molecular aspects of ovarian follicle ageing. *Human Reproduction Update*. 2008; **14**(2): 131–42.
13. Yin D, Chen K. The essential mechanisms of aging: Irreparable damage accumulation of biochemical side-reactions. *Experimental Gerontology*. 2005; **40**(6): 455–65.
14. Harman D. Free radical theory of aging: An update: Increasing the functional life span. *Annals of the New York Academy of Sciences*. 2006; **106**: 710–21.
15. Peppa M, Uribarri J, Vlassara H. Aging and glycoxidant stress. *Hormones*. 2008; **7**(2): 123–32.
16. Rabbani N, Thornalley PJ. The dicarbonyl proteome: Proteins susceptible to dicarbonyl glycation at functional sites in health, aging, and disease. *Annals of the New York Academy of Sciences*. 2008; **1126**: 124–7.
17. Chaplen FW, Fahl WE, Cameron DC. Evidence of high levels of methylglyoxal in cultured Chinese hamster ovary cells. *Proceedings of the National Academy of Sciences of the United States of America*. 1998; **95**(10): 5533–8.
18. Tatone C, Heizenrieder T, Di Emidio G, Treffon P, Amicarelli F, Seidel T, Eichenlaub-Ritter U. Evidence that carbonyl stress by methylglyoxal exposure induces DNA damage and spindle aberrations, affects mitochondrial integrity in mammalian oocytes and contributes to oocyte ageing. *Human Reproduction*. 2011; **26**(7): 1843–59.
19. Jinno M, Takeuchi M, Watanabe A, Teruya K, Hirohama J, Eguchi N, Miyazaki A. Advanced glycation end-products accumulation compromises embryonic development and achievement of pregnancy by assisted reproductive technology. *Human Reproduction*. 2011; **26**(3): 604–10.
20. Fujii EY, Nakayama M. The measurements of RAGE, VEGF, and AGEs in the plasma and follicular fluid of reproductive women: The influence of aging. *Fertility and Sterility*. 2010; **94**(2): 694–700.
21. Malickova K, Jarosova R, Rezabek K, Fait T, Masata J, Janatkova I, Zima T, Kalousova M. Concentrations of sRAGE in serum and follicular fluid in assisted reproductive cycles—A preliminary study. *Clinical Laboratory*. 2010; **56**(9–10): 377–84.
22. Tatone C, Amicarelli F. The aging ovary—The poor granulosa cells. *Fertility and Sterility*. 2013; **99**(1): 12–17.
23. Lin RY, Reis ED, Dore AT, Lu M, Ghodsi N, Fallon JT, Fisher EA, Vlassara H. Lowering of dietary advanced glycation endproducts (AGE) reduces neointimal formation after arterial injury in genetically hypercholesterolemic mice. *Atherosclerosis*. 2002; **163**(2): 303–11.

24. Vlassara H, Cai W, Crandall J, Goldberg T, Oberstein R, Dardaine V, Peppa M, Rayfield EJ. Inflammatory mediators are induced by dietary glycotoxins, a major risk factor for diabetic angiopathy. *Proceedings of the National Academy of Sciences of the United States of America*. 2002; **99**(24): 15596–601.
25. Zheng F, He C, Cai W, Hattori M, Steffes M, Vlassara H. Prevention of diabetic nephropathy in mice by a diet low in glycoxidation products. *Diabetes/Metabolism Research and Reviews*. 2002; **18**(3): 224–37.
26. Diamanti-Kandarakis E, Piperi C, Korkolopoulou P, Kandaraki E, Levidou G, Papalois A, Patsouris E, Papavassiliou AG. Accumulation of dietary glycotoxins in the reproductive system of normal female rats. *Journal of Molecular Medicine*. 2007; **85**(12): 1413–20.
27. Chang YJ, Chan WH. Methylglyoxal has injurious effects on maturation of mouse oocytes, fertilization, and fetal development, via apoptosis. *Toxicology Letters*. 2010; **193**(3): 217–23.
28. Diamanti-Kandarakis E, Piperi C, Kalofoutis A, Creatsas G. Increased levels of serum advanced glycation end-products in women with polycystic ovary syndrome. *Clinical Endocrinology*. 2005; **62**(1): 37–43.
29. Boutzios G, Livadas S, Piperi C, Vitoratos N, Adamopoulos C, Hassiakos D, Iavazzo C, Diamanti-Kandarakis E. Polycystic ovary syndrome offspring display increased oxidative stress markers comparable to gestational diabetes offspring. *Fertility and Sterility*. 2013; **99**(3): 943–50.
30. Diamanti-Kandarakis E, Piouka A, Livadas S, Piperi C, Katsikis I, Papavassiliou AG, Panidis D. Anti-mullerian hormone is associated with advanced glycosylated end products in lean women with polycystic ovary syndrome. *European Journal of Endocrinology / European Federation of Endocrine Societies*. 2009; **160**(5): 847–53.
31. Papachroni KK, Piperi C, Levidou G, Korkolopoulou P, Pawelczyk L, Diamanti-Kandarakis E, Papavassiliou AG. Lysyl oxidase interacts with AGE signalling to modulate collagen synthesis in polycystic ovarian tissue. *Journal of Cellular and Molecular Medicine*. 2010; **14**(10): 2460–9.
32. Christakou C, Economou F, Livadas S, Piperi C, Adamopoulos C, Marinakis E, Jdiamanti-Kandarakis E. Strong and positive association of endothelin-1 with AGEs in PCOS: A causal relationship or a bystander? *Hormones*. 2011; **10**(4): 292–7.
33. Kaya C, Erkan AF, Cengiz SD, Dunder I, Demirel OE, Bilgihan A. Advanced oxidation protein products are increased in women with polycystic ovary syndrome: Relationship with traditional and nontraditional cardiovascular risk factors in patients with polycystic ovary syndrome. *Fertility and Sterility*. 2009; **92**(4): 1372–7.
34. Tatone C, Carbone MC, Campanella G, Festuccia C, Artini PG, Talesa V, Focarelli R, Amicarelli F. Female reproductive dysfunction during ageing: Role of methylglyoxal in the formation of advanced glycation endproducts in ovaries of reproductively-aged mice. *Journal of Biological Regulators and Homeostatic Agents*. 2010; **24**(1): 63–72.
35. Abordo EA, Minhas HS, Thornalley PJ. Accumulation of alpha-oxoaldehydes during oxidative stress: A role in cytotoxicity. *Biochemical Pharmacology*. 1999; **58**(4): 641–8.
36. Kandaraki E, Chatzigeorgiou A, Piperi C, Palioura E, Palimeri S, Korkolopoulou P, Koutsilieris M, Papavassiliou AG. Reduced ovarian glyoxalase-I activity by dietary glycotoxins and androgen excess: A causative link to polycystic ovarian syndrome. *Molecular Medicine*. 2012; **18**: 1183–9.
37. Tantalaki E, Piperi C, Livadas S, Kollias A, Adamopoulos C, Koulouri A, Christakou C, Diamanti-Kandarakis E. Impact of dietary modification of advanced glycation end products (AGEs) on the hormonal and metabolic profile of women with polycystic ovary syndrome (PCOS). *Hormones (Athens)*. 2014; **13**(1):65–73.
38. Diamanti-Kandarakis E, Alexandraki K, Piperi C, Aessopos A, Paterakis T, Katsikis I, Panidis D. Effect of metformin administration on plasma advanced glycation end product levels in women with polycystic ovary syndrome. *Metabolism: Clinical and Experimental*. 2007; **56**(1): 129–34.
39. Diamanti-Kandarakis E, Katsikis I, Piperi C, Alexandraki K, Panidis D. Effect of long-term orlistat treatment on serum levels of advanced glycation end-products in women with polycystic ovary syndrome. *Clinical Endocrinology*. 2007; **66**(1): 103–9.
40. Diamanti-Kandarakis E, Piperi C, Alexandraki K, Katsilambros N, Kouroupi E, Papailiou J, Lazaridis S, et al. Short-term effect of orlistat on dietary glycotoxins in healthy women and women with polycystic ovary syndrome. *Metabolism: Clinical and Experimental*. 2006; **55**(4): 494–500.
41. Thornalley PJ. Protein and nucleotide damage by glyoxal and methylglyoxal in physiological systems—Role in ageing and disease. *Drug Metabolism and Drug Interactions*. 2008; **23**(1–2): 125–50.

12

Dietary AGEs and Diabetic Complications

Ma. Eugenia Garay-Sevilla, Armando Gómez-Ojeda, and Claudia Luevano-Contreras
University of Guanajuato Campus León
León, México

CONTENTS

KEY POINTS

- Exogenous advanced glycation end products (AGEs) in various foods, together with endogenous AGEs, are important contributors to the body pool of AGEs in diabetic and nondiabetic subjects.
- AGEs exert their biological effects by two mechanisms: one independent of receptors by damaging protein structure and one involving receptors which induce proinflammatory molecules that could contribute to cellular dysfunction and tissue damage.
- Dietary AGEs (dAGEs) suppress protective defenses such as AGER-1, SIRT-1, and PPARγ in diabetic subjects.
- Lowering the intake of AGEs decreases body AGE levels, thereby reducing their toxic effects and slowing down renal damage, decreases oxidative stress and inflammation markers, and improves insulin sensitivity.
- dAGE restriction studies seem to have identified an effective and promising therapeutic approach in diabetic subjects.

12.1 Introduction

Diabetes mellitus is characterized by chronic hyperglycemia and altered cellular homeostasis, which lead to diffuse vascular damage and multi-organ dysfunction (Nolan et al. 2011). In the long term, diabetic patients risk both microvascular and macrovascular complications, the former resulting in damaged retinal, renal, and neural tissues, which may cause blindness, end-stage renal disease, and nontraumatic lower limb amputations (Nolan et al. 2011). Chilelli et al. described that advanced glycation end products (AGEs) seem to be not actors but directors of the processes leading to the complications, for at least two main reasons: first, AGEs have several intracellular and extracellular targets, so they can seem as a bridge between intracellular and extracellular damage; second, whatever the level of hyperglycemia, AGE-related intracellular glycation of the mitochondrial respiratory chain proteins has been found to produce more reactive oxygen species, triggering a vicious cycle that amplifies AGE formation. Importantly, excessive formation of AGEs is regarded as the most important mechanism that triggers the pathophysiological cascades associated with the onset of diabetic complications, such as nephropathy, retinopathy, neuropathy, and diseases of the macrovasculature (atherosclerosis, stroke, peripheral disease) (Chilelli et al. 2013).

Recently, more attention has been paid to the exogenous AGEs in various foods. Together with endogenous AGEs, these compounds form the majority of free adducts, which represent the greater proportion of circulating AGEs in diabetic and nondiabetic subjects (Kanková 2008). It has been well documented that exogenous (dietary) AGEs are related directly to plasma levels of AGEs in healthy, diabetic, and renal disease individuals, contributing to the promotion of oxidative, inflammatory, and degenerative processes that underlie the pathogenesis of many chronic diseases such as diabetes (Uribarri et al. 2011) and progressively increasing the risk for both microvascular and macrovascular diseases. Lowering the intake of AGEs through the diet decreases body AGEs levels, thereby reducing their toxic effects.

12.2 AGEs in the Diet: Formation Modulators and Factors Affecting Formation, Absorption, and Elimination

Although there are other AGE formation pathways that have an important contribution to the formation of endogenous AGEs (polyol, glycoxidation, and lipid peroxidation, among others), the Maillard reaction is particularly important as a contributor to dietary AGEs (dAGEs) and their subsequent link to oxidative stress (OS) and inflammation markers.

There are *in vivo* therapeutic approaches to diminish AGE formation (Williams et al. 2007), but these approaches are considered risky and impractical to apply in foods. Avoiding AGE formation in foods by changing cooking techniques seems to be the most practical and promising approach.

Several factors may affect dAGE formation, including temperature, pH, substrates, moisture, and reaction time during cooking. High cooking temperatures applied for long periods of time lead to a higher AGE formation rate. The Maillard reaction has an optimum pH range around pH 10, and therefore, lowering the pH of foods marinating in lemon, vinegar, etc. may decrease AGE formation (Uribarri et al. 2010). Additionally, the rate of AGE formation is highly dependent on the type of food. Generally, animal-derived foods will produce higher AGE amounts compared to carbohydrates. The water content inversely influences the reaction; wet food or food prepared in an aqueous environment is less prone to AGE formation (Uribarri et al. 2010). All of these factors can combine in a synergistic manner, and individuals can control dAGE intake by either avoiding certain prepared foods or changing cooking methods, neither of which require reducing the quantity of the chosen food.

12.2.1 Intestinal Absorption of AGEs

Once dAGEs are ingested, two main factors contribute to their contribution to the body AGE pool, absorption and elimination. Approximately 10 % of dAGEs consumed are absorbed, and of these, only 30 % are excreted (Koschinsky et al. 1997). Chemical/physiological behavior of AGEs seems to be strongly influenced by whether or not they are bound to proteins (Bergmann et al. 2001). The intestinal absorption process and rate of a specific AGE seem to be dependent on size. This is exemplified by pentosidine and carboxymethyllysine (CML), which in the bound form are less and more slowly absorbed, while conversely, the free forms of both are highly and readily absorbed (Bergmann et al. 2001).

Due to the limited present knowledge on this subject, further studies are needed to better define AGE absorption factors.

12.2.2 Elimination of AGEs

Once absorbed, there are several mechanisms by which the body's defenses degrade and subsequently excrete AGEs. These defenses include enzymatic defense, either in deglycating proteins (fructosamine-3-kinase) or degrading AGEs and their precursors (glyoxalase systems); cell surface receptors that mediate uptake, degradation, and removal of AGEs such as AGE-receptor complex AGER (AGER-1, AGER-2, AGER-3), among others (Ott et al. 2014); antioxidant systems; and renal clearance.

Renal clearance is particularly important as AGEs are mostly cleared by the kidneys, and as previously stated, about 30% of absorbed AGEs are cleared by kidneys in healthy subjects. In renal disease (a common condition among type 2 diabetics), excreted AGE levels can decrease to even just 5% (Koschinsky et al. 1997), with a subsequent rise in AGE body levels. It is pertinent to underline that some recent researches showed diminished renal damage after dAGE restriction (Peppa et al. 2004a; Ueda et al. 2006). To gain a better understanding of this matter, this chapter will review the effect of dAGEs in animal and human studies.

12.3 Effect of a Low-AGE Diet on Serum AGEs, OS, and Inflammation

As previously reviewed, dAGE absorption is relatively modest, and AGEs are highly excreted. While this still generates controversy among experts, growing evidence suggests that dAGEs are absorbed into the circulation (Somoza et al. 2006). This is consistent with several studies that report on the role of dAGEs in increasing OS and inflammation in animals and humans.

Adverse health effects resulting from dAGEs may be in part due to their potential promotion of a low-grade inflammation state. This may be the primary link between dAGEs and several diabetic complications (Baynes and Thorpe 1999; Vlassara et al. 2002; Ramasamy et al. 2005; Uribarri et al. 2007, 2014). Underlying molecular mechanisms are not clearly understood, but AGEs cause damage through two primary mechanisms: they may bind to biomolecules, changing directly their molecular conformation and therefore their function (Figure 12.1). Furthermore, they may bind to the surface cell receptor RAGE that initiates intracellular signaling cascades, promoting OS and inflammation. All these effects are important in diabetic subjects (Cai et al. 2004).

Damage due to interaction of AGEs with RAGE is especially interesting. RAGE acts as a signal transduction receptor for AGEs, apparently, mostly CML. RAGE is a member of the Ig family, and its expression is upregulated by AGEs in a wide range of cells. Once RAGE is activated, activation of transcriptional nuclear factor-κB (NF-κB) is induced along with their target genes, making it a major regulator of inflammation and immune response (Kislinger et al. 1999). Expression of RAGE is enhanced in certain cells in diabetes and in inflammation. This way, the axis AGEs/RAGE is involved in the regulation of the inflammatory state and can be characterized by the expression of a variety of cytokines such as IL-6 and tumor necrosis factor-α (TNF-α). Additionally, this contributes to increasing OS through NADPH oxidase (Zhang et al. 2006), followed by subsequent signal cascading. RAGE action initiated by AGEs generates OS, which further potentiates formation and accumulation of AGEs, and this subsequent interaction with RAGE creates a positive feedback loop increasing OS.

Through these mechanisms, the dAGE/RAGE interaction seems to be related to several diabetic complications, depending on the cell type and where the interaction is expressed; this is supported by recent work in the field.

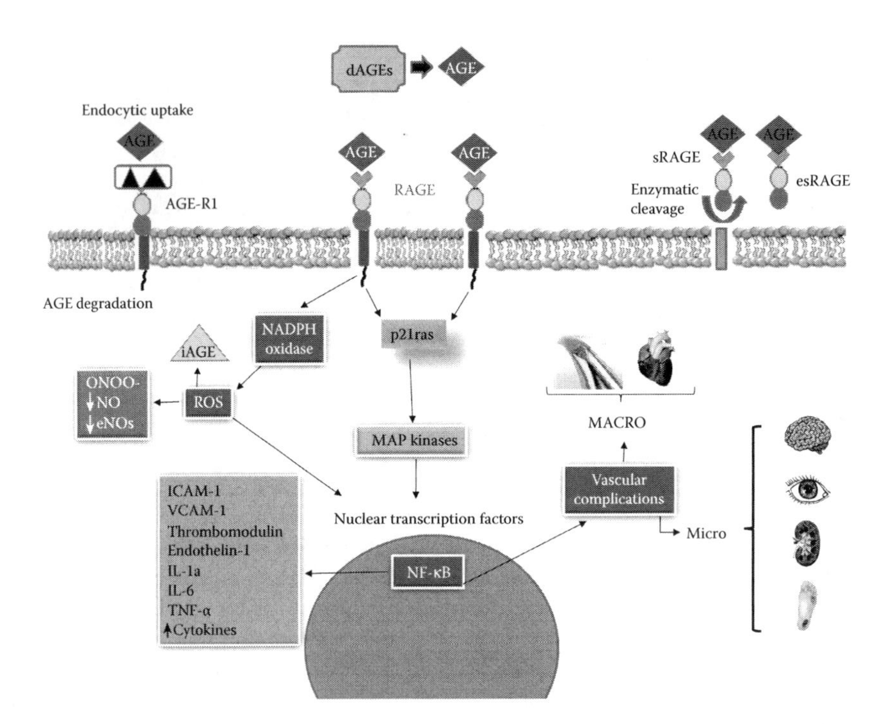

FIGURE 12.1 Representation of endogenous and exogenous AGEs mechanism of action. The mechanism of damage mediated by receptor includes two different types of receptors: the receptor responsible for AGE degradation, mainly AGE-R1 and the multiligand receptor for AGEs; receptor for AGE (RAGE), which mediates proatherogenic, inflammatory, and immune responses via activation of NF-κB, resulting in the increased expression and synthesis of proinflammatory cytokines, ROS production, and different marker of endothelial damage. sRAGE are present in the circulation and may act as decoy molecules or as surrogate biomarker. Thus, the damage occurs to the tissues and development of microvascular and macrovascular complications. dAGE, dietary advanced glycation end products; AGE-R, AGE-receptor 1; ROS, reactive oxygen species; VCAM-1, vascular cell adhesion molecule-1; IL-1a, interleukin 1a; TNF-α, tumor necrosis factor-alpha; NF-κB, nuclear factor kappa B; sRAGE, soluble receptor for advanced glycation end products; esRAGE, endogen secretor receptor for advanced glycation end products.

Several studies have noted that dAGEs induce inflammatory mediators. Evidence has shown an association between dAGEs and serum AGEs in diabetic patients (Vlassara et al. 2002), with dAGEs increasing several markers of OS and inflammation (mitogen-activated protein kinase [MAPK], NF-κB, vascular cell adhesion molecule-1 [VCAM-1], 8-isoprostane, and TNF-α, among others) (Baynes and Thorpe 1999; Vlassara et al. 2002; Negrean et al. 2007; Luévano-Contreras et al. 2013). dAGEs also seem to impair endothelial function (Negrean et al. 2007) in diabetic subjects, and furthermore, recent research has shown that dAGEs suppress protective defenses such as AGER-1, SIRT-1, and PPARγ in diabetic subjects (Uribarri et al. 2011, 2014).

In this regard, dAGE restriction studies seem to have identified an effective and promising therapeutic approach in diabetic subjects. Some effects of this dAGE restriction reported in several studies include slowed renal damage (Peppa et al. 2004; Ueda et al. 2006), decreased OS and inflammation markers, and improved insulin sensitivity (Uribarri et al. 2011, 2014; Luévano-Contreras et al. 2013).

Moreover, benefits of dAGE restriction are not limited to diabetic subjects or those with compromised renal function. Increasingly, studies have shown that the deleterious effects of dAGEs also occur in healthy subjects of different ages, including increased inflammation markers (Uribarri et al. 2011, 2014, 2015; Forbes et al. 2014; Mark et al. 2014) and an association with insulin resistance (IR). These results have been found in a number of different studies, which may imply that dAGEs are a modifiable risk factor for IR (Forbes et al. 2014; Mark et al. 2014; Uribarri et al. 2015). In the following sections, this chapter will describe how both endogenous and exogenous AGEs may contribute to the complications seen in diabetes.

12.3.1 Microvascular Complications in Diabetes

In patients with diabetes, microvascular damage in kidneys, retinas, and peripheral nerves can occur when endothelial cells from the microvascular beds are damaged, with subsequent capillary occlusion, ischemia, and organ damage (Luévano-Contreras et al. 2013).

12.3.1.1 Eye Diseases Associated with AGEs in Diabetes

Accumulation of AGEs has been observed in all different eye compartments, including the cornea, lens, retina, Bruch's membrane, sclera, and optic nerve, and it could be involved in eye diseases associated with diabetes such as cataracts, diabetic keratopathy, and diabetic retinopathy (Kandarakis et al. 2014).

AGE accumulation could be involved in the apoptosis and subsequent corneal alterations observed in diabetic keratopathy, which is characterized by delayed wound healing, and epithelial erosion. Kim et al. (2011) found that diabetic rats had higher accumulation of AGEs and higher expression of 8-hydroxyguanosine and NF-κB in corneal tissues in comparison to their controls, concluding that the pathogenesis of diabetic keratopathy may be associated in part with the accumulation of AGEs, OS, and activation of NF-κB.

Glycation of structural proteins, such as myelin, tubulin, and lens crystallins, as well as the accumulation of AGEs in lens epithelial cells, could be involved in cataract formation (Kandarakis et al. 2015). Kim et al. (2012) studied the effect of AGE accumulation on lens epithelial cells *in vitro* and *in vivo* and found an increased expression of apoptosis-related molecules including NF-κB, Bax, and Bcl-2. They found that cataractous lenses of diabetic rats had accumulation of argpyrimidine, a methylglyoxal-derived AGE, in lens epithelial cells; apoptosis in these cells was markedly increased.

Potentially, the most important eye complication in diabetes is diabetic retinopathy, which may lead to blindness in these patients. Diabetic retinopathy is characterized by proliferation of blood vessels, vascular occlusion, angiogenesis, increased permeability of capillaries, and progressive loss of retinal pericytes (elongated cells around and along endothelial cells) and endothelial cells (Singh et al. 2014). Accumulation of methylglyoxal-derived AGEs could be involved in the early and intermediate stages of the microvascular damage seen in retinopathy. A 20-fold increase in diabetic vitreous methylglyoxal has been seen in diabetic patients in comparison to controls (Kandarakis et al. 2014). The level of AGEs from retinal blood vessels has been found to correlate with the degree of retinopathy in subjects with type 2 diabetes mellitus (Huebschmann et al. 2006), leading to the hypothesis that AGEs could be involved in the damage seen in retinopathy. Additionally, the upregulation of vascular endothelial growth factor (VEGF) along with the interaction of AGEs with RAGE could potentially increase angiogenesis and neovascularization (characteristic of proliferative retinopathy) (Ahmed 2005).

There is not yet sufficient data to explain how dAGEs contribute to eye diseases. However, a recent study in animal models found that dAGEs upregulate RAGE and VEGF-A expression in ocular tissues. Kandarakis et al. (2015) studied young (4 weeks old) and adult (12 weeks old) Wistar rats that were fed a high- or low-AGE diet for 3 months and found that serum AGEs, fructosamine, and C-reactive protein (CRP) levels were significantly higher in animals with the high-AGE (H-AGE) diet in comparison to the low-AGE diet, independent of animal age ($p < 0.0001$). In addition, RAGE and VEGF-A expression was upregulated in ocular tissues of both young and adult animals fed the H-AGE diet. The authors concluded that dAGE intake affects the physiology of ocular tissues by upregulating RAGE and VEGF-A, contributing to enhanced inflammatory responses and pathologic neovascularization in normal organisms independent of aging.

12.3.1.2 Renal Disease

In healthy subjects with normal renal function, the kidneys clear circulating AGEs. However, patients with uremia and diabetic nephropathy have high levels of AGEs, in part the result of inadequate renal clearance (Dawnay 2003).

Failure to clear AGEs resulting from diabetic renal disease as well as the long-term effect of dAGE consumption has been well studied in animal models. For example, Coughlan et al. (2011) found that

CML was increased only 4 weeks after diabetes induction and progressively increased after 32 weeks in diabetic animals, concluding that urinary excretion of CML is a marker of progressive renal damage in experimental diabetic nephropathy. In another study, the long-term intake of dAGEs in rats led to an increase in proteinuria that over time could induce renal damage (Sebeková et al. 2005).

AGEs are associated with damages seen in renal disease such as glomerular basement membrane thickening, mesangial expansion, glomerulosclerosis, and tubulointerstitial fibrosis (Goh et al. 2008). Chronic kidney disease is characterized by a decline in glomerular filtration, which in part could be responsible for decreased AGE excretion. The higher systemic accumulation of AGEs will activate RAGE, with subsequent increases in inflammatory molecules, and OS that will in turn promote additional glomerulosclerosis and further renal decline (Gugliucci and Menini 2014).

Several studies have found higher serum AGE levels in both diabetic and nondiabetic kidney disease compared to controls (Poulsen et al. 2013). For instance, patients with end-stage renal damage and diabetes had higher AGE levels compared to healthy controls (Bucala et al. 1994). Patients with uremia on a reduced intake of dAGEs, both with and without diabetes, showed reduced levels of inflammatory molecules such as TNF-α and higher sensitivity to CRP (hsCRP) (Uribarri et al. 2003). Reduction of dAGEs in patients with chronic kidney disease ($n = 9$) resulted in lower levels of serum CML and methylglyoxal, as well as VCAM-1, TNF-α and reduced expression of RAGE in peripheral blood mononuclear cells. In contrast, AGER1 had an increased expression in comparison to the control group who consumed a regular diet (Vlassara et al. 2009).

12.3.1.3 Neuropathy

Diabetic neuropathy (DNO) is the most common complication of diabetes; almost 50% of patients with diabetes develop DNO. Sural, peroneal, and saphenous nerves of human diabetic subjects contain AGEs not only in the perineurium, endothelial cell, and pericytes of endoneurial microvessels but also in myelinated and unmyelinated fibers (Thornalley 2002). Some *in vitro* studies have found an increased glycation of myelin in diabetes (Nguyen et al. 2012). Nerve demyelination seen in DNO could be explained by phagocytosis of the glycated myelin by macrophages. In animal studies, when AGEs are injected in peripheral nerves, there is a reduction in sensory motor conduction velocities, nerve action potentials, and blood flow (Ahmed 2005). However, the mechanism by which AGEs could be involved in DNO is not clear.

12.3.2 Macrovascular Complications

Cardiovascular disease (CVD) is a long-term complication for people with diabetes mellitus, which often leads to reduced life span (Mercer et al. 2012) and is a main cause of mortality. Atherosclerosis constitutes the main pattern for the development of CVD and is characterized by the thickening of the intima with plaque and eventual occlusion of the arterial lumen (Vlassara et al. 1984). Abnormal levels of lipoprotein glycation are of great importance for the enhancement of atherogenesis in diabetes mellitus (Peppa et al. 2004).

In type 2 diabetic patients, elevated AGEs are associated with macrovascular abnormalities, including coronary atherosclerosis (Basta et al. 2004), and have been shown to be a biomarker of severity of this disease (Yeboah et al. 2004), independent from other well-known risk factors such as hypertension, hyperlipidemia, and smoking (Hegab et al. 2012). Additionally, serum AGEs were found to be elevated in diabetic patients with coronary heart disease (Kilhovd et al. 2005). AGEs were also found to be elevated in patients with obstructive coronary artery disease, and these results were correlated to the severity of coronary artery disease and the resulting adverse clinical outcomes (Kiuchi et al. 2001).

Chang et al. in 2011 found that AGEs were positively associated with total cholesterol, triglycerides, and low-density lipoprotein-C (LDL-C) and negatively correlated with high-density lipoprotein-C. These findings suggest that AGEs may be a marker for atherosclerosis. Previous *in vivo* studies in diabetic vascular atheromatosis have found CML and pentosidine in increased concentrations in both plasma and tissues in these patients (Chuyen et al. 2006).

Increased AGE accumulation is not just restricted to patients with diabetes but can also occur in renal failure, states of increased OS, and as a result of an increased intake of dAGEs. Therefore, AGEs may be involved in the development of heart failure in nondiabetic patients as well.

The numerous effects of AGEs on vessel wall function include the formation of chemical cross-links within and between connective tissue components or between the elements and plasma constituents. This can impair vasodilation and LDL removal (Huebschmann et al. 2006). Because AGE-LDL retained in the aortic wall increases the accumulation of foam cells, it is also considered to be an efficient proatherogenic substance. AGEs also affect the physical properties of arteries by decreasing their distensibility and elasticity (Vlassara and Striker 2007).

Stirban et al. (2013) recently reviewed the pathogenic mechanisms of AGEs on the vascular system and found that some mechanisms are associated with inflammation and OS (Cai et al. 2002), increased glycation of LDL and HDL (Duell et al. 1991), activation of the proinflammatory inducible nitric oxide (NO) synthase (iNOS) (Wever et al. 1998), and inhibition of NO availability (Xu et al. 2005).

Elevated serum levels of AGEs in patients with diabetes accelerate the development and progression of heart failure both indirectly through their vascular effects and directly through direct actions on the myocardium. AGEs exert their deleterious effect by receptor-mediated mechanisms and receptor-independent mechanisms of action that include the formation of cross-links with basic components in the basement membrane of the extracellular matrix, permanently modifying its structural characteristics (Ahmed 2005; Palimeri et al. 2015). AGE receptors are present on the surface of different cell types such as macrophages, adipocytes, endothelial cells, and vascular smooth muscle cells as well as several types of receptors such as RAGE, AGE-R1, AGE-R2, and AGE-R3 among others that have been described throughout this chapter (Stitt et al. 1999). AGEs induce a wide range of signaling pathways that trigger inflammation, atherogenesis, and vasoconstriction, leading to coronary dysfunction, atherosclerosis, and thrombosis (Hegab et al. 2012). In addition to higher expression in these conditions, RAGE has also been detected in carotid artery plaques and has been shown to be associated with increased inflammatory reactions (Cipollone et al. 2003). Levels of soluble RAGE (sRAGE) and endogenous secretory receptors (esRAGE) are elevated in type 2 diabetic patients with coronary artery disease or atherosclerotic burden (Fujisawa et al. 2013). Activation of RAGE could also result in fibrosis, impaired calcium metabolism, and vasoconstriction in the cardiovascular system (Hartog et al. 2007).

Formation and accumulation of AGEs play a central role in the vascular damage caused by diabetes. Inhibiting AGE formation, blocking the AGE–RAGE system, and restricting food-derived AGEs may become novel therapeutic strategies for treating the vascular complications of diabetes (Yamagishi 2011). Additionally, high levels of AGEs in the diet could play an important role in the causation of diabetes and resulting diabetic complications, as reducing the amount of AGEs in the diet of animals can ameliorate diabetes and its complications, regardless of glycemic levels (Vlassara and Striker 2007).

12.4 Studies in Animal Models

Lin et al. (2002) evaluated the association between dAGE content and neointimal formation after arterial injury in genetically hypercholesterolemic mice that were randomly assigned to receive either a H-AGE diet or a similar diet with 10-fold lower AGE content. These mice underwent femoral artery injury 1 week later and were maintained on their diets for an additional 4 weeks. At 4 weeks after injury, a significant decrease in neointimal formation was noted in the low-AGE (L-AGE) diet group, which correlated with a decrease in circulating AGE levels. Immunohistochemistry also showed a reduced deposition of AGEs in the endothelia, smooth muscle cell, and macrophages in neointimal lesions of L-AGE diet-fed mice.

This study evaluating the influence of diet-related AGE on atherosclerosis in diabetic and nondiabetic apoE (–/–) mice showed that the atherosclerosis lesions at the aortic root of the L-AGE group were smaller. Serum AGEs were also lower in the diabetic L-AGE than in the H-AGE mice, and immunohistochemical comparisons showed markedly suppressed tissue AGEs, AGE-receptor-1 and -2, and RAGE expression, reduced numbers of inflammatory cells, tissue factor, VCAM-1, and MCP-1 in the L-AGE diabetic group (Lin et al. 2003).

L-AGE diets in animal studies have been shown to reverse IR and chronic inflammation, inhibit the progression of atherosclerosis, and prevent experimental diabetic nephropathy and neuropathy (Uribarri et al. 2007).

12.5 Studies in Humans

In patients with diabetes, dAGE restriction has not been tested for an effect on diabetic complications. However, as AGEs correlate with indicators of OS, inflammation, and endothelial damage, changes that are directly influenced by the intake of dAGEs can suggest the effects of diets low in AGEs on diabetic complications in a variety of studies.

Vlassara et al. (2002) studied the effects of two diets, one with high AGE content (H-AGE) and the other with 5-fold lower AGE (L-AGE) content on inflammatory mediators of 24 diabetic subjects: 11 in a 2-week crossover and 13 in a 6-week parallel study. After 2 weeks on L-AGE, diabetic patients showed a significant reduction of serum AGEs as well as significant decreases of markers of endothelial function (VCAM-1), TNF-α, and CRP.

In another study on both healthy subjects and DM type 2 patients, a test beverage high in AGEs was created by concentrating to 1.8×10^6 AGE units, which contained neither carbohydrates nor lipids. This beverage was prepared from glucose and was caffeine-free. After the single oral challenge of high dAGE beverage, both DM patients and controls had elevated serum AGEs and signs of endothelial dysfunction as measured by flow-mediated dilatation (FMD) and plasminogen activator inhibitor-I (Uribarri et al. 2007).

In a crossover study with 20 subjects with type 2 DM, a H-AGE diet resulted in impaired FMD, elevated adhesion molecules, and higher levels of a marker for OS, leading to more pronounced microvascular and macrovascular dysfunctions and endothelial damage compared to a L-AGE diet. The authors concluded that chemical modifications of food by means of cooking play a major role in influencing the extent of postprandial vascular dysfunction (Negrean et al. 2007).

LDL modification by AGEs is thought to contribute to CVD in diabetes, and in one study, 24 diabetic subjects were randomized to either a standard diet (here called high-AGE or H-AGE) or a diet 5-fold lower in AGEs (L-AGE diet) for 6 weeks. It was shown that exposure to daily dietary glycoxidants enhances LDL-induced vascular toxicity via redox-sensitive MAPK activation (Cai et al. 2004).

Another study of diabetic patients who had similar degree of glycemic control and lipidemia showed that high AGE intake can transform the circulating macromolecules to a much greater extent and render a more proatherogenic lipid profile than those of subjects on a L-AGE diet (Cai et al. 2010).

12.6 Conclusions

AGEs are important in the development of the microvascular and macrovascular complications of diabetes. dAGEs are significant contributors to plasma AGEs in humans. Several studies have shown that a reduction in dAGE intake may result in effective suppression of different markers of inflammation, OS, and endothelial damage in diabetes, thereby leading to the prevention or delaying the complications of diabetes. As a result, prevention and treatment must focus not only on early glycemic control but also on reducing OS and in particular the dietary intake of exogenous AGEs.

In addition to other important aspects of treatment, common dietary principles should be recommended to all diabetic patients to attempt to prevent the development of diabetes complications. For example, preparing meals by steam cooking or boiling in water rather than grilling and frying foods and cooking at lower temperatures are important diet modifications that can reduce the intake of AGEs.

In diabetes as well as in all diseases, the most important thing is prevention.

REFERENCES

Ahmed, N. 2005. Advanced glycation end products: Role in pathology of diabetic complications. *Diabetes Res Clin Pract* 67:3–21.

Basta, G., Schmidt, AM., De Caterina, R. 2004. Advanced glycation end products and vascular inflammation: Implications for accelerated atherosclerosis in diabetes. *Cardiovasc Res* 63:582–92.

Baynes, J.W., Thorpe, S.R. 1999. Role of oxidative stress in diabetic complications: A new perspective on an old paradigm. *Diabetes* 48:1–9.

Bergmann, R., Helling, R., Heichert, C., et al. 2001. Radio fluorination and positron emission tomography (PET) as a new approach to study the in vivo distribution and elimination of the advanced glycation endproducts N-epsilon-carboxymethyllysine (CML) and N-epsilon-carboxyethyllysine (CEL). *Nahrung* 45:182–88.

Bucala, R., Makita, Z., Vega, G., et al. 1994. Modification of low density lipoprotein by advanced glycation end products contributes to the dyslipidemia of diabetes and renal insufficiency. *Proc Natl Acad Sci U S A* 91:9441–45.

Cai, W., Gao, Q.D., Zhu, L., Peppa, M., He, C., Vlassara, H. 2002. Oxidative stress-inducing carbonyl compounds from common foods: Novel mediators of cellular dysfunction. *Mol Med* 8:337–46.

Cai, W., He, J.C., Zhu, L., et al. 2004. High levels of dietary advanced glycation end products transform low-density lipoprotein into a potent redox-sensitive mitogen-activated protein kinase stimulant in diabetic patients. *Circulation* 110:285–91.

Cai, W., Torreggiani, M., Zhu, L., et al. 2010. AGER1 regulates endothelial cell NADPH oxidase-dependent oxidant stress via PKC-delta: Implications for vascular disease. *Am J Physiol Cell Physiol* 298:C624–34.

Chang, J.B., Chu, N.F., Syu, J.T., Hsieh, A.T., Hung, Y.R. 2011. Advanced glycation end products (AGEs) in relation to atherosclerotic lipid profiles in middle-aged and elderly diabetic patients. *Lipids Health Dis* 10:228.

Chilelli, N.C., Burlina, S., Lapolla, A. 2013. AGEs, rather than hyperglycemia, are responsible for microvascular complications in diabetes: A "glycoxidation-centric" point of view. *Nutr Metab Cardiovasc Dis* 23:913–19.

Chuyen, N.V. 2006. Toxicity of the AGEs generated from the Maillard reaction: On the relationship of food-AGEs and biological-AGEs. *Mol Nutr Food Res* 50:1140–9.

Cipollone, F., Iezzi, A., Fazia, M., et al. 2003. The receptor RAGE as a progression factor amplifying arachidonate-dependent inflammatory and proteolytic response in human atherosclerotic plaques: Role of glycemic control. *Circulation* 108:1070–77.

Coughlan, M.T., Forbes, J.M. 2011. Temporal increases in urinary carboxymethyllysine correlate with albuminuria development in diabetes. *Am J Nephrol* 34:9–17.

Dawnay, A. 2003. Renal clearance of glycation adducts: Anti-glycation defence in uraemia and dialysis. *Biochem Soc Trans* 31:1386–89.

Duell, P.B., Oram, J.F., Bierman, E.L. 1991. Nonenzymatic glycosylation of HDL and impaired HDL-receptor-mediated cholesterol efflux. *Diabetes* 40:377–84.

Forbes, J.M., Sourris, K.C., de Courten, M.P., et al. 2014. Advanced glycation endproducts (AGEs) are cross-sectionally associated with insulin secretion in healthy subjects. *Amino Acids* 46:321–26.

Fujisawa, K., Katakami, N., Kaneto, H., et al. 2013. Circulating soluble RAGE as a predictive biomarker of cardiovascular event risk in patients with type 2 diabetes. *Atherosclerosis* 227:425–28.

Goh, S.Y., Cooper, M.E. 2008. Clinical review: The role of advanced glycation end products in progression and complications of diabetes. *J Clin Endocrinol Metab* 93:1143–52.

Gugliucci, A., Menini, T. 2014. The axis AGE-RAGE-soluble RAGE and oxidative stress in chronic kidney disease. *Adv Exp Med Biol* 824:191–208.

Hartog, J.W., Voors, A.A., Bakker, S.J., Smit, A.J, van Veldhuisen, D.J. 2007. Advanced glycation end-products (AGEs) and heart failure: Pathophysiology and clinical implications. *Eur J Heart Fail* 9:1146–55.

Hegab, Z., Gibbons, S., Neyses, L., Mamas, M.A. 2012. Role of advanced glycation end products in cardiovascular disease. *World J Cardiol* 26:90–102.

Huebschmann, A.G., Regensteiner, J.G., Vlassara, H., Reusch, J.E. 2006. Diabetes and advanced glycoxidation end products. *Diabetes Care* 29:1420–32.

Kandarakis, S.A., Piperi, C., Moschonas, D.P., Korkolopoulou, P., Papalois, A., Papavassiliou, A.G. 2015. Dietary glycotoxins induce RAGE and VEGF up-regulation in the retina of normal rats. *Exp Eye Res* 137:1–10.

Kandarakis, S.A., Piperi, C., Topouzis, F., Papavassiliou, A.G. 2014. Emerging role of advanced glycation-end products (AGEs) in the pathobiology of eye diseases. *Prog Retin Eye Res* 42:85–102.

Kanková, K. 2008. Diabetic threesome (hyperglycaemia, renal function and nutrition) and advanced glycation end products: Evidence for the multiple-hit agent? *Proc Nutr Soc* 67:60–74.

Kilhovd, B.K., Juutilainen, A., Lehto, S., et al. 2005. High serum levels of advanced glycation end products predict increased coronary heart disease mortality in nondiabetic women but not in nondiabetic men: A population-based 18-year follow-up study. *Arterioscler Thromb Vasc Biol* 25:815–20.

Kim, J., Kim, O.S., Kim, C.S., Sohn, E., Jo, K., Kim, J.S. 2012. Accumulation of argpyrimidine, a methylglyoxal-derived advanced glycation end product, increases apoptosis of lens epithelial cells both in vitro and in vivo. *Exp Mol Med* 44:167–75.

Kim, J., Kim, C.S., Sohn, E., Jeong, I.H., Kim, H., Kim, J.S. 2011. Involvement of advanced glycation end products, oxidative stress and nuclear factor-kappa B in the development of diabetic keratopathy. *Graefes Arch Clin Exp Ophthalmol* 249:529–36.

Kislinger, T., Fu, C., Huber, B., et al., 1999. N(epsilon)(carboxymethyl)lysine modifications of proteins are ligands for RAGE that activate cell signaling pathways and modulate gene expression. *J Biol Chem* 274:31740–749.

Kiuchi, K., Nejima, J., Takano, T., Ohta, M., Hashimoto, H. 2001. Increased serum concentrations of advanced glycation end products: A marker of coronary artery disease activity in type 2 diabetic patients. *Heart* 85:87–91.

Koschinsky, T., He, C.J., Mitsuhashi, T., et al. 1997. Orally absorbed reactive glycation products (glycotoxins): An environmental risk factor in diabetic nephropathy. *Proc Natl Acad Sci U S A* 94:6474–79.

Lin, R.Y., Choudhury, R.P., Cai, W., et al. 2003. Dietary glycotoxins promote diabetic atherosclerosis in apolipoprotein E-deficient mice. *Atherosclerosis* 168:213–20.

Lin, R.Y., Reis, E.D., Dore, A.T., et al. 2002. Lowering of dietary advanced glycation endproducts (AGE) reduces neointimal formation after arterial injury in genetically hypercholesterolemic mice. *Atherosclerosis* 163:303–11.

Luévano-Contreras, C., Garay-Sevilla, M.E., Wrobel, K., Malacara, J.M., Wrobel, K. 2013. Dietary advanced glycation end products restriction diminishes inflammation markers and oxidative stress in patients with type 2 diabetes mellitus. *J Clin Biochem Nutr* 52:22–6.

Mark, A.B., Poulsen, M.W., Andersen, S., et al. 2014. Consumption of a diet low in advanced glycation end products for 4 weeks improves insulin sensitivity in overweight women. *Diabetes Care* 37:88–95.

Mercer, B.N., Morais, S., Cubbon, R.M., Kearney, M.T. 2012. Diabetes mellitus and the heart. *Int J Clin Pract* 66:640–7.

Negrean, M., Stirban, A., Stratmann, B., et al. 2007. Effects of low- and high-advanced glycation end product meals on macro- and microvascular endothelial function and oxidative stress in patients with type 2 diabetes mellitus. *Am J Clin Nutr* 85:1236–243.

Nguyen, D.V., Shaw, L.C., Grant, M.B. 2012. Inflammation in the pathogenesis of microvascular complications in diabetes. *Front Endocrinol* 3:170.

Nolan, C.J., Damm, P., Prentki, M. 2011. Type 2 diabetes across generations: From pathophysiology to prevention and management. *Lancet* 378:169–81.

Ott, C., Jacobs, K., Haucke, E., Navarrete Santos, A., Grune, T., Simm, A. 2014. Role of advanced end products in celular signaling. *Redox Biol* 2:411–29.

Palimeri, S., Palioura, E., Diamanti-Kandarakis, E. 2015. Current perspectives on the health risks associated with the consumption of advanced glycation end products: Recommendations for dietary management. *Diabetes Metab Syndr Obes* 8:415–26.

Peppa, M., Uribarri, J., Cai, W., Lu, M., Vlassara H. 2004. Glycoxidation and inflammation in renal failure patients. *Am J Kidney Dis* 43:690–95.

Peppa, M., Uribarri, J., Vlassara, H. 2004. The role of advanced glycation end products in the development of atherosclerosis. *Curr Diab Rep* 4:31–6.

Poulsen, M.W., Hedegaard, R.V., Andersen, J.M., et al. 2013. Advanced glycation endproducts in food and their effects on health. *Food Chem Toxicol* 60:10–37.

Ramasamy, R., Vannucci, S.J., Yan, S.S., Herold, K., Yan, S.F., Schmidt, A.M.2005. Advanced glycation end products and RAGE: A common thread in aging, diabetes, neurodegeneration, and inflammation. *Glycobiology* 15:16R–28R.

Sebeková, K., Hofmann, T., Boor, P., et al. 2005. Renal effects of oral maillard reaction product load in the form of bread crusts in healthy and subtotally nephrectomized rats. *Ann N Y Acad Sci* 1043:482–91.

Singh, V.P., Bali, A., Singh, N., Jaggi, A.S. 2014. Advanced glycation end products and diabetic complications. *Kor J Physiol Pharmacol* 18:1–14.

Somoza, V., Wenzel, E., Weiss, C., Clawin-Radecker, I., Grubel, N., Erbersdobler, H. 2006. Dose-dependent utilization of casein-linked lysine alanine, N(epsilon)-fructose lysine and N(epsilon)-carboxy methyl lysine in rats. *Mol Nutr Food Res* 50:833–41.

Stirban, A., Gawlowski, T., Roden, M. 2013. Vascular effects of advanced glycation endproducts: Clinical effects and molecular mechanisms. *Mol Metab* 3:94–108.

Stitt, A.W, He, C., Vlassara H. 1999. Characterization of the advanced glycation end-product receptor complex in human vascular endothelial cells. *Biochem Biophys Res Commun* 256:549–56.

Thornalley, P.J. 2002. Glycation in diabetic neuropathy: Characteristics, consequences, causes, and therapeutic options. *Int Rev Neurobiol* 50:37–57.

Ueda, S., Yamagishi, S., Takeuchi, M., et al. 2006. Oral adsorbent AST-120 decreases serum levels of AGEs in patients with chronic renal failure. *Mol Med* 12:180–84.

Uribarri, J., Cai, W., Peppa, M., et al. 2007. Circulating glycotoxins and dietary advanced glycation endproducts: Two links to inflammatory response, oxidative stress, and aging. *J Gerontol A Biol Sci Med Sci* 62:427–33.

Uribarri, J., Cai, W., Pyzik, R., et al. 2014. Suppression of native defense mechanisms, SIRT1 and PPARγ, by dietary glycoxidants precedes disease in adult humans; relevance to lifestyle-engendered chronic diseases. *Amino Acids* 46:301–09.

Uribarri, J., Cai, W., Ramdas, M., et al. 2011. Restriction of advanced glycation end products improves insulin resistance in human type 2 diabetes: Potential role of AGER1 and SIRT1. *Diabetes Care* 34:1610–16.

Uribarri, J., Cai, W., Woodward, M., et al. 2015. Eleveated serum advanced glycation end products in obese indicate risk for the metabolic syndrome: A link between healthy and unhealthy obesity? *J Clin Endocrinol Metab* 100:1957–66.

Uribarri, J., Peppa, M., Cai, W., et al. 2003. Restriction of dietary glycotoxins reduces excessive advanced glycation end products in renal failure patients. *J Am Soc Nephrol* 14:728–31.

Uribarri, J., Stirban, A., Sander, D., et al. 2007. Single oral challenge by advanced glycation end products acutely impairs endothelial function in diabetic and nondiabetic subjects. *Diabetes Care* 30:2579–82.

Uribarri, J., Woodruff, S., Goodman, S., et al. 2010. Advanced glycation end products in foods and a practical guide to their reduction in the diet. *J Am Diet Assoc* 110:911–16.

Vlassara, H., Brownlee, M., Cerami, A. 1984. Accumulation of diabetic rat peripheral nerve myelin by macrophages increases with the presence of advanced glycosylation endproducts. *J Exp Med* 160:197–207.

Vlassara, H., Cai, W., Crandall, J., Goldberg, T. 2002. Inflammatory mediators are induced by dietary glycotoxins, a major risk factor for diabetic angiopathy. *Proc Natl Acad Sci U S A* 99:15596–601.

Vlassara, H., Cai, W., Goodman, S., et al. 2009. Protection against loss of innate defenses in adulthood by low advanced glycation end products (AGE) intake: Role of the antiinflammatory AGE receptor-1. *J Clin Endocrinol Metab* 94:4483–91.

Vlassara, H., Palace, M.R. 2003. Glycoxidation: The menace of diabetes and aging. *Mt Sinai J Med* 70:232–41.

Vlassara, H., Striker, G. 2007. Glycotoxins in the diet promote diabetes and diabetic complications. *Curr Diab Rep* 7:235–41.

Wever, R.M., Lüscher, T.F., Cosentino, F., Rabelink, T.J. 1998. Atherosclerosis and the two faces of endothelial nitric oxide synthase. *Circulation* 97:108–12.

Williams, M.E., Bolton, W.K., Khalifah, R.G., Degenhardt, T.P., Schotzinger, R.J., McGill, J.B. 2007. Effects of pyridoxamine in combined phase 2 studies of patients with type 1 and type 2 diabetes and overt nephropathy. *Am J Nephrol* 27:605–14.

Xu, B., Ji, Y., Yao, K., Cao, YX., Ferro, A. 2005. Inhibition of human endothelial cell nitric oxide synthesis by advanced glycation end-products but not glucose: Relevance to diabetes. *Clin Sci* 109:439–46.

Yamagishi, S. 2011. Role of advanced glycation end products (AGEs) and receptor for AGEs (RAGE) in vascular damage in diabetes. *Exp Gerontol* 46:217–24.

Yeboah, F.K., Alli, I., Yaylayan, V.A., Yasuo, K., Chowdhury, S.F., Purisima, E.O. 2004. Effect of limited solid-state glycation on the conformation of lysozyme by ESI-MSMS peptide mapping and molecular modeling. *Bioconjug Chem* 15:27–34.

Zhang, M., Kho, A.L., Anilkumar, N., et al. 2006. Glycated proteins stimulate reactive oxygen species production in cardiac myocytes: Involvement of Nox2 (gp91phox)-containing NADPH oxidase. *Circulation* 113:1235–243.

13

Dietary AGEs and Aging

Claudia Luevano-Contreras, Ma. Eugenia Garay-Sevilla, and Armando Gomez-Ojeda
University of Guanajuato
Leon, Mexico

CONTENTS

KEY POINTS

- The endogenous production and accumulation of advanced glycation end products (AGEs), which increases in the body along with age, is one of the mechanisms implicated in normal aging.
- Dietary AGEs (dAGEs) may also have a role in aging through increasing circulating AGEs.
- High intake of dAGEs could lead to their accumulation in target tissues affected by chronic diseases common in aging.
- dAGEs measured by dietary records correlated with circulating levels of AGEs, inflammatory, and oxidative stress (OS) markers.
- In human intervention studies, restriction of dAGEs decreases circulating AGEs, insulin resistance, and inflammatory and OS markers, which are associated with chronic diseases common in aging.

13.1 Introduction

Life expectancy of women and men has increased linearly and has nearly doubled in the industrial nations (Oeppen and Vaupel 2002), with a visible change in the causes of death from infectious to degenerative diseases (most of them age-associated). Several mechanisms have been implicated in normal aging, one of them is the endogenous production and accumulation of advanced glycation end products (AGEs), a heterogeneous group of compounds with well-known prooxidant and proinflammatory features (Vlassara et al. 2008). The most well-described AGEs are carboxymethyllysine (CML), pentosidine, pyrraline, and methylglyoxal (MG, an α-oxaldehyde, and precursor of AGEs), which have been used as biomarkers for *in vivo* formation of AGEs (Ahmed 2005). Additionally, exogenous AGEs (the primary source is smoking and diet) could also accumulate and be involved in the molecular mechanisms implicated in aging. In this chapter, a brief description is given on how endogenous and dietary AGEs (dAGEs) could be associated with some age-associated chronic diseases and aging.

13.2 Hypotheses of Normal Aging

Aging is a natural and complex process characterized by a gradual decrease in some physiological functions. Endogenous, genetic, and environmental factors are involved in aging, which often is accompanied by several pathophysiological processes leading to the consequent reduction in the ability to cope with environmental stress (Uribarri et al. 2007, 2014). It is now believed that aging is induced by lifelong accumulation of molecular damage, which leads to tissue dysfunction, reduction of the functional reserve, disease, and eventually to death (Simm et al. 2015).

There are several aging hypotheses, and only a few of them will be briefly described here (Medvedev 1990). A popular theory attributes aging to endogenous reactive oxygen species (ROS), to the consequent oxidative stress (OS) and their harmful effects (Harman 2006). With aging, there is an increase in OS (Harman 2006) that coupled with a decrease in the antioxidant machinery (Hipkiss 2006) and the proteasomal system (Chondrogianni and Gonos 2005) leads to a progressive accumulation of macromolecular oxidative damage. The increase in OS and the decrease in the antioxidant defense system could lead to a gradual decline in some physiological functions.

The glycation theory of aging, partially influenced by Bjorksten theory of aging (cross-links impair cell and tissue function), proposed that glycation itself could be behind the diminished functions associated with aging (Cerami 1985). AGE production and accumulation increases in the body along with age, and whether this is a causal effect or a consequence of aging is still subject to debate (Brownlee 1995; Uribarri et al. 2014).

AGEs may be linked to aging by several mechanisms. For instance, another theory proposed a synergistic effect between OS and glycation (Kristal and Yu 1992), which suggests that aging is produced by the sum of the damage induced by free radicals, glycation, and their interaction. Although AGEs and ROS have different sites of actions and generation mechanism, they might interact to cause age-associated deterioration. The increase in the endogenous production of ROS favors endogenous AGE formation through several pathways (glycoxidation, the Maillard reaction, and lipid peroxidation) and can therefore lead to a higher AGE formation rate. Additionally, glycation of biomolecules could alter the structure and function of antioxidant enzymes (Levine 2002; Rabbani and Thornalley 2008). Finally, during AGE formation, there is a generation of ROS (Brownlee 1995) and reactive dicarbonyls, which contribute to increased OS in a positive feedback loop very well known in diabetes research (Levine 2002).

Aging is also associated with a chronic low-grade inflammatory status (Van Puyvelde et al. 2014). The so-called inflamm-aging theory involves the interaction of AGEs with the cell surface receptor, RAGE. AGEs/RAGE interaction could have a potential promotion of a low-grade inflammatory state (Franceschi et al. 2000; Ramasamy et al. 2005). This theory proposes that continuous inflammatory response could lead to progressive proinflammatory status, and an overload with antigens (among them food) is likely responsible for an inflammatory response. This will gradually lead to a low-grade inflammation and a decrease in physiological performance associated with aging (Franceschi et al. 2000; Ramasamy et al. 2005) (Figure 13.1).

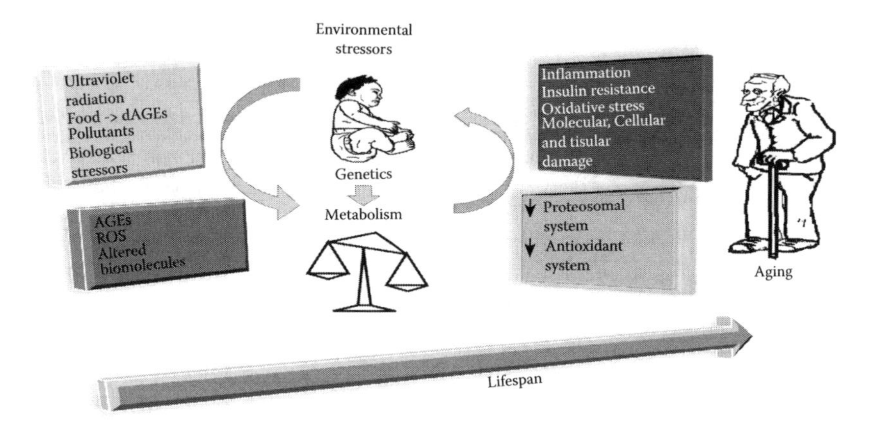

FIGURE 13.1 Aging is a complex process that involves genetics, environmental factors, and the complex interaction between them. The amount and length of exposure to environmental factors could decrease the ability to cope with environmental stress, leading to several pathophysiological processes, often present during aging.

13.3 Health Implications Associated with AGEs in the Elderly

It has been described that AGEs could contribute to chronic diseases such as sarcopenia, kidney disease, cancer, cardiovascular diseases, diabetes, Alzheimer's disease, rheumatoid arthritis, osteoporosis, cataracts, other degenerative ophthalmic diseases, Parkinson's disease, vascular dementia, and several other chronic diseases (Luevano-Contreras and Chapman-Novakofski 2010). A comprehensive review of these chronic diseases is out of the scope of this chapter, and only a few of them will be described here.

13.3.1 AGEs and Cardiovascular Aging

Cardiac aging, an independent risk factor for cardiovascular disease, is associated with structural remodeling and functional decline of the heart (Chiao 2013). Several reports have proposed that during the aging process, AGEs are a major cause of cardiac and vascular dysfunction, and they are involved in the prognosis and severity of heart failure and predict cardiovascular disease mortality in older adults (Campbell et al. 2012; Simm 2013). Some of the mechanisms described for vascular dysfunction are an increase in myocardial stiffening through the cross-linking of elastin and collagen with the subsequent development of cardiac fibrosis, and stimulation of inflammation and OS through activation of RAGE (Tikellis et al. 2008). Additionally, vascular stiffening, diastolic dysfunction, endothelial dysfunction, and atherosclerotic plaque formation have also been reported (Zieman and Kass 2004).

Regarding cardiovascular mortality, Semba et al. reported that women aged 65 and older (n = 559) followed by 4.5 years in the highest quartile of CML had higher risk of dying of cardiovascular disease (Semba et al. 2009b). Furthermore, a study with postmenopausal women (n = 106) found that after adjustment for age, body mass index, insulin resistance indices, fasting glucose, and insulin levels, a significant correlation was found between AGEs and testosterone and free androgen indices (Diamanti-Kandarakis et al. 2010). Hence, from these reports, it appears that high concentrations of AGEs could be a risk factor for cardiovascular disease in older women.

13.3.2 AGEs and Sarcopenia

Sarcopenia is common in older people, and it is associated with a progressive decline in muscle mass quality and strength, decrease in functional performance, higher risk of falls, and an increased mobility disability (Candow and Chilibeck 2005). In addition, reduced muscle mass in elderly individuals has been associated with decreased survival rates following critical illness. Muscle atrophy could result from a reduction in the size and number of muscle fibers due to several processes, such as physical inactivity, inadequate nutrition, OS, and hormonal changes (Sakuma et al. 2014). Sarcopenia could be at least partly explained by an upregulation of oxidative metabolism and an ensuing increase in abnormal ROS (Mosoni et al. 2004). The accumulation of ROS can induce higher rates of cellular damage to essential substances such as DNA, proteins, and lipid-containing structures (Fulle et al. 2004). Older adults have increased cross-linking of collagen and deposition of AGEs in skeletal muscle that also with glycation-related cross-linking of intramuscular connective tissue may contribute to altered muscle force transmission and muscle function with healthy aging. In aging animals, the increased muscle stiffness and the reduced muscle function are associated with cross-linking of collagen in muscle, tendons, and cartilages (Haus et al. 2007). AGEs may also play a role in sarcopenia through upregulation of inflammation and endothelial dysfunction in the microcirculation of skeletal muscle through RAGE (Semba et al. 2010). In older community-dwelling adults, elevated circulating CML was independently associated with low grip strength and greater muscle weakness (Dalal et al. 2009), and subjects with higher CML were at an increased risk of developing severe walking disability (Sun et al. 2012).

13.3.3 AGEs and Cancer

The incidence of some types of cancer exponentially increases with age, yet the reason is not fully understood. However, the evidence points toward an accumulation of genetic alterations (Adams et al. 2015). Some *in vitro* studies implied a potential role of AGEs in cancer proliferation, migration, and invasion of cell lines of breast, prostate, and lung cancer (Palimeri et al. 2015). Moreover, an epidemiological study found an association between the soluble AGEs receptors and the risk of pancreatic cancer (Jiao et al. 2011).

13.4 Dietary AGEs and Aging

In addition to endogenous AGEs, mainly formed by cellular metabolism, dAGEs may also have a role in aging to a greater or lesser extent by several mechanisms. dAGEs form during heat-enhanced cooking, which promotes the Maillard reaction, adding a desirable flavor, color, and aroma to foods. There is growing evidence that the average Western diet is a plentiful source of exogenous AGEs (Chao et al. 2009; Uribarri et al. 2010).

Dietary AGEs can have an impact on health through several systematic mechanisms. They could not only increase circulating AGEs and accumulate in tissues, but also add to the inflammatory status observed in aging by directly acting as ligands for RAGE and activate major signal transduction pathways (Zill et al. 2003; Somoza et al. 2005). The dAGEs–RAGE interaction could increase the level of soluble signals such as cytokines and free radicals (Kislinger et al. 1999; Ramasamy et al. 2005), thus indirectly contributing to increase the prooxidant status and the inflammatory response, to deplete antioxidant defenses, to affect endothelial function, and to promote insulin resistance (Uribarri et al. 2011, 2014; Forbes et al. 2014).

The effects of dAGEs have been described in studies with animal models, in cross-sectional studies, and clinical trials, with dietary manipulation of the amount of dAGEs. First, it is important to describe some cross-sectional studies showing that dAGEs are associated with the levels of circulating AGEs (cAGEs), mainly CML and MG. Uribarri et al. compared healthy older adults (60–80 years, $n = 56$) with younger adults (18–45 years, $n = 116$), and estimated the amount of dAGEs from 3 days food records using a database with the content of AGEs in certain foods. They found that older adults had higher levels of CML and MG, as well as inflammation and OS markers when compared with their younger counterparts. Serum AGEs correlated with the homeostatic model assessment (HOMA, a measure of insulin resistance), and with levels of 8-isoprostanes, a lipoxidation marker. Moreover, dAGEs correlated with CML, MG, and C-reactive protein (Uribarri et al. 2007). Furthermore, a study in healthy subjects (n = 325) and patients with kidney disease (n = 66) found a positive correlation between CML and dAGEs. Older participants (>60 years) had higher levels of CML and MG than the younger group (18–45 years) (Vlassara et al. 2009a). More recently, Uribarri et al. (2014) studied the influence of dAGEs in an older group (>60 years) (n = 67) and found that dAGEs directly correlated with cCML (r = 0.6), cMG (0.5), tumor necrosis factor alpha (TNF-alpha) (r = 0.5), vascular cellular adhesion molecule 1 (VCAM-1) (r = 0.46), 8-isoprostanes (r = 0.44), and mRNA RAGE (r = 0.45) and inversely correlated with adiponectin and inflammatory protein, (r = −0.3) (correlations had a p-value < 0.05). From these cross-sectional studies, it could be concluded that dAGEs measured by dietary records correlated with circulating levels of AGEs, inflammatory markers, OS markers, and mRNA RAGE, and that CML levels are higher in the older groups studied.

Besides these cross-sectional data, interventional and prospective studies have been conducted to evaluate the effect of low-AGE diets on chronic diseases associated with aging. For instance, a study with 18 nondiabetic patients with renal failure on maintenance peritoneal dialysis found a reduction of 34% in serum CML and 35% reduction in MG when dAGEs intake was reduced for 4 weeks. In contrast, the subjects with high dAGEs intake had an elevation of serum CML, MG, and CML-LDL by 29%, 26%, and 50%, respectively (Uribarri et al. 2003). In a similar study, a decrease in levels of cAGEs, MG, and C-reactive protein was observed in the low-AGE diet compared with the highAGE diet (approximately 35%, 44%, and 17%, respectively; $P < 0.03$) (Peppa et al. 2004). A long-term intervention on the effects of dAGEs (4 months) included subjects with diabetes and also an older healthy subjects group (n = 18) with an average age of 67 ± 1.7 years. The older group was randomized to follow either a low-AGEs diet or their usual dAGE intake, and the group with restricted dAGEs had lower levels of serum CML, MG, 8-isoprostanes, and TNF-alpha when compared with the subjects with the regular dAGE intake. Additionally, the group with restricted dAGEs and diabetes had a decrease in insulin resistance measured by the HOMA (Uribarri et al. 2011).

Regarding the role of dAGEs in cancer, a relationship between dAGEs and pancreatic cancer has been proposed in the NIH-AARP (National Health Institute-American Association for Retired Persons) Diet and Health Study, a prospective study in adults 50–70 years of age. Men in the fifth quintile of CML-AGE consumption had increased pancreatic cancer risk (hazards ratio [HR]: 1.43; 95% confidence interval [CI]: 1.06, 1.93, p = 0.003) but not women (HR: 1.14; 95% CI: 0.76, 1.72, p = 0.42). Additionally, men in the highest quintile of red meat consumption had a higher risk of pancreatic cancer (HR: 1.35; 95% CI: 1.07, 1.70). However, after adjustment for CML-AGE consumption, the HR decreased to 1.20 (95% CI: 0.95, 1.53) (Jiao et al. 2015). Even when the mechanism is not fully understood, it is important to further explore the relation of high dAGE intake and incidence of other types of cancers.

13.5 Accumulation of dAGEs, Role of Decline of Renal Function, and Impairment in AGE Detoxification System with Aging

In addition to the evidence showing that dietary manipulation modifies circulating AGEs, it is important to discuss a study by Roncero-Ramos et al. addressing tissue accumulation of dAGEs in an animal model. They fed weaning rats with different fractions and amounts of CML for 88 days. It was found that the heart and tail tendons of rats had a higher concentration of CML in the group with the higher intake of CML. The correlation between CML intake and the concentration in the heart was 0.41 (p = 0.02). Despite the use of an animal model, and following rats for only 3 months, these results support that high intake of dAGEs could lead to their accumulation in target tissues affected by chronic diseases common in aging (Roncero-Ramos et al. 2013). Other animal studies have also found an accumulation of dAGEs in liver, bladder, and kidneys (Germond et al. 1987). Moreover, Grossin et al. studied wild-type and RAGE knockout mice (used as a model of vascular aging) to observe the long-term effects of CML-enriched diet and RAGE in aortic aging. Mice followed either a control diet or CML-enriched diets (50, 100, or 200 μg CML/g of food) during 9 months. In the mice fed with CML diets, endothelium-dependent relaxation was reduced, RAGE and VCAM-1 expression were increased in the aortic wall, and the aortic pulse wave velocity was increased. The RAGE-knockout mice were protected against CML-enriched diet–induced endothelial dysfunction. The authors conclude that CML-enriched diets induced endothelial dysfunction and accelerated the development of arterial aging in a RAGE-dependent manner (Grossin et al. 2015).

13.5.1 Decline in Renal Function with Aging

Glomerular filtration rate (GFR, an index of kidney function) declines progressively with age by about 1 mL/min/year (Stevens et al. 2006). According to results from the Baltimore Longitudinal Study, which has one of the best descriptions of the course of renal function with aging, GFR declines 1.51 mL/min/1.73m^2 after the age of 80 years (Vlassara et al. 2009b). However, this decrease in the elderly is variable, with some retaining effective kidney clearance rates and others progressing to chronic kidney disease (CKD), which then impacts the quality of life and increases overall morbidity and mortality (Bonner et al. 2013). It is not clear if the accumulation of AGEs could be a consequence of the decline of renal function or a cause of such decline. It has been found that serum AGEs correlated directly with levels of inflammatory and OS markers, and inversely with serum creatinine (Linden et al. 2008). The kidney is the main site for the excretion of AGEs, and a mild decrease in renal function may be associated with the increased levels observed in the older population. Indeed, two important longitudinal studies, the Women's Health and Aging Study I in Baltimore and the InCHIANTI study in Tuscany found elevated plasma CML in subjects older than 64 years. CML levels were associated with CKD and the estimated GFR, at baseline and during follow-ups (Semba et al. 2009a, 2009c).

The accumulation of AGEs with the slowly progressive decrease in renal function in aging may induce a release of inflammatory mediators and the generation of ROS before the decrease in kidney function becomes clinically evident (Oberg et al. 2004). CKD in aging is also associated with increased levels of interleukin 6, C-reactive protein, and other markers of inflammation. Thus, the CKD of aging is associated with an inflammatory state, which may be associated with the general increase in OS noted with aging (Fried et al. 2006).

13.5.2 AGE Detoxification

A decreased renal function with aging could explain the increased OS found in older populations because it has been proposed that AGEs removal through AGE receptor-1 (AGER1) may depend on kidney excretion (Vlassara et al. 2012). Indeed, in nonobese diabetic mice, high tissue AGE levels and kidney disease were associated with low expression of AGER1 in the kidney (Huebschmann et al. 2006). Furthermore, human circulating mononuclear cells from subjects with diabetes and severe diabetes complications showed low expression of AGER1 and high serum AGEs (He et al. 2001). Supporting this evidence, Vlassara et al. found that dietary, serum, and urine AGEs correlated positively with peripheral mononuclear cell AGER1 levels in older healthy participants, and AGER1 was suppressed in CKD subjects, whereas receptors for AGE and TNF-alpha were increased. Therefore, it can be concluded that the defense mechanism exerted by AGER1 is lost in patients with diabetes mellitus and its efficiency decreased with aging and CKD (Vlassara and Striker 2011). The cause of AGER1 downregulation in aging remains to be elucidated; however, this effect is reversible by consumption of an AGE-restricted diet in both humans and mice (Cai et al. 2007, 2008; Vlassara et al. 2009a; Uribarri et al. 2011). Indeed, Cai et al. found a restored level of AGER1 by reducing dAGEs in an animal study, whereas in patients with type 2 diabetes, the suppressed expression and function of AGER1 increased after dAGEs restriction (Uribarri et al. 2011). Similarly, a study of healthy adults (18–45 and >60 years old) and CKD patients found that a moderate (30%–50%) reduction of dAGEs reduced the normal baseline levels of serum AGEs, OS, and inflammation and restored the levels of AGER1, in healthy and aging subjects and CKD patients (Vlassara et al. 2009a).

From this evidence, it is important to recognize that dAGEs contribute to the body's AGE pool, and that restriction of dAGEs could have a significant role in decreasing circulating AGEs. In addition, the function of AGER1, fundamental on the AGEs detoxification system, that could be affected in the older population is restored after a low-AGE diet. (Sebekova et al. 2001; Vlassara et al. 2002; Uribarri et al. 2005, 2007) (Figure 13.2).

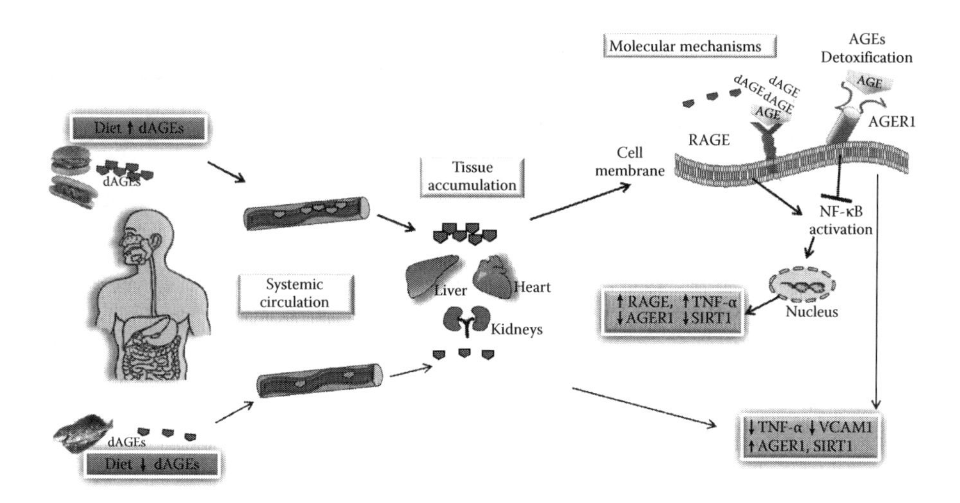

FIGURE 13.2 A high dAGEs intake could increase circulating AGEs and accumulate in tissues, also they could act as ligands for RAGE. dAGEs–RAGE interaction could increase the transcription levels of TNF-alpha and RAGE and decrease AGER1 and SIRT 1. A diet low in AGEs decreased the levels of inflammation markers and restores AGER1 and SIRT 1 values. TNF-alpha, tumor necrosis factor alpha; dAGEs, dietary advanced glycation end products; RAGE, receptor for advanced glycation end products; AGER1, advanced glycation end products receptor 1; SIRT 1, silent mating type information regulation 2 homolog 1.

13.6 Caloric Restriction or dAGE Restriction?

It seems clear that several intervention studies with the objective of reducing dAGEs have had successful results on decreasing inflammatory markers, OS markers, and insulin resistance, which are associated with chronic diseases common in aging, yet is not clear if reducing dAGEs could have an impact on lifespan. Some animal studies have shown promising results, but there is a lack of epidemiological studies showing similar results.

Calorie restriction (CR) increases lifespan in *Caenorhabditis elegans* and mice; several centenarian populations have been studied, and they have one thing in common: a lower calorie intake (Luevano-Contreras and Chapman-Novakofski 2010).

The mechanism by which CR (30%–40%) delays the aging process remains to be fully elucidated. It has been proposed that CR is involved in regulating cellular and systemic redox status and in modulating gene expression related to macromolecules and organelle turnover, energy metabolism, and cell death and survival. CR can reduce the incidence of mitochondrial abnormalities and attenuates OS, which could be considered as protective effects (Shimokawa 2008).

Positive effects of CR in mice could be explained in part by a decrease in the intake of AGEs and the concomitant decrease of OS (Cai et al. 2007). To prove this hypothesis, Cai et al. studied if reduction on CR would have an impact on reducing AGE intake and if this could explain benefits of CR in mice. They randomized mice to three different diets (n = 22 per group): regular, CR, and CR-high-AGE diet. The group with CR had a longer lifespan in comparison with the other two groups. Furthermore, mice in the CR-high-AGE diet had increased OS, accelerated aging-related cardiovascular and renal disease, and a shorter lifespan than mice in the regular diet (Cai et al. 2007). To further prove that AGEs restriction has similar effects than CR, they assigned mice to two different diets, a regular diet high in AGEs and a restricted diet in AGEs but with the same caloric intake. The mice in the low-AGE diet had a longer lifespan and also increased AGER1 expression, whereas mice in high-AGE diets developed insulin resistance, decreased AGER1, increased RAGE, fibrosis in the heart and kidney, a reduced glutathione/oxidized glutathione ratio, and increased serum 8-isoprostane (Cai et al. 2008). The mechanisms by which restriction of AGEs competes with CR effects remain to be fully elucidated.

Although there are a few human studies showing the effects of CR on circulating AGEs, two clinical studies have found that after a few months of CR, levels of circulating CML were reduced in overweight or obese subjects. For instance, Rodriguez et al. studied 47 overweight and obese premenopausal women who underwent CR (20 kcal/kg initial weight) with a Mediterranean-type diet for 3 months. They found reduced levels of CML and insulin resistance measured by HOMA in 17 women compliant to the diet (Rodriguez et al. 2015). Moreover, Gugliucci et al. studied 37 overweight and obese subjects undergoing a low-calorie diet for 2 months and also found a decrease in AGEs. However, dAGEs were not measured in the diets, and it is not possible to know if these results were due to CR or dAGE restriction (Gugliucci et al. 2009).

In contrast, Uribarri et al. reduced dAGEs and maintained calorie intake in a long-term (4 months) interventional study with 18 healthy participants (>60 years) who were randomized to either a low-dAGE diet or their usual diet (n = 8) without CR (Uribarri et al. 2014). Consistently with other studies, in the group with dAGE restriction, there was a decrease in circulating CML, MG, 8-isoprostanes, mononuclear cells TNF-alpha protein, full-length RAGE, and AGER1 mRNA. Of special interest was the increase in SIRT1 mRNA and mononuclear cells PPAR γ protein levels in the restricted dAGEs group. SIRT 1 had a negative correlation ($r = -0.510$, $p = 0.001$) with dAGEs independent of calories and other macronutrients. Also, the protein levels of the anti-inflammatory nuclear receptor PPARγ correlated negatively with dAGEs and circulating AGEs, and after dAGE restriction, these levels significantly increased by 50%. SIRT 1, a member of the sirtuin family, is a key regulator of signaling and transcription factors, including the insulin receptor and its substrates, which also regulates inflammatory responses in mononuclear cells and macrophages.

SIRT 1 activity is suppressed in OS conditions such as diabetes, cardiovascular disease, and aging. In patients with diabetes, a restriction in dAGEs also increases SIRT1 mRNA after 4 months of intervention (Uribarri et al. 2014). For this reason, it would be important to further explore whether the restriction of dAGEs alone is enough to restore SIRT 1, AGER1, and PPARγ levels in the elderly population as well as in subjects with chronic diseases associated with aging.

13.7 Conclusions

In summary, AGEs from dietary supply and endogenous production lead to increased circulatory levels of AGEs and their accumulation in tissues that together with impairment in the detoxification system may contribute to increased OS, an inflammatory status and a decrease in the defense systems (AGER1, SIRT1) observed in the elderly.

Nonetheless, at least one study restricting dAGEs in healthy elderly has not found changes in inflammatory or oxidation markers (Semba et al. 2014), although they found an association between the consumption of AGEs and their circulatory levels.

Therefore, until proper inhibitors of glycation are found, restricting dAGEs could be a promising intervention in chronic diseases associated with aging as well as a prevention tool for healthy elderly.

REFERENCES

Adams, P. D., H. Jasper, and K. L. Rudolph. 2015. Aging-induced stem cell mutations as drivers for disease and cancer. *Cell Stem Cell* 16 (6):601–12. doi: 10.1016/j.stem.2015.05.002.

Ahmed, N. 2005. Advanced glycation endproducts—Role in pathology of diabetic complications. *Diabetes Res Clin Pract* 67 (1):3–21. doi: 10.1016/j.diabres.2004.09.004.

Bonner, A., M. Caltabiano, and L. Berlund. 2013. Quality of life, fatigue, and activity in Australians with chronic kidney disease: A longitudinal study. *Nurs Health Sci* 15 (3):360–7. doi: 10.1111/nhs.12038.

Brownlee, M. 1995. Advanced protein glycosylation in diabetes and aging. *Annu Rev Med* 46:223–34. doi: 10.1146/annurev.med.46.1.223.

Cai, W., J. C. He, L. Zhu, X. Chen, S. Wallenstein, G. E. Striker, and H. Vlassara. 2007. Reduced oxidant stress and extended lifespan in mice exposed to a low glycotoxin diet: Association with increased AGER1 expression. *Am J Pathol* 170 (6):1893–902. doi: 10.2353/ajpath.2007.061281.

Cai, W., J. C. He, L. Zhu, X. Chen, F. Zheng, G. E. Striker, and H. Vlassara. 2008. Oral glycotoxins determine the effects of calorie restriction on oxidant stress, age-related diseases, and lifespan. *Am J Pathol* 173 (2):327–36. doi: 10.2353/ajpath.2008.080152.

Campbell, D. J., J. B. Somaratne, A. J. Jenkins, D. L. Prior, M. Yii, J. F. Kenny, A. E. Newcomb, C. G. Schalkwijk, M. J. Black, and D. J. Kelly. 2012. Diastolic dysfunction of aging is independent of myocardial structure but associated with plasma advanced glycation end-product levels. *PLoS One* 7 (11):e49813. doi: 10.1371/journal.pone.0049813.

Candow, D. G., and P. D. Chilibeck. 2005. Differences in size, strength, and power of upper and lower body muscle groups in young and older men. *J Gerontol A Biol Sci Med Sci* 60 (2):148–56.

Cerami, A. 1985. Hypothesis. Glucose as a mediator of aging. *J Am Geriatr Soc* 33 (9):626–34.

Chao, P.-C., C.-C. Hsu, and M.-C. Yin. 2009. Analysis of glycative products in sauces and sauce-treated foods. *Food Chemistry* 113 (1):262–6. doi: 10.1016/j.foodchem.2008.06.076.

Chiao, Y. A. 2013. MicroRNA-34a: A new piece in the cardiac aging puzzle. *Circ Cardiovasc Genet* 6 (4):437–8. doi: 10.1161/CIRCGENETICS.113.000277.

Chondrogianni, N., and E. S. Gonos. 2005. Proteasome dysfunction in mammalian aging: Steps and factors involved. *Exp Gerontol* 40 (12):931–8. doi: 10.1016/j.exger.2005.09.004.

Dalal, M., L. Ferrucci, K. Sun, J. Beck, L. P. Fried, and R. D. Semba. 2009. Elevated serum advanced glycation end products and poor grip strength in older community-dwelling women. *J Gerontol A Biol Sci Med Sci* 64 (1):132–7. doi: 10.1093/gerona/gln018.

Diamanti-Kandarakis, E., I. Lambrinoudaki, F. Economou, M. Christou, C. Piperi, A. G. Papavassiliou, and G. Creatsas. 2010. Androgens associated with advanced glycation end-products in postmenopausal women. *Menopause* 17 (6):1182–7. doi: 10.1097/gme.0b013e3181e170af.

Forbes, J. M., K. C. Sourris, M. P. de Courten, S. L. Dougherty, V. Chand, J. G. Lyons, D. Bertovic, et al. 2014. Advanced glycation end products (AGEs) are cross-sectionally associated with insulin secretion in healthy subjects. *Amino Acids* 46 (2):321–6. doi: 10.1007/s00726-013-1542-9.

Franceschi, C., M. Bonafe, S. Valensin, F. Olivieri, M. De Luca, E. Ottaviani, and G. De Benedictis. 2000. Inflamm-aging. An evolutionary perspective on immunosenescence. *Ann N Y Acad Sci* 908:244–54.

Fried, L. F., J. S. Lee, M. Shlipak, G. M. Chertow, C. Green, J. Ding, T. Harris, and A. B. Newman. 2006. Chronic kidney disease and functional limitation in older people: Health, aging and body composition study. *J Am Geriatr Soc* 54 (5):750–6. doi: 10.1111/j.1532-5415.2006.00727.x.

Fulle, S., F. Protasi, G. Di Tano, T. Pietrangelo, A. Beltramin, S. Boncompagni, L. Vecchiet, and G. Fano. 2004. The contribution of reactive oxygen species to sarcopenia and muscle ageing. *Exp Gerontol* 39 (1):17–24.

Germond, J. E., G. Philippossian, U. Richli, I. Bracco, and M. J. Arnaud. 1987. Rapid and complete urinary elimination of [14C]-5-hydroxymethyl-2-furaldehyde administered orally or intravenously to rats. *J Toxicol Environ Health* 22 (1):79–89. doi: 10.1080/15287398709531052.

Grossin, N., F. Auger, C. Niquet-Leridon, N. Durieux, D. Montaigne, A. M. Schmidt, S. Susen, et al. 2015. Dietary CML-enriched protein induces functional arterial aging in a RAGE-dependent manner in mice. *Mol Nutr Food Res* 59 (5):927–38. doi: 10.1002/mnfr.201400643.

Gugliucci, A., K. Kotani, J. Taing, Y. Matsuoka, Y. Sano, M. Yoshimura, K. Egawa, et al. 2009. Short-term low calorie diet intervention reduces serum advanced glycation end products in healthy overweight or obese adults. *Ann Nutr Metab* 54 (3):197–201. doi: 10.1159/000217817.

Harman, D. 2006. Free radical theory of aging: An update: Increasing the functional life span. *Ann N Y Acad Sci* 1067:10–21. doi: 10.1196/annals.1354.003.

Haus, J. M., J. A. Carrithers, S. W. Trappe, and T. A. Trappe. 2007. Collagen, cross-linking, and advanced glycation end products in aging human skeletal muscle. *J Appl Physiol (1985)* 103 (6):2068–76. doi: 10.1152/japplphysiol.00670.2007.

He, C. J., T. Koschinsky, C. Buenting, and H. Vlassara. 2001. Presence of diabetic complications in type 1 diabetic patients correlates with low expression of mononuclear cell AGE-receptor-1 and elevated serum AGE. *Mol Med* 7 (3):159–68.

Hipkiss, A. R. 2006. Accumulation of altered proteins and ageing: Causes and effects. *Exp Gerontol* 41 (5):464–73. doi: 10.1016/j.exger.2006.03.004.

Huebschmann, A. G., J. G. Regensteiner, H. Vlassara, and J. E. Reusch. 2006. Diabetes and advanced glycoxidation end products. *Diabetes Care* 29 (6):1420–32. doi: 10.2337/dc05-2096.

Jiao, L., R. Stolzenberg-Solomon, T. P. Zimmerman, Z. Duan, L. Chen, L. Kahle, A. Risch, et al. 2015. Dietary consumption of advanced glycation end products and pancreatic cancer in the prospective NIH-AARP diet and health study. *Am J Clin Nutr* 101 (1):126–34. doi: 10.3945/ajcn.114.098061.

Jiao, L., S. J. Weinstein, D. Albanes, P. R. Taylor, B. I. Graubard, J. Virtamo, and R. Z. Stolzenberg-Solomon. 2011. Evidence that serum levels of the soluble receptor for advanced glycation end products are inversely associated with pancreatic cancer risk: A prospective study. *Cancer Res* 71 (10):3582–9. doi: 10.1158/0008-5472.CAN-10-2573.

Kislinger, T., C. Fu, B. Huber, W. Qu, A. Taguchi, S. Du Yan, M. Hofmann, et al. 1999. N(epsilon)-(carboxymethyl)lysine adducts of proteins are ligands for receptor for advanced glycation end products that activate cell signaling pathways and modulate gene expression. *J Biol Chem* 274 (44):31740–9.

Kristal, B. S., and B. P. Yu. 1992. An emerging hypothesis: Synergistic induction of aging by free radicals and Maillard reactions. *J Gerontol* 47 (4):B107–14.

Levine, R. L. 2002. Carbonyl modified proteins in cellular regulation, aging, and disease. *Free Radic Biol Med* 32 (9):790–6.

Linden, E., W. Cai, J. C. He, C. Xue, Z. Li, J. Winston, H. Vlassara, and J. Uribarri. 2008. Endothelial dysfunction in patients with chronic kidney disease results from advanced glycation end products (AGE)-mediated inhibition of endothelial nitric oxide synthase through RAGE activation. *Clin J Am Soc Nephrol* 3 (3):691–8. doi: 10.2215/CJN.04291007.

Luevano-Contreras, C., and K. Chapman-Novakofski. 2010. Dietary advanced glycation end products and aging. *Nutrients* 2 (12):1247–65. doi: 10.3390/nu2121247.

Medvedev, Z. A. 1990. An attempt at a rational classification of theories of ageing. *Biol Rev Camb Philos Soc* 65 (3):375–98.

Mosoni, L., D. Breuille, C. Buffiere, C. Obled, and P. P. Mirand. 2004. Age-related changes in glutathione availability and skeletal muscle carbonyl content in healthy rats. *Exp Gerontol* 39 (2):203–10. doi: 10.1016/j.exger.2003.10.014.

Oberg, B. P., E. McMenamin, F. L. Lucas, E. McMonagle, J. Morrow, T. A. Ikizler, and J. Himmelfarb. 2004. Increased prevalence of oxidant stress and inflammation in patients with moderate to severe chronic kidney disease. *Kidney Int* 65 (3):1009–16. doi: 10.1111/j.1523-1755.2004.00465.x.

Oeppen, J., and J. W. Vaupel. 2002. Demography. Broken limits to life expectancy. *Science* 296 (5570):1029–31. doi: 10.1126/science.1069675.

Palimeri, S., E. Palioura, and E. Diamanti-Kandarakis. 2015. Current perspectives on the health risks associated with the consumption of advanced glycation end products: Recommendations for dietary management. *Diabetes Metab Syndr Obes* 8:415–26. doi: 10.2147/DMSO.S63089.

Peppa, M., J. Uribarri, W. Cai, M. Lu, and H. Vlassara. 2004. Glycoxidation and inflammation in renal failure patients. *Am J Kidney Dis* 43 (4):690–5.

Rabbani, N., and P. J. Thornalley. 2008. The dicarbonyl proteome: Proteins susceptible to dicarbonyl glycation at functional sites in health, aging, and disease. *Ann N Y Acad Sci* 1126:124–7. doi: 10.1196/annals.1433.043.

Ramasamy, R., S. J. Vannucci, S. S. Yan, K. Herold, S. F. Yan, and A. M. Schmidt. 2005. Advanced glycation end products and RAGE: A common thread in aging, diabetes, neurodegeneration, and inflammation. *Glycobiology* 15 (7):16R–28R. doi: 10.1093/glycob/cwi053.

Rodriguez, J. M., L. Leiva Balich, M. J. Concha, C. Mizon, D. Bunout Barnett, G. Barrera Acevedo, S. Hirsch Birn, et al. 2015. Reduction of serum advanced glycation end-products with a low calorie Mediterranean diet. *Nutr Hosp* 31 (6):2511–17. doi: 10.3305/nh.2015.31.6.8936.

Roncero-Ramos, I., C. Delgado-Andrade, F. J. Tessier, C. Niquet-Leridon, C. Strauch, V. M. Monnier, and M. P. Navarro. 2013. Metabolic transit of N(epsilon)-carboxymethyl-lysine after consumption of AGEs from bread crust. *Food Funct.* 4(7):1032–1039. doi: 10.1039/c3fo30351a.

Sakuma, K., W. Aoi, and A. Yamaguchi. 2014. The intriguing regulators of muscle mass in sarcopenia and muscular dystrophy. *Front Aging Neurosci* 6:230. doi: 10.3389/fnagi.2014.00230.

Sebekova, K., M. Krajcoviova-Kudlackova, R. Schinzel, V. Faist, J. Klvanova, and A. Heidland. 2001. Plasma levels of advanced glycation end products in healthy, long-term vegetarians and subjects on a western mixed diet. *Eur J Nutr* 40 (6):275–81.

Semba, R. D., L. Ferrucci, J. C. Fink, K. Sun, J. Beck, M. Dalal, J. M. Guralnik, and L. P. Fried. 2009a. Advanced glycation end products and their circulating receptors and level of kidney function in older community-dwelling women. *Am J Kidney Dis* 53 (1):51–8. doi: 10.1053/j.ajkd.2008.06.018.

Semba, R. D., L. Ferrucci, K. Sun, J. Beck, M. Dalal, R. Varadhan, J. Walston, J. M. Guralnik, and L. P. Fried. 2009b. Advanced glycation end products and their circulating receptors predict cardiovascular disease mortality in older community-dwelling women. *Aging Clin Exp Res* 21 (2):182–90.

Semba, R. D., J. C. Fink, K. Sun, S. Bandinelli, J. M. Guralnik, and L. Ferrucci. 2009c. Carboxymethyl-lysine, an advanced glycation end product, and decline of renal function in older community-dwelling adults. *Eur J Nutr* 48 (1):38–44. doi: 10.1007/s00394-008-0757-0.

Semba, R. D., S. K. Gebauer, D. J. Baer, K. Sun, R. Turner, H. A. Silber, S. Talegawkar, L. Ferrucci, and J. A. Novotny. 2014. Dietary intake of advanced glycation end products did not affect endothelial function and inflammation in healthy adults in a randomized controlled trial. *J Nutr* 144 (7):1037–42. doi: 10.3945/jn.113.189480.

Semba, R. D., E. J. Nicklett, and L. Ferrucci. 2010. Does accumulation of advanced glycation end products contribute to the aging phenotype? *J Gerontol A Biol Sci Med Sci* 65 (9):963–75. doi: 10.1093/gerona/glq074.

Shimokawa, I., Chiba, T., Yamaza, H., & Komatsu, T. 2008. Longevity genes: insights from calorie restriction and genetic longevity models. *Molecules & Cells*, Springer Science & Business Media BV, 26(5):427–435.

Simm, A. 2013. Protein glycation during aging and in cardiovascular disease. *J Proteomics* 92:248–59. doi: 10.1016/j.jprot.2013.05.012.

Simm, A., B. Muller, N. Nass, B. Hofmann, H. Bushnaq, R. E. Silber, and B. Bartling. 2015. Protein glycation - Between tissue aging and protection. *Exp Gerontol* 68:71–5. doi: 10.1016/j.exger.2014.12.013.

Somoza, V., M. Lindenmeier, T. Hofmann, O. Frank, H. F. Erbersdobler, J. W. Baynes, S. R. Thorpe, et al. 2005. Dietary bread crust advanced glycation end products bind to the receptor for AGEs in HEK-293 kidney cells but are rapidly excreted after oral administration to healthy and subtotally nephrectomized rats. *Ann N Y Acad Sci* 1043:492–500. doi: 10.1196/annals.1333.056.

Stevens, L. A., T. Greene, and A. S. Levey. 2006. Surrogate end points for clinical trials of kidney disease progression. *Clin J Am Soc Nephrol* 1 (4):874–84. doi: 10.2215/CJN.00600206.

Sun, K., R. D. Semba, L. P. Fried, D. A. Schaumberg, L. Ferrucci, and R. Varadhan. 2012. Elevated serum carboxymethyl-Lysine, an advanced glycation end product, predicts severe walking disability in older women: The women's health and aging study I. *J Aging Res* 2012:586385. doi: 10.1155/2012/586385.

Tikellis, C., M. C. Thomas, B. E. Harcourt, M. T. Coughlan, J. Pete, K. Bialkowski, A. Tan, A. Bierhaus, M. E. Cooper, and J. M. Forbes. 2008. Cardiac inflammation associated with a Western diet is mediated via activation of RAGE by AGEs. *Am J Physiol Endocrinol Metab* 295 (2):E323–30. doi: 10.1152/ajpendo.00024.2008.

Uribarri, J., W. Cai, M. Peppa, S. Goodman, L. Ferrucci, G. Striker, and H. Vlassara. 2007. Circulating glycotoxins and dietary advanced glycation endproducts: Two links to inflammatory response, oxidative stress, and aging. *J Gerontol A Biol Sci Med Sci* 62 (4):427–33.

Uribarri, J., W. Cai, R. Pyzik, S. Goodman, X. Chen, L. Zhu, M. Ramdas, G. E. Striker, and H. Vlassara. 2014. Suppression of native defense mechanisms, SIRT1 and PPARgamma, by dietary glycoxidants precedes disease in adult humans; relevance to lifestyle-engendered chronic diseases. *Amino Acids* 46 (2):301–9. doi: 10.1007/s00726-013-1502-4.

Uribarri, J., W. Cai, M. Ramdas, S. Goodman, R. Pyzik, X. Chen, L. Zhu, G. E. Striker, and H. Vlassara. 2011. Restriction of advanced glycation end products improves insulin resistance in human type 2 diabetes: Potential role of AGER1 and SIRT1. *Diabetes Care* 34 (7):1610–16. doi: 10.2337/dc11-0091.

Uribarri, J., W. Cai, O. Sandu, M. Peppa, T. Goldberg, and H. Vlassara. 2005. Diet-derived advanced glycation end products are major contributors to the body's AGE pool and induce inflammation in healthy subjects. *Ann N Y Acad Sci* 1043:461–6. doi: 10.1196/annals.1333.052.

Uribarri. J., M. Peppa, W. Cai, T. Goldberg, M. Lu, S. Baliga, J. A. Vassalotti, and H. Vlassara. 2003. Dietary glycotoxins correlate with circulating advanced glycation end product levels in renal failure patients. *Am J Kidney Dis* 42 (3):532–8.

Uribarri, J., S. Woodruff, S. Goodman, W. Cai, X. Chen, R. Pyzik, A. Yong, G. E. Striker, and H. Vlassara. 2010. Advanced glycation end products in foods and a practical guide to their reduction in the diet. *J Am Diet Assoc* 110 (6):911–16. doi: 10.1016/j.jada.2010.03.018.

Van Puyvelde, K., T. Mets, R. Njemini, I. Beyer, and I. Bautmans. 2014. Effect of advanced glycation end product intake on inflammation and aging: A systematic review. *Nutr Rev* 72 (10):638–50. doi: 10.1111/nure.12141.

Vlassara, H., W. Cai, X. Chen, E. J. Serrano, M. S. Shobha, J. Uribarri, M. Woodward, and G. E. Striker. 2012. Managing chronic inflammation in the aging diabetic patient with CKD by diet or sevelamer carbonate: A modern paradigm shift. *J Gerontol A Biol Sci Med Sci* 67 (12):1410–16. doi: 10.1093/gerona/gls195.

Vlassara, H., W. Cai, J. Crandall, T. Goldberg, R. Oberstein, V. Dardaine, M. Peppa, and E. J. Rayfield. 2002. Inflammatory mediators are induced by dietary glycotoxins, a major risk factor for diabetic angiopathy. *Proc Natl Acad Sci U S A* 99 (24):15596–601. doi: 10.1073/pnas.242407999.

Vlassara, H., W. Cai, S. Goodman, R. Pyzik, A. Yong, X. Chen, L. Zhu, et al. 2009a. Protection against loss of innate defenses in adulthood by low advanced glycation end products (AGE) intake: Role of the anti-inflammatory AGE receptor-1. *J Clin Endocrinol Metab* 94 (11):4483–91. doi: 10.1210/jc.2009-0089.

Vlassara, H., and G. E. Striker. 2011. AGE restriction in diabetes mellitus: A paradigm shift. *Nat Rev Endocrinol* 7 (9):526–39. doi: 10.1038/nrendo.2011.74.

Vlassara, H., J. Uribarri, W. Cai, and G. Striker. 2008. Advanced glycation end product homeostasis: Exogenous oxidants and innate defenses. *Ann N Y Acad Sci* 1126:46–52. doi: 10.1196/annals.1433.055.

Vlassara, H., J. Uribarri, L. Ferrucci, W. Cai, M. Torreggiani, J. B. Post, F. Zheng, and G. E. Striker. 2009b. Identifying advanced glycation end products as a major source of oxidants in aging: Implications for the management and/or prevention of reduced renal function in elderly persons. *Semin Nephrol* 29 (6):594–603. doi: 10.1016/j.semnephrol.2009.07.013.

Zieman, S. J., and D. A. Kass. 2004. Advanced glycation endproduct crosslinking in the cardiovascular system: Potential therapeutic target for cardiovascular disease. *Drugs* 64 (5):459–70.

Zill, H., S. Bek, T. Hofmann, J. Huber, O. Frank, M. Lindenmeier, B. Weigle, et al. 2003. RAGE-mediated MAPK activation by food-derived AGE and non-AGE products. *Biochem Biophys Res Commun* 300 (2):311–15.

14

AGEs and Erectile Dysfunction: Any Role of Dietary AGEs?

Delminda Neves
Instituto de Investigação e Inovação em Saúde (I3S) Rua Alfredo Allen
Porto, Portugal

CONTENTS

KEY POINTS

- Erectile dysfunction is an early sign of cardiovascular disease and its prevalence is highly increased in the elderly and in diabetic and chronic kidney disease patients.
- Endothelial nitric oxide synthase–derived nitric oxide is fundamental in the mechanism of penile erection.
- Advanced glycation end products (AGEs) provided from diet are absorbed in the intestine and interact nonspecifically with proteins in the body.
- AGEs preferentially accumulate in the erectile tissue increasing oxidative damage and degradation of nitric oxide.
- Food antioxidants mitigate cavernous nitric oxide degradation and preserve erectile function.

14.1 Erectile Dysfunction Epidemiology

Erectile dysfunction (ED), defined as the inability to develop and maintain an erection for satisfactory sexual intercourse, is a highly prevalent disease affecting millions of men worldwide with a tendency for widespread increase. The Massachusetts Male Aging Study reported a global prevalence of 52% considering any degree of ED (Feldman et al. 1994). Although the direct causes of ED remain poorly understood and likely to be multifactorial in origin, several epidemiological studies evidenced risk factors for ED development. Among these studies, a recent report demonstrated that increasing age is the independent variable most strongly associated with ED (Ghalayini et al. 2010). Besides aging, obesity (defined by body mass index), diabetes mellitus (DM), hypertension, chronic kidney disease (CKD), coronary heart disease, and also psychological causes constitute major risk factors for the development of ED (Navaneethan et al. 2010; Shaeer et al. 2012).

14.2 ED Is an Early Marker of Systemic Vascular Disease

Analysis of epidemiological data evidences that ED shares important risk factors with cardiovascular disease (CVD), which supports the common etiology of these diseases. In fact, ED is highly prevalent among CVD patients, and it has been recently recognized as an early marker of CVD (Cheitlin 2004). ED is the manifestation of a hard to identify condition, endothelial dysfunction described below, which precedes atherosclerosis formation, a chronic inflammatory disease that develops over years and evolves to CVD (Lusis 2000).

14.3 Physiology of Erection

Sexual arousal is activated in higher cortical centers, which then stimulate the medial preoptic and paraventricular nuclei of the hypothalamus. Descending signals through the parasympathetic nervous system activate terminations in the sacral area. The development of an erection is a complex event that involves not only psychological and neurological stimuli but also endocrine, vascular, and local anatomic systems, particularly the highly vascularized corpora cavernosa that constitutes the erectile tissue of the penis that fills with blood during erection highly increasing their volume. Human corpus cavernosum (CC) has a sponge-like texture, exhibiting a mesh of interconnected cavernous sinusoidal spaces, lined by endothelium and separated by trabeculae composed mainly of smooth muscle and connective tissue (collagen fibers and fibroblasts) (Figure 14.1).

Transmission electron microscopy observation demonstrated that the proportion of connective tissue to smooth muscle cells (SMC) changes along aging, with a marked decrease in SMC (Tomada et al. 2008) (Figure 14.2). Histological observation of erectile tissue of patients with CVD risk

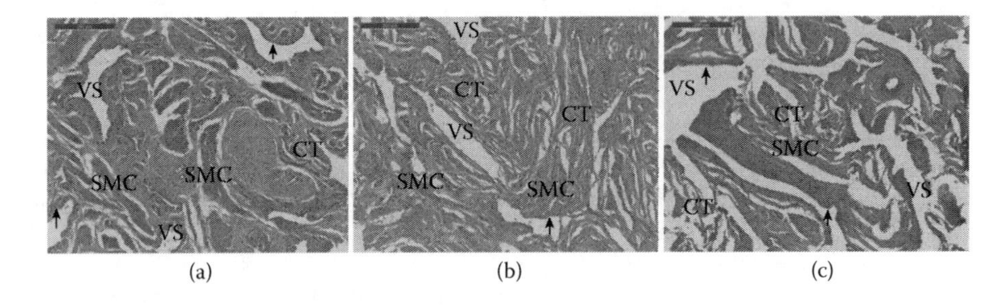

FIGURE 14.1 Hematoxylin and eosin staining of penile tissue from young (a), healthy aged (b) and patient with erectile dysfunction (c). Human cavernous tissue has a sponge-like structure, with cavernous vascular spaces (VS) lined by endothelium (arrow) and separated by trabeculae composed mainly of connective tissue (CT) and smooth muscle cells (SMC). Cavernous tissue from patients with erectile dysfunction presents structural disorganization and poorly limited VS.

factors and overt ED demonstrates structural disorganization and poorly limited vascular spaces (Figure 14.1).

The neuronal stimulus results in the inhibition of adrenergic tone and in the liberation of the nonadrenergic, noncholinergic neurotransmitter gaseous molecule nitric oxide (NO) from nerves synthesized by neuronal NO synthase (nNOS). Concomitantly, the increased blood flow on the luminal surface of the

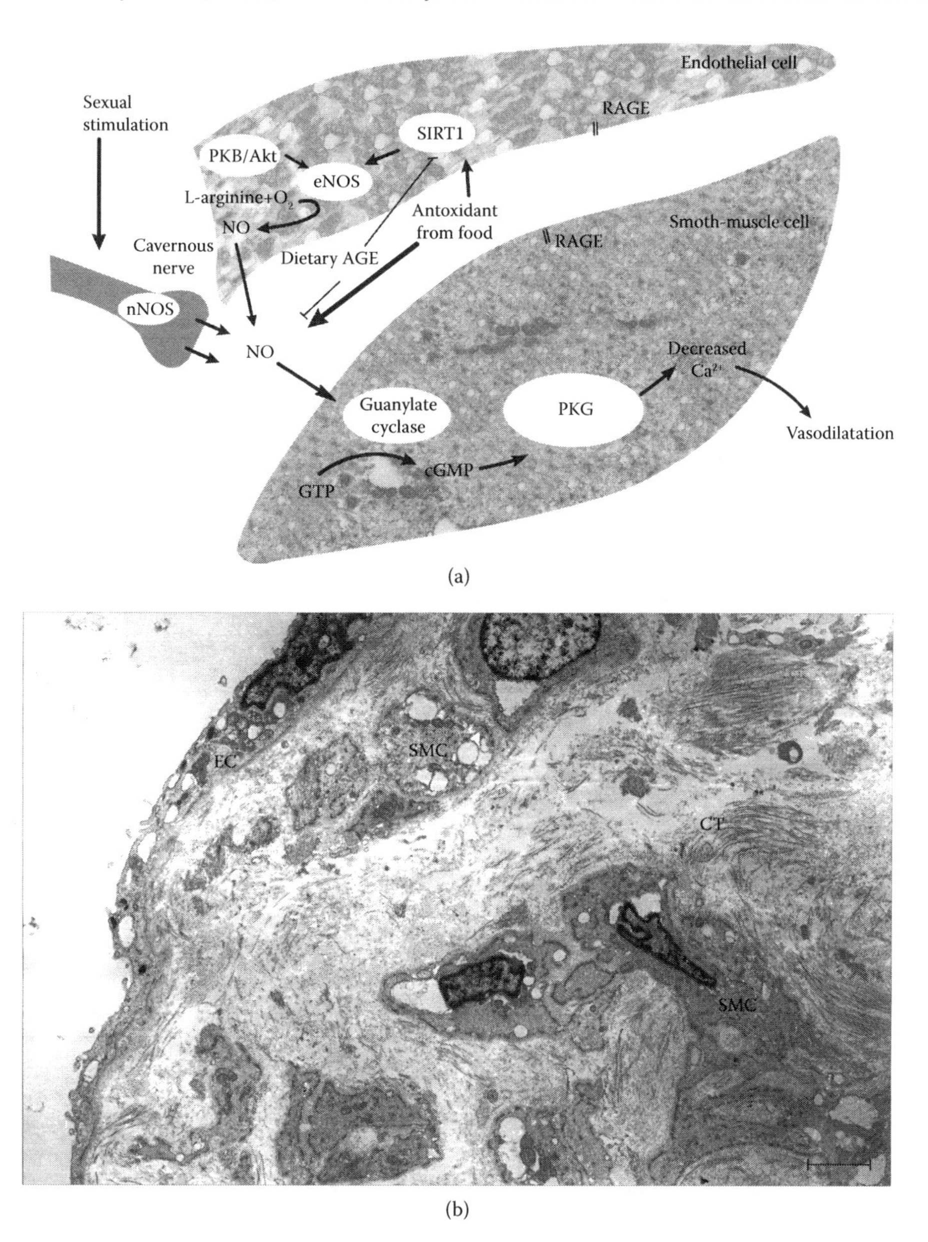

FIGURE 14.2 (a) Schematic representation of the erection mechanism. Sexual stimulus promotes synthesis of NO by nNOS. Concomitantly, PKB/Akt is activated and phosphorylates eNOS, promoting generation of NO. SIRT1 also activates eNOS by deacetylation. NO difuses to SMC, and thereby stimulates the conversion of GTP to cGMP by guanylate cyclase. cGMP activates PKG, further decreasing the intracellular calcium, which triggers the relaxation of smooth muscle, and ensuing vasodilatation. (b) Transmission electron microscopy image of the cavernous tissue of an aged healthy individual. Scale bar: 2 μm. cGMP, cyclic guanosine monophosphate; CT, connective tissue; EC, endothelial cell; GTP, guanosine triphosphate; eNOS, endothelial NO synthase; nNOS, neuronal NO synthase; NO, nitric oxide; PKB/Akt, protein kinase B; PKG, protein kinase G; RAGE, receptor of advanced glycation end products; SIRT1, Sirtuin1; SMC, smooth muscle cells.

penile vessels causes shear stress, which may lead to activation of protein kinase B (PKB/Akt) (Suzuki et al. 2014). This enzyme is the main activator of endothelial NO synthase (eNOS). Thus, while NO produced by nNOS initiates penile erection, NO generated by eNOS participates in the sustained erection required for normal sexual performance (Burnett et al. 1996). NO is easily diffusible to SMC, and NO stimulates the enzyme guanylate cyclase that converts guanosine triphosphate (GTP) to cyclic guanosine monophosphate (cGMP) (Figure 14.2). In turn, the increase in cGMP levels results in activation of protein kinase G and further decrease in intracellular calcium, which trigger the relaxation of both arterial and trabecular smooth muscle. Vasodilatation enhances arterial blood flow into the vascular spaces of the penis, and intracavernous pressure is further increased by blood entrapment in the corpora cavernosa by a veno-occlusion mechanism that results from the compression of the subtunical venules against the tunica albuginea (Ignarro et al. 1990).

14.4 Mechanisms of ED Onset

Endothelium and SMC strongly cooperate in the erectile process, while the former produces most of the NO, SMC support vasodilatation. Indeed, functional or structural modifications in endothelium, or loss of SMC, could result in ED. The most common form of ED presents vascular origin and directly results from vascular disease of the penile arteries, failure of the corporal veno-occlusive, or sinusoidal relax mechanisms. The last one is provoked by an endothelium-dependent inability to accomplish vasodilatation caused by impaired bioavailability of NO defined as endothelial dysfunction (Shamloul et al. 2013).

Among the risk factors for ED, most of them, in particular aging, DM, and CKD, constitute conditions that are strongly associated with an increase in oxidative stress (Stadtman 1992; Bonnefont-Rousselot et al. 2000), characterized by an imbalance between the production of reactive oxygen species (ROS) and the endogenous antioxidant defenses at cellular level. The increase in oxidative stress compromises NO bioavailability necessary to erectile function by direct reaction between ROS and NO. Prooxidative conditions also induce damage in the cavernous cells. In addition, it is now clear that oxidative stress promotes advanced glycation end products (AGEs) formation, and that in turn, AGEs induce oxidative stress, constituting a deleterious vicious cycle that highly compromises normal erectile function (Mohamed et al. 1999). AGEs primarily result from nonenzymatic glycation of proteins by the Maillard reaction that forms between free amino groups of amino acids and carboxylic groups of sugars. Glycated proteins further rearrange, dehydrate, condense, and cross-link through complex reactions. Degradation of these products could generate highly reactive carbonyl compounds (glyoxal and methylglyoxal), also formed during glycolysis or glucose auto-oxidation (Rabbani and Thornalley 2012). Not only proteins but also lipids and nucleic acids exposed to reducing sugars could suffer glycation or glycoxidation reactions. AGEs indeed constitute a chemically heterogeneous group of compounds, taking into account that the pattern of AGEs formed in any reaction is critically dependent on the precise conditions under which the reaction is occurring.

Diabetes is a condition that strongly favors AGE formation, particularly in the absence of glycemic control. Glucose is freely transported from blood to endothelial cells independently of insulin and provokes mitochondrial electron leakage and superoxide anion formation that ultimately results in increased methylglyoxal-derived AGE formation (Peyroux and Sternberg 2006).

In chronological aging, AGEs form slowly and predominantly on long-lived proteins, such as extracellular matrix proteins that present low rate of turnover. AGE-modified proteins resist proteolytic digestion and thus tend to accumulate along aging. In oxidative media such as that found in cells of aged tissues, proteins could also suffer irreversible oxidation that results in carbonyl groups formation and subsequent loss of protein function.

AGE accumulation in the vascular system, including the sinusoidal vessels of cavernous tissue, is deleterious and associates with loss of function (reviewed by Neves 2013) (Table 14.1). AGE cross-linking of collagen leads to vascular wall thickening and decreased extensibility of cavernous tissue. In addition, AGE-modified extracellular matrix proteins contribute to the accumulation of amorphous hyalinized material that is chemotactic for monocytes that secrete inflammatory molecules in the subendothelial space (Kirstein et al. 1990). In these conditions, proliferation of SMC and further atheroma formation are favored.

TABLE 14.1

Summary of the Effects of AGE/RAGE in Erectile Function

Effect	Type of Model	Study
↑ Oxidative stress	*In vitro*	Mohamed et al. 1999
↑ AGE accumulation in cavernous tissue ↓ Extensibility of cavernous tissue	Human CC	Seftel et al. 1997
↑ Accumulation of amorphous hyalinized material in subendothelial space ↑ Migration of monocytes to subendothelial space ↑ Secretion of inflammatory molecules	Human isolated monocytes	Kirstein et al. 1990
↓ NO ↓ cGMP ↓ Endothelium-dependent vasodilatation	Diabetic rats	Bucala et al. 1991
↑ Uncouple of eNOS ↓ eNOS mRNA expression	Diabetic mice	Su et al. 2008
↓ SIRT1 expression	Human peripheral blood cells	Uribarri et al. 2011
↑ Inflammatory response through NFkB activation	*In vitro*	Huttunen et al. 1999

Note: AGEs, advanced glycation end products; cGMP, cyclic guanosine monophosphate; eNOS, endothelial NO synthase; NFkB, nuclear factor kappaB; NO, nitric oxide; SIRT1, sirtuin1.

The amount of NO has been demonstrated to be directly reduced by AGEs, which compromises the extent of endothelium-dependent vasodilatation through decreased cGMP bioavailability (Bucala et al. 1991). It has also been demonstrated that AGEs reduce eNOS mRNA expression and induce uncoupling of eNOS that impedes NO synthesis (Su et al. 2008). AGEs also intervene in the regulation of activity of sirtuin 1 (SIRT1), which constitutes an additional mechanism in the control of erectile function. SIRT1 is a NAD-dependent deacetylase that belongs to the family of seven mammalian sirtuins, homologs of silent mating-type information regulator (SIR) 2 of yeast. It is known that SIRT1 prevents vascular cells senescence and improves endothelial function through eNOS activation synergistically with the Akt/PKB (Mattagajasingh et al. 2007). SIRT1 expression was demonstrated in the cytoplasm of SMC in the CC of human origin (Tomada et al. 2013). Interestingly, SIRT1 expression in blood cells of aged patients was inversely correlated not only with AGE levels in blood (Uribarri et al. 2011) (Table 14.1) but also with markers of inflammation and of oxidative stress (Uribarri et al. 2014).

Corroborating the notion that AGE formation and accumulation contribute to increased ED risk, it was demonstrated that levels of AGEs observed in cavernous tissue of diabetic patients were significantly higher than those observed in the serum, indicating that erectile tissue constitutes a preferential location for AGE accumulation (Seftel et al. 1997). A decrease in urinary excretion of AGEs has also been observed in patients with renal impairment. Indeed, the circulating AGE levels, and probably the AGE accumulation in erectile tissue, are proportional to the severity of kidney disease (Tessier et al. 2012).

14.5 Receptors of AGEs

Besides their participation in cross-linking of the proteins, AGEs interact on cells with AGE-affinity molecules, generally named AGE receptors (AGER). The main function of these molecules, expressed at cell surface mainly in monocytes and macrophages, is mediation of AGE cell uptake from blood and tissues. The first cell surface receptor found to be involved in endocytosis and degradation that contributes to suppression of AGE-mediated pathways was AGER1 (Lu et al. 2004). An additional class of AGE receptors expressed by macrophages and endothelial cells that intervenes in endocytosis and degradation of AGEs is galectin-3 or AGER3. However, the role of galectin-3 in AGE protection is far from being consensual, considering evidence of its proatherosclerotic effects in rodent experimental models. In line, a significant correlation between galectin-3 levels and risk factors of CVD was demonstrated in a cohort of 7,968 subjects (de Boer et al. 2012).

Other AGE receptors have also been identified that trigger inflammatory processes in tissues, instead of being involved in AGE effects mitigation. In fact, most of the deleterious effects normally attributed to AGEs occur after engagement and activation of the receptor of AGEs (RAGE) (a member of the immunoglobulin superfamily) expressed in a wide range of tissues including SMC and endothelium even in the absence of injury or inflammation (Brett et al. 1993). RAGE expression is highly increased in response to AGE formation, which amplifies outcomes initiated by AGEs. Besides being involved in several signaling cascades, and in particular in those associated with atherosclerotic processes (reviewed by Neves 2013), RAGE is a potent upregulator of nuclear factor kappaB (NF-κB), a transcription factor responsible for many key biological processes, such as inflammation, apoptosis, and stress response, that modulates gene transcription of endothelin-1, vascular endothelial growth factor, transforming growth factor β, proinflammatory cytokines, interleukins 1α and 6 and tumor necrosis factor α (TNF-α), and of the adhesion molecules, such as vascular cell adhesion molecule-1 (VCAM-1) and intercellular adhesion molecule-1 (ICAM-1) (Huttunen et al. 1999).

AGE levels modulate expression of their receptors. When AGEs are low, RAGE is downregulated and AGER1 upregulated, the latter one leading to AGE endocytosis and degradation. In this situation, SIRT1 is also activated, mitigating inflammatory response and oxidative stress in cells. A prolonged high-AGE burden increments RAGE signaling, represses AGER1-mediated AGE degradation, and increases SIRT1 ubiquitination and proteasome-mediated degradation, shortening its half-life, which together result in increased inflammation and oxidative stress (Poulsen et al. 2013; Huang et al. 2015). As far as we know, expression of RAGE or other classes of AGE receptors in CC has not been yet demonstrated in human.

14.5.1 Soluble RAGE

Besides RAGE expression in multiple cell types, soluble forms of RAGE (sRAGE) retain the ability to bind AGEs circulating in blood. At least two types of sRAGE forms can be distinguished, a form of sRAGE that results of proteolytic cleavage of cell surface RAGE and a novel splice variant expressed and secreted in human vascular cells, which is named endogenous secretory RAGE (esRAGE) and neutralizes AGE effects in endothelial cells (Yonekura et al. 2003).

Interestingly, soluble forms of RAGE seem to protect against atherosclerotic plaque formation and inflammation by AGE scavenging, which prevent their interaction with cell surface proinflammatory receptors. This assumption is supported by the observation of a strong negative correlation between esRAGE blood levels and subclinical atherosclerosis and CVD risk factors that in turn associates with ED (Koyama et al. 2005). Blood levels of esRAGE have been proposed as a novel biomarker for ED (Emanuele and Bertona 2006).

14.6 Contribution of Dietary AGEs to the ED Development

In addition to endogenously produced AGEs, this heterogeneous class of compounds could be provided from diet and further absorbed in the intestine and passed to the circulation. In fact, diet represents an important source of AGEs, and a strong correlation between AGE consumption and serum levels has been demonstrated (Semba et al. 2012). AGEs are often incorporated into foods for intensifying the natural flavors and the highest levels are found in browned or caramelized foodstuffs, such as coffee or cola drinks. Other foods contain a variable content of AGEs, dependent on food products and on processing parameters, for example, cooking temperature and water content. While dry heat cooking promotes dietary AGE formation, increasing humidity conditions in the process of cooking decreases AGE content (Uribarri et al. 2010). Reduction of AGEs in foods could be also achieved by modulation of pH and by the use of lemon juice or vinegar, taking into account that the rate of Maillard reaction that initiates AGE formation is considerably low at acidic pH. Maillard reaction leads to a decrease in the nutritional value of foods as a result of the degradation of the amino acids. Concomitantly, loss of nutrients such as vitamins, phenolic acids, and polyunsaturated fatty acids in foods may occur due to heat exposure (Tessier et al. 2012).

The global AGE content of Western diet significantly increased in the last 50 years, mostly due to the increase in high-heat-treated foods. Higher molecular weight (HMW) AGEs could be formed during cooking, however, low molecular weight (LMW) AGEs are predominantly absorbed after degradation in the intestine (Finot and Magnenat 1981). Dietary AGEs apparently impact on vascular function, as depicted in Table 14.2 that summarizes the most relevant findings on experimental models and patients. *In vitro* studies strongly suggest that exposure to food-derived AGEs increases oxidative stress, inhibits angiogenesis processes, and promotes TNFα and protein cross-linking formation in human umbilical vein endothelial cells or mouse peritoneal macrophages (Cai et al. 2002; Liu et al. 2013). The apparent deleterious role of AGEs on endothelial function was supported by several studies. Grossin et al. showed that chronic ingestion of carboxymethyllisine (CML), a dietary AGE, for 9 months, induced endothelial dysfunction and arterial stiffness in a RAGE-dependent manner in mice. Sena et al. demonstrated that methylglyoxal diminished NO-dependent vasorelaxation. Moreover, there is evidence that circulating AGEs from diet correlate with inflammatory marker high-sensitivity C-reactive protein blood levels (Uribarri et al. 2007b; Cai et al. 2008; Sena et al. 2012; Grossin et al. 2015). Others, however, found no correlation between circulating levels of CML and markers of endothelial activation or AGE content of diet, adopted for 6 weeks in middle-aged healthy adults (Sjögren et al. 2007; Semba et al. 2014). The discrepancy found among data could be attributed not only to the differences between populations and extension of treatments but also to the fact that all the measurements in human were done in blood samples collected after a 12-hour fast. AGE accumulation in vessel tissue, in particular in CC vasculature, was not investigated.

Among the studies carried out in healthy, obese, diabetic, or individuals with kidney disease, some of them observed the effect of a single administration or meal with high-level AGE content, comparatively with a low-level AGE counterpart, while others studied the effect of a dietary intervention that varied from 2 weeks to 4 months (Table 14.2). While a single oral dose of an AGE load seems to decrease flow-mediated dilation and reactive hyperemia and to increase blood markers of oxidative stress and endothelial dysfunction in diabetic patients (Negrean et al. 2007; Uribarri et al. 2007a; Stirban et al. 2008), no differences were found for inflammation or endothelial activation markers in obese healthy individuals that only manifested an increase in oxidative stress markers (Poulsen et al. 2014). These findings demonstrated that even an isolated dose of dietary AGEs induce a more deleterious effect in vascular function in diabetic than in nondiabetic patients. In line, Vlassara et al. evidenced that high-AGE diet for 2 or 6 weeks increased inflammatory markers in diabetic patients (Vlassara et al. 2002). On the contrary, when a 4-month low-AGE dietary intervention was tested in groups of diabetic and healthy individuals, data demonstrated that diabetic patients respond to the reduction in dietary AGE content, taking into account that marked differences in levels of AGEs, insulin, Homeostasis Model Assessment index, leptin, oxidative stress, and adiponectin were observed. Healthy subjects only showed a decrease in oxidative stress blood markers (Uribarri et al. 2011).

CKD patients also seem to be responsive to reduction of dietary content of AGEs, considering the decrease in oxidative stress markers, RAGE, and TNFα observed in this group of patients when treated with a low-AGE diet for 4 weeks. In addition, authors verified a recovery of AGER1 mRNA levels that otherwise were suppressed in CKD patients (Vlassara et al. 2009).

Dietary AGEs have been found to downregulate SIRT1 expression in peripheral mononuclear blood cells of old individuals (Uribarri et al. 2014), a population that is prone to develop CVD including ED, owning to the age-related increase in oxidative stress. In the mentioned study, a positive correlation between dietary AGEs and RAGE and AGER1 expression levels and TNFα and VCAM-1 levels in blood was also verified, supporting the notion that downregulation of SIRT1 induced by AGEs promotes inflammation and probably endothelial dysfunction.

Circulating mononuclear blood cells could infiltrate in tissues, particularly in those that accumulate AGEs in extracellular matrix, promoting secretion of inflammatory cytokines and atherosclerosis progression. All evidence supports a role for AGE cavernous deposition in the progression of ED, but the specific involvement of dietary AGEs comparatively with those spontaneously formed in cavernous

TABLE 14.2

Outcomes of Dietary AGEs on Vascular Function

Study	Diet	Type of Model	Outcome
Cai et al. 2002	Affinity-purified food-AGE extracts exposed to 250°C for 10 minutes	HUVECs	HUVECs exposed to food-derived AGEs presented depletion of cellular GSH and activation of GPx that increase oxidative stress.
		Mouse peritoneal macrophages	TNF-α and protein cross-linking formation are promoted in macrophages after exposure to animal products–derived AGE rich in lipid oxidation compounds.
Liu et al. 2013	CML	HUVECs	CML decreases HUVEC tube formation and in a dose-dependent fashion decreases proliferation rate and promotes apoptosis. NADPH oxidase is activated, ROS production increased, SHP-1 expression and activity are upregulated, and VEGFR-2 phosphorylation and kinase activity downregulated.
Cai et al. 2008	Methylglyoxal-BSA–supplemented diet for 6 months	C57BL/6J mice	Increase in markers of oxidative stress in animals treated with methylglyoxal-BSA.
	ER or high-AGE-ER diet prepared by brief heat treatment for 24 months		High AGE-ER–treated old mice developed shortened lifespan, insulin resistance, marked myocardial, and renal fibrosis, and high levels of 8-isoprostanes, AGEs, RAGE, and low AGER1 and GSH/GSSG levels than ER counterparts.
Sena et al. 2012	Methylglyoxal in drinking water (50–75 mg/kg/day) for 3 months	Male Wistar and spontaneously diabetic GK rats	NO bioavailability and NO-dependent vasorelaxation were significantly reduced in methylglyoxal-treated Wistar rats. An increase in the oxidative stress marker nitrotyrosine and in expression of RAGE were also observed. Equivalent changes were found in methylglyoxal-treated GK rats when compared with control diabetic rats.
Grossin et al. 2015	CML–BSA–enriched diet (50, 100, or 200 μg/g of food) versus BSA-enriched diet for 9 months	Wild-type and RAGE(-/-)male C57BL/6 mice	Wild-type, but not RAGE(–/–)animals, fed with higher dose of CML presented a decrease in endothelium-dependent relaxation and SIRT1 expression but an increase in RAGE and VCAM-1 levels, pulse wave velocity, and elastin disruption
Vlassara et al. 2002	Low- and high-AGE (5-fold CML content) meals prepared at different temperature for 2 weeks	11 diabetic patients (mean age 52 years)	High-AGE diet for 2 or 6 weeks increases TNF-α expression in blood cells and VCAM-1 in serum at 2 weeks. At 6 weeks of high-AGE diet, CRP in blood increases.
	6 weeks in identical regimen	13 diabetic patients (mean age 62 years)	
Negrean et al. 2007	Low- and high-AGE meals prepared with identical ingredients cooked at different temperature and time (2.750 vs. 15.100 kU AGE, respectively)	20 (14 male) type 2 diabetic patients (mean age 55 years)	After high-AGE meal, the flow-mediated dilation and reactive hyperemia decreased significantly more than after the low-AGE meal. Increase in serum methylglyoxal, thiobarbituric acid–reactive substances (marker of oxidative stress), ICAM-1, VCAM-1, and E-selectin (markers of endothelial dysfunction), but not on inflammation markers was found after high-AGE meal.

(Continued)

TABLE 14.2 ***(Continued)***

Outcomes of Dietary AGEs on Vascular Function

Study	Diet	Type of Model	Outcome
Uribarri et al. 2007a	Unique intake of an AGE-rich beverage (1800 kU AGE), no carbohydrates or lipids	44 (36 male) diabetic patients, 10 healthy individuals (5 men), mean age 50 years for diabetic and 43 years for healthy subjects	After AGE-rich beverage intake, serum AGEs and plasminogen activator 1 increased and flow-mediated dilation decreased in all individuals. No changes for glucose or VCAM-1.
Stirban et al. 2008	Low- and high-AGE meals prepared with identical ingredients cooked at different temperature and time (2.750 vs. 15.100 kU AGE, respectively)	20 (13 male) type 2 diabetic patients, mean age 56 years	After high-AGE meal, an increase in blood levels of methylglyoxal, E-selectin, VCAM-1, and thiobarbituric acid–reactive substances, as well as a decrease in adiponectin and leptin were found.
Vlassara et al. 2009	High-AGE diet (>13 AGE Eq/day) meals were prepared at home and dietary AGEs reduced (30%–50%) by modification of the cooking time and temperature without changing the quality or quantity of food (4 months).	30 healthy individuals divided according to age (18–45 years) and older than 60 years	Low-AGE diet reduces AGEs, oxidative stress markers, RAGE, and TNF-α in peripheral blood cells in normal and CKD patients. VCAM-1 levels were reduced in healthy patients with low-AGE diet. AGER1 was suppressed in CKD, whereas RAGE and TNF-α were increased. AGER1 mRNA levels in blood cells of CKD patients on the low-AGE diet were increased comparatively with those of patients on high-AGE diet.
	Equivalent dietary intervention, meals were prepared in the clinical research center and given to patients twice a week (4 weeks)	9 kidney disease patients	
Uribarri et al. 2011	4 months dietary intervention. Low-AGE diet was prepared by cooking procedures that avoid AGE formation. Total AGE content on diet was reduced to 50%	18 (4 male) diabetic patients, 18 healthy individuals (4 men), mean age 61 years for diabetic and 67 years for healthy subjects	AGE-restricted diet led to the reduction of levels of AGEs, insulin, HOMA index, leptin, and oxidative stress but increased levels of adiponectin on blood and a reduction in expression of SIRT1 and AGER1 in peripheral blood cells of diabetic patients. These changes, with exception o decrease in oxidative stress, were not verified in healthy subjects submitted to equivalent dietary pattern.
Poulsen et al. 2014	Low- and high-AGE meals prepared with identical ingredients cooked at different temperature and time (2.8 vs. 5.0 mg CML, respectively)	19 healthy, overweight individuals (3 men, mean age 37 years)	Glycemic response and urinary secretion of markers of oxidative stress increased after high-AGE meal. No differences in blood CML levels and markers of inflammation or endothelial activation.
Semba et al. 2014	Low- and high-AGE meals (3 meals/day and 1 evening snack only differ on preparation, isocaloric and nutrient equivalent). High-AGE diet was 4 times higher in AGEs than low-AGE diet (6 weeks)	24 healthy individuals (10 men, mean age 59 years)	No differences were found for inflammation and endothelium function markers, serum or urinary CML, and receptors for AGEs.

(Continued)

TABLE 14.2 ***(Continued)***

Outcomes of Dietary AGEs on Vascular Function

Study	Diet	Type of Model	Outcome
Uribarri et al. 2014	High-AGE diet group contains >15AGE Eq/day, low-AGE diet was prepared by cooking procedures that avoid AGE formation (4 months)	Observational study—67 healthy volunteers (27 men, age >60 years)Interventional study—18 healthy participants (5 male), mean age 64 years	Dietary AGE intake correlates with soluble CML, markers of inflammation and of oxidative stress. SIRT1 expression in peripheral mononuclear blood cells is lower in men and is inversely correlated with AGE levels in blood and markers of inflammation and of oxidative stress. Dietary AGE restriction lowered AGE levels in blood and markers of inflammation and oxidative stress, expression of RAGE and AGER1, and increased SIRT1 expression and PPAR-γ protein in peripheral mononuclear blood cells.

Note: AGE, advanced glycation end products; AGER1, advanced glycation end products receptor 1; BSA, bovine serum albumin; CKD, chronic kidney disease; CML, N(ε)carboxymethyllysine; CRP, C-reactive protein; ER, energy restriction; GPx, glutathione peroxidase; GSH, glutathione; GSSG, glutathione disulfide; HOMA, Homeostasis Model Assessment; HUVECs, human umbilical vein endothelial cells; ICAM-1, intercellular adhesion molecule 1; NADPH oxidase, nicotinamide adenine dinucleotide phosphate-oxidase; NO, nitric oxide; PPAR-γ, peroxisome proliferator–activated receptor-γ; RAGE, receptor of advanced glycation end-products; ROS, reactive oxygen species; SIRT1-sirtuin1; SHP-1, Src - homology 2 domain containing protein tyrosine phosphatase TNF-α, tumor necrosis factor-α; VCAM-1, vascular cell adhesion molecule-1; VEGFR-2, vascular endothelial growth factor receptor-2.

tissue in the erectile function remains to be elucidated. Among AGE species, peptide-bound AGEs (HMW AGE) are those that possess more extensive tissue retention and also present higher affinity to RAGE (Poulsen et al. 2013). On the contrary, LMW AGE adducts that are mostly absorbed from diet (free amine or amino acid–derived) presented a low affinity to RAGE (Penfold et al. 2010) and thus reduced deleterious effects on vascular function. Nevertheless, we should not exclude the possibility of HMW AGE formation in tissue when diet-derived LMW AGE are abundant. In addition, it is still uncertain if dietary AGEs are able to activate RAGE, taking into account that some AGE adducts do not bind to RAGE regardless of high-molecular weight.

Despite the lack of knowledge of the exact contribution of dietary AGEs on vascular disturbances and in particular on ED progression, reduction on AGE intake could represent a strategy to avoid AGE-related damage. Dietary AGE restriction might be difficult to maintain for a long term in humans, but benefits in the prevention of atherosclerosis and ED not only in diabetic or CKD patients but also in healthy individuals could be valuable. An additional strategy discussed in the next point could be the increment of intake of nutrients or foodstuffs that mitigate the deleterious effects of AGEs.

14.7 Effects of Nutrients that Could Interfere in AGE Formation or Activity in CC

Natural compounds available in food with antioxidant or antiglycating capability are accessible and safe and could exert protection of the effects of AGEs in the cardiovascular system, in particular in the erectile tissue. Among the diverse studies carried out to evaluate nutritional interference on erectile function, some employed single dietary compounds alone or in association with inhibitors of phosphodiesterase-5 (PDE-5), first-line treatment for ED. Others tested the effects of entire foodstuffs, fruit juices, beverages, or even diet patterns. In this last type of studies, the global effect could be due to multiple mechanisms, including natural antioxidant action of nutrients, such as polyphenols, vitamins, and spermidine that indirectly control AGE formation, or inhibition of AGE formation and reactivity as that recognized for carnosine, a dipeptide of beta-alanine and histidine, highly concentrated in muscle and brain. Table 14.3 summarizes the most important studies in this matter.

TABLE 14.3

List of Nutrients/Foods that Interfere in AGE Formation and Activity in the CC

Nutrient/ Food	Design	Effect	Study
Curcumin/ turmeric	Diabetic rats treated with single-dose 10 mg/kg or water-soluble 10 mg/kg/day pure curcumin for 12 weeks (n = 12/group)	Single-dose or water-soluble curcumin (higher effect) ameliorated ED through elevation in intracavernous pressure, cGMP levels, eNOS, and nNOS genes and decrease in NF-κB and iNOS genes.	Abdel et al. 2012
L-Carnitine/red meat, dairy products	90 patients were treated with propionyl-L-carnitine 2 g/day plus acetyl-L-carnitine 2 g/day (mean age 66 years) or placebo (mean age 63 years) for 6 months	L-carnitine significantly improved nocturnal penile tumescence and IIEF score.	Cavallini et al. 2004
	54 men (35–75 years) were treated for 3 month with propionyl-L-carnitine 250 mg/day, L-arginine 2.5g/day and niacin 20 mg/day	Ameliorated erectile function	Gianfrilli et al. 2012
	40 patients with DM-related ED (mean age 64 years) treated with inhibitor of PDE-5 supplemented or not with 250 mg/day propionyl-L-carnitine for 24 weeks	Mean scores of IIEF significantly improved in patients treated with propionyl-L-carnitine and inhibitor of PDE-5 comparatively with inhibitor of PDE-5 alone.	Gentile et al. 2004
	20 patients with DM-related ED (50- 60 years) treated with inhibitor of PDE-5 supplemented or not with 2 g/day propionyl-L-carnitine, L-arginine 2.5 g/day and nicotinic acid 20 mg/day for 12 weeks	Mean scores of IIEF significantly improved in patients treated with propionyl-L-carnitine, L-arginine, and nicotinic acid and inhibitor of PDE-5 comparatively with inhibitor of PDE-5 alone.	Gentile et al. 2009
α-lipoic/meat, broccoli, spinach, and γ-linolenic acids/ vegetable oils	Male diabetic rats were treated for 4 or 8 weeks with α-lipoic 28 mg/kg/day and γ-linolenic 35 mg/kg/day, or with each one alone (n = 9–16/group)	α-lipoic in association with γ-linolenic acid, but not the isolated fatty acids, resulted in an improvement in NO-mediated neural and endothelium-dependent relaxation of CC.	Keegan et al. 2001
Vitamin E/ vegetables, fish, plant oils, and seeds	Diabetic rats were treated with vitamin E 20 IU/day, PDE-5 inhibitor, or both for 3 weeks (n = 5/group)	Vitamin E increments PDE-5 inhibitor action, leading to increase in intracavernous pressure and in nNOS levels.	De Young et al. 2003
	Aged rats (18 months) were treated with vitamin E 80 IU/day associated or not with PDE-5 inhibitor for 3 weeks (n = 7–8/group)	Both vitamin E and PDE-5 inhibitor when used alone increased intracavernous pressure, incremented circulating NO levels, and reduced oxidative stress.	Helmy and Senbel 2012
	9 patients (46–74 years) low responders to PDE-5 inhibitors were treated with PDE-5 inhibitor and vitamin E (300 mg/day α-tocopherol) for at least 1 month	IIEF-5 score increased in an average of 3.3 points.	Kondoh et al. 2008
Caffeine/coffee	Control and diabetic rats treated with caffeine 20 mg/kg/day for 8 weeks (n = 8–9/group)	Caffeine increases intracavernous pressure and upregulates cGMP synthesis.	Yang et al. 2008
	3724 men (mean age 49 years) representative of the civilian population were subjected to a survey that assessed informative data relative to nutrition habits including caffeine consumption, ED, and health conditions	An inverse correlation between caffeine consumption and prevalence of ED in healthy, obese/overweight, and hypertensive individuals, but not in diabetic patients, was found.	Lopez et al. 2015

(Continued)

TABLE 14.3 ***(Continued)***

List of Nutrients/Foods that Interfere in AGE Formation and Activity in the CC

Nutrient/ Food	Design	Effect	Study
Ginseng	Rats with diabetes-induced ED were intraperitoneally injected with panax notoginseng saponins 50, 100, or 150 mg/kg/day of for 4 weeks (n = 6/group)	Ginseng treatment mitigates AGE levels; increments intracavernous pressure, NO, eNOS, and cGMP levels; and decreases cell apoptosis.	Lin et al. 2013
EGCG/Green tea	Rats were treated for 6 months with green tea (833 mg of total catechin/L) or catechin extract excluding EGCG (200 mg of total catechin /L) until complete 18 months (n = 10/group)	VEGF and VEGFR2 expression and perivascular lipid deposition in the CC were reduced.	Neves et al. 2008
	Aged diabetic rats (2 years) were treated with green tea, EGCG (7.6 mg/L) solution or EGCG solution and PDE-5 inhibitor for 8 weeks (n = 19–22/group)	EGCG treatment increased eNOS and cGMP levels and exerted antioxidant effects.	Mostafa et al. 2013
Resveratrol/Red wine	Rats were treated for 6 months with red wine or ethanol solution until complete 12 months (n = 6/group)	VEGF and VEGFR2 expression were reduced and compensated by an increase in angiopoietins 1 and 2 in the CC of rats treated with red wine.	Neves et al. 2010
	Diabetic rats were treated with resveratrol (5 mg/kg/day)alone or in association with a PDE-5 inhibitor for 4 weeks (n = 4/group)	Resveratrol associated with a PDE-5 inhibitor incremented cavernous vasorelaxation.	Fukuhara et al. 2011
	Diabetic rats were treated with resveratrol (5 mg/kg/day) or saline for 8 weeks (n = 17/group)	Resveratrol treatment reduced apoptosis, upregulated the expression of SIRT1, mitigated oxidative stress, and increased intracavernous pressure.	Yu et al. 2013
cyanidin-3-O-β-D-glucopyranoside/ Pomegranate juice	Diabetic rats were treated with cyanidin-3-O-β-D-glucopyranoside (10 mg/kg/day) for 8 weeks (n = 12/group)	Cyanidin-3-O-β-D-glucopyranoside treatment reduced oxidative stress and cell apoptosis, increased expression of eNOS and nNOS, and increased intracavernous blood flow.	Ha et al. 2012
	53 ED patients were divided into two groups that consumed pomegranate juice (1.5 mmol/day total polyphenol) or placebo for 28 days. Each patient participated in the study with the opposite beverage after	Pomegranate juice consumption tended to improve erections.	Forest et al. 2007
Mediterranean diet	2 years of consumption of Mediterranean diet by men with metabolic syndrome (mean age 44 years) (n = 35) control group (n = 30)	Serum concentrations of CRP significantly reduced and endothelial function score improved in the patients treated with Mediterranean diet. IIEF score strongly ameliorated in men in the intervention group, where about one-third of men regained a normal sexual function.	Esposito et al. 2006

Note: CC, corpus cavernosum; cGMP, cyclic guanosine monophosphate; CRP, C-reactive protein; DM, diabetes mellitus; ED, erectile dysfunction; EGCG, epigallocatechin-3-gallate; eNOS, endothelial nitric oxide synthase; IIEF, International Index of Erectile Function; iNOS, inducible nitric oxide synthase; nNOS, neuronal nitric oxide synthase; NF-κB, nuclear factor kappaB; PDE-5, phosphodiesterase-5; SIRT1, sirtuin 1; VEGF, vascular endothelial growth factor; VEGFR2, vascular endothelial growth factor receptor 2.

14.7.1 Curcumin

Curcumin is a polyphenol abundant in turmeric powder that inhibits AGE effects, apparently by direct trapping of methylglyoxal. When orally administrated for 8 weeks to diabetic rats, curcumin reduced AGEs and cross-linking of collagen (Sajithlal et al. 1998). Curcumin dietary supplementation lowers oxidative stress and improves vascular function including erectile function in a rat model of diabetes through increase in expression of eNOS and nNOS, and repression of inflammatory genes and iNOS (Abdel et al. 2012). Other polyphenols such as resveratrol, quercetin, and epigallocatechin-3-gallate (EGCG) might also inhibit AGE-induced vascular damage (reviewed by Neves 2013).

14.7.2 L-Carnitine

L-Carnitine is a small peptide constituted by lysine and methionine available in red meat and dairy products that possess antiglycating effects. L-carnitine treatment reduces the levels of methylglyoxal and glycated hemoglobin in blood, and collagen cross-linking in tissues of rats fed with high-fructose diet (Rajasekar and Anuradha 2007). Administration of L-carnitine seems promissory to ED patients, considering that it significantly improved nocturnal penile tumescence and International Index of Erectile Function (IIEF) score (Cavallini et al. 2004). When associated with niacin and L-arginine, it also ameliorated erectile function in ED patients (Gianfrilli et al. 2012). Derivatives of L-carnitine have also been employed as adjuvants of inhibitors of PDE-5 with very promissory results for DM-related ED (Gentile et al. 2004, 2009).

14.7.3 Fatty Acids

Alpha-lipoic acid prevents formation of AGE-modified products, mitigates oxidative stress, and blocks inflammatory responses induced by AGEs in endothelial cells (Bierhaus et al. 1997). In association with γ-linolenic acid, an improvement in NO-mediated neural and endothelium-dependent relaxation of CC in streptozotocin-induced diabetes rat was verified, suggesting that the combination of these fatty acids naturally present in food might be employed in the treatment of diabetes-related ED (Keegan et al. 2001).

14.7.4 Vitamin E

Vitamin E is a blanket term for eight different compounds abundant in vegetables, fish, plant oils, and sunflower seeds with recognized antioxidant properties. Regarding antiglycating properties, data from different studies are not consensual.

Vitamin E is known to enhance endothelial function through an increment of circulating NO levels and ameliorate ED when combined with a PDE-5 inhibitor in experimental rat models of diabetic and aged rats that presented increase in intracavernous pressure and nNOS levels after treatment (De Young et al. 2003; Helmy and Senbel 2012). Also in men, vitamin E administration to nine low responders to PDE-5 inhibitors for at least 1 month was shown to increase the IIEF-5 score to an average of 3.3 points (Kondoh et al. 2008).

14.7.5 Caffeine

Caffeine is a crystalline xanthine alkaloid that increases intracavernous pressure and upregulates cGMP synthesis in diabetic rats when orally administrated for 8 weeks (Yang et al. 2008). Coffee is the main source of caffeine; however, this beverage is also particularly rich in not only AGE adducts, in particular methylglyoxal, but also melanoidins, compounds formed by Maillard reaction that confer beneficial antioxidant and anti-inflammatory effects. The final effect of regular coffee consumption in terms of glycative action remains to be clarified, but a recent report of data of the National Health and Nutrition Examination Survey (NHANES) 2001–2004 that enrolled 3,724 patients indicated an inverse correlation between caffeine consumption and prevalence of ED in healthy, obese/overweight, and hypertensive individuals, but not in diabetic patients (Lopez et al. 2015).

14.7.6 Ginseng

Ginseng is a natural product prepared from the roots of *Panax*, which is rich in saponins that may be included in drinks. Several evidence support that ginseng not only mitigates AGE levels but also increments erectile function (Lin and Gou 2013). Several clinical trials demonstrated that ginseng significantly improved erectile function in men, by an equivalent but slow fashion as PDE-5 inhibitors do (reviewed by Moyad and Park 2012).

14.7.7 Beverages with Polyphenols

The consumption of food naturally rich in polyphenols owning to their potent antioxidant capacities has been demonstrated to be beneficial to the vascular system and specifically to the cavernous tissue. Chronic administration of polyphenols extract from fruits with antiglycating activity to rats caused significant increases in intracavernous blood flow and SMC relaxation, probably through increment in NO bioavailability (Ha et al. 2012). Moreover, pomegranate juice consumption tended to improve erections in a cohort of 53 men with mild to moderate ED. (Forest et al. 2007). Other beverages, such as red wine or green tea, naturally rich in polyphenols (SIRT1-activator resveratrol and EGCG, respectively) apparently diminished atherosclerosis progression in cavernous tissue of the rat and activated protective mechanisms of cavernous tissue vascularization when consumed for 6 months (Neves et al. 2008, 2010). In line, orally administrated resveratrol alone or in association with a PDE-5 inhibitor incremented cavernous vasorelaxation in animal models (Fukuhara et al. 2011; Yu et al. 2013), and EGCG exerted antioxidant effects (Mostafa et al. 2013).

14.7.8 Mediterranean Diet

Mediterranean diet is a low-AGE diet pattern (Uribarri et al. 2010) rich in whole grain, fruits, vegetables, legumes, walnut, and olive oil. Adoption of Mediterranean diet by men with metabolic syndrome and ED for 2 years significantly improved endothelial and erectile functions, together with a significant reduction of systemic vascular inflammation (Esposito et al. 2006).

14.8 Conclusions

High levels of dietary AGEs are associated with loss of defense mechanisms for inflammation and oxidative stress, which may raise susceptibility to chronic metabolic diseases and ED. A low-AGE diet rich in antioxidants can thus preserve or restore such defenses, averting ED in those individuals that present an increased risk, such as diabetics, aged men, and patients with CKD. A particular recommendation to reduce dietary AGEs should be given to diabetic patients due to their incremented inflammatory, oxidative stress, and endothelial activation responses. As well, patients with any degree of renal failure should be instructed to reduce intake of dietary AGEs due to their reduced excretory capacity. Low-AGE dietary intervention or anti-AGE nutrient or food consumption could also be associated with current treatments with PDE-5 inhibitors, ameliorating responses of refractory patients, and reducing doses, which minimizes side effects or complications of these medications.

ACKNOWLEDGMENT

The author thanks Sérgio Evangelista from Laboratório de Iconografia, Faculdade de Medicina da Universidade do Porto-Portugal, for artwork in Figure 14.2.

REFERENCES

Abdel, A.M.T., T. Motawi, A. Rezq, et al. 2012. Effects of a water-soluble curcumin protein conjugate vs. pure curcumin in a diabetic model of erectile dysfunction. *J Sex Med* 9:1815–33.

Bierhaus, A., S. Chevion, M. Chevion, et al. 1997. Advanced glycation end product-induced activation of NF-kappaB is suppressed by alpha-lipoic acid in cultured endothelial cells. *Diabetes* 46:1481–90.

Bonnefont-Rousselot, D., J.P. Bastard, M.C. Jaudon, and J. Delattre. 2000. Consequences of the diabetic status on the oxidant/antioxidant balance. *Diabetes Metab* 26:163–76.
Brett, J., A.M. Schmidt, S.D. Yan, et al. 1993. Survey of the distribution of a newly characterized receptor for advanced glycation end products in tissues. *Am J Pathol* 143:1699–712.
Bucala, R., K.J. Tracey, and A. Cerami. 1991. Advanced glycosylation products quench nitric oxide and mediate defective endothelium-dependent vasodilatation in experimental diabetes. *J Clin Invest* 87:432–8.
Burnett, A.L., R.J. Nelson, D.C. Calvin, et al. 1996. Nitric oxide-dependent penile erection in mice lacking neuronal nitric oxide synthase. *Mol Med* 2:288–96.
Cai, W., Q.D. Gao, L. Zhu, M. Peppa, C. He, and H. Vlassara. 2002. Oxidative stress-inducing carbonyl compounds from common foods: Novel mediators of cellular dysfunction. *Mol Med* 8:337–46.
Cai, W., J.C. He, L. Zhu, et al. 2008. Oral glycotoxins determine the effects of calorie restriction on oxidant stress, age-related diseases, and lifespan. *Am J Pathol* 173:327–36.
Cavallini, G., S. Caracciolo, G. Vitali, F. Modenini, and G. Biagiotti. 2004. Carnitine versus androgen administration in the treatment of sexual dysfunction, depressed mood, and fatigue associated with male aging. *Urology* 63:641–6.
Cheitlin, C.M.D. 2004. Erectile dysfunction: The earliest sign of generalized vascular disease? *J Am Coll Cardiol* 43:185–6.
De Boer, R.A., D.J. van Veldhuisen, R.T. Gansevoort, et al. 2012. The fibrosis marker galectin-3 and outcome in the general population. *J Intern Med* 272:55–64.
De Young, L., D. Yu, D. Freeman, and G.B. Brock. 2003. Effect of PDE5 inhibition combined with free oxygen radical scavenger therapy on erectile function in a diabetic animal model. *Int J Impot Res* 15:347–54.
Emanuele, E. and M. Bertona. 2006. Endogenous secretory RAGE as a potential biochemical screening tool for erectile dysfunction. *Med Hypotheses* 67:668–9.
Esposito, K., M. Ciotola, F. Giugliano, et al. 2006. Mediterranean diet improves erectile function in subjects with the metabolic syndrome. *Int J Impot Res* 18:405–10.
Feldman, H.A., I. Goldstein, D.G. Hatzichristou, R.J. Krane, and J.B. McKinlay. 1994. Impotence and its medical and psychosocial correlates: Results of the Massachusetts Male Aging Study. *J Urol* 151:54–61.
Finot, P.A. and E. Magnenat. 1981. Metabolic transit of early and advanced Maillard products. *Prog Food Nutr Sci* 5:193–207.
Forest, C.P., H. Padma-Nathan, and H.R. Liker. 2007. Efficacy and safety of pomegranate juice on improvement of erectile dysfunction in male patients with mild to moderate erectile dysfunction: A randomized, placebo-controlled, double-blind, crossover study. *Int J Impot Res* 19:564–7.
Fukuhara, S., A. Tsujimura, H. Okuda, et al. 2011. Vardenafil and resveratrol synergistically enhance the nitric oxide/cyclic guanosine monophosphate pathway in corpus cavernosal smooth muscle cells and its therapeutic potential for erectile dysfunction in the streptozotocin-induced diabetic rat: Preliminary findings. *J Sex Med* 8:1061–71.
Gentile, V., G. Antonini, M. Antonella Bertozzi, et al. 2009. Effect of propionyl-L-carnitine, L-arginine and nicotinic acid on the efficacy of vardenafil in the treatment of erectile dysfunction in diabetes. *Curr Med Res Opin* 25:2223–8.
Gentile, V., P. Vicini, G. Prigiotti, A. Koverech, and F. Di Silverio. 2004. Preliminary observations on the use of propionyl-L-carnitine in combination with sildenafil in patients with erectile dysfunction and diabetes. *Curr Med Res Opin* 20:1377–84.
Ghalayini, I.F., M.A. Al-Ghazo, R. Al-Azab, et al. 2010. Erectile dysfunction in a Mediterranean country: Results of an epidemiological survey of a representative sample of men. *Int J Impot Res* 22:196–203.
Gianfrilli, D., R. Lauretta, C. Di Dato, et al. 2012. Propionyl-L-carnitine, L-arginine and niacin in sexual medicine: A nutraceutical approach to erectile dysfunction. *Andrologia* 44:600–4.
Grossin, N., F. Auger, C. Niquet-Leridon, et al. 2015. Dietary CML-enriched protein induces functional arterial aging in a RAGE-dependent manner in mice. *Mol Nutr Food Res* 59:927–38.
Ha, U.S., J.S. Koh, H.S. Kim, et al. 2012. Cyanidin-3-O-β-D-glucopyranoside concentrated materials from mulberry fruit have a potency to protect erectile function by minimizing oxidative stress in a rat model of diabetic erectile dysfunction. *Urol Int* 88:470–6.
Helmy, M.M. and A.M. Senbel. 2012. Evaluation of vitamin E in the treatment of erectile dysfunction in aged rats. *Life Sci* 90:489–94.

Huang, K.P., C. Chen, J. Hao, J.Y. Huang, P.Q. Liu, and H.Q. Huang. 2015. AGEs-RAGE system down-regulates Sirt1 through the ubiquitin-proteasome pathway to promote FN and TGF-β1 expression in male rat glomerular mesangial cells. *Endocrinology* 156:268–79.

Huttunen, H.J., C, Fages, and H. Rauvala. 1999. Receptor for advanced glycation end products (RAGE)-mediated neurite outgrowth and activation of NF-kappaB require the cytoplasmic domain of the receptor but different downstream signaling pathways. *J Biol Chem* 274:19919–24.

Ignarro, L.J., P.A. Bush, G.M. Buga, K.S. Wood, J.M. Fukuto, and J. Rajfer. 1990. Nitric oxide and cyclic GMP formation upon electrical field stimulation cause relaxation of corpus cavernosum smooth muscle. *Biochem Biophys Res Commun* 31:843–50.

Keegan, A., M.A. Cotter, and N.E. Cameron. 2001. Corpus cavernosum dysfunction in diabetic rats: Effects of combined alpha-lipoic acid and gamma-linolenic acid treatment. *Diabetes Metab Res Rev* 17:380–6.

Kirstein, M., J. Brett, S. Radoff, S. Ogawa, D. Stern, and H. Vlassara. 1990. Advanced protein glycosylation induces transendothelial human monocyte chemotaxis and secretion of platelet-derived growth factor: Role in vascular disease of diabetes and aging. *Proc Natl Acad Sci U S A* 87:9010–14.

Kondoh, N., Y. Higuchi, T. Maruyama, M. Nojima, S. Yamamoto, and H. Shima. 2008. Salvage therapy trial for erectile dysfunction using phosphodiesterase type 5 inhibitors and vitamin E: Preliminary report. *Aging Male* 11:167–70.

Koyama, H., T. Shoji, H. Yokoyama, et al. 2005. Plasma level of endogenous secretory RAGE is associated with components of the metabolic syndrome and atherosclerosis. *Arterioscler Thromb Vasc Biol* 25:2587–93.

Lin, F. and X. Gou. 2013. Panax notoginseng saponins improve the erectile dysfunction in diabetic rats by protecting the endothelial function of the penile corpus cavernosum. *Int J Impot Res* 25:206–11.

Liu, S.H., W.H. Sheu, M.R. Lee, et al. 2013. Advanced glycation end product Nε-carboxymethyllysine induces endothelial cell injury: The involvement of SHP-1-regulated VEGFR-2 dephosphorylation. *J Pathol* 230:215–27.

Lopez, D.S., R. Wang, K.K. Tsilidis, et al. 2015. Role of caffeine intake on erectile dysfunction in US Men: Results from NHANES 2001–2004. *PLoS One* 10:e0123547.

Lu, C., J.C. He, W. Cai, H. Liu, L. Zhu, and H. Vlassara. 2004. Advanced glycation endproduct (AGE) receptor 1 is a negative regulator of the inflammatory response to AGE in mesangial cells. *Proc Nat Acad Sci* 101:11767–72.

Lusis, A.J. 2000. Atherosclerosis. *Nature* 407:233–41.

Mattagajasingh, I., C.S. Kim, A. Naqvi, et al. 2007. SIRT1 promotes endotheliumdependent vascular relaxation by activating endothelial nitric oxide synthase. *Proc Natl Acad Sci U S A* 104:14855–60.

Mohamed, A.K., A. Bierhaus, S. Schiekofer, H. Tritschler, R. Ziegler, and P.P. Nawroth. 1999. The role of oxidative stress and NF-kappaB activation in late diabetic complications. *Biofactors* 10:157–67.

Mostafa, T., D. Sabry, A.M. Abdelaal, I. Mostafa, and M. Taymour. 2013. Cavernous antioxidant effect of green tea, epigallocatechin-3-gallate with/without sildenafil citrate intake in aged diabetic rats. *Andrologia* 45:272–7.

Moyad, M.A. and K. Park. 2012. What do most erectile dysfunction guidelines have in common? No evidence-based discussion or recommendation of heart-healthy lifestyle changes and/or Panax ginseng. *Asian J Androl* 14:830–41.

Navaneethan, S.D., M. Vecchio, and D.W. Johnson. 2010. Prevalence and correlates of self-reported sexual dysfunction in CKD: A meta-analysis of observational studies. *Am J Kidney Dis* 56:670–85.

Negrean, M., A. Stirban, B. Stratmann, et al. 2007. Effects of low- and high-advanced glycation endproduct meals on macro- and microvascular endothelial function and oxidative stress in patients with type 2 diabetes mellitus. *Am J Clin Nutr* 85:1236–43.

Neves, D. 2013. Advanced glycation end-products: A common pathway in diabetes and age-related erectile dysfunction. *Free Radic Res* 47:49–69.

Neves, D., M. Assunção, F. Marques, J.P. Andrade, and H. Almeida. 2008. Does regular consumption of green tea influence VEGF and its receptors expression in aged rat erectile tissue? Possible implications in vasculogenic erectile dysfunction progression. *AGE* 30:217–28.

Neves, D., I. Tomada, M. Assunção, F. Marques, H. Almeida, and J.P. Andrade. 2010. Effects of chronic red wine consumption on the expression of vascular endothelial growth factor, angiopoietin 1, angiopoietin 2 and its receptors in rat erectile tissue. *J Food Sci* 75:H79–86.

Penfold, S.A., M.T. Coughlan, S.K. Patel, et al. 2010. Circulating high-molecular-weight RAGE ligands activate pathways implicated in the development of diabetic nephropathy. *Kidney Int* 78:287–95.

Peyroux, J. and M. Sternberg. 2006. Advanced glycation endproducts (AGEs): Pharmacological inhibition in diabetes. *Pathologie Biologie* 54:405–19.

Poulsen, M.W., M.J. Bak, and J.M. Andersen. 2014. Effect of dietary advanced glycation end products on postprandial appetite, inflammation, and endothelial activation in healthy overweight individuals. *Eur J Nutr* 53:661–72.

Poulsen, M.W., R.V. Hedegaard, J.M. Andersen, et al. 2013. Advanced glycation endproducts in food and their effects on health. *Food Chem Toxicol* 60:10–37.

Rabbani, N. and P.J. Thornalley. 2012. Glycation research in aminoacids: A place to call home. *Aminoacids* 42:1087–96.

Rajasekar, P. and C.V. Anuradha. 2007. L-Carnitine inhibits protein glycation in vitro and in vivo: Evidence for a role in diabetic management. *Acta Diabetol* 44:83–90.

Sajithlal, G.B., P. Chithra, and G. Chandrakasan. 1998. Effect of curcumin on the advanced glycation and cross-linking of collagen in diabetic rats. *Biochem Pharmacol* 56:1607–14.

Seftel, A.D., N.D. Vaziri, Z. Ni, et al. 1997. Advanced glycation end products in human penis: Elevation in diabetic tissue, site of deposition, and possible effect through iNOS or eNOS. *Urology* 50:1016–26.

Semba, R.D., A. Ang, S. Talegawkar, et al. 2012. Dietary intake associated with serum versus urinary carboxymethyl-lysine, a major advanced glycation end product, in adults: The Energetics Study. *Eur J Clin Nutr* 66:3–9.

Semba, R.D., S.K. Gebauer, D.J. Baer, et al. 2014. Dietary intake of advanced glycation end products did not affect endothelial function and inflammation in healthy adults in a randomized controlled trial. *J Nutr* 144:1037–42.

Sena, C.M., P. Matafome, J. Crisóstomo, et al. 2012. Methylglyoxal promotes oxidative stress and endothelial dysfunction. *Pharmacol Res* 65:497–506.

Shaeer, O. and K. Shaeer. 2012. The Global Online Sexuality Survey (GOSS): The United States of America in 2011. Chapter I: Erectile Dysfunction among English-Speakers. *J Sex Med* 9:3018–27.

Shamloul, R. and H. Ghanem. 2013. Erectile dysfunction. *Lancet* 381:153–65.

Sjögren, P., G. Basta, R. de Caterina, et al. 2007. Markers of endothelial activity are related to components of the metabolic syndrome, but not to circulating concentrations of the advanced glycation end-product N epsilon-carboxymethyl-lysine in healthy Swedish men. *Atherosclerosis* 195:e168–75.

Stadtman, E.R. 1992. Protein oxidation and aging. *Science* 257:1220–4.

Stirban, A., M. Negrean, C. Götting, et al. 2008. Dietary advanced glycation endproducts and oxidative stress: In vivo effects on endothelial function and adipokines. *Ann N Y Acad Sci* 1126:276–9.

Su, J., P.A. Lucchesi, R.A. Gonzalez-Villalobos, et al. 2008. Role of advanced glycation end products with oxidative stress in resistance artery dysfunction in type 2 diabetic mice. *Arterioscler Thromb Vasc Biol* 28:1432–8.

Suzuki, E., H. Nishimatsu, S. Oba, M. Takahashi, and Y. Homma. 2014. Chronic kidney disease and erectile dysfunction. *World J Nephrol* 3:220–9.

Tessier, F.J. and I. Birlouez-Aragon. 2012. Health effects of dietary Maillard reaction products: The results of ICARE and other studies. *Amino Acids* 42:1119–31.

Tomada, I., N. Tomada, H. Almeida, and D. Neves. 2013. Androgen depletion in humans leads to cavernous tissue reorganization and upregulation of Sirt1-eNOS axis. *Age* 35:35–47.

Tomada, N., R. Oliveira, I. Tomada, P. Vendeira, and D. Neves. 2008. Comparative ultrastructural study of human corpus cavernosum during ageing. *Microsc Microanal* 14:S3152–5.

Uribarri, J., W. Cai, M. Peppa, et al. 2007b. Circulating glycotoxins and dietary advanced glycation endproducts: Two links to inflammatory response, oxidative stress, and aging. *J Gerontol A Biol Sci Med Sci* 62:427–33.

Uribarri, J., W. Cai, R. Pyzik, et al. 2014. Suppression of native defense mechanisms, SIRT1 and PPARγ, by dietary glycoxidants precedes disease in adult humans; relevance to lifestyle-engendered chronic diseases. *Amino Acids* 46:301–9.

Uribarri, J., W. Cai, M. Ramdas, et al. 2011. Restriction of advanced glycation end products improves insulin resistance in human type 2 diabetes: Potential role of AGER1 and SIRT1. *Diabetes Care* 34:1610–16.

Uribarri, J., A. Stirban, D. Sander, et al. 2007a. Single oral challenge by advanced glycation end products acutely impairs endothelial function in diabetic and nondiabetic subjects. *Diabetes Care* 30:2579–82.

Uribarri, J., S. Woodruff, S. Goodman, et al. 2010. Advanced glycation end products in foods and a practical guide to their reduction in the diet. *J Am Diet Assoc* 110:911–16.

Vlassara, H. and W. Cai, S. 2009. Protection against loss of innate defenses in adulthood by low advanced glycation end products (AGE) intake: Role of the antiinflammatory AGE receptor-1. *J Clin Endocrinol Metab* 94:4483–91.

Vlassara, H., W. Cai, and J. Crandall. 2002. Inflammatory mediators are induced by dietary glycotoxins, a major risk factor for diabetic angiopathy. *Proc Natl Acad Sci U S A* 99:15596–601.

Yang, R., J. Wang, Y. Chen, Z. Sun, R. Wang, and Y. Dai. 2008. Effect of caffeine on erectile function via up-regulating cavernous cyclic guanosine monophosphate in diabetic rats. *J Androl* 29:586–91.

Yonekura, H., Y. Yamamoto, S. Sakurai, et al. 2003. Novel splice variants of the receptor for advanced glycation end-products expressed in human vascular endothelial cells and pericytes, and their putative roles in diabetes-induced vascular injury. *Biochem J* 370:1097–109.

Yu, W., Z. Wan, X.F. Qiu, Y. Chen, and Y.T. Dai. 2013. Resveratrol, an activator of SIRT1, restores erectile function in streptozotocin-induced diabetic rats. *Asian J Androl* 15:646–51.

15

Biological Implications of Diet-Derived Advanced Glycation End Products on Carcinogenesis

David P. Turner and Victoria J. Findlay
Medical University of South Carolina
Charleston, SC

CONTENTS

KEY POINTS

- Environmental and lifestyle behavioral factors are thought to contribute to the majority of cancer cases. With this in mind, there is a growing emphasis upon lifestyle alteration as a strategy for cancer prevention and treatment.
- While it has long been recognized that diet and exercise produce health benefits, the scientific literature lacks a clear understanding of the specific biological mechanisms by which nutritional change can produce these health benefits.
- Increasing evidence supports a role for dietary-associated advanced glycation end products (AGEs) in the carcinogenic process.
- AGEs may represent a group of nutrient-associated biomarkers that are linked to patterns of food consumption, leading to increased risk of cancer and recurrence in cancer survivors.
- AGEs may be critical molecular tools with which to correlate epidemiological, interventional, and tumor biology in order to better assess the effects of diet on cancer risk.

15.1 Introduction

An increasing number of scientific studies provide compelling evidence that the majority of cancers are preventable through behavioral and environmental change. While genetic mutation remains a significant contributor to the carcinogenic process (Couzin-Frankel 2015), interrelated lifestyle factors such as poor diet, lack of exercise, and obesity function to amplify that risk (Wu et al. 2016). With this in mind, there is a growing emphasis upon lifestyle alteration as a strategy for cancer prevention and treatment. While the deleterious effects of poor diet and obesity on cancer etiology are now widely accepted, our basic mechanistic understanding of the molecular effects of poor nutrition on the inherent biology of tumors is severely lacking. What we eat can have significant effects on cancer onset, growth, progression, and treatment; however, we do not yet fully understand how a healthy lifestyle can alter tumor biology to improve prognosis and overall survival. Such an understanding is critical if we are to establish lifestyle intervention as a frontline strategy for the prevention of cancer.

Advanced glycation end products (AGEs) are reactive metabolites that irreversibly accumulate in tissues and organs as we grow older (Turner 2015, 2017). They are produced endogenously in the body during normal metabolism and by the oxidation of biological macromolecules (Foster et al. 2014; Turner 2015, 2017). AGEs accumulate in our tissues and organs over time and contribute to the development and complications associated with diseases of advancing age, including diabetes, cardiovascular disease, renal failure, arthritis, and neurodegenerative disorders (Peppa et al. 2003; Thornalley 2003a; Uribarri et al. 2005, 2010; Cho et al. 2007; Ansari and Rasheed 2008; Noordzij et al. 2008; Ansari and Rasheed 2010). AGE pathogenic effects include modification of protein function, genetic fidelity, cellular signaling, and stress responses. AGEs are emerging as a unifying biological consequence of poor nutrition and lifestyle that may contribute to the onset and progression of cancer. In addition to their endogenous production as part of normal energy metabolism, diet represents a significant external source of AGEs, which contributes to the AGE accumulation pool and disease complications. It is estimated that 10%–30% of AGEs are derived from exogenous sources such as diet (Uribarri et al. 2010). Therefore, both normal metabolism and lifestyle factors contribute to the AGE accumulation pool in the body; interrelated biological pathways associated with glucose metabolism such as glycolysis and hyperglycemia, as well as oxidative and inflammatory stress responses, increase the formation of AGE precursor levels and the overall endogenous AGE accumulation. In a potential feedback loop, these AGEs may in turn alter the regulation of glucose flux: for example, in adipocyte cell lines, AGE modification of albumin increases the production of reactive oxygen species (ROS), which can inhibit glucose uptake (Singh et al. 2014). Additionally, AGE treatment in muscle cells impairs insulin receptor signaling to alter glycogen synthase activity and glucose uptake (Miele et al. 2003) and the activation of stress response pathways to perpetuate the pathogenic cycle further (Figure 15.1a). Also, contributing to the AGE levels in the body is their exogenous intake resulting from an unhealthy diet high in sugar and fat, drinking alcohol, and smoking. Additionally, a sedentary lifestyle perpetuates these dietary effects (Figure 15.1b). Exogenous factors contribute to the accumulation pool by increasing both precursor and preformed AGEs as well as affecting the biological pathways associated with endogenous AGE formation (Figure 15.1c). The resulting increase in AGE formation may result in a pro-tumorigenic microenvironment conducive to cancer onset and/or recurrence.

15.2 Diet and Cancer

Environmental and lifestyle risk factors are now thought to contribute to as much as 80% of all cancer cases in developed countries (World Health Organization [WHO]). Worldwide each year, around 14 million new cancer cases are diagnosed, and almost 9 million cancer deaths are recorded. The cost to the world economy caused by premature death and disability from cancer is estimated to be around 1 trillion dollars and is rising. The number of new cancer cases is expected to be more than 20 million per year by 2030 with 13 million cancer deaths. Therefore, environmental and lifestyle risk factors represent

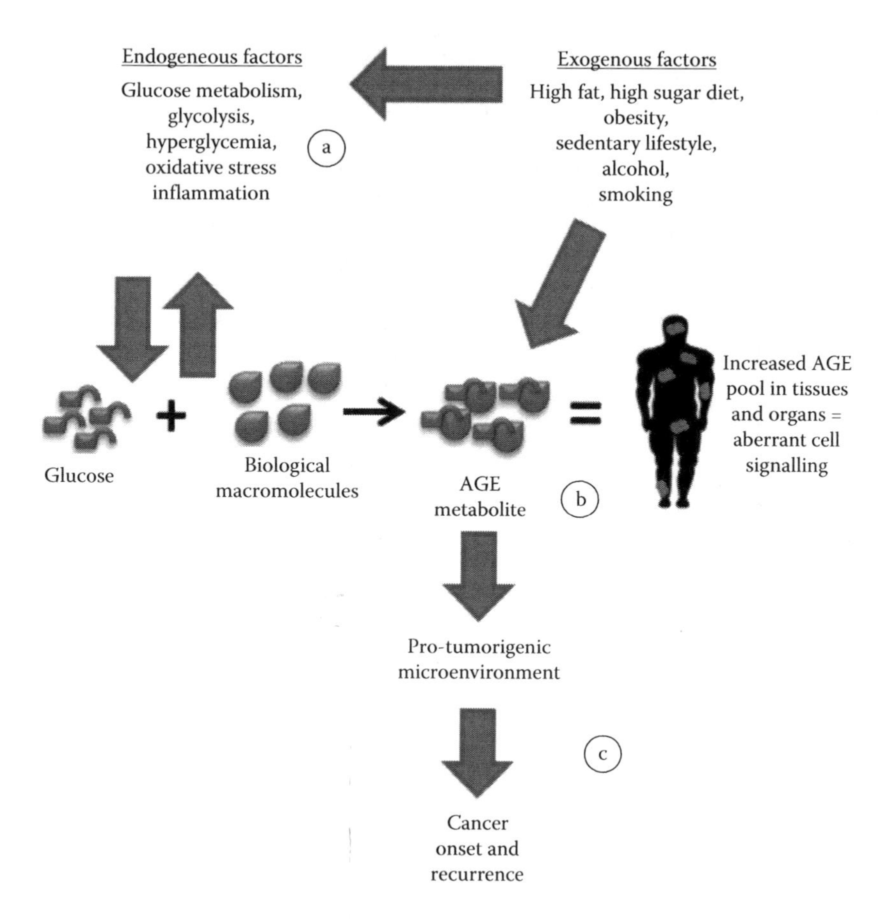

FIGURE 15.1 Endogenous and exogenous factors combine to increase the AGE accumulation pool. Endogenous and exogenous factors combine to increase the formation of AGE precursor levels and increase overall AGE accumulation in the body. In a potential feedback loop, the pathogenic effects of AGEs may increase the activation of stress response pathways that can alter the regulation of glucose uptake and flux to perpetuate the pathogenic cycle further (a). This results in an increase in AGE accumulation through the generation of both AGE precursors and AGE metabolites, the pathogenic effects of which alter biological pathways to promote disease complications (b). The resulting increase in AGE formation may result in a pro-tumorigenic inflammatory microenvironment conducive to cancer onset and/or recurrence (c).

a critical area for the development of cancer prevention strategies aimed at reducing their exposure in order to significantly reduce the burden of cancer. Modifiable risk factors, as defined by the WHO, include:

- Tobacco use (cigarettes and smokeless tobacco)
- Being overweight or obese
- Unhealthy diet (high fat and high sugar with low fruit and vegetable intake)
- Sedentary lifestyle
- Alcohol consumption
- Ionizing/ultraviolet radiation
- Human papilloma virus infection
- Air pollution

It is estimated that around 30% of the most commonly occurring cancers can be prevented by adopting a healthier lifestyle of healthy eating, maintaining a healthy weight, and exercising regularly (WHO).

15.2.1 Diet and Cancer Risk/Survival

A recent review concisely documents the issues and challenges faced by investigators attempting to relate what we eat to overall cancer risk (Mayne et al. 2016). Issues such as study design, data collection, and additional confounding factors have made such analyses difficult and have often led to inconsistent data. Despite these challenges, a clear link between nutrition and cancer biology is generally accepted, and individuals consuming an unhealthy diet are now thought to be at higher risk of developing cancer. Several epidemiological studies have shown that people with a healthier eating regimen have lower incidence for breast, lung, colon, and stomach cancer. Additionally, being overweight or obese, often a consequence of poor diet, is also strongly associated with increased risk of postmenopausal breast, colon, rectal, kidney, pancreatic, esophageal, and endometrial cancers (Key et al. 2004; Parkin 2011).

In addition to cancer risk, diet also has significant implications for cancer survivors. Improved treatment of cancer has led to increases in the number of people surviving cancer, and currently there are 32 million (5-years post-diagnosed) cancer survivors. For these survivors, the effects of treatment often lead to a myriad of unique physical and psychosocial issues that impact their long-term health-related quality of life (HRQOL) and potentially survival outcomes (Skolarus et al. 2014). Weight gain is a common occurrence in cancer survivors whether it is a consequence of their treatment or changes in lifestyle habits. The time after cancer diagnosis has been shown to be a key period for diet change (Fassier et al. 2017). Although research relating to nutrition and surviving cancer is in its infancy, evidence indicates that avoiding weight gain after diagnosis or treatment can reduce the risk of recurrence. Zhang et al. (2015) examined dietary intake and quality in 1,500 cancer survivors who were matched by age, sex, and race/ethnicity to 3,000 individuals with no cancer history. Results showed that dietary intake patterns for cancer survivors were worse than those in the control group.

The number of cancer survivors in the United States who are obese has risen from almost 18 million in 1992 to just over 33 million in 2015 (https://progressreport.cancer.gov/after/obesity). Meta-analysis studies show that four out of five observational studies show a positive correlation between loss of weight and reduced mortality in overweight or obese cancer survivors. The remaining study showed no change (Jackson et al. 2017). Central to most evidence-based lifestyle cancer prevention strategies, preventing either tumor onset or recurrence, is a well-balanced and healthy diet. Eating healthily can have multiple beneficial effects with relation to the carcinogenic process. Eating a well-balanced diet can help to prevent the development of known cancer risk factors such as being overweight or obese and associated disease comorbidities such as diabetes and insulin resistance. Eating vegetables, fruits, wholegrain foods, and pulses, and avoiding sugary drinks, processed and red meats, and other high calorie foods such as fast foods are likely to prevent weight gain and its associated consequences. A similar dietary pattern is also recommended by the WHO as a cancer prevention strategy to reduce both its risk and its recurrence in cancer survivors:

- Eat at least five portions/servings of non-starchy vegetables and fruits each day.
- Eat relatively unprocessed cereals and/or pulses with every meal.
- Limit refined starchy foods.
- Limit consumption of red meat to less than 500 g a week.
- Limit the consumption of processed foods significantly.
- Limit or avoid alcoholic drinks.
- Avoid salt-preserved, salted, or salty foods. Limit intake to less than 2.4 g sodium a day.

15.2.2 Diet and Tumor Biology

As our understanding of tumor biology advances, it is becoming increasingly clear that lifestyle factors such as poor nutrition can have distinct molecular consequences on the biological makeup of individuals, altering cell signaling events and gene expression profiles to promote tumor growth, decreasing overall HRQOL, and contributing to disease progression (Turner 2015). The majority of studies aimed at gaining a better mechanistic understanding of the effects of diet on carcinogenesis, examining the impact of a particular food, food group, or nutrient compound on tumor onset and growth. However, as patterns of food consumption vary greatly and are highly individualized, this is a linearized approach, which contributes to the inconsistent data surrounding diet and cancer risk. Dietary patterns consist of a complex series of macronutrients and micronutrients (a particular food or nutrient[s] is not digested alone) that may undergo a complex set of interactions with multiple biological processes to affect tumor biology. Molecular assessment of dietary patterns is, therefore, more effective but is faced with its own methodological challenges. The identification of nutrient-associated biomarkers that are linked to patterns of food consumption may represent critical molecular tools with which to correlate epidemiological, interventional, and tumor biology in order to better assess the effects of diet on cancer risk.

15.3 Dietary AGEs and Cancer

Many of the modifiable cancer risk factors defined by the WHO are also associated with increased levels of AGE metabolites. AGE accumulation is exacerbated by the same social and environmental factors contributing to health disparity; poor diet, obesity, and a lack of exercise are interrelated lifestyle factors that not only contribute to cancer risk and progression but also significantly increase the AGE accumulation pool in the body. As discussed throughout this book, the typical Western diet, high in sugar, protein, and fat and low in fruit, grains, and vegetables, is particularly AGE-laden, contributing as much as 30% of the AGEs accumulated within the body (Uribarri et al. 2005, 2007, 2010; Vlassara 2005). AGEs are naturally present in uncooked meats, however, frying, grilling, or roasting (i.e., dry heat) accelerates AGE formation in foods by around 10-fold (Figure 15.2). Food processing and manufacturing are also major sources of exogenous AGEs. The pathogenic consequences of elevated AGE levels include protein dysfunction, protein cross-linking, decreased genetic fidelity, and aberrant cell signaling. AGEs function as ligand activators for the transmembrane receptor for AGE (RAGE). AGE activation of RAGE is a potent inducer of active, persistent, immune-mediated inflammation and oxidative stress often through the upregulation of key master transcriptional regulators leading to differential cytokine and chemokine profiles (Turner 2015). Elevated AGE levels as a consequence of diet and lifestyle may lead to the oncogenic activation of RAGE, leading to a proinflammatory microenvironment conducive to tumor onset, growth, and progression.

Compared to other chronic diseases, the link between dietary AGEs and cancer is an emerging field of research. The majority of cancer-associated studies (as discussed below) have centered on levels of carboxymethyllysine (CML). CML is often used as an indicator of overall AGE levels within the context of food and has been extensively studied in animal models of chronic disease (Ames 2008; Han et al. 2013).

Raw chicken
~800 AGE
kU/100g
Poached chicken
~1,000 AGE
kU/100g
Fried chicken
~7,000 AGE
kU/100g
Raw carrots
~10 AGE kU/100g
Boiled carrots
~25 AGE kU/100g
Grilled carrots
~220 AGE kU/100g

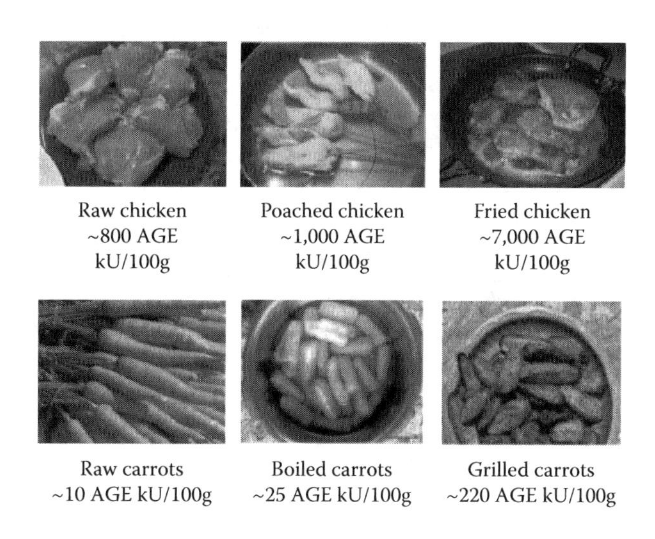

FIGURE 15.2 How we cook food can increase exogenous AGE content. AGEs are naturally present in all foods, however, frying, grilling, or roasting (i.e., high and/or dry heat) greatly accelerates AGE formation in foods compared to poaching and boiling (i.e., low and/or moist heat). (From Uribarri et al. *J Am Diet Assoc*. 110(6):911–916, 2010.)

While the study of AGE levels in different tumor types has been restricted to relatively small cohorts, overall, the data indicate that higher levels of AGEs do correlate with cancer risk and tumor biology.

15.3.1 Breast Cancer

CML levels are elevated in breast tumor tissue independent of tumor stage and type (Bachmeier et al. 2008). Mass spectrometry analysis of breast tumor tissue identified several AGE-modified proteins with functional significance to breast cancer progression (Korwar et al. 2012). Tesarova et al. (2007) examined CML levels in 86 breast cancer patients stratified by stage and histological staining. Compared to 14 healthy controls, breast cancer patients had higher serum AGE concentrations ($p < 0.01$) at the early (Stages I and II) stages of disease and even higher levels at late stages of the disease (Stages III and IV). Highest levels of AGEs were also accompanied by high levels of AGE precursors. One study investigating the levels of the methylglyoxyl-derived Arg-pyrimidine AGE adduct in breast cancer subtypes found its levels increased in cancer cells compared to adjacent non-cancer tissue. Significantly, comparison among subtypes revealed that triple-negative breast cancer tissue, while often being the most aggressive, had the lowest Arg-pyrimidine levels compared to other subtypes. Accompanying the lower Arg-pyrimidine levels in triple-negative tumors was an increased expression of the methylglyoxyl-detoxifying enzyme glyoxylase 1. This suggests that cells may be able to mount an orchestrated defense to higher AGE levels in aggressive tumors (Chiavarina et al. 2014).

AGEs, endogenous or exogenous, also alter breast tumor biology. Exogenous treatment with AGEs increases the growth, migratory, and invasive properties of breast cancer cell lines (Sharaf et al. 2015). Expression of RAGE is elevated in advanced-stage and triple-negative breast tumors and node-positive tissues compared with other tissues ($p < 0.001$) (Nankali et al. 2016). Additionally, a positive association between RAGE expression and tumor size has also been reported ($p = 0.029$).

15.3.2 Prostate Cancer

Yang et al. (2015) examined CML levels and oxidative stress biomarkers in 24 cases of prostate cancer and 24 controls. Higher levels of plasma CML were positively associated with increased risk of prostate cancer (relative risk 1.79; 95% confidence interval, 1.00–3.21). Significantly, markers of oxidative stress were not associated with increased risk. Another study identified a race-specific, tumor-dependent pattern of AGE accumulation (Foster et al. 2014). AGE levels were significantly elevated in both serum and tumor from prostate cancer patients, with highest accumulation occurring in the more aggressive tumors. When examined in a paired cohort of patients, high AGE levels in the serum correlated with high AGE accumulation in cancer tissue. Significantly, when the data were stratified by race, AGE metabolite levels were significantly higher in serum from African American when compared to European American prostate cancer patients. Similar to that observed in a breast cancer background, exogenous AGE treatment of prostate cancer cells promotes cell growth, migration, and invasion. AGE-mediated cross-linking of modified basement membrane promotes the invasive properties of prostate epithelial cells and correlates with decreased overall survival (Rodriguez-Teja et al. 2014). Reduced RAGE expression inhibits prostate-specific antigen expression and cell proliferation in prostate cancer cell lines and tumor growth in Nude mice (Elangovan et al. 2012). Affinity studies indicate that RAGE preferentially interacts with AGEs on prostate cancer cells over other potential ligands (Allmen et al. 2008), and the AGE-RAGE signaling axis has been shown to promote prostate cancer cell proliferation by increasing retinoblastoma phosphorylation and degradation (Bao et al. 2015).

15.3.3 Pancreatic Cancer

In the largest study examining AGE levels in a cancer cohort, Jiao et al. (2015) estimated CML consumption in the NIH-AARP Diet and Health Study to examine the association between CML levels and pancreatic cancer. Using a cohort of 2,193 pancreatic cancer cases, dietary-derived CML was associated with an increased risk of pancreatic cancer in men (HR: 1.43; 95% CI: 1.06, 1.93, $p = 0.003$) but not women (HR: 1.14; 95% CI: 0.76, 1.72, $p = 0.42$). Significantly, men who eat the most red meat (often a significant source of dietary AGEs) had the highest risk of pancreatic cancer (HR: 1.35; 95% CI: 1.07, 1.70, $p = 0.003$).

This may explain, at least in part, the positive association between red meat and pancreatic cancer. However, a previous study in a cohort of 454 patients with exocrine pancreatic cancer found that CML levels were associated with a reduction in pancreatic risk (OR = 0.57; 95% CI, 0.32–1.01) (Grote et al. 2012).

15.3.4 Other Cancers

Studies investigating the association between dietary AGEs and other cancers apart from breast, prostate, and pancreas are lacking; however, a mechanistic role for AGEs in pathogenesis of both colorectal cancer and melanoma has been reported, which have been recently reviewed (Yamagishi et al. 2015; Turner 2017).

15.4 Sugar-Derived AGEs

The consumption of refined carbohydrates, often in the form of sugar and high-fructose corn syrup, is a major factor in the obesity and diabetes epidemics in the Western world. Fructose is common in today's modern diet, particularly in the form of high-fructose corn syrup, and is thought to play a causative role in the increasing rates of cardiovascular disease, hypertension, diabetes, and cancer (Levi and Werman 1998; Tokita et al. 2005; Takeuchi et al. 2010). Whether sugar alone can directly cause cancer is controversial and requires further study. However, sugar does promotes obesity and diabetes, which are recognized as cancer risk factors. Meta-analysis studies have identified a link between dietary glycemic index, glycemic load, and risk of breast (Dong and Qin 2011; Romieu et al. 2012), prostate (Vidal et al. 2015), colorectal (Gnagnarella et al. 2008), lung (Melkonian et al. 2016), and endometrial (Gnagnarella et al. 2008) cancers. Additionally, a recent study of MD Anderson found that the direct consumption of sucrose by mice, at comparable levels to that often consumed on a typical Western diet, resulted in increased breast tumor growth and lung metastasis compared to mice fed a starch control diet (Jiang et al. 2016). The high-sucrose diet resulted in dysregulated bioactive lipid metabolism, altering membrane function as well as intracellular signaling. This study is one of the first to demonstrate the biological potential of increased sugar intake to directly influence tumor-associated pathways to promote cancer growth. The molecular and pathogenic links between AGEs, lifestyle, and sugar metabolism are extensively documented for diabetes and cardiovascular disease. However, a potential contribution to the development and progression of cancer is lacking (Turner 2015). Carbohydrates such as fructose and glucose are processed by specific molecular pathways to produce essential metabolites that are required for energy production (Uribarri et al. 2005, 2010). These essential metabolites produce carbohydrate intermediates, which react with free amino groups to generate reactive carbonyl species (RCS). RCS are AGE precursors which in turn react non-enzymatically with macromolecules such as proteins, lipids, and DNA to produce AGEs (Thornalley 2003a, 2003b, 2008; Uribarri et al. 2005, 2010; Ansari and Rasheed 2008). RCSs can undergo further oxidation, dehydration, and polymerization to give rise to the formation of alternative AGE metabolites. AGEs are also produced by the direct oxidation of glycolytic intermediates, proteins, and other biological macromolecules (Thornalley 2003a, 2003b, 2008; Uribarri et al. 2005, 2010; Ansari and Rasheed 2008; Turner 2015).

15.4.1 Glucose Metabolism and Cancer

The reprogramming of glucose metabolism and the increased uptake of glucose are critical to the tumorigenic process, especially aerobic glycolysis where glucose is converted to lactate even in the presence of oxygen (often termed the Warburg effect) (Kritikou 2008; Palsson-McDermott and O'Neill 2013). Increased glucose metabolism promotes several of the hallmarks of cancer including inhibition of apoptosis, oncogenesis, and chemotherapy resistance (Ward and Thompson 2012; Yoshida 2015). Epidemiological studies indicate a positive correlation between blood glucose levels and tumor growth *in vivo*, and hyperglycemia is positively associated with increased risk of cancer and decreased overall survival for several tumor types including prostate (Jee et al. 2005; Xu et al. 2005; Pelicano et al. 2006; Ikeda et al. 2009). Decreases in circulating glucose levels via calorie restriction can reduce tumor growth in animal models (Santisteban et al. 1985; Seyfried et al. 2003; Xu et al. 2005; Pelicano et al. 2006).

Evidence suggests that abnormal glucose uptake may occur earlier in African American cancer patients who often present with aggressive disease (Seewaldt et al. 2012).

15.4.2 AGE Biology and Glucose Metabolism

Increased glucose metabolism as a consequence of increased sugar intake is also a unifying biological consequence, which links poor lifestyle and cancer with AGEs. Sugar-related disease states such as dyslipidemia, hypertension, and hyperglycemia along with poor diet play a fundamental role in increasing AGE levels in the body. Stress response is a critical regulator of glucose flux and is intrinsically linked with AGE signaling; immune-mediated activation of macrophages and dendritic cells causes a switch from oxidative phosphorylation toward glycolysis (Kelly and O'Neill 2015; O'Neill 2016). Through the activation of RAGE-mediated transcriptional regulation, AGEs increase the stimulatory effect of glucose on macrophages to potentially promote atherosclerosis. AGEs also modulate lymphoid cell function (Coughlan et al. 2011) as well as increase macrophage polarization into an inflammatory M1 phenotype through the RAGE/NF-κB signaling pathway (Jin et al. 2015). Antioxidants inhibit AGE-induced changes in glucose consumption (de Arriba et al. 2003), and increases in RCS lead to increased AGE formation. In cancer cells, high ROS levels can result from increased metabolic activity and mitochondrial dysfunction and can promote cancer progression toward an aggressive phenotype (Hanahan and Weinberg 2011; Policastro et al. 2012). Eating the same foods that increase AGE levels in our bodies such as red meats, high fat, and high carbohydrates can also increase oxidative stress and RCS/ROS, promoting chronic disease (Vetrani et al. 2013).

As shown in Figure 15.3, AGEs accumulate and are significantly elevated in tumor tissue (green fluorescence) compared to non-cancerous tissue. Elevated AGE levels in tumors would be expected to

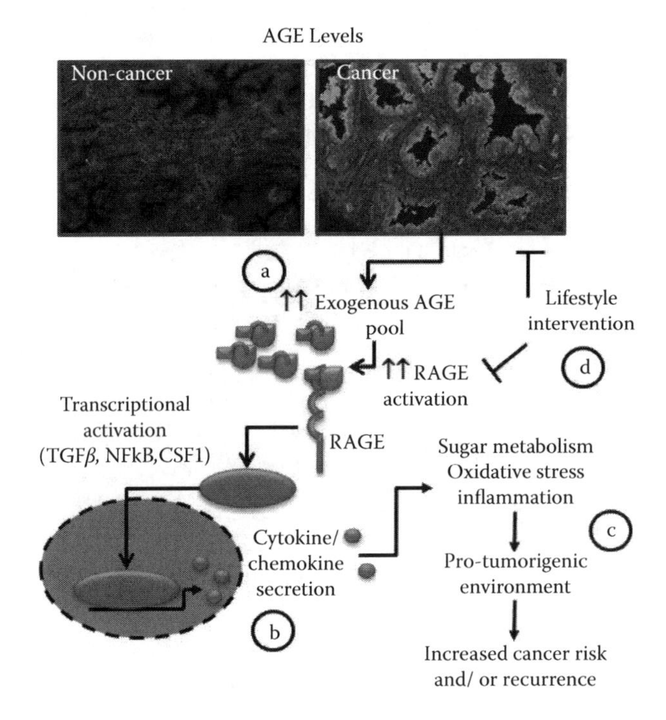

FIGURE 15.3 AGE activation of RAGE can promote a pro-tumorigenic microenvironment. AGE accumulation levels are significantly elevated in tumor tissue (green fluorescence) compared to non-cancerous tissue. Elevated AGE levels in tumors would be expected to increase the AGE accumulation pool and in turn the activation of the AGE cognate transmembrane receptor RAGE (a). RAGE activation alters the transcriptional program of a number of master transcriptional regulators to alter chemokine/cytokine secretion profiles (b). AGE-mediated changes in transcriptional activity can have profound effects on biological pathways involved in sugar metabolism and stress response pathways to create a pro-tumorigenic environment (c). Lifestyle intervention such as reduced dietary intake of AGE may be a viable cancer prevention strategy by at least in part inhibiting this pathway (d).

increase the AGE accumulation pool and in turn the activation of the AGE cognate transmembrane receptor RAGE (Figure 15.3a). RAGE activation alters the transcriptional program of a number of master transcriptional regulators such as NF-κB (nuclear factor kappa-light-chain-enhancer of activated B cells), CSF (Colony stimulating factor 1), and TGFβ (Transforming growth factor beta), which in turn regulate chemokine/cytokine secretion (Figure 15.3b). Such aberrant transcriptional activity has profound effects on biological pathways involved in sugar metabolism and stress response pathways to create a pro-tumorigenic environment conducive to increased cancer risk and/or recurrence (Figure 15.3c). Lifestyle interventions such as reduced dietary intake of AGEs may be a viable cancer prevention strategy by at least in part inhibiting this pathway (Figure 15.3d).

15.5 Conclusions

As discussed, it is estimated that by living a healthier lifestyle, at least one in every three cancer cases may be preventable. While epidemiological links between lifestyle factors such as diet and cancer have been well documented, their molecular effects on the biological makeup of tumors remain largely unexplored. AGE accumulation in the body is a direct result of (1) their endogenous production during cellular metabolism and (2) their exogenous intake as a consequence of poor diet and other lifestyle and environmental factors. The specific contribution of endogenous and exogenous sources of AGE to either tumor onset or progression has not been delineated. However, the biological consequences of both endogenous and exogenous AGE accumulation are intrinsically linked to glucose metabolism, chronic inflammation, and oxidative stress. All these processes can alter the cellular microenvironment of normal cells to promote tumor initiation or alter the tumor microenvironment to create a pro-tumorigenic niche that promotes tumor growth and progression. In pre-cancerous lesions, a constant state of inflammation and increased ROS production can cause both genetic and epigenetic alterations to increase cancer risk (Schumacker 2015). In established tumors, inflammation mediates cross talk between cancer epithelial and stromal cells, resulting in the active recruitment of immune cells to the tumor microenvironment and increased oxidative stress. The inflammatory milieu created contributes to tumor onset and progression by promoting genetic instability, cell survival, growth, and metastasis (Tafani et al. 2016).

Systematic and meta-analysis reviews indicate that healthy nutrition reduces the risk of developing cancer and potentially mortality among cancer survivors. The original concept that AGEs may represent a biological consequence of poor lifestyle is a novel approach to explain the increased incidence and mortality figures observed within specific populations affected by cancer health disparity. Compared to other chronic diseases, the existence of AGE metabolites and their connections with disease biology and lifestyle are unfamiliar to the general public as well as the cancer research community. A greater understanding of the interplay between risk factors such as diet and the molecular mechanisms associated with cancer and cancer recurrence will significantly impact quality of life and overall survival. Studies are needed that define the impact of diet on cancer-associated pathways and to delineate mechanistically how lifestyle interventions may influence quality of life and overall survival. Such a mechanistic understanding may represent a unique cancer risk factor associated with disease onset and/or recurrence. This would allow for intensive risk reduction and improved identification of high-risk patients requiring defined dietary and physical activity intervention aimed at reducing prognostic biomarker levels. It may also lead to innovative insights for pharmacologic and lifestyle adjustment and identify protective factors that may underlie differences in health outcomes observed between minority populations. To this end, AGEs may represent a ubiquitous group of nutrient-associated biomarkers that are linked to patterns of food consumption, which may be used to correlate epidemiological and interventional data with biological pathways involved in tumor biology.

Significantly, dietary and lifestyle intervention studies may have greatest impact on outcomes for health disparity populations who tend to have lower HRQOL, highest cancer burden, and lowest overall cancer survival and where a lack of exercise, poor diet, and rates of obesity are often most prevalent (Reams et al. 2009; Martin et al. 2013; Kinseth et al. 2014). Lifestyle intervention therefore may prove to be a practical and powerful strategy for all health care providers, institutions, and communities seeking to improve quality of life among cancer survivors across wide racial/ethnic, geographic, and socioeconomic strata.

ACKNOWLEDGMENTS

DPT's and VJF's work was supported in part by grants from the National Institute of Health/National Cancer Institute (CA176135-Turner, CA194469-Turner and CA157071-Ford).

REFERENCES

Allmen, E. U., M. Koch, G. Fritz, and D. F. Legler. 2008. V domain of RAGE interacts with AGEs on prostate carcinoma cells. *Prostate* 68 (7):748–58. doi: 10.1002/pros.20736.

Ames, J. M. 2008. Determination of N epsilon-(carboxymethyl)lysine in foods and related systems. *Ann N Y Acad Sci* 1126:20–4. doi: 10.1196/annals.1433.030.

Ansari, N. A., and Z. Rasheed. 2008. Non-enzymatic glycation of Proteins: From diabetes to cancer. *Biomed Chem* 3 (4):335–342.

Ansari, N. A., and Z. Rasheed. 2010. Non-enzymatic glycation of proteins: From diabetes to cancer. *Biomed Khim* 56 (2):168–78.

Bachmeier, B. E., A. G. Nerlich, H. Rohrbach, E. D. Schleicher, and U. Friess. 2008. Maillard products as biomarkers in cancer. *Ann N Y Acad Sci* 1126:283–7. doi: 10.1196/annals.1433.057.

Bao, J. M., M. Y. He, Y. W. Liu, Y. J. Lu, Y. Q. Hong, H. H. Luo, Z. L. Ren, S. C. Zhao, and Y. Jiang. 2015. AGE/RAGE/Akt pathway contributes to prostate cancer cell proliferation by promoting Rb phosphorylation and degradation. *Am J Cancer Res* 5 (5):1741–50.

Chiavarina, B., M. J. Nokin, F. Durieux, E. Bianchi, A. Turtoi, O. Peulen, P. Peixoto, et al. 2014. Triple negative tumors accumulate significantly less methylglyoxal specific adducts than other human breast cancer subtypes. *Oncotarget* 5 (14):5472–82. doi: 10.18632/oncotarget.2121.

Cho, S. J., G. Roman, F. Yeboah, and Y. Konishi. 2007. The road to advanced glycation end products: A mechanistic perspective. *Curr Med Chem* 14 (15):1653–71.

Coughlan, M. T., F. Y. Yap, D. C. Tong, S. Andrikopoulos, A. Gasser, V. Thallas-Bonke, D. E. Webster, et al. 2011. Advanced glycation end products are direct modulators of beta-cell function. *Diabetes* 60 (10):2523–32. doi: 10.2337/db10-1033.

Couzin-Frankel, J. 2015. Biomedicine. The bad luck of cancer. *Science* 347 (6217):12. doi: 10.1126/science.347.6217.12.

de Arriba, S. G., C. Loske, I. Meiners, G. Fleischer, M. Lobisch, K. Wessel, H. Tritschler, R. Schinzel, and G. Munch. 2003. Advanced glycation endproducts induce changes in glucose consumption, lactate production, and ATP levels in SH-SY5Y neuroblastoma cells by a redox-sensitive mechanism. *J Cereb Blood Flow Metab* 23 (11):1307–13. doi: 10.1097/01.WCB.0000090622.86921.0E.

Dong, J. Y., and L. Q. Qin. 2011. Dietary glycemic index, glycemic load, and risk of breast cancer: Meta-analysis of prospective cohort studies. *Breast Cancer Res Treat* 126 (2):287–94. doi: 10.1007/s10549-011-1343-3.

Elangovan, I., S. Thirugnanam, A. Chen, G. Zheng, M. C. Bosland, A. Kajdacsy-Balla, and M. Gnanasekar. 2012. Targeting receptor for advanced glycation end products (RAGE) expression induces apoptosis and inhibits prostate tumor growth. *Biochem Biophys Res Commun* 417 (4):1133–8. doi: 10.1016/j.bbrc.2011.12.060.

Fassier, P., L. Zelek, L. Lecuyer, P. Bachmann, M. Touillaud, N. Druesne-Pecollo, P. Galan, et al. 2017. Modifications in dietary and alcohol intakes between before and after cancer diagnosis: Results from the prospective population-based NutriNet-Sante cohort. *Int J Cancer* 141 (3):457–70. doi: 10.1002/ijc.30704.

Foster, D., L. Spruill, K. R. Walter, L. M. Nogueira, H. Fedarovich, R. Y. Turner, M. Ahmed, et al. 2014. AGE metabolites: A biomarker linked to cancer disparity? *Cancer Epidemiol Biomarkers Prev* 23 (10):2186–91. doi: 10.1158/1055-9965.epi-14-0564.

Gnagnarella, P., S. Gandini, C. La Vecchia, and P. Maisonneuve. 2008. Glycemic index, glycemic load, and cancer risk: A meta-analysis. *Am J Clin Nutr* 87 (6):1793–801.

Grote, V. A., A. Nieters, R. Kaaks, A. Tjonneland, N. Roswall, K. Overvad, M. R. Nielsen, et al. 2012. The associations of advanced glycation end products and its soluble receptor with pancreatic cancer risk: A case-control study within the prospective EPIC Cohort. *Cancer Epidemiol Biomarkers Prev* 21 (4):619–28. doi: 10.1158/1055-9965.epi-11-1139.

Han, L., L. Li, B. Li, D. Zhao, Y. Li, Z. Xu, and G. Liu. 2013. Review of the characteristics of food-derived and endogenous ne-carboxymethyllysine. *J Food Prot* 76 (5):912–18. doi: 10.4315/0362-028X.JFP-12-472.

Hanahan, D., and R. A. Weinberg. 2011. Hallmarks of cancer: The next generation. *Cell* 144 (5):646–74. doi: 10.1016/j.cell.2011.02.013.

Ikeda, F., Y. Doi, K. Yonemoto, T. Ninomiya, M. Kubo, K. Shikata, J. Hata, et al. 2009. Hyperglycemia increases risk of gastric cancer posed by Helicobacter pylori infection: A population-based cohort study. *Gastroenterology* 136 (4):1234–41. doi: 10.1053/j.gastro.2008.12.045.

Jackson, S. E., M. Heinrich, R. J. Beeken, and J. Wardle. 2017. Weight loss and mortality in overweight and obese cancer survivors: A systematic review. *PLoS One* 12 (1):e0169173. doi: 10.1371/journal.pone.0169173.

Jee, S. H., H. Ohrr, J. W. Sull, J. E. Yun, M. Ji, and J. M. Samet. 2005. Fasting serum glucose level and cancer risk in Korean men and women. *JAMA* 293 (2):194–202. doi: 10.1001/jama.293.2.194.

Jiang, Y., Y. Pan, P. R. Rhea, L. Tan, M. Gagea, L. Cohen, S. M. Fischer, and P. Yang. 2016. A sucrose-enriched diet promotes tumorigenesis in mammary gland in part through the 12-lipoxygenase pathway. *Cancer Res* 76 (1):24–9. doi: 10.1158/0008-5472.CAN-14-3432.

Jiao, L., R. Stolzenberg-Solomon, T. P. Zimmerman, Z. Duan, L. Chen, L. Kahle, A. Risch, et al. 2015. Dietary consumption of advanced glycation end products and pancreatic cancer in the prospective NIH-AARP Diet and health study. *Am J Clin Nutr* 101 (1):126–34. doi: 10.3945/ajcn.114.098061.

Jin, X., T. Yao, Z. Zhou, J. Zhu, S. Zhang, W. Hu, and C. Shen. 2015. Advanced glycation end products enhance macrophages polarization into M1 phenotype through activating RAGE/NF-kappaB pathway. *Biomed Res Int* 2015:732450. doi: 10.1155/2015/732450.

Kelly, B., and L. A. O'Neill. 2015. Metabolic reprogramming in macrophages and dendritic cells in innate immunity. *Cell Res* 25 (7):771–84. doi: 10.1038/cr.2015.68.

Key, T. J., A. Schatzkin, W. C. Willett, N. E. Allen, E. A. Spencer, and R. C. Travis. 2004. Diet, nutrition and the prevention of cancer. *Public Health Nutr* 7 (1A):187–200.

Kinseth, M. A., Z. Jia, F. Rahmatpanah, A. Sawyers, M. Sutton, J. Wang-Rodriguez, D. Mercola, and K. L. McGuire. 2014. Expression differences between African American and Caucasian prostate cancer tissue reveals that stroma is the site of aggressive changes. *Int J Cancer* 134 (1):81–91. doi: 10.1002/ijc.28326.

Korwar, A. M., H. S. Bhonsle, A. D. Chougale, S. S. Kote, K. R. Gawai, V. S. Ghole, C. B. Koppikar, and M. J. Kulkarni. 2012. Analysis of AGE modified proteins and RAGE expression in HER2/neu negative invasive ductal carcinoma. *Biochem Biophys Res Commun* 419 (3):490–4. doi: 10.1016/j.bbrc.2012.02.039.

Kritikou, E. 2008. Metabolism: Warburg effect revisited. *Nat Rev Cancer* 8 (4):247.

Levi, B., and M. J. Werman. 1998. Long-term fructose consumption accelerates glycation and several age-related variables in male rats. *J Nutr* 128 (9):1442–9.

Martin, D. N., A. M. Starks, and S. Ambs. 2013. Biological determinants of health disparities in prostate cancer. *Curr Opin Oncol* 25 (3):235–41. doi: 10.1097/CCO.0b013e32835eb5d1.

Mayne, S. T., M. C. Playdon, and C. L. Rock. 2016. Diet, nutrition, and cancer: Past, present and future. *Nat Rev Clin Oncol* 13 (8):504–15. doi: 10.1038/nrclinonc.2016.24.

Melkonian, S. C., C. R. Daniel, Y. Ye, J. A. Pierzynski, J. A. Roth, and X. Wu. 2016. Glycemic index, glycemic load, and lung cancer risk in non-hispanic whites. *Cancer Epidemiol Biomarkers Prev* 25 (3):532–9. doi: 10.1158/1055-9965.epi-15-0765.

Miele, C., A. Riboulet, M. A. Maitan, F. Oriente, C. Romano, P. Formisano, J. Giudicelli, F. Beguinot, and E. Van Obberghen. 2003. Human glycated albumin affects glucose metabolism in L6 skeletal muscle cells by impairing insulin-induced insulin receptor substrate (IRS) signaling through a protein kinase C alpha-mediated mechanism. *J Biol Chem* 278 (48):47376–87. doi: 10.1074/jbc.M301088200.

Nankali, M., J. Karimi, M. T. Goodarzi, M. Saidijam, I. Khodadadi, A. N. Razavi, and F. Rahimi. 2016. Increased expression of the receptor for advanced glycation end-products (RAGE) is associated with advanced breast cancer stage. *Oncol Res Treat* 39 (10):622–628. doi: 10.1159/000449326.

Noordzij, M. J., J. D. Lefrandt, and A. J. Smit. 2008. Advanced glycation end products in renal failure: An overview. *J Ren Care* 34 (4):207–12. doi: 10.1111/j.1755-6686.2008.00038.x.

O'Neill, L. A. 2016. A metabolic roadblock in inflammatory macrophages. *Cell Rep* 17 (3):625–626. doi: 10.1016/j.celrep.2016.09.085.

Palsson-McDermott, E. M., and L. A. O'Neill. 2013. The Warburg effect then and now: From cancer to inflammatory diseases. *Bioessays* 35 (11):965–73. doi: 10.1002/bies.201300084.

Parkin, D. M. 2011. 9. Cancers attributable to inadequate physical exercise in the UK in 2010. *Br J Cancer* 105 Suppl 2:S38–41. doi: 10.1038/bjc.2011.482.

Pelicano, H., D. S. Martin, R. H. Xu, and P. Huang. 2006. Glycolysis inhibition for anticancer treatment. *Oncogene* 25 (34):4633–46. doi: 10.1038/sj.onc.1209597.

Peppa, M., J. Uribarri, and H. Vlassara, 2003. Glucose, advanced glycation end products, and diabetes complications: What is new and what works. *Clin Diabetes* 21 (4):186–7.

Policastro, L. L., I. L. Ibanez, C. Notcovich, H. A. Duran, and O. L. Podhajcer. 2012. The tumor microenvironment: Characterization, redox considerations, and novel approaches for reactive oxygen species-targeted gene therapy. *Antioxid Redox Signal.* 19 (8):854–95. doi: 10.1089/ars.2011.4367.

Reams, R. R., D. Agrawal, M. B. Davis, S. Yoder, F. T. Odedina, N. Kumar, J. M. Higginbotham, T. Akinremi, S. Suther, and K. F. Soliman. 2009. Microarray comparison of prostate tumor gene expression in African-American and Caucasian American males: A pilot project study. *Infect Agent Cancer* 4 Suppl 1:S3. doi: 10.1186/1750-9378-4-S1-S3.

Rodriguez-Teja, M., J. H. Gronau, C. Breit, Y. Z. Zhang, A. Minamidate, M. P. Caley, A. McCarthy, et al. 2014. AGE-modified basement membrane cooperates with Endo180 to promote epithelial cell invasiveness and decrease prostate cancer survival. *J Pathol.* 235 (4):581–92. doi: 10.1002/path.4485.

Romieu, I., P. Ferrari, S. Rinaldi, N. Slimani, M. Jenab, A. Olsen, A. Tjonneland, et al. 2012. Dietary glycemic index and glycemic load and breast cancer risk in the European Prospective Investigation into Cancer and Nutrition (EPIC). *Am J Clin Nutr* 96 (2):345–55. doi: 10.3945/ajcn.111.026724.

Santisteban, G. A., J. T. Ely, E. E. Hamel, D. H. Read, and S. M. Kozawa. 1985. Glycemic modulation of tumor tolerance in a mouse model of breast cancer. *Biochem Biophys Res Commun* 132 (3):1174–9.

Schumacker, P. T. 2015. Reactive oxygen species in cancer: A dance with the devil. *Cancer Cell* 27 (2):156–7. doi: 10.1016/j.ccell.2015.01.007.

Seewaldt, V., A. Hoffman, and C. Ibarra-Drendall. 2012. Abstract P1-03-01: Evidence for the Warburg effect in mammary atypia from high-risk African American women. *Cancer Res* 72 (24 Supplement):P1-03-01. doi: 10.1158/0008-5472.sabcs12-p1-03-01.

Seyfried, T. N., T. M. Sanderson, M. M. El-Abbadi, R. McGowan, and P. Mukherjee. 2003. Role of glucose and ketone bodies in the metabolic control of experimental brain cancer. *Br J Cancer* 89 (7):1375–82. doi: 10.1038/sj.bjc.6601269.

Sharaf, H., S. Matou-Nasri, Q. Wang, Z. Rabhan, H. Al-Eidi, A. Al Abdulrahman, and N. Ahmed. 2015. Advanced glycation endproducts increase proliferation, migration and invasion of the breast cancer cell line MDA-MB-231. *Biochim Biophys Acta* 1852 (3):429–41. doi: 10.1016/j.bbadis.2014.12.009.

Singh, V. P., A. Bali, N. Singh, and A. S. Jaggi. 2014. Advanced glycation end products and diabetic complications. *Kor J Physiol Pharmacol* 18 (1):1–14. doi: 10.4196/kjpp.2014.18.1.1.

Skolarus, T. A., A. M. Wolf, N. L. Erb, D. D. Brooks, B. M. Rivers, W. Underwood, 3rd, A. L. Salner, et al. 2014. American Cancer Society prostate cancer survivorship care guidelines. *CA Cancer J Clin* 64 (4):225–49. doi: 10.3322/caac.21234.

Tafani, M., L. Sansone, F. Limana, T. Arcangeli, E. De Santis, M. Polese, M. Fini, and M. A. Russo. 2016. The interplay of reactive oxygen species, hypoxia, inflammation, and sirtuins in cancer initiation and progression. *Oxid Med Cell Longev* 2016:3907147. doi: 10.1155/2016/3907147.

Takeuchi, M., M. Iwaki, J. Takino, H. Shirai, M. Kawakami, R. Bucala, and S. Yamagishi. 2010. Immunological detection of fructose-derived advanced glycation end-products. *Lab Invest* 90 (7):1117–27. doi: 10.1038/labinvest.2010.62.

Tesarova, P., M. Kalousova, B. Trnkova, J. Soukupova, S. Argalasova, O. Mestek, L. Petruzelka, and T. Zima. 2007. Carbonyl and oxidative stress in patients with breast cancer—Is there a relation to the stage of the disease? *Neoplasma* 54 (3):219–24.

Thornalley, P. J. 2003a. The enzymatic defence against glycation in health, disease and therapeutics: A symposium to examine the concept. *Biochem Soc Trans* 31 (Pt 6):1341–2. doi: 10.1042/.

Thornalley, P. J. 2003b. Protecting the genome: Defence against nucleotide glycation and emerging role of glyoxalase I overexpression in multidrug resistance in cancer chemotherapy. *Biochem Soc Trans* 31 (Pt 6):1372–7. doi: 10.1042/.

Thornalley, P. J. 2008. Protein and nucleotide damage by glyoxal and methylglyoxal in physiological systems—Role in ageing and disease. *Drug Metabol Drug Interact* 23 (1–2):125–50.

Tokita, Y., Y. Hirayama, A. Sekikawa, H. Kotake, T. Toyota, T. Miyazawa, T. Sawai, and S. Oikawa. 2005. Fructose ingestion enhances atherosclerosis and deposition of advanced glycated end-products in cholesterol-fed rabbits. *J Atheroscler Thromb* 12 (5):260–7.

Turner, D. P. 2015. Advanced glycation end-products: A biological consequence of lifestyle contributing to cancer disparity. *Cancer Res* 75 (10):1925–9. doi: 10.1158/0008-5472.can-15-0169.

Turner, D. P. 2017. The role of advanced glycation end-products in cancer disparity. *Adv Cancer Res* 133:1–22. doi: 10.1016/bs.acr.2016.08.001.

Uribarri, J., W. Cai, M. Peppa, S. Goodman, L. Ferrucci, G. Striker, and H. Vlassara. 2007. Circulating glycotoxins and dietary advanced glycation endproducts: Two links to inflammatory response, oxidative stress, and aging. *J Gerontol A Biol Sci Med Sci* 62 (4):427–33.

Uribarri, J., W. Cai, O. Sandu, M. Peppa, T. Goldberg, and H. Vlassara. 2005. Diet-derived advanced glycation end products are major contributors to the body's AGE pool and induce inflammation in healthy subjects. *Ann N Y Acad Sci* 1043:461–6. doi: 1043/1/461 [pii]10.1196/annals.1333.052.

Uribarri, J., S. Woodruff, S. Goodman, W. Cai, X. Chen, R. Pyzik, A. Yong, G. E. Striker, and H. Vlassara. 2010. Advanced glycation end products in foods and a practical guide to their reduction in the diet. *J Am Diet Assoc* 110 (6):911–16 e12. doi: 10.1016/j.jada.2010.03.018.

Vetrani, C., G. Costabile, L. Di Marino, and A. A. Rivellese. 2013. Nutrition and oxidative stress: A systematic review of human studies. *Int J Food Sci Nutr* 64 (3):312–26. doi: 10.3109/09637486.2012.738651.

Vidal, A. C., C. D. Williams, E. H. Allott, L. E. Howard, D. J. Grant, M. McPhail, K. N. Sourbeer, et al. 2015. Carbohydrate intake, glycemic index and prostate cancer risk. *Prostate* 75 (4):430–9. doi: 10.1002/pros.22929.

Vlassara, H. 2005. Advanced glycation in health and disease: Role of the modern environment. *Ann N Y Acad Sci* 1043:452–60. doi: 10.1196/annals.1333.051.

Ward, P. S., and C. B. Thompson. 2012. Metabolic reprogramming: A cancer hallmark even warburg did not anticipate. *Cancer Cell* 21 (3):297–308. doi: 10.1016/j.ccr.2012.02.014.

Wu, S., S. Powers, W. Zhu, and Y. A. Hannun. 2016. Substantial contribution of extrinsic risk factors to cancer development. *Nature* 529 (7584):43–7. doi: 10.1038/nature16166.

Xu, R. H., H. Pelicano, Y. Zhou, J. S. Carew, L. Feng, K. N. Bhalla, M. J. Keating, and P. Huang. 2005. Inhibition of glycolysis in cancer cells: A novel strategy to overcome drug resistance associated with mitochondrial respiratory defect and hypoxia. *Cancer Res* 65 (2):613–21.

Yamagishi, S., T. Matsui, and K. Fukami. 2015. Role of receptor for advanced glycation end products (RAGE) and its ligands in cancer risk. *Rejuvenation Res* 18 (1):48–56. doi: 10.1089/rej.2014.1625.

Yang, S., S. M. Pinney, P. Mallick, S. M. Ho, B. Bracken, and T. Wu. 2015. Impact of oxidative stress biomarkers and carboxymethyllysine (an Advanced Glycation End Product) on prostate cancer: A prospective study. *Clin Genitourin Cancer* 13 (5):e347–51. doi: 10.1016/j.clgc.2015.04.004.

Yoshida, G. J. 2015. Metabolic reprogramming: The emerging concept and associated therapeutic strategies. *J Exp Clin Cancer Res* 34:111. doi: 10.1186/s13046-015-0221-y.

Zhang, F. F., S. Liu, E. M. John, A. Must, and W. Demark-Wahnefried. 2015. Diet quality of cancer survivors and noncancer individuals: Results from a national survey. *Cancer* 121 (23):4212–21. doi: 10.1002/cncr.29488.

16

Advanced Glycation End Products and Their Receptors in Aspiration-Induced Acute Respiratory Distress Syndrome

Julie Ottosen
University of Minnesota
Minneapolis, MN

Peter Smit
Wake Forest University
Winston-Salem, NC

Weidun Alan Guo
University at Buffalo
Buffalo, NY

CONTENTS

KEY POINTS

- Gastric aspiration results in a heterogeneous pulmonary inflammatory response.
- Dietary advanced glycation end products (AGEs) upregulate RAGE and promote pulmonary inflammatory response.
- Epithelial low pH injury serves as a second-hit for aspiration-induced acute respiratory distress syndrome.
- An AGE-restricted diet helps reduce pulmonary inflammatory response.
- Decreasing RAGE activation helps reduce pulmonary inflammatory response.

16.1 Introduction

Acute respiratory distress syndrome (ARDS) is a rapidly developing, severe, and often life-threatening condition characterized by widespread inflammation of the lung. It has previously been referred to as "shock lung," "wet lung," or "Da Nang lung," but was first described in its current name by Ashbaugh et al. in 1967 (1). Until recently, milder forms of ARDS were referred to as "acute lung injury." However, throughout this chapter, we will use the newer term ARDS, as defined by the Berlin criteria in 2012 (2).

Clinically, gastric aspiration is a significant cause of pneumonitis and ARDS. This is particularly true in patients with altered levels of consciousness due to head injury, sedation, or underlying disease processes. While aspiration events in hospitalized patients are relatively common, we continue to have limited understanding of the pathophysiology. Furthermore, treatment for these patients remains largely supportive. Although advances in critical care, including widespread implementation of lung protective ventilation strategies and patient proning, have shown a benefit, the morbidity and mortality associated with ARDS remain dishearteningly high. Identifying risk factors and developing targeted therapies for the management of patients with aspiration-induced lung injury and ARDS are essential to improving outcomes.

Advanced glycation end products (AGEs) and their receptor, the receptor for advanced glycation end products (RAGE), have been implicated in a number of disease processes, including diabetes mellitus, cardiovascular disease, chronic renal failure, and neurodegenerative disorders. Accumulation of AGEs has also been linked to the accelerated multisystem functional decline that occurs with aging (3). Germane to our work, AGEs/RAGE have been shown to play a significant role in pulmonary disease. Consequently, AGEs/RAGE has become potential targets for directed therapy against pulmonary inflammatory processes, including aspiration pneumonitis and ARDS.

This chapter will focus on the role of AGEs/RAGE in gastric aspiration-induced pulmonary inflammatory response. We will describe how a high-AGE diet has been implicated as a risk factor for severe pulmonary inflammatory disease. We then will explain the characteristics of interaction between AGEs and RAGE and signaling pathways in the pathogenesis of aspiration-induced ARDS. Finally, we will speculate on what this might mean for future preventative and therapeutic strategies.

16.2 Pathophysiology of ARDS in Relation to AGEs/RAGE

The pathophysiology of aspiration and subsequent ARDS is related to endothelial injury and increased vascular permeability. It may be broken into three overlapping stages: exudative, proliferative, and fibrotic. Although indirect causes have been linked to ARDS, direct injury from aspiration is one of the prominent triggers of disease. The first phase is exudative. This is an acute inflammatory stage, typified by release of proinflammatory cytokines, influx of neutrophils, and impaired endothelial cell barrier function. Respiratory failure during the exudative phase is attributed to accumulation of protein-rich fluid in distal airspaces and to decreased surfactant production by type II epithelial cells. These early events are followed by the proliferative phase, which develops 2 to 7 days after initiation of lung injury. This phase is characterized by the proliferation of type 2 pneumocytes, early fibrotic changes, and intimal thickening of the pulmonary capillaries. Some individuals will then progress to the third stage, the fibrotic stage, with increased collagen deposition, prolonged ventilation–perfusion mismatching, and diminished lung compliance.

The clinical manifestations of an aspiration vary widely, ranging from subclinical signs such as dry cough or dysphonia to fulminant life-threatening respiratory failure. A question that arises when considering the great variability in response to aspiration is "Why is it that some patients recover without serious sequelae, whereas others develop severe pulmonary disease?"

16.2.1 High-AGE Diet and Aspiration-Induced ARDS

Recent studies have demonstrated that AGEs play a significant role in the pathogenesis of aspiration-induced lung injury and ARDS. The hypothesis is that pre-injury accumulation of AGEs due to high dietary intake upregulates RAGE and primes the lung for a more robust inflammatory response.

AGEs are a heterogeneous group of compounds that derive from nonenzymatic glycation and oxidation of lipids and proteins. Classically, endogenous forms are found in the setting of chronic hyperglycemia as a result of the "Maillard reaction." But AGEs may also be acquired from diet. These exogenous AGEs are generated during the heating process of many foods. It has been demonstrated that Western fast food is high in AGEs. The average Western diet is rich in these compounds. Once ingested, dietary AGEs contribute significantly to the body's AGE pool and are indistinguishable from endogenous forms in both structure and function. As shown in Figure 16.1, AGE–RAGE interaction activates NF-κB, which in turn transduces a variety of inflammatory and apoptotic signals in the cell. Additionally, AGEs are directly linked to increased generation of reactive oxygen species by their suppressive effects on superoxide dismutase and catalase, diminished glutathione stores, and activation of protein kinase C.

As described elsewhere in this book, food-derived AGEs add substantially to overall AGE burden, predisposing individuals to oxidative stress, inflammation, and a number of chronic diseases (4). These include diabetes mellitus, atherosclerosis, coronary artery occlusion, cardiac fibrosis, and neurodegenerative diseases, including Alzheimer's, chronic renal failure, and cystic fibrosis. Given the high constitutive levels of the AGE receptor, RAGE, in the lung, makes sense that this organ could be particularly susceptible to AGE-mediated injury.

Previous work by Guo et al. examined the pulmonary inflammatory response to aspiration in mice who had been fed a diet either high or low in AGEs (5). The high-AGE diet was prepared by autoclaving standard feed at 125°C for 30 minutes. This method produced 110 ng of AGEs per milligram of feed in the high-AGE diet versus 23 ng in the low-AGE diet. Mice were randomized to either a high- or low-AGE diet for 4 weeks, after which aspiration was induced with intratracheal instillation of acidified gastric particles, adjusted to a pH of 1.25, to mimic true aspirate contents. Bronchoalveolar lavage (BAL), pulmonary function testing, and lung harvesting were then performed. Compared to mice fed

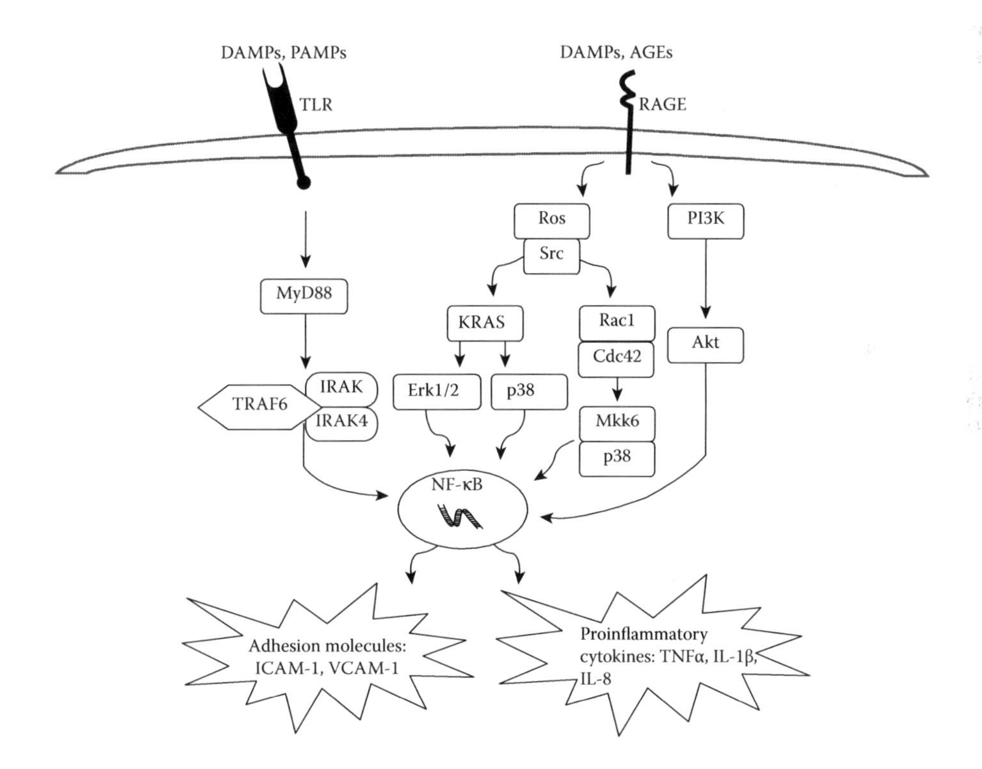

FIGURE 16.1 The cell membrane receptors (TLR and RAGE) and their ligands. The interaction between the receptors and ligands (DAMPs, PAMPs, and AGEs) leads to the activation of the NF-κB pathway and the ultimate release of adhesion molecules and proinflammatory cytokines. (With kind permission from Springer Science+Business Media: *J. Intensive Care Med.*, The receptor for advanced glycation end products and acute lung injury/acute respiratory distress syndrome, 38(10), 1588–1598, 2012, Guo, W. A., et al., copyright 2012.)

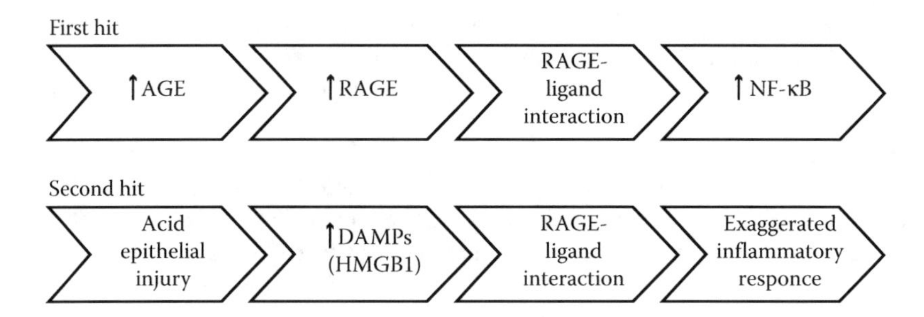

FIGURE 16.2 The "two-hit" model of gastric aspiration-induced ARDS. The "first hit" is the prime event of AGE accumulation and RAGE upregulation, while the "second hit" is the acidic injury to the epithelial cell of the airway due to gastric aspiration. The "first hit" appears to predispose to an exaggerated pulmonary inflammatory response after gastric aspiration, while the "second hit" promotes the release of DAMPs that can interact with RAGE and other pattern recognition receptors (PRRs).

a low-AGE diet, mice fed a high-AGE diet had multiple markers of greater pulmonary injury. This included increased lung tissue resistance, higher BAL albumin concentrations, greater polymorphonuclear (PMN) cell counts, and elevated lung myeloperoxidase activity (MPO) following gastric aspiration.

In 2001, Schmidt et al. hypothesized a "two-hit model" of tissue inflammation and injury mediated by RAGE and its ligands (6). Smit and colleagues (7) subsequently applied this "two-hit model" to aspiration-induced lung injury to explain the pathogenesis of this exaggerated pulmonary inflammatory response (Figure 16.2). They posited that upregulation of RAGE in the lung and accumulation of plasma AGEs by a high-AGE diet constituted the "first hit." Some patients may present with a preexisting high blood levels of AGEs before the clinical gastric aspiration occurs. The "second hit" was the alveolar epithelial injury due to aspiration of acidified gastric particles, releasing a variety of endogenous damage-associated molecular patterns or DAMPs (discussed in detail later in this chapter). Lung tissue injury resulted in a rise in HMGB-1. Once such proinflammatory DAMP released upon cell necrosis, they could bind to the pulmonary RAGE and propagate an exaggerated inflammatory response. The authors were able to demonstrate that a diet high in AGEs led to increased pulmonary RAGE levels, augmenting the inflammatory response to aspiration in the presence of endogenous DAMPs (7). This suggests that pre-injury diet, by affecting AGE and RAGE stores, may factor significantly in the evolution of direct lung injury leading to ARDS after aspiration.

16.2.2 RAGE in the Lung

RAGE is a transmembrane pattern recognition receptor of the immunoglobulin superfamily that was first characterized by Neeper et al. in 1992 (8). Through its ability to recognize a common structural motif, RAGE can bind with multiple ligands. AGEs are a prototypic ligand. However, RAGE also has the ability to recognize a number of other molecules as listed in Table 16.1. As shown in Figure 16.1, the interaction between RAGE and its ligands results in proinflammatory gene activation, activation of NADP oxidase leading to reactive oxygen species (ROS) formation, and activation of the NF-κB pathway resulting in oxidative stress and inflammation. In addition to sharing ligands, RAGE also shares a number of signaling pathways with certain members of the toll-like receptor (TLR) family. Here, it plays an immune role by detecting danger signals, including pathogen-associated molecular patterns (PAMPs) and endogenous damage-associated molecular patterns (DAMPS), or Alarmins (9). PAMPs are a diverse set of microbial molecules with shared motifs that are recognized by cells of the innate immune system and alert the host to invading pathogens (10). DAMPs, conversely, are endogenous equivalents of PAMPs. They are pleiotropic intracellular proteins released during cell death, initiating, and perpetuating noninfectious inflammatory processes.

The lung, continuously exposed to the external environment, is constantly flooded with a range of infectious pathogens, foreign antigens, PAMPs, and DAMPs. This makes it a particularly susceptible organ for injury and may explain why RAGE, although expressed in endothelial cells throughout the body, is found at its highest concentrations in the lung. Perhaps, these high concentrations, even during

TABLE 16.1

RAGE Ligands

Ligand	Description	Location	Clinical Implications
HMGB1 (Amphoterin)	Chromosomal DNA–binding proteins induce inflammatory signaling	Expressed at their highest level in the CNS during embryonic development; elevated in the CNS in response to injury	Antibodies may confer protection against damage and tissue injury during arthritis, colitis, ischemia, sepsis, endotoxemia, and SLE; proposed target for nonsmall-cell lung cancer therapy
S100/calgranulins: S100B, S100A7 (psoriasin), S100P, S100A8/A9 complex (calprotectin)	Closely related family of proteins characterized for role in intracellular calcium binding	Highly expressed in brain/CNS, especially astrocytes	At low concentrations, stimulate neurite outgrowth, NO release; at high concentrations, proinflammatory; targeted for the treatment of atherosclerosis and arthritis
Amyloid-β-protein	Peptide fragment 40–42 amino acids in length, formed from proteolytic cleavage of B-amyloid precursor protein. Promotes oxidative stress, neuron death	Abundantly expressed in the brain	Forms the main component of amyloid plaques in Alzheimer's dementia; Aggregates in cerebral blood vessels to cause cerebral amyloid angiopathy; Contributes to Lewy Body dementia and inclusion body myositis
Mac-1(macrophage 1 antigen)	β2 integrin classically regarded as a proinflammatory molecule because of its ability to promote phagocyte cytotoxic functions	Expressed on the cell surface of immune cells, including monocytes, granulocytes, macrophages, and natural killer cells	Mediates inflammation by regulating leukocyte adhesion; involved in phagocytosis, cell-mediated cytotoxicity, chemotaxis, and cellular activation; implicated in SLE

Note: CNS, central nervous system; NO, nitric oxide; SLE, systemic lupus erythematosus.

normal physiologic state, evolved to allow RAGE to function as a sensor for environmental cues. While located primarily on the basement membrane of type I pneumocytes, RAGE is also expressed on type II pneumocytes, bronchiolar epithelium, alveolar macrophages, and vascular endothelial cells. As mentioned above, interaction of RAGE with its ligands, including advance glycation end products, PAMPS and DAMPs, leads to a proinflammatory cascade that results in loss of alveolar–endothelial integrity and the hallmark findings of ARDS. Recent genome studies have identified multiple loci for RAGE acting as an important determinant of pulmonary function. RAGE coupling with ICAM1 has been linked to leukocyte recruitment and adhesion during the acute posttraumatic pulmonary inflammatory response. These findings suggest that the lung responds to RAGE ligands that are identified as potential dangers, augmenting immune response. However, while this may be protective, excessive, and persistent inflammation resulting from RAGE-ligand interaction may result in harmful effects, including ARDS.

16.2.3 RAGE as a Biomarker

A biomarker is a clinical parameter that is measured with the intention of providing information about a disease process. Aside from being a diagnostic tool, biomarkers may help predict which patients are at risk for respiratory failure and ARDS following aspiration, who might progress to pulmonary fibrosis and require long-term mechanical ventilation, and who are most likely to suffer long-term morbidity and mortality.

The soluble form of RAGE (sRAGE) is a cleaved form of the receptor that can be measured in plasma, and has been proposed as a biomarker for type I alveolar cell injury. Plasma RAGE levels have been shown to be elevated in samples from patients with acute lung injury as compared to healthy controls and those with hydrostatic pulmonary edema (11). Calfee et al. subsequently measured sRAGE levels in 676 patients enrolled in the ARMA study both at entry into the study and after 3 days of mechanical ventilation. Higher sRAGE levels at entry were associated with more prominent radiographic findings as well as higher physiologic indices of pulmonary injury and higher APACHE III scores (12). These data suggest that sRAGE may be measured as marker of disease severity. However, this theory must be addressed with caution, as subjects with higher baseline sRAGE who were treated with lung protective mechanical ventilation did not fare differently in terms of ventilator-free days, organ failure–free days, or mortality.

16.3 AGEs/RAGE as Therapeutic Targets in Aspiration-Induced ARDS

Survival after ARDS has improved since it was first described in 1967, but remains unacceptably low. ARDS associated with aspiration pneumonitis is associated with 30% mortality and is a substantial cause of death in critically ill and injured patients. Current management strategies for aspiration-induced lung injury have been primarily supportive, with the use of aggressive pulmonary toilet, O_2 supplementation, mechanical ventilation, prone positioning to improve ventilation-perfusion mismatch, inhaled pulmonary vasodilators such as nitric oxide and epoprostenol, and the use of extracorporeal membrane oxygenation (ECMO). Newer measures to combat ARDS have shifted toward preventative practices which include upright positioning with head of bed elevation 30 degrees to prevent ongoing aspiration events: aggressive pulmonary toilet: and low tidal volume (lung protective) ventilation to prevent progression to the fibroproliferative phase of ARDS (13). Understanding the characteristics and interaction between AGEs and RAGE may bring a new perspective in the search for the prevention and treatment of aspiration-induced ARDS.

16.3.1 Advanced Glycation End Products

Application of an AGE-restricted diet has been shown to reduce not only the systemic levels of AGEs but also the levels of markers of oxidative stress and inflammation in the setting of diabetes. In the first human study in 2002, Vlassara et al. compared patients fed low and regular AGE diets for a period of 6 weeks. Meals with specific AGE content were prepared in the clinical research unit and patients picked them up twice a week for the duration of the study. Subjects in the low-AGE diet group demonstrated decreased levels of circulating AGEs as well as decreased markers of endothelial function and inflammation such as VCAM-1, hsCRP, and TNF-α. Prior to this study, high serum AGE levels in diabetic patients were thought to result exclusively from hyperglycemia-induced endogenous overproduction. The ability to reduce circulating AGEs by as much as 40% emphasized the importance of dietary modification in regulating their levels and curbing their deleterious effects (14). Low-AGE diets have also been shown to be beneficial in the setting of neurodegenerative disease. High dietary AGEs were associated with a decline in memory in the elderly when studied by Vlassara et al. in 2009 (15). A subsequent 2014 study examined the role of AGE in mice. After feeding the creatures three different types of diets—one low in AGEs, one high in AGEs, and a "normal" diet—those mice who were eating the least amount of AGEs enjoyed improved cognitive function. In an observation study, Perrone et al. were subsequently able to demonstrate a similar benefit in humans (16).

If a low-AGE diet is beneficial in the setting of diabetes and dementia, could it also be beneficial in the setting of aspiration and ARDS? In a murine model, Guo et al. demonstrated that high dietary AGEs lead to pre-injury accumulation and a more robust pulmonary inflammatory response after gastric aspiration (5). Mice fed a low-AGE diet fared better. This implies that a diet high in AGEs is a risk factor for progression to ARDS after aspiration, and that diet modification may be an effective strategy for mitigating that risk.

Dietary AGEs represent a potential modifiable risk factor as a strategy to attenuate pulmonary inflammation. Two large databases now exist that quantify the content of carboxymethylcellulose, a commonly measured AGE, in >500 food items. This makes it possible not only to estimate daily dietary AGE intake but also to design diets with a specific AGE content. Although practitioners have little control over what patients consume outside of the hospital, inpatient diets can be regulated, especially in critically ill individuals receiving tube feeds. Providing a low-AGE source of nutrition may be beneficial in preventing progression to severe pulmonary inflammatory disease.

16.3.2 Receptor for Advanced Glycation End Products

To date, only reduction of mechanical ventilation–induced lung injury (VILI) through the use of lung protective ventilation strategies and ECMO has been shown to decrease mortality. However, before full-blown ARDS develops, it is not possible to deploy these strategies. Therefore, novel approaches to treatment are needed. Since ARDS is associated with upregulation of RAGE expression on pulmonary epithelial cells, decreasing RAGE activation could be instrumental in decreasing the severity of lung injury following gastric aspiration.

16.3.2.1 RAGE-Ligand Interference

Alagebrium, or ALT-711, is a compound that breaks cross-linkages in AGEs, rendering them innocuous by inhibiting their ability to bind RAGE. Some studies suggest that alagebrium is renoprotective in diabetes. In a murine model of gastric aspiration, Guo et al. demonstrated that the administration of ALT-711 at the time of direct lung injury attenuated the pulmonary inflammatory response as evidence by decreased bronchoalveolar neutrophils and myeloperoxidase activity (5).

Pyridoxamine and aminoguanidine are agents that prevent the formation of endogenous N-E-carboxymethyllysine (CML), a well-studied AGE compound. They have also been shown to significantly reduce glomerular lesions in CD1 mice with end stage renal disease (17). Presumably, these agents, by lowering levels of circulating AGEs, might confer protection against other RAGE mediated inflammatory processes, including lung injury and ARDs.

Although the above agent seems promising, it is important to remember that RAGE is a receptor with multiple ligands and is expressed robustly in the lung. Thus limiting one potential ligand, AGEs, may not effectively abrogate the overwhelming inflammatory response in the lung following aspiration. Development of agents that target other RAGE ligands, such as high motility group box 1 (HMGB-1), S100 proteins, serum amyloid A (SAA), and heat shock proteins, is the focus of ongoing research.

16.3.2.2 Anti-RAGE Antibody

In a model of sepsis, RAGE knockout mice (RAGE -/-) had improved survival over controls following cecal ligation and puncture. Since that study, a neutralizing antibody to the RAGE receptor was developed. Using a similar model of sepsis, Lutterloh et al. were able to demonstrate that anti-RAGE monoclonal antibody effectively decreased mortality when compared to controls, even when administration was delayed for 24 hours (18). A recent study also showed that humanized anti-RAGE antibody conferred a survival advantage in mice with pneumococcal pneumonia (19). These studies all suggest that RAGE blocking agents may be promising therapeutic agents, inhibiting RAGE ligation with disruption of the subsequent inflammatory signaling pathways.

16.3.2.3 Soluble RAGE as a Decoy Receptor

In addition to its role as a biomarker, soluble RAGE (sRAGE) may also serve as a decoy receptor, as it fully retains its ability to bind RAGE ligands, but does not result in the downstream signaling that activates the NF-κB proinflammatory pathway. In one study looking at mice with LPS-induced lung injury, treatment with sRAGE significantly attenuated neutrophil infiltration, lung permeability, and proinflammatory cytokine production (20). It is reasonable to extrapolate that sRAGE administration may have similar beneficial effects after aspiration-induced lung injury.

16.4 Conclusions

AGEs and RAGE play an important role in the sequela of gastric aspiration, which is common among hospitalized patients and a significant cause of respiratory failure and ARDS. These conditions carry high rates of morbidity and mortality and contribute significantly to health care costs. Response to aspiration is heterogeneous, and identifying patients who are at greatest risk for ensuing pulmonary complications would prove useful to their management. High circulating levels of AGEs, as well as upregulation of RAGE receptors in the lung, appear to predispose to a more severe pulmonary inflammatory response following gastric aspiration, and may be viewed as both risk factors and biomarkers for acute lung injury. Additionally, RAGE-ligand signaling pathways set off a proinflammatory cascade that contributes significantly to lung injury following aspiration. Targeting this axis is an essential strategy for developing novel and directed therapies for aspiration pneumonitis and ARDS.

REFERENCES

1. Ashbaugh, D. G, Bigelow, D. B., Petty T. L., and Levin, B. E. Acute respiratory distress in adults. *Lancet* 2 (7511): 319–23, 1967.
2. Ranieri, V. M., Rubenfeld, G. D., Thompson, B. T., Ferguson, N. D., Caldwell, N. E., Fan, E., Camporota, L., and Slutsky, A. S. Acute respiratory distress syndrome: The Berlin definition. *JAMA* 307(23): 2526–33, 2012.
3. Semba, R., Nicklett, E. J., and Ferrucci, L. Does accumulation of advanced glycation end products contribute to the aging phenotype? *J Gerontol A Biol Sci Med Sci* 65(9): 963–75, 2010.
4. Uribarri, J., del Castillo, M. D., de la Maza, M. P., Filip, R., Garay-Sevilla, M. E., Luevano-Contreras, M., Macias-Cervantes, M. H., et al. Dietary advanced glycation end productts and their role in health and disease. *Adv Nutr* 451–472, 2014.
5. Guo, W. A., Davidson, B. A., Ottosen, J., Ohtake, P., Rhagavendran, K., Mullan, B. A., Dayton, M. T., Knigh, P. R., 3rd. Effect of high advanced glycation end-product diet on pulmonary inflammatory response and pulmonary function following gastric aspiration. *Shock Dec* 38 (6):677–84, 2012.
6. Schmidt, A. M., Yan, S. D., Yan, S. F., and Stern, D. M. The multiligand receptor RAGE as a progression factor amplifying immune and inflammatory responses. *J Clin Investig* 108: 949–55, 2001.
7. Smit, P., Guo, W. A., Davidson, B. A., Mullan, B. A., Helinski, J. D., Knight, III P. R. Deitary AGE-Associated RAGE and HMGB-1 in aspiration lung injury. *J Surg Res* 191(1): 214–223, 2014.
8. Neeper, M., Sshmidt, A. M., Brett, J., Yan, S. D., Wang, F., Pan, Y. C., Elliston, K., Stern, D., and Shaw, A. Cloning and expression of a cell surface receptor for advanced glycosylation end products of proteins. *J Biol Chem* 267(21): 14998–15004, 1992.
9. Guo, W. A., Knight, P. R., Raghavendran, K. The receptor for advanced glycation end products and acute lung injury/acute respiratory distress syndrome. *J Intensive Care Med* 38(10): 1588–1598, 2012.
10. Janeway, C. A., and Medzhitov, R. Innate immune recognition. *Ann Rev Immunol* 20: 197–216, 2002.
11. Uchida, T., S. M., Ware, L. B., Kojima, K., Hata, Y., Makita, K., Mednick, G., Matthay, Z. A., Matthay, M. A. Receptor for advanced glycation end products is a marker of type I cell injury in acute lung injury. *Am J Respir Crit Care Med* 173: 1008–15, 2006.
12. Calfee, C. S., W. L., Eisner, M. D., Parsons, P. E., Thompson, B. T., Wickersham, N., Matthay, M. A. NHLBI ARDS Network. Plasma receptor for advanced glycation end-products and clinical outcomes in acute lung injury. *Thorax* 63: 1083–9, 2008.
13. Litell, J. M., Gong, M. N., Talmor, D., and Gajic, O. Acute lung injury: Preventnion may be the best medicine. *Respir Care* 56: 1546, 2011.
14. Vlassara, H., Cai, W., Crandall, J., Goldberg, T., Oberstein, R., Dardaine, V., Peppa, M., and Rayfield, E. J. Inflammatory mediators are induced by dietary glycotoxins, a major risk factor for diabetic angiopathy. *Proc Natl Acad Sci U S A* 99(24): 15596–15601, 2002.

15. Vlassara, H., Cai, W., Goodman, S., Pyzik, R., Yong, A., Chen, X., Zhu, L., et al. Protection against loss of innate defenses in adulthood by low advanced glycation end products (AGE) intake: Role of the antiinflammatory AGE receptor-1. *J Clin Endocrinol Metab* 94(11): 4483–4491, 2009.
16. Perrone, L., and Grant, W. B. Observational and ecological studies of dietary advanced glycation end products in national diets and Alzheimer's disease incidence and prevalence. *J Alzheimer's Dis* 45(3): 965–979, 2015.
17. Furukawa, M., Gohda, T., Tanimoto, M., Tomino, Y. Pathogenesis and novel treatment from the mouse model of type 2 diabetic nephropathy. *Scientific World J* 2013: 928197, 2013.
18. Lutterloh, E. C., Opal, S. M., Pittman, D., Keith, J. C., Jr, Tan, X. Y., Clancy, B. M., Palmer, H., et al. Inhibition of the RAGE products increases survival in experimental models of severe sepsis and systemic infection. *Crit Care* 11(6): R122, 2007.
19. Christaki, E., Opal, S. M., Keith, J. C., Jr, Kessimian, N., Palardy, J. E., Parejo, N. A., Tan, X. Y., et al. A monoclonal antibody against RAGE alters gene expression and is protective in experimental models of sepsis and pneumococcal pneumonia. *Shock* 35(5): 492–498, 2011.
20. Zhang, H., Tasaka, S., Shiraishi, Y., Fukunaga, K., Yamada, W., Seki, H., Ogawa, Y., et al. Role of soluble receptor for advanced glycation end products on endotoxin-induced lung injury. *Am J Respir Crit Care Med* 178(4): 356–62, 2007.

17

Dietary AGEs in the Development and Progression of Chronic Kidney Disease

Amelia K. Fotheringham and Linda A. Gallo
Mater Research – UQ
Woolloongabba, Australia

Josephine M. Forbes
Baker IDI Heart and Diabetes Institute
Melbourne, Australia

CONTENTS

KEY POINTS

- Chronic kidney disease is highly prevalent with one in three people at risk.
- Kidney function is an accurate predictor of lifespan.
- AGEs, including those from the diet, are excreted by the kidneys.
- AGE accumulation can damage kidneys, leading to chronic kidney disease.
- Novel interventions such as decreasing dietary AGEs and/or intestinal absorption of AGEs can combat chronic kidney disease.

17.1 A Snap Shot of Kidney Function

The kidneys filter around 200 L of blood each day, with 1–2 L of waste leaving the body as urine. This is an essential homeostatic process that, together with the reabsorption and secretion of molecules, regulates nutrient, water, and waste balance in the body. They also produce and/or regulate several hormones and enzymes, which help to maintain blood pressure and bone health, and manufacture red blood cells. When blood glucose levels are low, the kidneys also function as a gluconeogenic organ, rapidly releasing glucose into the blood. Antigen–antibody complexes are also cleaved and processed for elimination in the kidneys. Hence, the kidneys not only present an extremely sophisticated waste disposal system but also are critical for a range of other homeostatic processes.

Each kidney is divided into two visually distinct regions: a granular outer cortex and striated inner medulla, owing to the highly organized array of the functional units of the kidney known as nephrons. Each human kidney contains about one million nephrons at birth, but this number steadily declines with age [1]. The glomerulus, the major vascular component of each nephron, is a fenestrated endothelial capillary tuft encompassed by a basement membrane (extracellular proteins and collagen) and epithelial contractile cells (podocytes and pedicels), and serves as the renal filtration barrier. This molecular sieve forms a size and charge exclusion strainer of sorts, retaining red blood cells and other large molecules while water and small neutral or cationic molecules (such as glucose, ions, and amino acids) are able to pass. This is a high throughput system where 600–650 mL of plasma enters the glomerulus each minute, of which 20% is filtered into the tubular component, beginning at the Bowman's capsule. This sets the average healthy adult glomerular filtration rate (GFR) at ~125 mL/min. The filtrate passes through the continuous tubular lumen, which is divided into segments based on structure and function—the proximal tubule, loop of Henle, distal tubule, and collecting duct. The newly formed urine from each nephron drains into renal calyces, the renal pelvis, and, via a single ureter from each kidney, into the bladder.

Urine is generally low in essential nutrients such as sodium, glucose, and water, but high in waste products such as urea, creatinine, and phenol. Fine-tuning of the urinary filtrate involves a highly coordinated effort by the different nephron segments and extensive peritubular capillary network. A number of different transporters are located on tubular epithelial cell membranes for reabsorption of important substances and secretion of any wastes that escaped filtration. Transepithelial transport involves penetration of five barriers for reabsorption from the tubular lumen: apical membrane, cytosol, basolateral membrane, interstitial fluid, and peritubular capillary wall (in reverse order for secretion). Many of these processes are highly energy-dependent, making the kidney one of the highest consumers of oxygen per gram of tissue in the body [2].

17.2 Classification of Chronic Kidney Disease and Worldwide Burden

Chronic kidney disease (CKD) is defined as either kidney damage or decreased kidney function for a duration that is equal to, or greater than, 3 months [3]. Kidney damage is determined by markers such as proteinuria (increased urinary excretion of albumin or any other protein) and abnormalities in urine and blood chemistry, while decreased kidney function is determined by a decline in estimated GFR (eGFR). There are five stages of progressive CKD, as outlined in Table 17.1. End-stage renal disease (ESRD) describes patients who are at Stage 5 of CKD and are being treated with dialysis or kidney transplantation. As many as one in three people are at risk of developing CKD, due to a range of factors including diabetes, high blood pressure, being of 60 years of age or older having a family history of CKD, obesity, and smoking [4]. The worldwide prevalence of CKD is between 8% and 16% [5]. Globally, diabetes is noted as the single most common cause of ESRD followed by hypertension or glomerulonephritis (Figure 17.1). In the developing world, infections, herbal and environmental toxins, pesticides, and some food additives also contribute significantly to the prevalence of kidney failure but a large proportion of causes remain unknown or not reported.

In 2012, total health care expenditure for ESRD in the United States alone was almost $30 billion [6]. An individual with CKD has a greater risk of cardiovascular death before progression to ESRD [7]. Thus, the impact of CKD on quality of life and financial burden extends well beyond that of ESRD. Indeed, therapeutic (blockade of the renin–angiotensin–system) and/or lifestyle interventions (diet salt and protein intake, and exercise) can slow the progression of CKD but the only option for Stage 5 CKD is renal replacement therapy (dialysis or kidney transplant).

TABLE 17.1

Classification and Treatment Plan for CKD

Stage	Description	GFR (mL/min/1.73 m²)	Treatment Plan
1	Kidney damage[a] (e.g., albuminuria) with normal or ↑ GFR	≥90	Observation and risk reduction
2	Kidney damage[a] (e.g., albuminuria) with mild ↓ GFR	60–89	Estimate progression and minimize risk factors
3	Moderately ↓ GFR	30–59	Evaluate and treat complications
4	Severely ↓ GFR	15–29	Prepare for renal replacement therapy
5	Kidney failure	<15 or dialysis	Renal replacement therapy (end-stage renal disease)

Note: GFR, glomerular filtration rate.

[a] Kidney damage is defined as albuminuria, hematuria, structural, or pathological abnormalities.

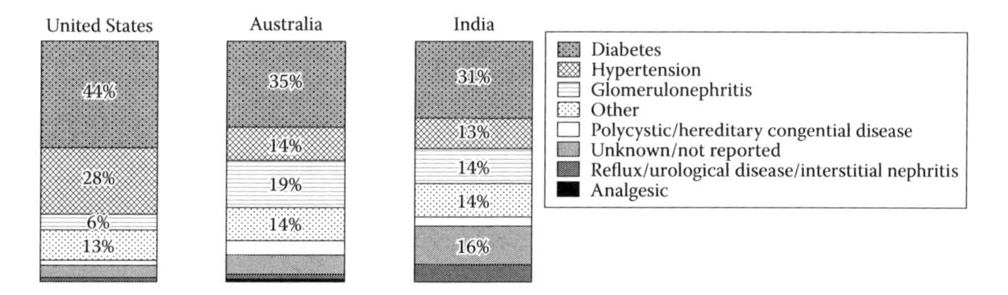

FIGURE 17.1 Causes of kidney failure. Diabetes continues to be the leading cause of ESRD in developed (e.g., US and Australia) and many developing (e.g., India) nations. (Modified from ANZDATA Report 2013; US Renal Data System 2013; Jha, V., et al. *Lancet (London, England)*, 382(9888), 260–272, 2013.)

17.3 Cellular Handling of AGEs by the Kidney

Evidence for how the kidneys handle AGEs in both humans and rodents is discussed in Chapters 4 and 5, and briefly outlined here. In healthy rats, intravenously injected low-molecular weight AGE-peptides, but not AGE-BSA, were freely filtered at the glomerulus and detected in urine [8]. AGEs, both free- and protein-bound, appear to bind to and/or enter proximal tubule cells *in vivo* and *in vitro* [8–12] and protein-bound AGEs have also been demonstrated to enter podocytes *in vitro* [13]. While renal proximal tubule cells can degrade AGE-modified albumin, this was at a limited capacity and resulted in increased cellular accumulation when compared to nonglycated albumin [11]. This was associated with slowed exocytosis of albumin peptide fragments via basolateral and apical membranes, suggesting abnormal processing of modified proteins by the renal tubule. Indeed, the transport of free- and/or protein-bound AGEs across the renal filtration barrier and tubular cells may depend on the degree and residue site(s) of glycation.

17.4 The Varied Effects of Exogenous AGEs on Kidney Function

In overweight, but otherwise healthy, individuals, a randomized cross-over study showed that high-AGE dietary intake over 2 weeks was associated with systemic inflammation, albuminuria, and decreased eGFR as well as increased AGE flux into the urine and reduced circulating levels [14]. This reduction in circulating AGEs has been seen in individuals with obesity [15–17], where there was evidence of renal hyperfiltration [15] suggesting increased urinary AGE flux. Indeed, individuals with the lowest serum N-ε-carboxymethyllysine (CML) levels had the highest eGFR, and the inverse relationship between serum CML and total fat mass was lost when corrected for eGFR [16]. However, there is also evidence of "trapping" or deposition of AGEs in human adipose tissue which might also explain, in part, the reduction in circulating AGEs in obesity [17], particularly when eGFR is reduced in some cases [14] (Figure 17.2).

There is a paucity of studies in humans examining the effects of dietary AGEs on renal function *per se* although AGEs have been shown to influence a number of its determinants. In healthy individuals and in those with diabetes, a single oral AGE challenge resulted in acute endothelial dysfunction [18], which is a known risk factor for CKD. Similarly, in individuals with diabetes, both a 2- and 6-week dietary intervention of high-AGEs increased inflammatory mediators compared to a diet that was 5-fold lower in AGE content [19]. However, in healthy adults, a 6-week diet that was either low or high in AGEs did not affect endothelial function or markers of inflammation compared to baseline [20]. While serum and urinary CML levels were reduced by the low-AGE diet, they were not elevated by the high-AGE diet; the AGE content of the latter was similar to that of a typical Western diet and may have been insufficient to induce changes to cardiovascular and kidney disease risk factors. In a randomized cross-over study in healthy individuals, 4 weeks' consumption of high heat–treated foods increased circulating and urinary CML levels, which was associated with elevated plasma cholesterol and triglycerides, and decreased insulin sensitivity [21]. While these changes would significantly alter the risk for kidney dysfunction, there were confounding differences in dietary macronutrients between interventions.

In healthy rats, chronic intravenous administration of AGE–RSA for 5 months resulted in albuminuria and glomerular structural injury, both of which were reduced by co-treatment with the AGE cross-link breaker, aminoguanidine [22]. In another study, subcutaneous infusion of AGE–RSA for 4 weeks in normal rats promoted kidney growth and renal expression of renin–angiotensin system components, and decreased GFR but did not affect albumin excretion [23]. AGE–RSA intraperitoneally administered to healthy rats for 4 months altered renal mitochondrial function but did not affect urinary albumin

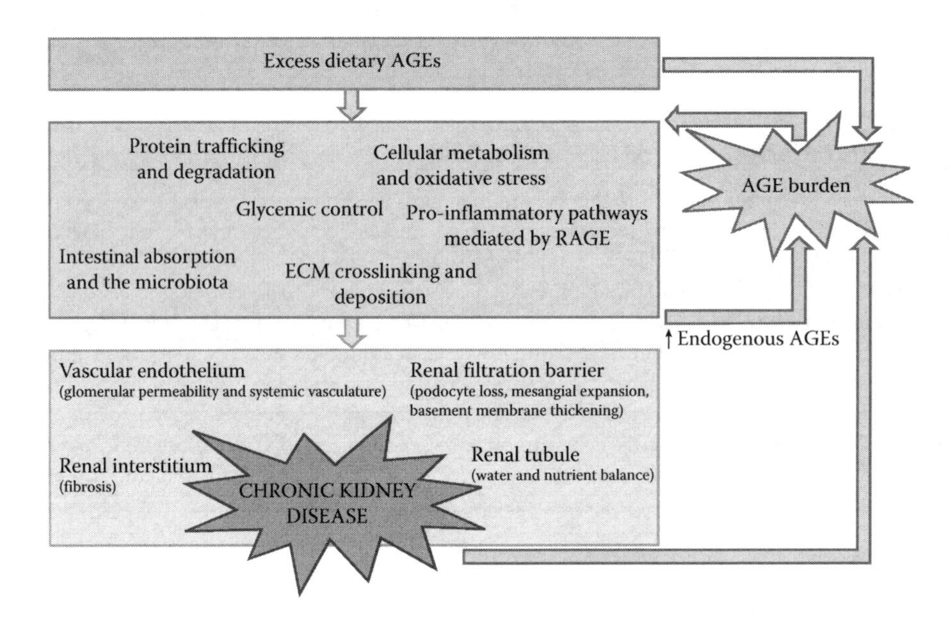

FIGURE 17.2 Hypothesized effects of excess dietary AGEs on the development and progression of CKD. Based on studies to date, chronic consumption of AGEs may adversely affect a number of processes in the body that, via direct or indirect pathways, modify compartments within the kidney and vasculature, and contribute to CKD. Further to this, proinflammatory and metabolic pathways that are modified by excess dietary AGEs may encourage the production of endogenous AGEs and contribute to the total AGE burden within the body. Together, these factors perpetually interrupt physiological processes and the overall kidney function.

excretion or GFR [24]. Other studies using diets high in AGE content in both healthy and 5/6th nephrectomized rats for 6 weeks revealed increased proteinuria, although GFR remained unaffected [25,26]. A more recent study in Wistar rats fed a diet that was high in fat and AGEs for 4 weeks, however, did identify increases in serum creatinine associated with enhanced kidney CML deposition [27]. Discrepancy between studies with regard to effects on the kidney could lie within different administration routes and/or differences in the timing and duration of AGE challenge. It is worth noting that, in healthy rats, orally ingested radioactive-labeled AGEs for 5 days followed by a 3-day washout period was able to increase the tissue burden of AGEs including within the kidney [28].

17.5 Evidence for a Link between AGEs and CKD

A number of clinical studies reported that circulating AGEs accumulate with a progressive decline in renal function, even in the absence of diabetes [29–31], and with markers of inflammation and oxidative stress in uremic patients [32]. Furthermore, a study conducted in individuals with at least 50 years of insulin-dependent diabetes identified that serum CEL and pentosidine levels were elevated in those suffering from any complication, including nephropathy [33]. In individuals with type 1 diabetes, with or without nephropathy, high serum AGEs (including CEL, pentosidine, and total AGE score) were predictive of cardiovascular disease and all-cause mortality [34]. Indeed, cardiovascular disease is an independent risk factor for CKD. Interestingly, unlike other AGEs, serum CML levels do not appear to correlate with CKD, cardiovascular disease, or mortality, in individuals with type 1 or type 2 diabetes and nephropathy [34,35]. It is worth noting that elevated circulating concentrations of soluble RAGE (sRAGE; secreted or cleaved circulating isoforms of RAGE) are also associated with, and predictive of, CKD [36,37]. In agreement with this, a larger study using individuals with type 2 diabetes from the ADVANCE study identified that circulating sRAGE and AGEs were associated with new or progressive kidney disease [38]. However, it remains unclear as to whether impaired renal clearance in CKD results in the accumulation of total body AGEs and/or exogenous AGE sources, such as those from the diet, contributing to CKD. *In vitro,* AGEs and reactive precursors formed at a rapid rate in serum from uremic patients [39], suggesting that circulating factors may stimulate the production of endogenous AGEs in individuals with impaired kidney function.

HbA_{1C}, a glycated marker of long-term glycemic control, is an accurate predictor of disease progression and mortality in CKD populations, even in the absence of diabetes [40]. Similarly, deterioration of glycemic control (increases in HbA_{1C}), including decreases in insulin sensitivity, is common in nondiabetic CKD patients [41,42]. Given the effects of dietary AGEs on glycemic control, it would be tempting to speculate that changes in cellular utilization of metabolic fuels could, at least in part, explain the detrimental effects of dietary AGEs on kidney function. Indeed, the relationship between strict glycemic control and improved renal outcomes and mortality rates is well established [43–46].

Many clinical studies have focused on the relationship between AGEs and kidney parameters using changes in skin collagen, which is a marker of endogenous AGE production. Skin collagen fluorescence is increased in nondiabetic CKD [47–49] and predicts those individuals with progressive CKD [47,50]. In a large clinical cohort of patients with type 1 diabetes, the Diabetes Control and Complications Trial (DCCT) and its follow-up study, Epidemiology of Diabetes Interventions and Complications (EDIC), skin collagen CML concentrations predicted individuals who developed nephropathy and cardiovascular disease, independent of their glycemic control [51,52]. In individuals with diabetes, increases in skin autofluorescence are associated with reductions in eGFR [53,54] and an increased incidence of CKD [54] and mortality [55].

A prospective study following a cohort of patients with type 1 diabetes showed that increased urinary CML clearance during hyperfiltration in early diabetic nephropathy, representing an increase in AGE burden, was associated with future rapid GFR decline. In that study, there were decreases in circulating AGE concentrations at the time of hyperfiltration, likely due to the increased clearance of AGEs into the urine (Perkins-BA; Abstract #0097; International Diabetes Federation Melbourne, Australia 2013). This is in agreement with a cross-sectional study, which demonstrated that elevated urinary excretion of protein-bound AGEs was associated with worsening degrees of CKD in both type 1 and type

2 diabetes [56]. This study also found that circulating AGEs were increased with worsening CKD in type 2 diabetes. Taken together, these data suggest that early tissue accumulation of AGEs, perhaps independently of glycemic control, is one of the most potent risk factors for progressive CKD. Further, there may be decreases in circulating AGE levels early in disease in Type 1 diabetes or obesity or with increases in dietary intake as a result of increased renal or hepatic clearance. This may be a compensatory response to combat the increased tissue burden of AGEs.

In those with ESRD, hemo- and peritoneal dialysis do not effectively remove AGEs, with circulating CML and methylglyoxal levels remaining well above that of healthy controls [57]. Short daily peritoneal dialysis and hemofiltration, however, have greater efficacy than hemodialysis in the removal of circulating AGEs, although the reasons for this are not apparent [58–60]. Although early studies with heat-treated dialysates showed an accumulation of AGEs [61], particularly in the peritoneal cavity [62], peritoneal dialysis is more effective at removing AGEs from the circulation [57,63]. The accumulation of AGEs has been correlated with the development of ESRD, such as dialysis-related amyloidosis [30]. Not surprisingly, renal transplantation lowers both tissue and circulating AGEs to a greater extent than dialysis [64].

17.6 Pathological Pathways Activated by Exogenous AGEs and Contributions to CKD

Increased exposure to exogenous AGEs, from sources such as diet, initiates a cascade of cellular effects in the body that affects renal structure and function, and may contribute to the development and progression of CKD (Figure 17.2).

Given the evidence for alterations to renal processing and clearance of AGE-modified proteins and peptides [11], renal cells may be exposed to abnormal types and quantities of modified proteins that ultimately interfere with their function. For example, increased AGE modification of proteins affects rates of proteolysis in retinal cells, via effects on the ubiquitin proteasome [65]. Further to this, AGEs also affect the autophagy–lysosome pathways in the human proximal tubule cell line, HK-2 [66], and appear to decrease the capacity of renal proximal tubule cells to degrade AGE-modified albumin [11]. This breakdown in cellular maintenance can lead to accumulation of damaged proteins and activation of inflammatory pathways [67] and is a likely contributor to renal decline.

Excess dietary AGEs are known to affect glycemic control. Briefly, an increase in blood glucose levels is known to promote intracellular and extracellular AGE formation, resulting in the accumulation of extracellular matrix (ECM) components [68], and disrupting matri–matrix [69], cell–cell [10], or matrix–cell [70] interactions, including in the kidney [71]. This may occur as a result of intracellular modification of ECM proteins, altering their secretory properties and folding. AGE modification of collagens such as type IV, a basement membrane glycoprotein, impairs endothelial cell adhesion, protein and cellular interactions, cell proliferation [72], ECM breakdown, and remodeling [73,74], and likely contributes to the thickening of glomerular and tubular basement membranes and expansion of the mesangial matrix. *In vitro*, glycation of the ECM brings about an increase in protein permeability of the glomerular basement membrane [75]. Further to this, glycation of circulating proteins appears to, at least *in vitro*, affect their relative permeability across the glomerular basement membrane [76].

As mentioned above, it is no great leap to imagine that AGE-induced alterations to glycemic control would change the distribution of various metabolic fuels, facilitating further intracellular formation of AGEs. Intracellular posttranslational modification of proteins by advanced glycation alters protein function, trafficking, and breakdown [68], especially given that intracellular formation of AGEs happens at an accelerated rate when compared with extracellular and *ex vivo* modeling. Although it is widely appreciated that increased glucose uptake and flux through glycolytic and pentose phosphate pathways is a major reason for the increased rate of intracellular AGE formation, any metabolic imbalance leading to excess generation of glycolytic intermediates or reactive oxygen species (ROS) can result in excessive modification of intracellular proteins by advanced glycation within cells [77]. Modification of DNA by AGEs has also been suggested as a contributor to the development of CKD [78].

Pathological effects induced by AGEs may be mediated by interaction with receptors, such as the receptor for advanced glycation end products (RAGE). RAGE is a multi-ligand pattern recognition receptor involved in the amplification of immune and inflammatory responses, primarily via activation of NF-κB and JAK-STAT pathways, and production of IL-1β and TNFα [79,80]. AGE–RAGE binding also stimulates NADPH oxidase and mitochondrially derived ROS [24,81], accumulation of ECM proteins, and the induction of cytokines including monocyte chemoattractant protein (MCP-1), transforming growth factor (TGF-β1), connective tissue growth factor (CTGF), and vascular endothelial growth factor (VEGF) [74,82–86]. These aforementioned pathways have been well described in the development and progression of diabetic complications in both humans and animal models.

Finally, another pathway by which excess consumption of AGEs could contribute to the development and progression of CKD is via effects on the gut microbiota. This area of research is in its relative infancy; however, disturbances to the gut are becoming increasingly recognized in CKD patients (reviewed in 87). Recently, the intestinal-derived uremic toxin, indoxyl sulfate, was shown to positively correlate with circulating AGEs in hemodialysis patients [88]. Although the links here remain unclear, human colonies of the microbiota do have the capacity to degrade some glycated amino acids [89]. Certainly, the impact of dietary AGEs on the gut microbiota and its relationship to CKD remain to be established.

17.7 Interventions to Decrease the Burden of Dietary AGEs in CKD

Dietary modulation of AGEs may be a simple, cost-effective, and complementary treatment option for CKD. Indeed, a low-AGE diet, which lowered serum and kidney AGE levels, protected against diabetic nephropathy in spontaneous mouse models of both type 1 and type 2 diabetes [90]. However, this was not evident in the STZ-induced diabetic mouse, whereby low-AGE feeding did not affect the AGE burden [91]. In a cross-sectional human study, a low-AGE diet versus high-AGE diet over 4 weeks reduced serum AGEs and surrogate markers of inflammation and oxidative stress in ESRD patients who were undergoing dialysis [57]. Similar findings were observed in a small, cross-sectional study conducted in individuals with Stage 3 CKD following 4 weeks of low-AGE dietary consumption [92]. However, in both of these studies, kidney function was not reported.

Another mode by which the impact of excess dietary AGEs could be minimized is via interference of gastrointestinal absorption. Sevelamer is a nonabsorbed phosphate-binder often prescribed to late-stage CKD patients for the reduction of blood phosphate levels. In hemodialysis patients, 12 months treatment with sevelamer prevented increases in plasma pentosidine levels and slowed the progression of coronary artery calcification compared to a calcium-based binder [93]. In individuals with Stage 2–4 diabetic CKD, 8 weeks' administration of sevelamer carbonate reduced plasma triglycerides and cholesterol levels, and markers of inflammation and oxidative stress, and improved long-term glycemic control determined by HbA_{1C} [94]. Indeed, circulating AGEs were reduced and *in vitro* data suggested that sevelamer binds AGE–BSA. These findings were recently confirmed by a larger study where sevelamer improved inflammatory profiles and reduced the AGE burden in individuals with diabetes and Stage 2–4 CKD [95]. There were no overall benefits to renal function in any of these studies, although subanalyses identified that albuminuria was reduced in both younger and non-Caucasian individuals but increased in Caucasians [95]. These interesting findings certainly warrant follow-up.

17.8 Conclusions

Within this chapter, we have reviewed the evidence for excess consumption of AGEs contributing to the development and progression of CKD. There is some compelling evidence that exogenous AGEs, such as those absorbed from the diet, alter aspects of kidney function and result in structural abnormalities that are characteristic of CKD. Specifically, exogenous AGEs affect glomerular filtration, urinary albumin, ion and water reabsorption, and can affect systemic glycemic control. Less clear, however, is whether a reduction in dietary AGEs, or their absorption into the circulation, could prevent the development and/or progression of CKD. At the very least, current evidence suggests that a reduction in consumption, and perhaps the absorption of dietary AGEs, can reduce risk factors for CKD and cardiovascular disease. Hence, this relatively straightforward and cost-effective approach to reduce kidney and cardiovascular risk factors is worthy of further consideration in basic science and large-scale clinical trials.

REFERENCES

1. Hoy WE, Douglas-Denton RN, Hughson MD, Cass A, Johnson K, Bertram JF. A stereological study of glomerular number and volume: Preliminary findings in a multiracial study of kidneys at autopsy. *Kidney Int Suppl.* 2003(83):S31–7.
2. Donough AAM, Thomson SC. Metabolic basis of solute transport. In *The Kidney* 9th ed. Taal MW, Chertow GM, Marsden PA, Skorecki K, Yu ASL, Brenner BM (Eds.), Philadelphia, PA: Elsevier Saunders; 2012. pp. 139–157.
3. Levey AS, Coresh J, Balk E, Kausz AT, Levin A, Steffes MW, et al. National Kidney Foundation practice guidelines for chronic kidney disease: Evaluation, classification, and stratification. *Ann Intern Med.* 2003;139(2):137–47.
4. Chadban SJ, Briganti EM, Kerr PG, Dunstan DW, Welborn TA, Zimmet PZ, et al. Prevalence of kidney damage in Australian adults: The AusDiab kidney study. *J Am Soc Nephrol.* 2003;14(7 Suppl 2):S131–8.
5. Jha V, Garcia-Garcia G, Iseki K, Li Z, Naicker S, Plattner B, et al. Chronic kidney disease: Global dimension and perspectives. *Lancet (London, England).* 2013;382(9888):260–72.
6. Saran R, Li Y, Robinson B, Ayanian J, Balkrishnan R, Bragg-Gresham J, et al. US Renal Data System 2014 Annual Data Report: Epidemiology of kidney disease in the United States. *Am J Kidney Dis.* 2015;65(6 Suppl 1):A7.
7. Keith DS, Nichols GA, Gullion CM, Brown JB, Smith DH. Longitudinal follow-up and outcomes among a population with chronic kidney disease in a large managed care organization. *Arch Intern Med.* 2004;164(6):659–63.
8. Gugliucci A, Bendayan M. Renal fate of circulating advanced glycated end products (AGE): Evidence for reabsorption and catabolism of AGE-peptides by renal proximal tubular cells. *Diabetologia.* 1996;39(2):149–60.
9. Miyata T, Ueda Y, Horie K, Nangaku M, Tanaka S, de Strihou CY, et al. Renal catabolism of advanced glycation end products: The fate of pentosidine. *Kidney Int.* 1998;53(2):416–22.
10. Oldfield MD, Bach LA, Forbes JM, Nikolic-Paterson D, McRobert A, Thallas V, et al. Advanced glycation end products cause epithelial-myofibroblast transdifferentiation via the receptor for advanced glycation end products (RAGE). *J Clin Investig.* 2001;108(12):1853–63.
11. Ozdemir AM, Hopfer U, Rosca MV, Fan XJ, Monnier VM, Weiss MF. Effects of advanced glycation end product modification on proximal tubule epithelial cell processing of aAlbumin. *Am J Nephrol.* 2008;28(1):14–24.
12. Gallicchio MA, Bach LA. Uptake of advanced glycation end products by proximal tubule epithelial cells via macropinocytosis. *Biochim Biophys Acta.* 2013;1833(12):2922–32.
13. Rüster C, Bondeva T, Franke S, Förster M, Wolf G. Advanced glycation end-products induce cell cycle arrest and hypertrophy in podocytes. *Nephrol Dial Transplant.* 2008;23(7):2179–91.
14. Harcourt BE, Sourris KC, Coughlan MT, Walker KZ, Dougherty SL, Andrikopoulos S, et al. Targeted reduction of advanced glycation improves renal function in obesity. *Kidney Int.* 2011;80(2):190–8.
15. Sebekova K, Somoza V, Jarcuskova M, Heidland A, Podracka L. Plasma advanced glycation end products are decreased in obese children compared with lean controls. *Int J Pediatr Obes.* 2009;4(2):112–18.
16. Semba RD, Arab L, Sun K, Nicklett EJ, Ferrucci L. Fat mass is inversely associated with serum carboxymethyl-lysine, an advanced glycation end product, in adults. *J Nutr.* 2011;141(9):1726–30.
17. Gaens KHJ, Goossens GH, Niessen PM, van Greevenbroek MM, van der Kallen CJH, Niessen HW, et al. Nε-(Carboxymethyl)lysine-Receptor for advanced glycation end product axis is a key modulator of obesity-induced dysregulation of adipokine expression and insulin resistance. *Arterioscler, Thromb, Vasc Biol.* 2014;34(6):1199–208.

18. Uribarri J, Stirban A, Sander D, Cai W, Negrean M, Buenting CE, et al. Single oral challenge by advanced glycation end products acutely impairs endothelial function in diabetic and nondiabetic subjects. *Diabetes Care*. 2007;30(10):2579–82.
19. Vlassara H, Cai W, Crandall J, Goldberg T, Oberstein R, Dardaine V, et al. Inflammatory mediators are induced by dietary glycotoxins, a major risk factor for diabetic angiopathy. *Proc Natl Acad Sci*. 2002;99(24):15596–601.
20. Semba RD, Gebauer SK, Baer DJ, Sun K, Turner R, Silber HA, et al. Dietary intake of advanced glycation end products did not affect endothelial function and inflammation in healthy adults in a randomized controlled trial. *J Nutr*. 2014;144(7):1037–42.
21. Birlouez-Aragon I, Saavedra G, Tessier FJ, Galinier A, Ait-Ameur L, Lacoste F, et al. A diet based on high-heat-treated foods promotes risk factors for diabetes mellitus and cardiovascular diseases. *Am J Clin Nutr*. 2010;91(5):1220–6.
22. Vlassara H, Striker LJ, Teichberg S, Fuh H, Li YM, Steffes M. Advanced glycation end products induce glomerular sclerosis and albuminuria in normal rats. *Proc Natl Acad Sci U S A*. 1994;91(24):11704–8.
23. Thomas MC, Tikellis C, Burns WM, Bialkowski K, Cao Z, Coughlan MT, et al. Interactions between renin angiotensin system and advanced glycation in the kidney. *J Am Soc Nephrol*. 2005;16(10):2976–84.
24. Coughlan MT, Thorburn DR, Penfold SA, Laskowski A, Harcourt BE, Sourris KC, et al. RAGE-Induced Cytosolic ROS promote mitochondrial superoxide generation in diabetes. *J Am Soc Nephrol*. 2009;20(4):742–52.
25. Sebekova K, Hofmann T, Boor P, Sebekova K Jr., Ulicna O, Erbersdobler HF, et al. Renal effects of oral maillard reaction product load in the form of bread crusts in healthy and subtotally nephrectomized rats. *Ann N Y Acad Sci*. 2005;1043:482–91.
26. Sebekova K, Faist V, Hofmann T, Schinzel R, Heidland A. Effects of a diet rich in advanced glycation end products in the rat remnant kidney model. *Am J Kidney Dis*. 2003;41(3 Suppl 1):S48–51.
27. de Assis AM, Rech A, Longoni A, da Silva Morrone M, de Bittencourt Pasquali MA, Perry ML, et al. Dietary n-3 polyunsaturated fatty acids revert renal responses induced by a combination of 2 protocols that increase the amounts of advanced glycation end product in rats. *Nutr Res. (New York, NY)*. 2015;35(6):512–22.
28. He C, Sabol J, Mitsuhashi T, Vlassara H. Dietary glycotoxins: Inhibition of reactive products by aminoguanidine facilitates renal clearance and reduces tissue sequestration. *Diabetes*. 1999;48(6):1308–15.
29. Miyata T, Ueda Y, Shinzato T, Iida Y, Tanaka S, Kurokawa K, et al. Accumulation of albumin-linked and free-form pentosidine in the circulation of uremic patients with end-stage renal failure: Renal implications in the pathophysiology of pentosidine. *J Am Soc Nephro*. 1996;7(8):1198–206.
30. Hou FF, Ren H, Owen WF Jr., Guo ZJ, Chen PY, Schmidt AM, et al. Enhanced expression of receptor for advanced glycation end products in chronic kidney disease. *J Am Soc Nephrol*. 2004;15(7):1889–96.
31. Semba RD, Fink JC, Sun K, Windham BG, Ferrucci L. Serum carboxymethyl-lysine, a dominant advanced glycation end product, is associated with chronic kidney disease: The Baltimore longitudinal study of aging. *J Renal Nutr*. 2010;20(2):74–81.
32. Witko-Sarsat V, Friedlander M, Capeillere-Blandin C, Nguyen-Khoa T, Nguyen AT, Zingraff J, et al. Advanced oxidation protein products as a novel marker of oxidative stress in uremia. *Kidney Int*. 1996;49(5):1304–13.
33. Sun JK, Keenan HA, Cavallerano JD, Asztalos BF, Schaefer EJ, Sell DR, et al. Protection from retinopathy and other complications in patients with type 1 diabetes of extreme duration: The Joslin 50-year medalist study. *Diabetes Care*. 2011;34(4):968–74.
34. Nin JW, Jorsal A, Ferreira I, Schalkwijk CG, Prins MH, Parving H-H, et al. Higher plasma levels of advanced glycation end products are associated with incident cardiovascular disease and all-cause mortality in type 1 diabetes: A 12-year follow-up study. *Diabetes Care*. 2011;34(2):442–7.
35. Busch M, Franke S, Wolf G, Brandstädt A, Ott U, Gerth J, et al. The advanced glycation end product Nε-Carboxymethyllysine is not a predictor of cardiovascular events and renal outcomes in patients with type 2 diabetic kidney disease and hypertension. *Am J Kidney Dis*. 2006;48(4):571–9.
36. Dalal M, Semba RD, Sun K, Crasto C, Varadhan R, Bandinelli S, et al. Endogenous secretory receptor for advanced glycation end products and chronic kidney disease in the elderly population. *Am J Nephrol*. 2011;33(4):313–18.
37. Rebholz CM, Astor BC, Grams ME, Halushka MK, Lazo M, Hoogeveen RC, et al. Association of plasma levels of soluble receptor for advanced glycation end products and risk of kidney disease: The atherosclerosis risk in communities study. *Nephrol Dial Transplant*. 2015;30(1):77–83.

38. Thomas MC, Woodward M, Neal B, Li Q, Pickering R, Marre M, et al. The relationship between levels of advanced glycation end-products and their soluble receptor and adverse outcomes in adults with type 2 diabetes. *Diabetes Care.* 2015;38(10):1891–7.
39. Weiss MF, Erhard P, Kader-Attia FA, Wu YC, Deoreo PB, Araki A, et al. Mechanisms for the formation of glycoxidation products in end-stage renal disease. *Kidney Int.* 2000;57(6):2571–85.
40. Trivin C, Metzger M, Haymann JP, Boffa JJ, Flamant M, Vrtovsnik F, et al. Glycated Hemoglobin level and mortality in a nondiabetic population with CKD. *Clin J Am Soc Nephrol.* 2015;10(6):957–64.
41. Chen J, Muntner P, Hamm LL, Fonseca V, Batuman V, Whelton PK, et al. Insulin resistance and risk of chronic kidney disease in nondiabetic US adults. *J Am Soc Nephrol.* 2003;14(2):469–77.
42. Fliser D, Pacini G, Engelleiter R, Kautzky-Willer A, Prager R, Franek E, et al. Insulin resistance and hyperinsulinemia are already present in patients with incipient renal disease. *Kidney Int.* 1998;53(5):1343–7.
43. The Diabetes Control and Complications Trial/Epidemiology of Diabetes Interventions and Complications Research Group. Retinopathy and nephropathy in patients with type 1 diabetes four years after a trial of intensive therapy. *N Eng J Med.* 2000;342(6):381–9.
44. Perkovic V, Heerspink HL, Chalmers J, Woodward M, Jun M, Li Q, et al. Intensive glucose control improves kidney outcomes in patients with type 2 diabetes. *Kidney Int.* 2013;83(3):517–23.
45. Bilous R. Microvascular disease: What does the UKPDS tell us about diabetic nephropathy? *Diabetic Med.* 2008;25 Suppl 2:25–9.
46. Patel A, MacMahon S, Chalmers J, Neal B, Billot L, Woodward M, et al. Intensive blood glucose control and vascular outcomes in patients with type 2 diabetes. *N Eng J Med.* 2008;358(24):2560–72.
47. McIntyre NJ, Fluck RJ, McIntyre CW, Taal MW. Skin autofluorescence and the association with renal and cardiovascular risk factors in chronic kidney disease stage 3. *Clin J Am Soc Nephrol.* 2011;6(10):2356–63.
48. Tanaka K, Tani Y, Asai J, Nemoto F, Kusano Y, Suzuki H, et al. Skin autofluorescence is associated with renal function and cardiovascular diseases in pre-dialysis chronic kidney disease patients. *Nephrol Dial Transplant.* 2011;26(1):214–20.
49. Smit AJ, Gerrits EG. Skin autofluorescence as a measure of advanced glycation endproduct deposition: A novel risk marker in chronic kidney disease. *Curr Opin Nephrol Hypertens.* 2010;19(6):527–33.
50. Tanaka K, Nakayama M, Kanno M, Kimura H, Watanabe K, Tani Y, et al. Skin autofluorescence is associated with the progression of chronic kidney disease: A prospective observational study. *PLoS One.* 2013;8(12):e83799.
51. Yu Y, Thorpe S, Jenkins A, Shaw J, Sochaski M, McGee D, et al. Advanced glycation end-products and methionine sulphoxide in skin collagen of patients with type 1 diabetes. *Diabetologia.* 2006;49(10):2488–98.
52. Orchard TJ, Lyons TJ, Cleary PA, Braffett BH, Maynard J, Cowie C, et al. The Association of skin intrinsic fluorescence with type 1 diabetes complications in the DCCT/EDIC study. *Diabetes Care.* 2013;36(10):3146–53.
53. Genevieve M, Vivot A, Gonzalez C, Raffaitin C, Barberger-Gateau P, Gin H, et al. Skin autofluorescence is associated with past glycaemic control and complications in type 1 diabetes mellitus. *Diabetes Metabol.* 2013;39(4):349–54.
54. Sugisawa E, Miura J, Iwamoto Y, Uchigata Y. Skin autofluorescence reflects integration of past long-term glycemic control in patients with type 1 diabetes. *Diabetes Care.* 2013;36(8):2339–45.
55. Meerwaldt R, Hartog JWL, Graaff R, Huisman RJ, Links TP, den Hollander NC, et al. Skin autofluorescence, a measure of cumulative metabolic stress and advanced glycation end products, predicts mortality in hemodialysis patients. *J Am Soc Nephrol.* 2005;16(12):3687–93.
56. Coughlan MT, Patel SK, Jerums G, Penfold SA, Nguyen TV, Sourris KC, et al. Advanced glycation urinary protein-bound biomarkers and severity of diabetic nephropathy in man. *Am J Nephrol.* 2011;34(4):347–55.
57. Peppa M, Uribarri J, Cai W, Lu M, Vlassara H. Glycoxidation and inflammation in renal failure patients. *Am J Kidney Dis.* 2004;43(4):690–5.
58. Fagugli RM, Vanholder R, De Smet R, Selvi A, Antolini F, Lameire N, et al. Advanced glycation end products: Specific fluorescence changes of pentosidine-like compounds during short daily hemodialysis. *Int J Artif Organs.* 2001;24(5):256–62.

59. Gerdemann A, Wagner Z, Solf A, Bahner U, Heidland A, Vienken J, et al. Plasma levels of advanced glycation end products during haemodialysis, haemodiafiltration and haemofiltration: Potential importance of dialysate quality. *Nephrol Dial Transplant.* 2002;17(6):1045–9.
60. Lin CL, Huang CC, Yu CC, Yang HY, Chuang FR, Yang CW. Reduction of advanced glycation end product levels by on-line hemodiafiltration in long-term hemodialysis patients. *Am J Kidney Dis.* 2003;42(3):524–31.
61. Lamb EJ, Cattell WR, Dawnay AB. In vitro formation of advanced glycation end products in peritoneal dialysis fluid. *Kidney Int.* 1995;47(6):1768–74.
62. Mahiout A, Ehlerding G, Brunkhorst R. Advanced glycation end-products in the peritoneal fluid and in the peritoneal membrane of continuous ambulant peritoneal dialysis patients. *Nephrol Dial Transplant.* 1996;11 Suppl 5:2–6.
63. Friedlander MA, Wu YC, Schulak JA, Monnier VM, Hricik DE. Influence of dialysis modality on plasma and tissue concentrations of pentosidine in patients with end-stage renal disease. *Am J Kidney Dis.* 1995;25(3):445–51.
64. Crowley LE, Johnson CP, McIntyre N, Fluck RJ, McIntyre CW, Taal MW, et al. Tissue advanced glycation end product deposition after kidney transplantation. *Nephron Clin Pract.* 2013;124(1–2):54–9.
65. Uchiki T, Weikel KA, Jiao W, Shang F, Caceres A, Pawlak D, et al. Glycation-altered proteolysis as a pathobiologic mechanism that links dietary glycemic index, aging, and age-related disease (in nondiabetics). *Aging Cell.* 2012;11(1):1–13.
66. Liu WJ, Shen TT, Chen RH, Wu H-L, Wang YJ, Deng JK, et al. Autophagy-lysosome pathway in renal tubular epithelial cells is disrupted by advanced glycation end products in diabetic nephropathy. *J Biol Chem.* 2015;290(33):20499–510.
67. Ott C, Jacobs K, Haucke E, Navarrete Santos A, Grune T, Simm A. Role of advanced glycation end products in cellular signaling. *Redox Biol.* 2014;2:411–29.
68. Brownlee M. Advanced protein glycosylation in diabetes and aging. *Ann Rev Med.* 1995;46:223–34.
69. Raabe HM, Höpner JH, Notbohm H, Sinnecker GHG, Kruse K, Müller PK. Biochemical and biophysical alterations of the 7S and NC1 domain of collagen IV from human diabetic kidneys. *Diabetologia.* 1998;41(9):1073–9.
70. Anderson SS, Kim Y, Tsilibary EC. Effects of matrix glycation on mesangial cell adhesion, spreading and proliferation. *Kidney Int.* 1994;46(5):1359–67.
71. Forbes JM, Cooper ME, Oldfield MD, Thomas MC. Role of advanced glycation end products in diabetic nephropathy. *J Am Soc Nephrol.* 2003;14 Suppl 3:S254–S8.
72. Kalfa TA, Gerritsen ME, Carlson EC, Binstock AJ, Tsilibary EC. Altered proliferation of retinal microvascular cells on glycated matrix. *Invest Ophthalmol Vis Sci.* 1995;36(12):2358–67.
73. Mott JD, Khalifah RG, Nagase H, Shield CF 3rd, Hudson JK, Hudson BG. Nonenzymatic glycation of type IV collagen and matrix metalloproteinase susceptibility. *Kidney Int.* 1997;52(5):1302–12.
74. Shimizu F, Sano Y, Haruki H, Kanda T. Advanced glycation end-products induce basement membrane hypertrophy in endoneurial microvessels and disrupt the blood-nerve barrier by stimulating the release of TGF-beta and vascular endothelial growth factor (VEGF) by pericytes. *Diabetologia.* 2011;54(6):1517–26.
75. Walton HA, Byrne J, Robinson GB. Studies of the permeation properties of glomerular basement membrane: Cross-linking renders glomerular basement membrane permeable to protein. *Biochim Biophys Acta.* 1992;1138(3):173–83.
76. Daniels BS, Hauser EB. Glycation of albumin, not glomerular basement membrane, alters permeability in an in vitro model. *Diabetes.* 1992;41(11):1415–21.
77. Hamada Y, Araki N, Koh N, Nakamura J, Horiuchi S, Hotta N. Rapid formation of advanced glycation end products by intermediate metabolites of glycolytic pathway and polyol pathway. *Biochem Biophys Res Commun.* 1996;228(2):539–43.
78. Stopper H, Schupp N, Bahner U, Sebekova K, Klassen A, Heidland A. Genomic damage in end-stage renal failure: Potential involvement of advanced glycation end products and carbonyl stress. *Sem Nephrol.* 2004;24(5):474–8.
79. Bierhaus A, Schiekofer S, Schwaninger M, Andrassy M, Humpert PM, Chen J, et al. Diabetes-associated sustained activation of the transcription factor nuclear factor-kappaB. *Diabetes.* 2001;50(12):2792–808.

80. Schmidt AM, Hori O, Chen JX, Li JF, Crandall J, Zhang J, et al. Advanced glycation endproducts interacting with their endothelial receptor induce expression of vascular cell adhesion molecule-1 (VCAM-1) in cultured human endothelial cells and in mice. A potential mechanism for the accelerated vasculopathy of diabetes. *J Clin Invest.* 1995;96(3):1395–403.
81. Wendt TM, Tanji N, Guo J, Kislinger TR, Qu W, Lu Y, et al. RAGE drives the development of glomerulosclerosis and implicates podocyte activation in the pathogenesis of diabetic nephropathy. *Am J Pathol.* 2003;162(4):1123–37.
82. Li JH, Huang XR, Zhu HJ, Oldfield M, Cooper M, Truong LD, et al. Advanced glycation end products activate Smad signaling via TGF-beta-dependent and independent mechanisms: Implications for diabetic renal and vascular disease. *Faseb J.* 2004;18(1):176–8.
83. Cooper ME. Pathogenesis, prevention, and treatment of diabetic nephropathy. *Lancet.* 1998;352(9123):213–19.
84. Sourris KC, Harcourt BE, Forbes JM. A new perspective on therapeutic inhibition of advanced glycation in diabetic microvascular complications: Common downstream endpoints achieved through disparate therapeutic approaches? *Am J Nephrol.* 2009;30(4):323–35.
85. Twigg SM, Chen MM, Joly AH, Chakrapani SD, Tsubaki J, Kim HS, et al. Advanced glycosylation end products up-regulate connective tissue growth factor (insulin-like growth factor-binding protein-related protein 2) in human fibroblasts: A potential mechanism for expansion of extracellular matrix in diabetes mellitus. *Endocrinology.* 2001;142(5):1760–9.
86. Isoda K, Folco E, Marwali MR, Ohsuzu F, Libby P. Glycated LDL increases monocyte CC chemokine receptor 2 expression and monocyte chemoattractant protein-1-mediated chemotaxis. *Atherosclerosis.* 2008;198(2):307–12.
87. Ramezani A, Raj DS. The gut microbiome, kidney disease, and targeted Interventions. *J Am Soc Nephrol.* 2014;25(4):657–70.
88. Lin CJ, Lin J, Pan CF, Chuang CK, Liu HL, Sun FJ, et al. Indoxyl sulfate, not P-cresyl sulfate, is associated with advanced glycation end products in patients on long-term hemodialysis. *Kidney Blood Pres Res.* 2015;40(2):121–9.
89. Hellwig M, Bunzel D, Huch M, Franz CMAP, Kulling SE, Henle T. Stability of individual maillard reaction products in the presence of the human colonic microbiota. *J Agric Food Chem.* 2015;63(30):6723–30.
90. Zheng F, He C, Cai W, Hattori M, Steffes M, Vlassara H. Prevention of diabetic nephropathy in mice by a diet low in glycoxidation products. *Diabetes/Metabol Res Rev.* 2002;18(3):224–37.
91. Tan ALY, Sourris KC, Harcourt BE, Thallas-Bonke V, Penfold S, Andrikopoulos S, et al. Disparate effects on renal and oxidative parameters following RAGE deletion, AGE accumulation inhibition, or dietary AGE control in experimental diabetic nephropathy. 2010;298(3):F763–70.
92. Vlassara H, Cai W, Goodman S, Pyzik R, Yong A, Chen X, et al. Protection against loss of innate defenses in adulthood by low Advanced Glycation End Products (AGE) intake: Role of the antiinflammatory AGE Receptor-1. *J Clin Endocrinol Metabol.* 2009;94(11):4483–91.
93. Kakuta T, Tanaka R, Hyodo T, Suzuki H, Kanai G, Nagaoka M, et al. Effect of sevelamer and calcium-based phosphate binders on coronary artery calcification and accumulation of circulating advanced glycation end products in hemodialysis patients. *Am J Kidney Dis.* 2011;57(3):422–31.
94. Vlassara H, Uribarri J, Cai W, Goodman S, Pyzik R, Post J, et al. Effects of sevelamer on HbA1c, inflammation, and advanced glycation end products in diabetic kidney disease. *Clin J Am Soc Nephrol.* 2012;7(6):934–42.
95. Yubero-Serrano EM, Woodward M, Poretsky L, Vlassara H, Striker GE, Group oboA-lS. Effects of sevelamer carbonate on advanced glycation end products and antioxidant/Pro-Oxidant status in patients with diabetic kidney disease. *Clin J Am Soc Nephrol.* 2015;10(5):759–66.

18

Dietary AGEs May Have Different Effects in People with Vegetarian versus Omnivorous Eating Patterns

Katarina Šebeková
Comenius University
Bratislava, Slovakia

Katarína Brouder Šebeková
John Radcliffe Hospital
Oxford, United Kingdom

CONTENTS

KEY POINTS

- Advanced glycation end products (AGEs) are implicated in pathophysiology of aging and different noncommunicable diseases.
- Vegetarians, presenting generally better cardiometabolic characteristics and lower risk for many chronic degenerative diseases in comparison with omnivores, paradoxically present higher circulating AGE levels.
- High intake of Maillard reaction products (MRPs) containing plant foods, high intake of fructose, and metabolic changes induced by lower protein intake of mainly plant origin might contribute to higher AGE levels in vegetarians.

- High levels of natural antioxidants and phytochemicals, healthy lifestyle, and factors not completely understood yet (e.g., vegetarian diet–induced changes in gut microbiota) might ameliorate or postpone the negative health effects of elevated circulating AGEs in vegetarians.
- Currently available limited data neither support the assumption that dietary MRPs have different effects in omnivores than in vegetarians, nor that plant-protein-derived MRPs exert different health effects from those of meat origin.

18.1 Vegetarian Diet

Vegetarians are typically considered as individuals who do not eat any meat, poultry, or fish, but consume only plant-based foods, that is, fruits, vegetables, pulses, cereals, sprouts, whole grains, and nuts. However, vegetarian diets vary in consumed and excluded foods, and vegetarians can be subclassified as vegans (V) not consuming any animal products; lacto-ovo-vegetarians (LOV) who eat also dairy products and/or eggs; and semi-vegetarians, who in addition to plant-based foods, diary, and eggs, consume also fish and shellfish, and some even very limited amounts of white meat. Omnivores (O) consume also red meat in addition to all the aforementioned compounds.

With regard to nutrients intake, well-balanced vegetarian diet–consuming vegetarians can meet the recommended daily allowance (RDA) for intake of all nutrients except for vitamin B_{12}, as there is no plant source of vitamin B_{12} (Bederova et al. 2000; Key et al. 2006; McEvoy et al. 2012; Sabate 2003). In comparison with omnivorous diet, vegetarian diets are usually rich in carbohydrates, n-6 fatty acids, dietary fiber, and vitamins (carotenoids, folic acid, vitamin C, and vitamin E), and poorer in proteins, saturated fat, long-chain n-3 fatty acids, and retinol. Except for vitamin B_{12}, common nutritional deficiencies in vegetarians include iron, calcium, zinc, omega-3 fatty acids, vitamin D, and iodine.

18.2 Health Effects of Vegetarian Diet

Vegetarians consuming balanced vegetarian diets generally present lower body mass index (BMI), lower BP values, more favorable lipid profile, lower levels of atherogenic risk factors (cholesterol, low-density lipoprotein cholesterol, atherogenic index, saturated fatty acids, lower lipid peroxidation products), higher levels of factors with antiatherogenic effect (HDL-to-cholesterol ratio, polyunsaturated fatty acids, vitamin E/cholesterol ratio, vitamin C), higher insulin sensitivity, and better antioxidant status, if compared with their omnivorous counterparts (Bederova et al. 2000; Key et al. 2006; McEvoy et al. 2012; Sabate 2003). Comparison of cardiometabolic characteristics of omnivores and vegetarians from our studies is given in Table 18.1 (Krajcovicova-Kudlackova et al. 2002; Sebekova et al. 2001a, 2003, 2006). Except for high intake of vitamins and fiber, the aforementioned benefits might also be on the account of indoles, thiocyanates, cumarins, phenols, flavonoids, terpenes, protease inhibitors, phytosterols, and other phytochemicals contained in a plant-based diet (Sabate 2003).

In comparison with meat, plant proteins contain lower amounts of essential amino acids (AA, mainly methionine and lysine), and they are richer in nonessential AAs (mainly arginine, serine, and glycine) (Krajcovicova-Kudlackova et al. 2005). Thus, even vegetarians meeting the RDA of protein intake consume less essential AAs, crucial for proper protein synthesis. Lower protein synthesis rate induced by plant-based diet consumption is reflected by lower plasma protein concentration not only in vegetarians but also in omnivores and experimental animals (Caso et al. 2000; Krajcovicova-Kudlackova et al. 1993; Thalacker-Mercer and Campbell 2008). To minimize changes in plasma albumin concentration, lower protein synthesis rate is compensated by lower albumin degradation rate and reduced renal fractional excretion of albumin (Caso et al. 2000).

Health benefits of vegetarian diet are associated with low rates of obesity, metabolic syndrome (MetS), type 2 diabetes, cardiovascular (CV) diseases, some types of cancers, and increased longevity (Craig 2010;

TABLE 18.1

Data on Standard and Nonstandard Cardiometabolic Risk Factors in Omnivores and Vegetarians

	Omnivores (n = 83)	Vegetarians (n = 153)	p
Age (years)	38.1 ± 12.2	38.1 ± 13.2	0.99
BMI (kg/m^2)	24.6 ± 4.3	22.5 ± 3.1	**<0.001**
SBP (mm Hg)	116 ± 15	111 ± 11	**0.004**
DBP (mm Hg)	74 ± 10	70 ± 7	**<0.001**
FPG (mmol/L)	4.4 ± 0.5	4.3 ± 0.5	0.14
FPI (μIU/mL)	6.9 ± 4.5	5.0 ± 2.3	**<0.001**
HOMA	1.42 ± 1.03	0.98 ± 0.46	**<0.001**
Cholesterol (mmol/L)	4.6 ± 0.9	4.6 ± 1.0	0.99
HDL-cholesterol (mmol/L)	1.5 ± 0.5	1.7 ± 0.5	**0.004**
LDL-cholesterol (mmol/L)	2.5 ± 0.9	2.4 ± 0.9	0.42
TAG (mmol/L)	1.3 ± 0.6	1.2 ± 0.7	0.27
Albumin (g/L)	48 ± 6	44 ± 3	**<0.001**
hsCRP (mg/l)	1.0 ± 1.5	0.5 ± 0.6	**<0.001**
Leukocyte counts (x.10^9/L)	5.8 ± 1.5	5.0 ± 1.4	**<0.001**
Uric acid (μmol/L)	280 ± 93	250 ± 75	**0.008**
Cystatin C (mg/L)	0.86 ± 0.13	0.87 ± 0.12	0.55

Sources: Pooled data from Sebekova, K., et al., *Mol. Nutr. Food Res.*, 50, 858–868, 2006; Sebekova, K., et al., *Clin. Chem.*, 49, 983–986, 2003; Sebekova, K., et al., *Eur. J. Nutr.*, 40, 275–281, 2001a.

Note: BMI, body mass index; SBP, systolic blood pressure; DBP, diastolic blood pressure; FPG, fasting plasma glucose; FPI, fasting plasma insulin; HOMA, the homeostasis model assessment of insulin sensitivity; HDL, high-density lipoprotein; LDL, low-density lipoprotein; TAG, triacylglycerols; hsCRP, high-sensitivity C-reactive protein; significant p in Student's t-test is given in **bold**.

Key et al. 2006; McEvoy et al. 2012; Sabate 2003; Turner-McGrievy and Harris 2014). These benefits are generally attributed to the absence of meat in the diet, and abundant consumption of fruits, vegetables, legumes, unrefined cereals, and nuts, as their consumption is consistently associated with a lower risk for many chronic degenerative diseases, and increased longevity (Sabate 2003). High intake of arginine decreases hypercholesterolemic effects of essential AAs; lower intake of methionine and lysine associates with decreased secretion of apoB-containing lipoproteins; and essential AAs are relatively more effective in releasing insulin, while the nonessential AAs (particularly arginine) preferentially induce release of glucagon (Krajcovicova-Kudlackova et al. 2005; Sanchez and Hubbard 1991). These mechanisms might contribute to preventive effects of plant proteins in the development of cardiometabolic diseases. However, vegetarianism is usually not restricted to plant-based diet, and is associated with healthy lifestyle. Vegetarians are often nonsmokers, abstain from alcohol, and exercise regularly.

18.3 Formation of Maillard Reaction Products/Advanced Glycation End Products

Pathways leading to formation of brownish substances in foods during thermal processing at high temperatures (such as roasting, frying, and baking), rendering foods attractive color, taste, and odor, were described more than 100 years ago by the French chemist C.L. Maillard (Maillard 1912). Maillard reaction products (MRPs) are formed spontaneously via nonenzymatic glycation, that is, reaction between carbonyl groups of reducing carbohydrates (fructose, glucose, etc.) and free amino groups of AAs, peptides, and proteins. Lysine and arginine represent preferential targets of Maillard reaction, as ε-amino-groups of AAs are more prone to glycation than α-amino-groups. Initially formed labile Schiff bases undergo spontaneous rearrangement yielding more stable but still reversible Amadori products. These undergo complex reactions leading to formation of a heterogeneous group of stable and irreversible

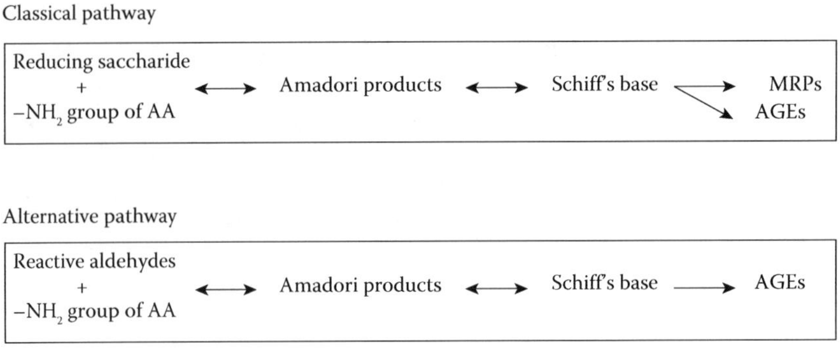

FIGURE 18.1 Classical and alternative pathways of Maillard reaction products (MRPs) and advanced glycation end products (AGEs) formation.

MRPs (Figure 18.1). In foods processed under high temperatures, MRPs are formed within seconds to few hours. Final products of Maillard reaction are insoluble melanoidins, abundant particularly in coffee, bakery products, cocoa, roasted potatoes, pulses and seeds, soy sauces, or black beer (Adams et al. 2005; Vitaglione et al. 2008).

Seven decades later, it has been revealed that analogous substances to MRPs—advanced glycation end products (AGEs)—are formed naturally in living organisms (Brownlee et al. 1984). Except for classical pathway, they are formed under enhanced oxidative stress and carbonyl stress, utilizing reactive aldehydes formed during lipid peroxidation and auto-oxidation of glucose. AGEs were in turn implicated in the pathophysiology of aging, and different noncommunicable diseases, as AGE-modification alters the structure and thus the function of proteins (Thorpe and Baynes 1996). Discovery of specific cell-surface receptor for AGEs–RAGE enabled to characterize the indirect harmful pathways leading to enhanced oxidative stress, and proinflammatory, diabetogenic, and atherogenic effects (Schmidt et al. 1996) (Figure 18.1).

In classical Maillard reaction, MRPs and AGEs are formed nonenzymatically by the reaction of reducing sugars with free amino groups ($-NH_2$) of AA. Labile Amadori products are rearranged into more stabile but still reversible Schiff's bases, which are converted into stabile irreversible MRPs (in foods) or AGEs (*in vivo* analogues of MRPs). During heat treatment of foods at temperatures above 100°C, MRPs occur within seconds to hours. Formation of AGEs *in vivo* via classical pathway under constant low temperature (37°C) requires weeks to months.

In vivo, interaction of AGEs with their specific cell-surface receptor RAGE activates down-stream pathways, such as that of nuclear factor kappa-B (NF-κB), resulting, among others, in production of reactive oxygen species. Lipooxidation-derived and glucose autooxidation-derived reactive aldehydes may augment formation of AGEs via alternative pathways. Through this pathway, AGEs might be formed within few days.

18.4 Skin Autofluorescence

Skin autofluorescence (SAF) is a noninvasive method enabling to approximate the tissue accumulation of glycemic-, oxidative-, and carbonyl stress–derived AGEs (Mulder et al. 2006). Degree of modification of skin collagen by various AGEs correlates well with SAF (Meerwaldt et al. 2005). In humans, SAF increases by aging and in the presence of diseases associated with elevated AGE levels (Klenovics et al. 2014; Koetsier et al. 2010). In diabetes and chronic renal failure, SAF is an independent predictor of major complications and mortality (Bos et al. 2011; Noordzij et al. 2008).

18.4.1 Effects of MRPs Consumption on Skin Autofluorescence

In healthy subjects and diabetics, intake of a single meal with a medium MRP content resulted in a significant increase (by 8.7% and 11.6%, respectively) in SAF 2 hours postprandially (Stirban et al. 2008).

Thus, the authors suggest that measurements of SAF should be performed in the fasting state. In elderly subjects, SAF did not correlate with dietary MRPs intake calculated from 3-day food diaries using the database of Goldberg et al., while it showed significant negative association with consumption of wine, proteins, and saturated fats (Goldberg et al. 2004; Jochemsen et al. 2009). Infant formulas contain hundreds-fold higher N^{ε}-carboxymethyl(lysine) levels (CML, a widely used indicator of MRPs formation in foods and the most abundant AGE in human body) in comparison with breast milk (Sebekova et al. 2008). During the first 6 months of life, formula-fed infants present higher SAF in comparison with breast-milk-fed infants (by 40% in 1- to -3-month olds and by 31% in 4-to-6-month olds). This difference gradually diminishes after the introduction of diversified diet (Sebekova et al. 2010).

18.4.2 Skin Autofluorescence in Vegetarian Hemodialyzed Patients

In comparison with omnivorous patients, vegetarian hemodialyzed patients present significantly lower SAF (by 22%) (Nongnuch and Davenport 2015). Regardless of dietary regimen, Caucasians displayed the highest and the African Afro-Caribbeans the lowest SAF levels. Vegetarian and omnivorous African Afro-Caribbeans differed in SAF only by 3%. Since the metabolic and nutritional characteristics of the patients according to their dietary regimen and ethnicity have not been reported, it remains unclear whether the observed differences in SAF between Caucasian, South Asian, and African Afro-Caribbean patients could be attributed to different ethnicities, dietary regimen, or disease-related factors. SAF reference values for Dutch and Chinese do not differ significantly (Koetsier et al. 2010; Yue et al. 2011). Lower protein content of vegetarian diets is contradictory to the high protein diet guideline for chronic dialysis patients (Kopple 2001). Vegetarian patients on maintenance hemodialysis present lower BMI and normalized protein catabolic rate in comparison with nonvegetarians (Wu et al. 2011).

18.5 Health Effects of Dietary MRPs

By the end of the last century, Koshinsky et al. suggested that ingested dietary MRPs are partially absorbed into circulation, where they might exert negative health effects (Koschinsky et al. 1997). Dietary MRPs are major contributors to the body's pool of AGEs (Uribarri et al. 2005). Two- to six-week-long human studies on the effects of high versus low dietary MRPs load were performed in parallel or cross-over design in healthy volunteers and in diabetic or chronic renal failure patients. Dietary MRPs content of the diets differed from 1.5- to 4.4-fold. Lower dietary intake of MRPs was generally reflected by lower levels of circulating AGEs and lower urinary excretion of AGEs. Intake of low versus high MRPs diet is associated with better indices of glucose homeostasis, lower oxidative stress, and inflammatory markers, and in some studies with lower body weight, improvement of lipid profile, renal function, and circulating adipokines is seen (reviewed in Delgado-Andrade 2014; Kellow and Savige 2013; Poulsen et al. 2013; Sebekova and Somoza 2007). Increased levels of circulating CML and those of AGE-associated fluorescence of plasma (AGE-Fl, a coarse estimate of accumulation of fluorescent AGEs [Munch et al. 1997]) imposed by infant formulas consumption during first 6 months of life seemed not to play a role in formula-consumption-associated insulin resistance, either directly or indirectly by induction of oxidative stress, microinflammation, or hyperleptinemia (Klenovics et al. 2013). Healthy rats consuming bread crusts containing MRPs-rich diet, i.e. diet enriched exclusively by plant-proteins-based MRPs, gained body and organ weights, for example,Healthy rats consuming bread crusts containing MRPs-rich diet, i.e. diet enriched exclusively by plant-proteins-based MRPs, gained body and organ weights, for example, developed proteinuria, and manifested insulin resistance, hyperleptinemia, and hyperadiponectinemia, and changes in leptin-induced central signaling of anorexigenic/orexigenic hormones, as well as in the neuronal activity in the central nervous system (Sebekova et al. 2005, 2012). Chronic oral administration of pure CML to rats were associated with its accumulation in kidneys, heart, liver, and lungs, and impaired markers of kidney and liver function, while fasting glycemia remained within the normal range (Li et al. 2015).

Difference in MRPs content of diets in clinical studies is most often achieved by adjustments of heating temperatures and/or changes in culinary methods. Extensive heating may lead to generation of toxic

Maillard reaction compounds (acrylamide, heterocyclic aromatic amines, and 5-hydroxymethylfurfural); it might affect the content of heat-sensitive nutrients, or even produce compounds with potentially beneficial health effects, such as melanoidins (Felton et al. 2007; Gokmen and Palazoglu 2008; Morales et al. 2012; Murkovic and Pichler 2006). These facts complicate the interpretation of the observed health effects of MRPs-rich diets.

18.6 Vegetarian Diet and Dietary MRPs

Typical domestic culinary processing of foods at high dry heat (such as baking, broiling, grilling, frying, and roasting used to prepare meat) results in abundant formation of MPRs. Plant-based foods are usually prepared by boiling, stewing, or steam-cooking—culinary methods requiring lower temperatures and cooking times in comparison to preparation of (particularly red) meat. Moreover, thermal processing of foods with low protein and/or carbohydrate content or high water content yields low or even negligible amounts of MRPs (Hull et al. 2012). From this point of view, consumption of vegetarian diet should impose lower MRPs load in comparison with omnivorous diet.

On the contrary, recently published databases on the levels of various MRPs in different foods and beverages quote that certain heat-processed plant-based food items contain high amounts of MRPs (Goldberg et al. 2004; Hull et al. 2012; Scheijen et al. 2016; Takeuchi et al. 2015; Uribarri et al. 2010). Thus, dark, whole meal, and currant bread, particularly if toasted; knäckebröd, rusks, biscuits, and cereal products; nuts, seeds (particularly if roasted), and dry-heat processed snacks containing seeds, nuts, dried berries, and soft fruits; dried cereals; fried or marinated tofu; dark chocolate; canned fish; lactic acid bacteria beverages particularly if sugar sweetened; fruit juices and drinks containing high amounts of reducing carbohydrates and/or soybean flour; sports and carbonated drinks; items which are or might be consumed in high amounts by vegetarians, might contribute to high dietary MRPs load. Different analytical methods used to determine MRPs content in foods yield in some cases contradictory results, and differences in the ingredient profiles and industrial or domestic culinary processing are also to be considered (Goldberg et al. 2004; Hull et al. 2012; Scheijen et al. 2016; Takeuchi et al. 2015; Uribarri et al. 2010).

Recent data suggest that MRPs occur during the lifetime of crop plants, particularly if grown under stress conditions, such as high light, drought, and metal stress (Bilova et al. 2015). Contemporary climate change in Central Europe, characterized by (formerly unusual) hot sunny summers with long periods of droughts alternating with short periods of heavy rains, might favor the stress-induced formation of MRPs in locally cultivated crop plants. However, the impact of consumption of stressed plants on AGE levels remains to be elucidated in further experimental and human studies.

18.7 AGE Levels in Vegetarians

Our group studied the levels of circulating AGEs in healthy vegetarians versus their age-matched omnivorous counterparts by the end of the last century (Krajcovicova-Kudlackova et al. 2002; Sebekova et al. 2001a, 2003, 2006). We hypothesized that lower cooking temperatures and time to prepare vegetarian food in comparison with that needed for preparation of meat should be reflected by lower levels of circulating AGEs in vegetarians (Sebekova et al. 2001a). Surprisingly, we revealed that CML as well as AGE-Fl levels were significantly higher (by 24% and 25%, respectively) in vegetarians when compared with omnivores (Figure 18.2). In comparison with the omnivores, vegans, lacto-ovo-vegetarians, and semi-vegetarians presented AGE-Fl levels higher by 15%, 32%, and 22%, respectively, while those of CML were higher by 24%, 26%, and 20%, respectively (Figure 18.3). In the whole group, both markers of advanced glycation correlated directly ($r = 0.745$, $p < 0.001$). Elevation of circulating AGEs in vegetarians was higher than that observed in Slovak type 1 diabetic children, displaying 17% higher AGE-Fl levels in comparison with their healthy counterparts (Jakus et al. 2012), but moderate if compared with a

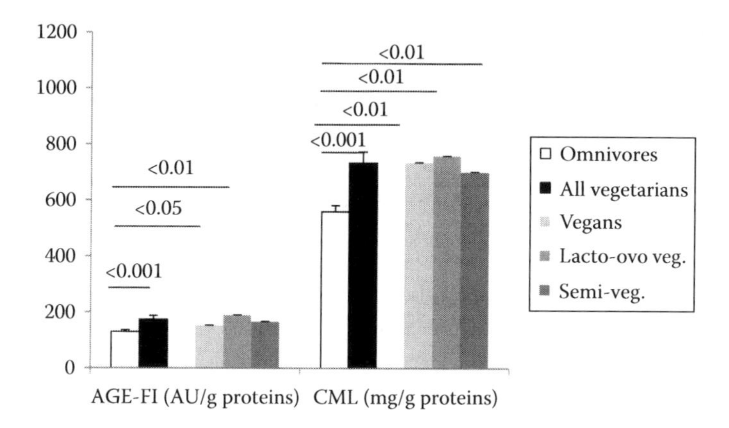

FIGURE 18.2 Plasma levels of N^ε^-(carboxymethyl)lysine and advanced glycation end products–associated fluorescence of plasma in omnivores and vegetarians. AGE-Fl, advanced glycation end products–associated fluorescence of plasma; AU, arbitrary units; CML, N^ε^-(carboxymethyl)lysine; veg., vegetarians. (Modified from Sebekova, K., et al., *Eur. J. Nutr.*, 40, 275–281, 2001a.)

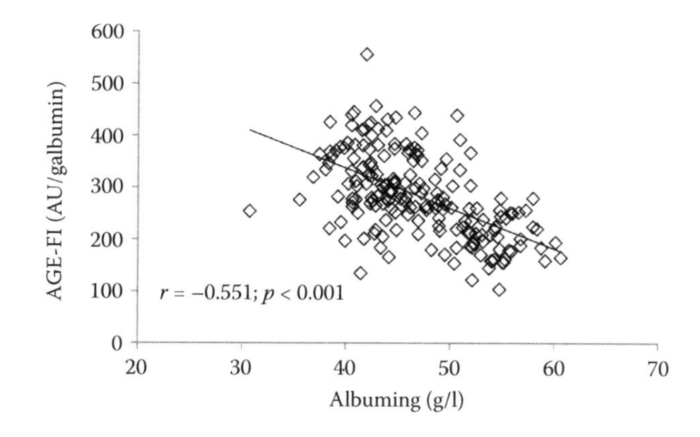

FIGURE 18.3 Relationship between advanced glycation end products–associated fluorescence of plasma and albuminemia in vegetarians. AGE-Fl, advanced glycation end products–associated fluorescence of plasma; AU, arbitrary units. (Pooled data from Sebekova, K., et al., Mol. *Nutr. Food Res.*, 50, 858–868, 2006; Sebekova, K., et al., *Clin. Chem.*, 49, 983–986, 2003; Sebekova, K., et al., *Eur. J. Nutr.*, 40, 275–281, 2001a.)

2-fold rise in AGE-Fl and CML levels in Slovak conservatively treated children with chronic renal insufficiency versus healthy controls (Sebekova et al. 2001b).

18.8 Potential Role of Nonalimentary Factors in Increased Circulating AGE Levels of Vegetarians

Aging, decreased renal function, persistent hyperglycemia, enhanced oxidative stress, microinflammation, and smoking represent major nonalimentary factors contributing to increased AGE production and/or accumulation. However, our vegetarians and omnivores were of similar age, nonsmokers, and presented similar renal function and fasting glycemia. Enhanced microinflammation as endogenous source of AGE production could also be excluded (Table 18.1). A direct significant correlation between cystatine C (a marker of renal function) and plasma AGE-Fl levels observed in both cohorts (Table 18.2) suggests that even in subjects with normal renal function, kidney is a key modulator of plasma AGE levels.

TABLE 18.2

Pearson Correlation Coefficients between Advanced Glycation End Products Associated Fluorescence of Plasma and Standard and Nonstandard Cardiometabolic Risk Factors in Omnivores and Vegetarians

	Omnivores (*n* = 83)		Vegetarians (*n* = 153)		r-to-z (Fischer)
	r	p	r	p	p
Age	0.389	**<0.001**	0.104	0.10	**0.027**
BMI	0.066	0.28	0.195	**0.008**	0.34
SBP	0.057	0.30	0.164	**0.021**	0.44
DBP	0.047	0.34	0.101	0.11	0.70
FPG	0.179	0.053	0.194	**0.008**	0.91
FPI	0.169	0.063	0.199	**0.007**	0.83
HOMA	0.133	0.12	0.190	**0.009**	0.67
Cholesterol	0.507	**<0.001**	0.072	0.19	**0.004**
HDL-cholesterol	−0.092	0.20	−0.162	**0.023**	0.61
LDL-cholesterol	0.382	**<0.001**	0.154	**0.029**	0.07
TAG	0.357	**<0.001**	0.289	**<0.001**	0.58
hsCRP	0.174	0.058	0.119	0.071	0.68
Leukocyte counts	0.121	0.14	0.269	**<0.001**	0.27
Uric acid	0.109	0.16	0.182	**0.012**	0.59
Cystatin C	0.271	**0.007**	0.366	**<0.001**	0.45

Sources: Pooled data from Sebekova, K., et al., *Mol. Nutr. Food Res.*, 50, 858–868, 2006; Sebekova, K., et al., *Clin. Chem.*, 49, 983–986, 2003; Sebekova, K., et al., *Eur. J. Nutr.*, 40, 275–281, 2001a.

Note: Fischer's r-to-z transformation; BMI, body mass index; SBP, systolic blood pressure; DBP, diastolic blood pressure; FPG, fasting plasma glucose; FPI, fasting plasma insulin; HOMA, the homeostasis model assessment of insulin sensitivity; HDL, high-density lipoprotein; LDL, low-density lipoprotein; TAG, triacylglycerols; hsCRP, high-sensitivity C-reactive protein; significant Pearson's correlation coefficients and significant difference in Pearson's correlation coefficients between the groups are given in bold.

18.9 Potential Role of Alimentary Factors in Enhanced Endogenous Production of AGEs in Vegetarians

18.9.1 Carbohydrates Intake

Dietary intake of carbohydrates was similar in omnivores and vegetarians (Sebekova et al. 2006). However, high intake of fruits and vegetables by vegetarians results in higher intake of fructose in comparison with that of glucose. Fructose is approximately an 8-fold more potent glycating agent in comparison with glucose, but its plasma concentration is approximately 14-fold lower. Thus, the contribution of extracellular glycation by fructose is generally considerably less than that by glucose (Schalkwijk et al. 2004). Our vegetarians consumed 3-to 5-fold more fruits and foodstuffs containing higher amounts of fructose in comparison to that of glucose (Krajcovicova-Kudlackova et al. 2002). Mean lysine and arginine intake of vegetarians represented approximately 54% and 60%, respectively, of that of omnivores. Increased fructose/lysine and fructose/arginine ratio could create a milieu favoring glycation of protein residues *in situ* in the intestine, or postprandially (DeChristopher et al. 2015). Thus, nutritional regimen in vegetarians might at least partially contribute to observed higher circulating AGE levels.

In rats, effects of chronic high dietary fructose intake on accumulation of AGEs are contradictory. Accumulation in tissues differs between the strains; is tissue-specific; depends on the concentration of dietary fructose, duration of the study, and age of the animals (Levi and Werman 1998; Lingelbach et al. 2000; Mikulikova et al. 2008). Experimental data regarding the effects of high fructose intake on plasma or tissue AGE levels in humans have not been reported yet.

18.9.2 Protein Intake

In our studies, all subjects met the RDA of protein intake, but vegetarians consumed less proteins (by 23% to 28%) in comparison with omnivores, reflected by significantly lower BMI and concentration of albumin (Table 18.1) (Sebekova et al. 2001a). Plasma AGE-Fl levels correlated inversely with albuminemia in vegetarians (Figure 18.3), but not in omnivores ($r = -0.010$, NS). Whether this might reflect longer explosion of albumin to intrinsic glycation due to slower protein turnover under consumption of plant protein–based diet remains unclear (Caso et al. 2000).

Higher protein intake in the omnivores in comparison with vegetarians could induce postprandial rise in glomerular filtration rate due to a protein-induced hyperfiltration (Desanto et al. 1995), resulting in increased renal excretion of low molecular weight (LMW) AGEs for several hours after meat meal ingestion. This mechanism could contribute to lower AGE levels in omnivores. On the contrary, the lower BMI associated lower metabolic turnover in vegetarians could result in a lower metabolic activity of the kidney—a key organ responsible for the excretion of AGEs (Gugliucci and Bendayan 1996). However, to justify these assumptions, urinary excretion of AGEs should be determined.

18.9.3 Oxidative Status

Antioxidative profile of vegetarians differed from that of omnivores: our vegetarians presented slightly but significantly lower plasma levels of major nonvitamin antioxidants—albumin by 8% and uric acid by 12% (Table 18.1). Consumption of vegetarian diet was reflected by significantly higher folate (1.2-fold) and β-carotene (3.4-fold) concentration, while the levels of vitamin C, E, and A were similar in both groups (Sebekova et al. 2006). A direct significant relationship between AGE-Fl/Alb levels and vitamin A (V: $r = 0.348$, $p < 0.001$; O: $r = 0.683$, $p < 0.001$) and vitamin E (V: $r = 0.168$, $p < 0.05$; O: $r = 0.469$, $p < 0.001$) suggests a potential link between alimentary absorption of lipophylic vitamins and AGE residues. Endogenous production of AGEs should be suppressed under high levels of circulating antioxidants.

18.9.4 Gut Microbiota

Gut microbiota modulates host metabolism, affecting energy homeostasis, inflammation and development of MetS, obesity, and CV diseases (Cani et al. 2012). Vegetarian diet affects the quantity and the profile of fecal bacteria; it is associated with a reduced abundance of pathobionts and a greater abundance of protective species (Glick-Bauer and Yeh 2014). In adolescent omnivores, 14-day long administration of MRPs-rich diet did not affect total fecal bacterial counts but resulted in significant decreases in lactobacilli, enterobacteria, escherichia, and Shigella groups, probably linked to the chemical structure and amounts of the dietary Maillard reaction derived compounds (Seiquer et al. 2014). Whether changes in fecal bacteria composition affect intestinal degradation of MRPs, and thus the absorption of LMW AGEs, remains unclear.

18.10 Contradiction between High Circulating AGEs and Favorable Cardiometabolic Profile in Vegetarians

Higher circulating AGE levels are generally considered to be associated with negative health effects, but vegetarians present more favorable cardiometabolic profile in comparison with age-matched omnivores (Krajcovicova-Kudlackova et al. 2002; Sebekova et al. 2003, 2006). However, hyperhomocysteinemia is also considered an independent risk factor for the development of CV diseases (Nygard et al. 1999), and vegetarians frequently present with hyperhomocysteinemia due to lack of dietary vitamin B_{12} (Craig 2010; McEvoy et al. 2012; Sabate 2003; Sebekova et al. 2003). In our cohort, correlations between circulating AGE-Fl levels and cardiometabolic risk factors were more frequently significant in vegetarians in comparison with omnivores (Table 18.2). However, correlation coefficients were generally weak, and Fischer's r-to-z transformation revealed that only those with age and total cholesterol differed significantly between vegetarians and omnivores. These data do not support the assumption that dietary MRPs have different effects in vegetarians than omnivores. Based on our cross-sectional data, we only might speculate that in lean, normotensive, insulin-sensitive vegetarians with normal lipid profile, renal function, and not presenting markers of inflammation, elevated circulating AGEs exert limited impact on aggravation of cardiometabolic risk factors. This might stem from protective actions of high levels of natural plant antioxidants and phytochemicals, ameliorating, or postponing negative health effects of elevated circulating AGEs in vegetarians. Moreover, melanoidins in thermally processed foods may act as antioxidant dietary fiber; as antimicrobial-, anti-inflammatory, or chelating agents; as modulators of phase I and phase II detoxification enzyme activities; and are used by microbiota to modify the equilibria among species in the gut environment (Morales et al. 2012). At least but not at last, negative health effects of thermally processed foods might rather result from additive effects of ingested different heat-processing-derived substances than from the intake of dietary AGEs *per se*.

Another question is whether plant-proteins-derived MRPs would exert different health effects from those derived from meat protein. At least in healthy rodents, consumption of bread-crusts-based MRPs-rich diet exerted negative metabolic effects (Sebekova et al. 2005, 2012).

Lower skin accumulation of AGEs in dialyzed vegetarian subjects in comparison with omnivores virtually contradicts our data on circulating AGEs in healthy vegetarians. However, plasma AGE levels mirror cumulative endogenous production of AGEs on circulating proteins, AGEs liberated during catabolism of tissue proteins, the recent dietary load of MRPs, as well as renal excretion of AGE peptides (Poulsen et al. 2013; Schinzel et al. 2001; Sebekova et al. 2008). Only LMW alimentary MRPs are absorbed into circulation, and those are unlikely to incorporate into the tissue matrix, including skin collagen (Poulsen et al. 2013). In healthy or hypertensive subjects, type 1 and 2 diabetics, no significant relationship between plasma CML or AGE-FL levels and SAF has been revealed (Sebekova et al. 2015; Stürmer et al. 2015). Neither comparative data on SAF in healthy vegetarians versus omnivores, nor those on plasma levels of AGEs in vegetarian and omnivorous hemodialyzed patients have been published to date.

18.11 Conclusions and Future Directions

The sources of increased circulating AGE levels in vegetarians if compared with omnivores are not completely clear. Current data suggest that it might be due to the high dietary intake of plant-food-derived MRPs, and lower and particularly plant protein intake–contributed changes in metabolic pathways. The role of vegetarian-diet-induced changes in gut microbiota profile with regard to production and absorption of dietary MRP-modified peptides has not been elucidated yet. Available data do not support an assumption that dietary plant-protein-derived MRPs induce different health effects in comparison with MRPs derived from meat protein. However, high levels of natural plants–derived antioxidants and phytochemicals in vegetarians might exert protective role and mitigate the negative health effects of elevated circulating AGEs.

Composition of used ingredients and the industrial or domestic culinary processing of foods might differ substantially. Additional studies are needed to elucidate whether vegetarians living in different geographical areas likewise present higher circulating AGE levels, and whether vegetarians of different ethnicity living in the same geographical area differ with regard to circulating AGEs. Data on SAF could elucidate the potential association of tissue glycometabolic memory with plasma AGEs and nutritional and metabolic status in vegetarians. To assess the circulating or tissue AGEs' associated risk of development of cardiometabolic diseases, longitudinal studies in vegetarians are definitely needed. Whether increased circulating AGE levels may negate the CV disease prevention benefits of vegetarian diets remains to be confirmed in aimed longitudinal studies.

REFERENCES

Adams, A., R. C. Borrelli, V. Fogliano, and N. De Kimpe. 2005. Thermal degradation studies of food melanoidins. *J Agric Food Chem* 53:4136–42.

Bederova, A., M. Kudlackova, R. Simoncic, et al. 2000. Comparison of nutrient intake and corresponding biochemical parameters in adolescent vegetarians and non-vegetarians [Article in Slovak]. *Cas Lek Cesk* 139:396–400.

Bilova, T., G. Paudel, E. Lukasheva, et al. 2015. Plant protein glycation: Possible effects on physiology and food quality. In *12th International Symposium on the Maillard Reaction*. Tokyo, p. 93. September 1–4, 2015, International Maillard Reaction Society and Japan Maillard Society, Tokyo

Bos, D. C., W. L. de Ranitz-Greven, and H. W. de Valk. 2011. Advanced glycation end products, measured as skin autofluorescence and diabetes complications: A systematic review. *Diabetes Technol Ther* 13:773–9.

Brownlee, M., H. Vlassara, and A. Cerami. 1984. Nonenzymatic glycosylation and the pathogenesis of diabetic complications. *Ann Intern Med* 101:527–37.

Cani, P.D., M. Osto, L. Geurts, and A. Everard. 2012. Involvement of gut microbiota in the development of low-grade inflammation and type 2 diabetes associated with obesity. *Gut Microbes* 3:279–88.

Caso, G., L. Scalfi, M. Marra, et al. 2000. Albumin synthesis is diminished in men consuming a predominantly vegetarian diet. *J Nutr* 130:528–33.

Craig, W. J. 2010. Nutrition concerns and health effects of vegetarian diets. *Nutr Clin Pract* 25:613–20.

DeChristopher, L.R., J. Uribarri, K.L. Tucker. 2015. Intakes of apple juice, fruit drinks and soda are associated with prevalent asthma in US children aged 2–9 years. *Public Health Nutr* 10:1–8.

Delgado-Andrade, C. 2014. Maillard reaction products: Some considerations on their health effects. *Clin Chem Lab Med* 52:53–60.

Desanto, N. G., P. Anastasio, M. Cirillo, et al. 1995. Sequential-analyses of variation in glomerular filtration rate to calculate the hemodynamic response to a meat meal. *Nephrol Dial Transplant* 10:1629–36.

Felton, J. S., M. G. Knize, R. W. Wu, et al. 2007. Mutagenic potency of food-derived heterocyclic amines. *Mutat Res* 616:90–4.

Glick-Bauer, M., and M. Yeh. 2014. The health advantage of a Vegan Diet: Exploring the gut microbiota connection. *Nutrients* 6:4822–4838.

Gokmen, V., and T. K. Palazoglu. 2008. Acrylamide formation in foods during thermal processing with a focus on frying. *Food Bioprocess Technol* 1:35–42.

Goldberg, T., W. J. Cai, M. Peppa, et al. 2004. Advanced glycoxidation end products in commonly consumed foods. *J Am Diet Assoc* 104:1287–91.

Gugliucci, A., and M. Bendayan. 1996. Renal fate of circulating advanced glycated end products (AGE): Evidence for reabsorption and catabolism of AGE-peptides by renal proximal tubular cells. *Diabetologia* 39:149–60.

Hull, G. L. J., J. V. Woodside, J. M. Ames, and G. J. Cuskelly. 2012. N-epsilon-(carboxymethyl)lysine content of foods commonly consumed in a Western style diet. *Food Chem* 131:170–4.

Jakus, V., M. Sapak, and J. Kostolanska. 2012. Circulating TGF-beta 1, glycation, and oxidation in children with diabetes mellitus type 1. *Exp Diabetes Res* 2012:510902.

Jochemsen, B. M., D. J. Mulder, J. J. Van Doormaal, et al. 2009. Relation between food and drinking habits, and skin autofluorescence and intima media thickness in subjects at high cardiovascular risk. *J Food Nutr Res* 48:51–8.

Kellow, N. J., and G. S. Savige. 2013. Dietary advanced glycation end-product restriction for the attenuation of insulin resistance, oxidative stress and endothelial dysfunction: A systematic review. *Eur J Clin Nutr* 67:239–48.

Key, T. J., P. N. Appleby, and M. S. Rosell. 2006. Health effects of vegetarian and vegan diets. *Proc Nutr Soc* 65:35–41.

Klenovics, K.S., P. Boor, V. Somoza, et al. 2013. Advanced glycation end products in infant formulas do not contribute to insulin resistance associated with their consumption. *PLoS One* 8:e53056.

Klenovics, K. S., R. Kollarova, J. Hodosy, P. Celec, and K. Sebekova. 2014. Reference values of skin autofluorescence as an estimation of tissue accumulation of advanced glycation end products in a general Slovak population. *Diabet Med* 31:581–5.

Koetsier, M., H. L. Lutgers, C. de Jonge, et al. 2010. Reference values of skin autofluorescence. *Diabetes Technol Ther* 12:399–403.

Kopple, J. D. 2001. National Kidney Foundation K/DOQI clinical practice guidelines for nutrition in chronic renal failure. *Am J Kidney Dis* 37:S66–70.

Koschinsky, T., C. J. He, T. Mitsuhashi, et al. 1997. Orally absorbed reactive glycation products (glycotoxins): An environmental risk factor in diabetic nephropathy. *Proc Natl Acad Sci U S A* 94:6474–9.

Krajcovicova-Kudlackova, M., K. Babinska, and M. Valachovicova. 2005. Health benefits and risks of plant proteins. *Bratisl Lek Listy* 106:231–4.

Krajcovicova-Kudlackova, M., L. Ozdin, and P. Bobek. 1993. Protein synthesis in growing and adult rats on casein and gluten nutrition. *Physiol Res* 42:17–22.

Krajcovicova-Kudlackova, M., K. Sebekova, R. Schinzel, and J. Klvanova. 2002. Advanced glycation end products and nutrition. *Physiol Res* 51:313–16.

Levi, B. and M. J. Werman. 1998. Long-term fructose consumption accelerates glycation and several age-related variables in male rats. *J Nutr* 128:1442–9.

Li, M., M. M. Zeng, Z. Y. He, et al. 2015. Increased accumulation of Protein-Bound N-epsilon-(Carboxymethyl) lysine in tissues of healthy rats after chronic oral N-epsilon-(Carboxymethyl)lysine. *J Agric Food Chem* 63:1658–63.

Lingelbach, L. B., A. E. Mitchell, R. B. Rucker, and R. B. McDonald. 2000. Accumulation of advanced glycation endproducts in aging male Fischer 344 rats during long-term feeding of various dietary carbohydrates. *J Nutr* 130:1247–55.

Maillard, L.C. 1912. Action des acides aminés sur les sucres: Formation des mélanoidines par voie méthodique. *C.R. Acad. Sci.* 154:66–8.

McEvoy, C. T., N. Temple, and J. V. Woodside. 2012. Vegetarian diets, low-meat diets and health: A review. *Public Health Nutr* 15:2287–94.

Meerwaldt, R., T. Links, R. Graaff, et al. 2005. Simple noninvasive measurement of skin autofluorescence, in *Maillard Reaction: Chemistry at the Interface of Nutrition, Aging, and Disease*, vol. 1043, Pp. 290–298, *Annals of the New York Academy of Sciences,* edited by J.W.Baynes, V. M.Monnier, J. M.Ames, S. R.Thorpe. The New York Academy of Sciences, New York.

Mikulikova, K., A. Eckhardt, J. Kunes, J. Zicha, and I. Miksik. 2008. Advanced glycation end-product pentosidine accumulates in various tissues of rats with high fructose intake. *Physiol Res* 57:89–94.

Morales, F. J., V. Somoza, and V. Fogliano. 2012. Physiological relevance of dietary melanoidins. *Amino Acids* 42:1097–109.

Mulder, D. J., T. Van de Water, H. L. Lutgers, et al. 2006. Skin autofluorescence, a novel marker for glycemic and oxidative stress-derived advanced glycation endproducts: An overview of current clinical studies, evidence, and limitations. *Diabetes Technol Ther* 8:523–35.

Munch, G., R. Keis, A. Wessels, et al. 1997. Determination of advanced glycation end products in serum by fluorescence spectroscopy and competitive ELISA. *Eur J Clin Chem Clin Biochem* 35:669–77.

Murkovic, M., and N. Pichler. 2006. Analysis of 5-hydroxymethylfurfual in coffee, dried fruits and urine. *Mol Nutr Food Res* 50:842–846.

Nongnuch, A., and A. Davenport. 2015. The effect of vegetarian diet on skin autofluorescence measurements in haemodialysis patients. *Br J Nutr* 113:1040–3.

Noordzij, M.J., J.D. Lefrandt, and A.J. Smit. 2008. Advanced glycation end products in renal failure: An overview. *J Ren Care* 34:207–12.

Nygard, O., S. E. Vollset, H. Refsum, L. Brattstrom, and P. M. Ueland. 1999. Total homocysteine and cardiovascular disease. *J Intern Med* 246:425–54.

Poulsen, M. W., R. V. Hedegaard, J. M. Andersen, et al. 2013. Advanced glycation endproducts in food and their effects on health. *Food Chem Toxicol* 60:10–37.

Sabate, J. 2003. The contribution of vegetarian diets to health and disease: A paradigm shift? *Am J Clin Nutr* 78:502S–7S.

Sanchez, A., and R.W. Hubbard. 1991. Plasma amino acids and the insulin/glucagon ratio as an explanation for the dietary protein modulation of atherosclerosis. *Med Hypotheses* 36:27–32.

Sebekova, K., P. Boor, M. Valachovicova, et al. 2006. Association of metabolic syndrome risk factors with selected markers of oxidative status and microinflammation in healthy omnivores and vegetarians. *Mol Nutr Food Res* 50:858–68.

Sebekova, K., T. Hofmann, P. Boor, et al. 2005. Renal effects of oral maillard reaction product load in the form of bread crusts in healthy and subtotally nephrectomized rats. *Ann N Y Acad Sci* 1043:482–91.

Sebekova, K., K. S. Klenovics, P. Boor, et al. 2012. Behaviour and hormonal status in healthy rats on a diet rich in Maillard reaction products with or without solvent extractable aroma compounds. *Physiol Behav* 105:693–701.

Sebekova, K., M. Krajcovicova-Kudlackova, P. Blazicek, et al. 2003. Functional hyperhomocysteinemia in healthy vegetarians: No association with advanced glycation end products, markers of protein oxidation, or lipid peroxidation after correction with vitamin B-12. *Clin Chem* 49:983–6.

Sebekova, K., M. Krajcovicova-Kudlackova, R. Schinzel, et al. 2001a. Plasma levels of advanced glycation end products in healthy, long-term vegetarians and subjects on a western mixed diet. *Eur J Nutr* 40:275–81.

Sebekova, K., L. Podracka, P. Blazicek, et al. 2001b. Plasma levels of advanced glycation end products in children with renal disease. *Pediatr Nephrol* 16:1105–112.

Sebekova, K., G. Saavedra, K. Klenovicsova, P. Boor, and I. Birlouez-Aragon. 2010. AGEs fluorescence of plasma, urine and skin reflects dietary exposure to Maillard products in formula-fed infants, in *Maillard Reaction: Interface between Aging, Nutrition and Metabolism*, edited by M. C. Thomas and J. Forbes. Cambridge, Great Britain, RSC Publishing, pp. 180–7.

Sebekova, K., G. Saavedra, C. Zumpe, et al. 2008. Plasma concentration and urinary excretion of N epsilon-(carboxymethyl)lysine in breast milk- and formula-fed infants. *Ann N Y Acad Sci* 1126:177–80.

Sebekova, K., and V. Somoza. 2007. Dietary advanced glycation endproducts (AGEs) and their health effects-PRO. *Mol Nutr Food Res* 51:1079–84.

Sebekova, K., M. Sturmer, G. Fazeli, et al. 2015. Is Vitamin D deficiency related to accumulation of advanced glycation end products, markers of inflammation, and oxidative stress in diabetic subjects? *Biomed Res Int*:2015:958097.

Seiquer, I., L.A. Rubio, M. J. Peinado, C. Delgado-Andrade, M.P. Navarro. 2014. Maillard reaction products modulate gut microbiota composition in adolescents. *Mol Nutr Food Res* 58:1552–60.

Schalkwijk, C. G., C. D. A. Stehouwer, and V. W. M. van Hinsbergh. 2004. Fructose-mediated non-enzymatic glycation: Sweet coupling or bad modification. *Diabetes Metab Res Rev* 20:369–82.

Scheijen, J.L., E. Clevers, L. Engelen, et al. 2016. Analysis of advanced glycation endproducts in selected food items by ultra-performance liquid chromatography tandem mass spectrometry: Presentation of a dietary AGE database. *Food Chem* 190:1145–50.

Schinzel, R., G. Munch, A. Heidland, and K. Sebekova. 2001. Advanced glycation end products in end-stage renal disease and their removal. *Nephron* 87:295–303.

Schmidt, A. M., O. Hori, R. Cao, et al. 1996. RAGE: A novel cellular receptor for advanced glycation end products. *Diabetes* 45 Suppl 3:S77–80.

Stirban, A., S. Nandrean, M. Negrean, T. Koschinsky, and D. Tschoepe. 2008. Skin autofluorescence increases postprandially in human subjects. *Diabetes Technol Ther* 10:200–5.

Stürmer, M., K. Šebeková, G. Fazeli, et al. 2015. 25-Hydroxyvitamin D and advanced glycation end products in healthy and hypertensive subjects: Are there interactions? *J Renal Nutr* 25:209–16.

Takeuchi, M., J. Takino, S. Furuno, et al. 2015. Assessment of the concentrations of various advanced glycation end-products in beverages and foods that are commonly consumed in Japan. *PLoS One* 10:e0118652.

Thalacker-Mercer, A. E., and W. W. Campbell. 2008. Dietary protein intake affects albumin fractional synthesis rate in younger and older adults equally. *Nutr Rev* 66:91–5.

Thorpe, S. R., and J. W. Baynes. 1996. Role of the maillard reaction in diabetes mellitus and diseases of aging. *Drugs Aging* 9:69–77.

Turner-McGrievy, G., and M. Harris. 2014. Key elements of plant-based diets associated with reduced risk of metabolic syndrome. *Curr Diab Rep* 14:524.

Uribarri, J., W. Cai, O. Sandu, et al. 2005. Diet-derived advanced glycation end products are major contributors to the body's AGE pool and induce inflammation in healthy subjects. *Ann N Y Acad Sci* 1043:461–6.

Uribarri, J., S. Woodruff, S. Goodman, et al. 2010. Advanced glycation end products in foods and a practical guide to their reduction in the diet. *J Am Diet Assoc* 110:911–16 e12.

Vitaglione, P., A. Napolitano, and V. Fogliano. 2008. Cereal dietary fibre: A natural functional ingredient to deliver phenolic compounds into the gut. *Trends Food Sci Technol* 19:451–63.

Wu, T. T., C. Y. Chang, W. M. Hsu, et al. 2011. Nutritional status of vegetarians on maintenance haemodialysis. *Nephrology* 16:582–7.

Yue, X., H. Hu, M. Koetsier, R. Graaff, and C. Han. 2011. Reference values for the Chinese population of skin autofluorescence as a marker of advanced glycation end products accumulated in tissue. *Diabet Med* 28:818–23.

19

Effects of Dietary AGEs in the Gut Microbiota Composition

Sergio Pérez-Burillo, Silvia Pastoriza, and José Ángel Rufián-Henares
Universidad de Granada
Granada, Spain

Cristina Delgado-Andrade
Estación Experimental del Zaidín (EEZ-CSIC)
Granada, Spain

CONTENTS

KEY POINTS

- Microbiota modulators are molecules, which pass through the gastrointestinal tract totally or partially intact.
- Advanced glycation end products (AGEs), largely present in the Western diet, are structures with decreased digestibility, thus potential modulators of colon microbiota.
- Human and animal trials demonstrate AGEs are able to modulate the intestinal microbiota composition.
- The specific effects are associated with their particular chemical structure and dietary amounts.
- Negative actions seem to be essentially linked to their ability to activate proinflammatory routes within the enterocyte, leading to different pathological processes.

19.1 Introduction

As it is well-established, advanced glycation end products (AGEs) are formed via the Maillard reaction and lipid oxidation, a complex network of nonenzymatic reactions involving the carbonyl groups of reducing sugars and lipid by-products, which react with the amino groups of proteins (Henle 2005). AGEs are inherent part of the Western diet since they are commonly found in thermally processed and stored foods. However, their great singularity is the fact that they are also produced in living beings as a normal consequence of physiological processes and different metabolic pathways. AGE formation is exacerbated under conditions of glucose levels chronically increased and in the presence of oxidative stress (Brownlee 2001; Folli et al. 2011). Overproduction of reactive oxygen species (ROS) can lead to a maladaptive response, causing the alteration of cellular glycolysis and generation of highly reactive dicarbonyl compounds which are the seeds for the rapid formation of AGEs (Thornalley 2005).

Traditionally, the value of food has been measured by its ability to provide energy and nutrients to the host. However, dietary habits are increasingly being regarded as one of the main factors contributing to health by influencing the diversity and composition of the human gut microbiota (De Filippo et al. 2010). As a consequence, the implication of dietary habits on the intestinal microbiota composition and health is currently a subject of paramount importance in human nutritional studies. Thus, there is growing evidence that bacteria within the colon play an important role in maintaining health, providing energy for the host, educating the immune system, and maybe even protecting against colon cancer (Tuohy et al. 2006; Flint 2012). The gut microbiota has been shown to affect several key physiological processes including, for example, lipid metabolism and energy homeostasis, development of the immune system, and fat storage regulation including related pathologies such as cardiovascular diseases or diabetes (Nicholson et al. 2012). On the contrary, the colonic microbiota derives its energy from dietary compounds, which escape digestion in the stomach and small intestine, and endogenous substrates such as mucins, secreted by the host. Thus, the human colonic microbiota may be viewed as an anaerobic digester, which acts mainly on material recalcitrant to digestion in the upper gut using an array of anaerobic metabolic pathways (Nicolson et al. 2005). From that point of view, participation of proteins in the glycation reactions gives rise to a less digestible product able to reach the final parts of the large intestine, which could be presented to different microorganisms belonging to the gut microbiota as substrate to obtain energy and nutrients.

The impact of the Maillard reaction products (MRP) on gut microbiota has been studied for the past 60 years (Helou et al. 2014), but the specific interest in the effects of AGEs on the intestinal bacterial population have risen in recent decades due to a significant increase to AGE exposure in the Western diet. In this review, special attention is paid to the last studies focused on AGE ability to act as microbiota modulators.

19.2 AGE Absorption and Their Role as Substrate for Gut Microbiota

Once AGEs are ingested in the diet, the gastrointestinal tract represents a first barrier to their penetration into the organism. After the gastric step, the intestinal barrier filters the compounds that will reach the internal media. Regardless of the exact mechanism, several factors will affect the absorption rate of AGEs. One of them is their solubility after the gastrointestinal digestion, since this is often the first component determining the bioavailability of a compound. The molecular weight and the free or protein-bound form of AGEs in the foodstuff play a significant part, probably because the protein-bound form impairs the proteolytic breakdown, leading to an impaired protein digestibility and a lower absorption rate (Delgado-Andrade 2015). In this context, our own research team recently established that the administration to adult rats of diets containing complex protein-bound forms of the AGE carboxymethyl-lysisne (CML) coming from bread crust led to a higher rate of CML excretion in feces than the administration of the simpler CML form present in the LMW fraction (<5 KDa) extracted from that bread crust (40.5% vs. 27.9%, respectively) (Roncero-Ramos et al. 2013). In the same line, but referred to the advanced fluorescent compound pentosidine, Förster et al. (2005) demonstrated its better absorption when administered from coffee brew (free) than when ingested in bakery products (protein-bound). Moreover, AGE consumption is not only isolated in the diet but also is accompanied by different MRP. The inhibitory actions of some of those compounds on specific and unspecific proteases have been described, a fact also resulting in the decrease of protein digestibility (Pintauro and Lucchina 1987).

Regarding the absorption mechanism of dietary AGEs, the exact pathway remains unclear, but free CML is most probably absorbed by simple diffusion rather than transported across the epithelium (Grunwald et al. 2006). Nevertheless, the absorption of CML as a dipeptide seems to use peptide transporters, especially PEPT1 (Hellwig et al. 2011). Thus, after the gastrointestinal transit, nonbioavailable AGEs will be excreted in feces in an intake-dependent manner, as established in the study by Delgado-Andrade et al. (2012) in which healthy adolescents aged 11–14 years were fed a diet low or high in AGEs.

These authors confirmed that CML absorption and fecal excretion are strongly influenced by dietary CML levels, whereas the urinary elimination, although also related to intake, appears to reach a saturation stage. Similarly to these results, Alamir et al. (2013) documented that a great part of the ingested CML from a diet based on extruded protein was eliminated in rats mainly in feces but also in urine (a final total excretion rate around 60%).

As a consequence of a worse digestibility of glycated proteins, AGEs, or even their metabolites, are able to reach the colon and act as possible substrate for microbiota metabolism there. In this sense, Mester et al. (1983) showed that early intermediate glycation products stimulate bacterial growth. Some investigations have documented that glycated pea proteins increased the lactobacilli and bifidobacteria populations in *in vitro* assays developed on the intestinal bacteria of a healthy human subject (Swiatecka et al. 2011). Recently, some researchers have stated that the use of *in vitro* digested glycoconjugated proteins (coming from the initial stage of the Maillard reaction) induced the growth of *Lactobacillus* and/or *Bifidobacterium* in a similar way as traditional prebiotics (Corzo-Martínez et al. 2012, 2013). Moreover, Laparra et al. (2011) observed an inhibition of the adhesion of *Escherichia coli* to mucin in the presence of Maillard-type glycoconjugated proteins.

The effects associated with AGEs, however, seem to have a more negative aspect, since in the opinion of some authors dietary undigested AGEs eventually enter the colon and act as a growth substrate for detrimental bacteria (Kellow et al. 2014). Thus, it is conceivable that the current Western diet, in which large amounts of AGEs come from highly processed foods, may adversely alter the colonic microbial composition, potentially promoting the risk for the appearance of metabolic and gastrointestinal diseases (Nakamura and Omaye 2012).

19.3 Studies Supporting the Ability of AGEs to Act as Microbiota Modulators

There is a significant amount of literature, which supports the ability of AGEs to interact with gut microbiota, alter its equilibrium, and definitively modify-its composition. Lanciotti et al. (1999) reported that AGEs induced an extension in the lag phase of *Bacillus stearothermophilus* and a reduction in the growth rate and final bacterial population in *in vitro* assays. Interestingly, the recent study by Helou et al. (2014) focused, among others, on the particular effect of the AGE CML on the growth of three different model strains of *E. coli*. It was observed that the use of a CML-enriched medium had no effect on the bacterial growth of all three *E. coli* strains studied. For their part, the extensive studies from Prof. Ames' group have shown a decrease in the bifidobacteria species and lactic flora in ulcerative colitis patients and an increase in clostridia and bacteroides species for both healthy subjects and ulcerative colitis patients with high AGE levels. The final result is a more detrimental community structure with significant increases in putatively harmful bacteria and decreases in dominant and assumed as beneficial bacteria (Ames et al. 2005; Tuohy et al. 2006; Ames 2008; Mills et al. 2008).

Our research group has recently joined this research line focused on the interactions between MRP, AGE, and the gut microbiota. Taking into account the important amount of studies performed *in vitro*, we aimed at the development of *in vivo* trials, moreover comparing animal models and human studies. On this base, two experiments were conducted. In experiment 1 (Figure 19.1), a group of male adolescents (11–14 years old) consumed diets either high or low in MRP in a 2-period cross-over trial; in experiment 2 (Figure 19.2), rats were fed diets supplemented or not with MRP model systems. Intestinal microbiota composition in fecal (adolescents) or cecal (rat) samples were assessed by qPCR analysis. Negative correlations were found in the human assay between lactobacilli numbers and dietary advanced MRP ($r = -0.418$ and -0.387, for hydroxymethylfurfural [HMF] and CML respectively, $p < 0.05$), whereas bifidobacteria counts were negatively correlated with Amadori compounds intake. Enterobacteria and *Escherichia/Shigella* counts significantly decreased after consumption of the high MRP diet by the boys, and these populations were also negatively correlated with HMF and CML intake ($p < 0.05$). The lack of concordance between this result and the findings from the study by Helou et al. (2014) on the growth of *E. coli* might be due to the fact that in a bacterial consortium, such as complete feces, a strong competition could exit between the different bacterial populations, leading to the inhibition of the growth of Enterobacteria and *Escherichia/Shigella* groups in our study. In experiment 2, the rat assay,

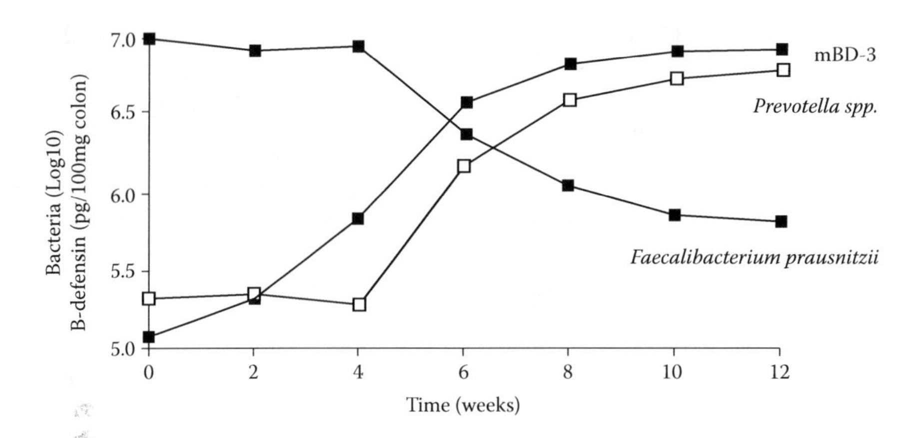

FIGURE 19.1 Monitorization of defensin mBD-3 and some bacterial species during long-term intake of CML in the diet of healthy WT mice.

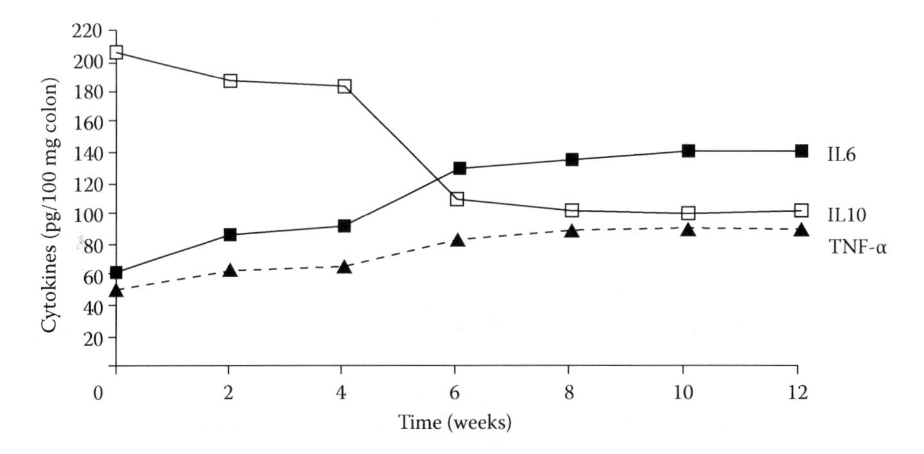

FIGURE 19.2 Monitorization of proinflammatory (IL6 and TNF-α) and anti-inflammatory cytokines (IL10) during long-term intake of CML in the diet of healthy WT mice.

total bacteria, and lactobacilli were negatively correlated with MRP intake (r = −0.674, −0.675, and −0.676, for Amadori compounds, HMF, and CML, respectively, $p < 0.05$), but no correlations were found with bifidobacteria, Enterobacteria, and *Escherichia/Shigella*. Our conclusion was that AGEs are able to modulate *in vivo* the intestinal microbiota composition both in humans and rats, and the specific effects are likely to be linked to the chemical structure and dietary amounts of the different browning compounds, since AGEs were administered together with different MRP in the diet (Seiquer et al. 2014).

Trying to find the mechanism responsible for the results observed and determining the specific effect of AGE consumption on microbiota composition, a new experiment was conducted. This time we focused on the effects of long-term consumption of large amounts of CML (3 months), using as source glycated bovine serum albumin in the diet of healthy WT mice, on different gut health parameters including microbiota population. Among those markers, β-defensin mBD-3, an antimicrobial peptide inducted by inflammatory or infectious stimulus, was measured. It is an antimicrobial peptide implicated in the resistance of intestinal epithelium to pathogenic colonization and the tolerance of the normal microbiota (Voss et al. 2006; Ramasundara et al. 2009). The mBD-3 defensin increased from the beginning of our assay, especially during the first 6 weeks. Parallelly, the presence of some species of the microbiota was modified during that period: *Faecalibacterium prausnitzii*, a microorganism associated with anti-inflammatory effects due to its role as producer of short chain fatty acids like butyric and propionic acids, strongly decreased; whereas the family *Prevotellaceae*, able to alter the barrier function in the gut due to the-production of mucin-degrading sulfatases (Wright et al. 2000), greatly increased in the microbiota of mice after CML consumption (Pastoriza 2013). The monitorization of the β-defensin mBD-3, *Faecalibacterium prausnitzii* and *Prevotella spp.* in the colon of these animals throughout the experimental period is depicted in Figure 19.1. As a consequence of these actions on gut microbiota, harmful effects on gut health could be triggered leading to systemic actions, due to the well-known participation of gastrointestinal flora on the individual health status (Nicholson et al. 2005).

19.4 Linkage between Microbiota Modulation by AGEs and Gastrointestinal Diseases

The possible imbalance induced by excessive and prolonged AGE consumption on gut microbiota might be connected with the appearance or aggravation of some gastrointestinal disorders involving inflammatory processes. This is plausible since AGEs, and more specifically CML, is known to bind the receptor for AGEs (RAGE), the which can be expressed by enterocytes (Anton et al. 2012). Several authors have established that RAGE stimulation leads to the activation of different intracellular proinflammatory mechanisms such as MAP kinase or NF-κβ, and even modulating RAGE expression, resulting in the sustenance and amplification of the signal (Schmidt et al. 2000; Zill et al. 2003).

Taking into account this premise and returning to our study focused on the effects of long-term consumption of CML in the diet of healthy mice, the increase detected in the colonic expression of the proinflammatory receptor RAGE can be better understood (unpublished data). The activation of RAGE by dietary CML was manifested in the elevation of proinflammatory cytokines such as TNF-α and IL6 to the detriment of the anti-inflammatory one IL10 (Figure 19.2). In summary, the results of our assay point out that long-term and constant CML consumption in the diet could promote unfavorable microbiota changes that, together with the activation of RAGE, would lead to a proinflammatory state in the gut epithelia of healthy animals.

From these findings, it can be deduced that AGEs could play a key role in the appearance and/or aggravation of inflammatory bowel diseases (IBD) such as Crohn's disease, ulcerative colitis, or irritable bowel syndrome. These disorders are related both with genetic predisposition and environmental factors like diet, also accompanied by microbiota alterations and deregulation of the immune response (Gassull et al. 2002). In this sense, increased urinary excretion and tissue deposits of the fluorescent AGE pentosidine has been observed in patients affected by Crohn's disease and ulcerative colitis during the periods of reactivation or the acute stage of the disorder (Kato et al. 2008). However, it is worthy to mention that Anton et al. (2012), after feeding mice affected by experimental colitis on highly heated chows rich in MRP concluded that the increased exposure to CML did not contribute to the aggravation of the inflammatory reaction or induce any gut inflammation on healthy mice, a fact that authors attributed to a reasonable level of CML exposure in the chows. Additionally, it must be considered that in this chow, a pool of MRP was present, not only CML, so that a joint effect could happen, modulating the final results.

19.5 Conclusions

Although much remains to be investigated, it seems clear that a significant and prolonged AGE intake can introduce imbalances in the composition of the intestinal microbiota, which would trigger pathological processes affecting not only gut integrity but also the overall health of the individual. Since these compounds activate specific proinflammatory receptors in the enterocytes, a cascade of biochemical mediators of inflammation can add to the microbiota alterations, leading to a proinflammatory state of the intestinal epithelium in healthy individuals or worsening symptoms in individuals affected by IBD. However, it must be taken into account that AGEs are consumed in the diet together with other MRP whose actions on the intestinal epithelium have been documented as positive—this is the case of melanoidins (Anton et al. 2012). Further studies should be conducted to better understand the global effect of the dietary MRP pool on the microbiota composition and thus establishing their joint action on gastrointestinal health.

REFERENCES

Alamir, I., Niquet-Leridon, C., Jacolot, P., Rodriguez, C., Orosco, M., Anton, P.M. and Tessier, F.J. 2013. Digestibility of extruded proteins and metabolic transit of N (epsilon)-carboxymethyllysine in rats. *Amino Acids.* 44: 1441–9.

Ames, J.M. 2009. Dietary Maillard reaction products: Implications for human health and disease. *Czech. J. Food Sci.* 27: S66–9.

Ames, J.M., Hinton, D., Crabbe, J., Tuohy, T. and Gibson, G. R. 2005. Glycated proteins: analysis and implications of dietary forms for human health and disease. In Eklund, T., Schwarz, M., Steinhart, H., Their, H. P. and Winterhalter, P. (eds.). *Macromolecules and their degradation products in food,* Gesellschaft Deutscher Chemiker, Frankfurt, pp. 316–323.

Anton, P.M., Craus, A., Niquet-Léridon, C. and Tessier, F.J. 2012. Highly heated food rich in Maillard reaction products limit an experimental colitis in mice. *Food Func.* 9: 941–9.

Brownlee, M. 2001. Biochemistry and molecular cell biology of diabetic complications. *Nature* 414: 813–20.

Corzo-Martínez, M., Ávila, M., Moreno, F.J., Requena, T. and Villamiel, M. 2012. Effect of milk protein glycation and gastrointestinal digestion on the growth of bifidobacteria and lactic acid bacteria. *Int. J. Food Microbiol.* 153: 420–7.

Corzo-Martínez, M., Hernandez-Hernandez, O., Villamiel, M., Rastall, R.A. and Moreno, F.J. 2013. In vitro bifidogenic effect of Maillard-type milk protein–galactose conjugates on the human intestinal microbiota. *Int. Dairy J.* 31: 127–31.

De Filippo, C., Cavalieri, D., Di Paola, M., Ramazzotti, M., Poullet, J.B., Massart, S., Collini, S., Pieraccini, G. and Lionetti, P. 2010. Impact of diet in shaping gut microbiota revealed by a comparative study in children from Europe and rural Africa. *PNAS* 107: 14691–6.

Delgado-Andrade, C. 2015. Carboxymethyl-lysine: Thirty years of investigation in the field of AGE formation. *Food Func.* 7(1): 46–57. doi: 10.1039/C5FO00918A.

Delgado-Andrade, C., Tessier, F.J., Niquet-Léridon, C., Seiquer, I. and Navarro, M.P. 2012. Study of the urinary and faecal excretion of Nε-carboxymethyllysine in young human volunteers. *Amino Acids* 43: 595–602.

Flint, H.J. 2012. The impact of nutrition on the human microbiome. *Nutr. Rev.* 70: S10–13.

Folli, F., Corradi, D., Fanti, P., Davalli, A., Paez, A., Giaccari, A., Perego, C. and Muscogiuri, G. 2011. The role of oxidative stress in the pathogenesis of type 2 diabetes mellitus micro- and macrovascular complications: Avenues for a mechanistic-based therapeutic approach. *Curr. Diabetes Rev.* 7: 313–24.

Förster, A., Kühne, Y. and Henle, T. 2005. Studies on absorption and elimination of dietary Maillard reaction products. *Ann. N.Y. Acad. Sci.* 1043: 474–81.

Gassull, M.A., Gomollón, F., Obrador, A. and Hinojosa, J. 2002. *Enfermedad inflamatoria intestinal.* Madrid: Ediciones Ergon.

Grunwald, S., Krause, R., Bruch, M., Henle, T. and Brandsch, M. 2006. Transepithelial flux of early and advanced glycation compounds across Caco-2 cell monolayers and their interaction with intestinal amino acid and peptide transport systems. *Br. J. Nutr.* 95: 1221–8.

Hellwig, M., Geissler, S., Matthes, R., Peto, A., Silow, C., Brandsch, M. and Henle, T. 2011. Transport of free and peptide-bound glycated amino acids: Synthesis, transepithelial flux at Caco-2 cell monolayers, and interaction with apical membrane transport proteins. *ChemBioChem.* 12: 1270–9.

Helou, C., Marier, D., Jacolot, P., Abdennebi-Najar, L., Niquet-Léridon, C., Tessier, F.J. and Gadonna-Widehem, P. 2014. Microorganisms and Maillard reaction products: A review of the literature and recent findings. *Amino Acids.* 46: 267–77.

Henle, T. 2005. Protein-bound advanced glycation endproducts (AGEs) as bioactive amino acid derivatives in foods. *Amino Acids.* 29: 313–22.

Kato, S., Itoh, K., Ochiai, M., Iwai, A., Park, Y., Hata, S., Takeuchi, K., et al. 2008. Increased pentosidine, an advanced glycation end-product, in urine and tissue reflects disease activity in inflammatory bowel diseases. *Gastroenterol Hepatol.* 23: S140–5.

Kellow, N.J., Coughlan, M.T., Savige, G.S. and Reid, C.M. 2014. Effect of dietary prebiotic supplementation on advanced glycation, insulin resistance and inflammatory biomarkers in adults with pre-diabetes: A study protocol for a double-blind placebo-controlled randomised crossover clinical trial. *BMC Endocr Disord.* 14: 55.

Lanciotti, R., Anese, M., Sinigaglia, M., Severini, C. and Massini, R. 1999. Effects of heated glucose-fructose-glutamic acid solutions on the growth of Bacillus stearothermophilus. *LWT Food Sci. Technol.* 32: 223–30.

Laparra, M.J., Corzo-Martinez, M., Villamiel, M., Moreno, F.J. and Sanz, Y. 2011. Maillard-type glycoconjugates from dairy proteins inhibit adhesion of Escherichia coli to mucin. *Food Chem.* 129: 1435–43.

Mester, L., Szabados, L. and Mester, M. 1983. Maillard reactions of therapeutic interest. In *The Maillard reaction in foods and nutrition*, ed. G.R. Waller and M.S. Feather, vol. 215, pp. 451–463. ACS Symposium Series. American Chemical Society, Washington, D.C.

Mills, D.J., Tuohy, K.M., Booth, J., Buck, M., Crabbe, M.J., Gibson, G.R. and Ames, J.M. 2008. Dietary glycated protein modulates the colonic microbiota towards a more detrimental composition in ulcerative colitis patients and non-ulcerative colitis subjects. *J. Appl. Microbiol.* 105: 706–14.

Nakamura, Y.K. and Omaye, S.T. 2012. Metabolic diseases and pro- and prebiotics: Mechanistic insights. *Nutr. Metab. (London)* 9: 60.

Nicholson, J.K., Holmes, E., Kinross, J., Burcelin, R., Gibson, G., Jia, W. and Pettersson, S. 2012. Host-gut microbiota metabolic interactions. *Science.* 336: 1262–7.

Nicholson, J.K., Holmes, E. and Wilson, I.D. 2005. Gut microorganisms, mammalian metabolism and personalized health care. *Nat. Rev. Microbiol.* 3: 431–8.

Pastoriza, S. 2013. Efecto de la ingesta de compuestos avanzados de la reacción de Maillard sobre el metabolismo gastrointestinal. http://hera.ugr.es/tesisugr/21915076.pdf (accessed October 16, 2015).

Pintauro, S.J. and Lucchina, L.A. 1987. Effects of Maillard browned egg albumin on drug-metabolizing enzyme systems in the rat. *Food Chem. Toxicol.* 25: 369–72.

Ramasundara, M., Leach, S.T., Lemberg, D.A. and Day, A.S. 2009. Defensins and inflammation: The role of defensins in inflammatory bowel disease. *J. Gastroenterol. Hepatol.* 24: 202–8.

Roncero-Ramos, I., Delgado-Andrade, C., Tessier, F.J., Niquet-Léridon, C., Strauch, C., Monnier, V.M. and Navarro, M.P. 2013. Metabolic transit of N(ε)-carboxymethyl-lysine after consumption of AGEs from bread crust. *Food Funct.* 4: 1032–9.

Schmidt, A.M., Yan, D.S., Yan, S.F. and Stern, D.M. 2000. The biology of the receptor for advanced glycation end products and its ligands. *Biochim. Biophys. Acta* 1498: 99–111.

Seiquer, I., Rubio, L.A., Peinado, M.J., Delgado-Andrade, C. and Navarro, M.P. 2014. Maillard reaction products modulate gut microbiota composition in adolescents. *Mol. Nutr. Food Res.* 58: 1552–60.

Swiatecka, D., Narbad, A., Ridgway, K.P. and Kostyra, H. 2011. The study on the impact of glycated pea proteins on human intestinal bacteria. *Int. J. Food Microbiol.* 145: 267–72.

Thornalley, P.J. 2005. Dicarbonyl intermediates in the maillard reaction. *Ann. N.Y. Acad. Sci.* 1043: 111–17.

Tuohy, K.M., Hinton, D.J.S., Davies, S.J., Crabbe, M.J.C., Gibson, G.R. and Ames, J.M. 2006. Metabolism of Maillard reaction products by the human gut microbiota – implications for health. *Mol. Nutr. Food Res.* 50: 847–57.

Voss, E., Wehkamp, J., Wehkamp, K., Stange, E.F., Schroder, J.M. and Harder, J. 2006. NOD2/CARD15 mediates induction of the antimicrobial peptide human beta-defensin-2. *J. Biol. Chem.* 281: 2005–11.

Wright, D.P., Rosendale, D.I. and Robertson, A.M. 2000. Prevotella enzymes involved in mucin oligosaccharide degradation and evidence for a small operon of genes expressed during growth on mucin. *FEMS Microbiol. Lett.* 190: 73–9.

Zill, H., Bek, S., Hofmann, T., Huber, J., Frank, O., Lindenmeier, M., Weigle, B., Erbersdobler, H.F., Scheidler, S., Busch A.E. and Faist, V. 2003. RAGE-mediated MAPK activation by food-derived AGE and non-AGE products. *Biochem. Biophys. Res. Commun.* 300, 311–15.

20

Associations of Circulating AGE Levels and Cardiovascular Disease—Incidence and Outcome

Kristian F. Hanssen and Kari Anne Sveen
University of Oslo
Oslo, Norway

CONTENTS

KEY POINTS

- We do not know in detail the mechanism for the increased incidence of cardiovascular disease (CVD) in diabetes.
- Advanced glycation end products (AGEs) are a probable mechanism.
- AGEs are associated with the development and progression of CVD disease in humans.
- AGEs are measured by principally three different methods: Immunoassay, LC-MS/MS, or fluorescence. However, standardization of these methods is needed.
- Further research in the field is needed to develop inhibitors of AGE activity in humans.

20.1 Introduction

Cardiovascular disease (CVD) is 2–3 times more common in diabetes type 2 (Laakso 2010) and 3–8 times more common in type 1 diabetes than in the general population (Retnakaran and Zinman 2008). The reasons for these increased incidence and prevalence are multifactorial in which traditional risk factors (smoking, hypertension, lipid changes, and age) are important, especially in type 2. However, hyperglycemia or factors closely associated with it are also major factors involved in the increased prevalence of CVD in both type 1 and type 2 diabetes. There are several biochemical factors altered in hyperglycemia that might be important (Brownlee 2001). However, it is extremely difficult to tease out which one, among the "myriad" of biochemical factors associated with hyperglycemia, is the real culprit since many of the factors are associated with each other. Among the "suspects", glycation of proteins (advanced glycation end products, AGEs) stands out as one of the most probable candidates. However, there are more than a hundred different modifications of proteins made by glucose or intermediary products in the metabolism of glucose or other reducing sugars (Ahmed and Thornalley 2007).

TABLE 20.1

Differences between Methods to Measure AGEs

	Specificity	Sensitivity	Recovery	What Is Measured?
Immunoassay	Variable	Variable	High	Total protein glycated
LC MS/MS	High	High	Variable	Amino acids glycated
Fluorescence	Low	Low	High	Fluorescence

20.2 Methods

In which tissue should AGEs be measured? Ideally in the tissue affected by the disease, this means that it should be measured in the heart or vascular tissues in case of CVD. This has proven difficult in humans so we rely heavily in animal data. However, data from blood and biopsies in human skin (Genuth et al. 2015) together with fluorescence data from human skin (AGE reader) (Mulder et al. 2006) are readily available.

There are mostly three different methods to measure AGEs at the present time. All of them have their strengths and weaknesses (Table 20.1).

The first method is an immunological method (Makita et al. 1992). This method is generally fraught with all the weaknesses of immunoassays (specificity, recovery, sensitivity, etc.). The quality and characterization of the antibody are very important. However, most antibodies used are "in house made," and there is no agreed standardization of AGE measurements using antibodies. Some of the antibodies have a specific epitope, but others have more broad AGE specificities recognizing a composite of AGEs ("total AGEs"). Therefore, one has to know the quality of the individual assay to be able to evaluate it. Some of the assays do not have acceptable recovery or dilution curves or coefficient of variation making the method uncertain. Mass spectrometry is a much more specific and sensitive method and some call it "the gold standard." However, when this method is used for large modified proteins, as most AGEs are, it has its own set of problems complicating the procedure. You have to extract the modified proteins from serum or plasma and subsequent harsh enzymatic or acid hydrolysis treatment to release the modified peptides. The recovery and total coefficient of variation of this treatment are often not included in the method section.

There are very few studies comparing simultaneous measurement of different AGEs in serum by immunoassay and LC MS/MS. One of them measured carboxymethyllysine (CML) by both immunoassay and MS/MS in 10 specimens with an r of 0.82 (Baynes JW per personal communication) (n = 10). We have recently compared measurements of serum MG-H1 (Methylglyoxal—Hydroimidazolone-1) by immunoassay and LC MS/MS (Sveen et al. 2014) and found a positive correlation between the two methods ($p = 0.041$; $n = 32$).

The third method to measure AGEs is measurement of fluorescence either in serum or in skin. At least two different skin readers (SAF) have been developed to measure skin fluorescence noninvasively (AGE Reader and SCOUT). The measurements of SAF have been interpreted as a measurement of AGEs. There are problems, however, with this interpretation (Thornalley and Rabbani 2014): (1) most AGEs are not fluorescent—particularly the quantitatively important hydroimidazolone (MG-H1), CML (Carboxymethyllysine) and CEL (Carboxyethyllysine); (2) fluorescence characteristics used in this assay are not specific for fluorescent AGEs; (3) fluorescence in proteins is due to multiple fluorophores which compete for the same excitation energy in the detection and hence there may be no direct relationship between concentration of the adduct and fluorescence; and (4) main components of SAF spectra are thought to be due to nicotinamide adenine dinucleotide, flavin adenine dinucleotide, and porphyrin.

20.3 Clinical Studies

In humans, several clinical studies have shown the association between serum AGEs and CVD, particularly in patients with diabetes mellitus. Kiuchi reported higher serum "total" AGEs measured by immunoassay in type 2 diabetes patients with coronary artery disease (CAD) than in patients without obstructive CAD and higher than in normoglycemic patients with and without obstructive CAD (Kiuchi et al. 2001). Similar results were reported by other authors also using immunoassays (Kilhovd et al. 1999) (Aso et al. 2000). Moreover, serum AGEs have been found to be associated with the degree of CAD in patients with type 2 diabetes and obstructive CAD. Of note, elevation of serum AGEs as measured by fluorescent spectrophotometry in patients undergoing percutaneous coronary intervention was identified as an independent risk factor for restenosis in diabetes mellitus (Choi et al. 2005).

Prospective studies also support the association between AGEs and cardiovascular disease (CVD). In a 12-year follow-up study of type 1 diabetes, circulating AGEs measured by LC MS/MS were associated with incident fatal and nonfatal CVD as well as all-cause mortality (Nin et al. 2011).

In female, but not in male type 2 diabetes patients, elevated serum "total" AGEs predicted mortality due to CAD during a follow-up of more than 18 years (Kilhovd et al. 2007). These authors reported a similar gender-specific pattern, in that serum levels of "total" AGEs predicted both total and CAD-induced mortality in normoglycemic women (Kilhovd et al. 2005).

A recent paper (Hanssen et al. 2015) showed that a composite of different plasma AGEs measured by LC MS/MS predicted the development of CVD in type 2 diabetes. However, the relationship was complicated with many confounding factors, especially BMI, which in itself was inversely associated with AGEs.

Dicarbonyl stress brought about by metabolites of glucose, especially a highly reactive metabolite, methylglyoxal, modifies proteins in several ways, especially by creating methylglyoxal-modified hydroimidazolone (MG-H1). By studying vulnerable plaques from coronary arteries from humans by LC MS/MS, an increased amount of MG-H1 was discovered (Hanssen et al. 2014). However, we did not find increased serum levels of HG-H1 in patients with coronary heart disease (unpublished).

Heart failure is common in both type 1 (Rosengren et al. 2015) and type 2 diabetes (Lind et al. 2012). The association between "total" serum AGEs and diastolic dysfunction in type 1 diabetes (Berg et al. 1999) is interesting, perhaps pointing to "stiff heart" as a consequence of increased glycation of proteins in the heart leading to subsequent heart failure. Further support for this notion is the association between a potent cross-linker AGE, glucosepane, and oxidative markers in skin and arterial stiffness and intima-media thickness in long-term type 1 diabetes (Sveen et al. 2015). In addition, impaired left ventricular function and myocardial blood flow reserve is associated with protein glycation, perhaps increasing the risk of heart failure (Sveen et al. 2014). A recent paper (Monnier et al. 2015) investigated skin collagen AGEs and their correlations to long-term subclinical CVD measurements such as coronary artery calcium score (CAC), changes carotid intima-media thickness (IMT) and cardiac MRI parameters in a subset of the DCCT/EDIC study. In type 1 diabetes, multiple AGEs were associated with IMT progression in spite of adjustment for Hemoglobin A1c implying a likely participatory role of glycation and AGE-mediated cross-linking on matrix accumulation in carotid arteries. This may also apply to functional cardiac MRI outcomes, especially left ventricular mass. The same authors have identified a fluorescent factor in skin, LW-1, which predicts cardiovascular surrogate end points (Sell et al. 2016).

Noninvasive measurements have shown that skin autofluorescence (SAF) is increased in people with increased cardiovascular risk such as people with carotid artery stenosis and peripheral artery disease, independent of the presence of diabetes (Noordzij et al. 2012). An association of SAF with the 1-year incidence of major adverse cardiac events has also been reported (Mulder et al. 2009). SAF also provides additional information on the UK Prospective Diabetes Study (UKPDS) risk score for the estimation of cardiovascular prognosis in people with type 2 diabetes mellitus (Lutgers et al. 2009).

The aforementioned studies linked high AGEs in serum and skin to cardiac disease and its outcome. But these studies could not prove a causal relationship, so the question remains unsolved whether AGEs are innocent bystanders or contribute to the development of CVD. It has been demonstrated that changing the cooking method alone (and thereby changing the amount of ingested AGEs) has a transient impact on postprandial microvascular and macrovascular endothelial function in persons with type 2 diabetes mellitus (Negrean et al. 2007). In addition, it was reported that acute oral administration of AGEs alone transiently impairs endothelial function as an early marker of atherosclerosis, supporting the concept that nutritional AGEs may have a direct detrimental effect on vasculature in humans (Stirban et al. 2013).

20.4 Conclusions

Thus, there is ample evidence for a strong association between different AGEs in serum and skin and cardiovascular parameters whether measured by immunological, MS/MS methods, or by fluorescence. However, it is quite uncertain if changes in serum AGEs brought about by different manipulations, for example, changes in food content of AGEs, will subsequently be reflected in changes in CVD. Therefore, the crucial question of whether these correlations are in some way causally related to CVD is still not proven. One way to prove this causality would be to inhibit the formation of AGEs in humans and study its outcome. This approach has proved to be successful in animal studies (Forbes et al. 2004). However, no study in humans has shown any convincing effect of glycation inhibition except, of course, for the studies (DCCT/EDIC) lowering blood glucose and subsequent AGEs (Monnier et al. 1999; Genuth et al. 2015). Thus, although much effort has been put into the field for the past 30 years, no definitive proof has emerged so far.

REFERENCES

Ahmed, N., and P. J. Thornalley. 2007. Advanced glycation endproducts: What is their relevance to diabetic complications? *Diabetes Obes Metab* 9 (3):233–45. doi: 10.1111/j.1463-1326.2006.00595.x.

Aso, Y., T. Inukai, K. Tayama, and Y. Takemura. 2000. Serum concentrations of advanced glycation endproducts are associated with the development of atherosclerosis as well as diabetic microangiopathy in patients with type 2 diabetes. *Acta Diabetol* 37 (2):87–92.

Berg, T. J., O. Snorgaard, J. Faber, P. A. Torjesen, P. Hildebrandt, J. Mehlsen, and K. F. Hanssen. 1999. Serum levels of advanced glycation end products are associated with left ventricular diastolic function in patients with type 1 diabetes. *Diabetes Care* 22 (7):1186–90.

Brownlee, M. 2001. Biochemistry and molecular cell biology of diabetic complications. *Nature* 414 (6865): 813–20. doi: 10.1038/414813a.

Choi, E. Y., H. M. Kwon, C. W. Ahn, G. T. Lee, B. Joung, B. K. Hong, Y. W. Yoon, et al. 2005. Serum levels of advanced glycation end products are associated with in-stent restenosis in diabetic patients. *Yonsei Med J* 46 (1):78–85.

Forbes, J. M., L. T. Yee, V. Thallas, M. Lassila, R. Candido, K. A. Jandeleit-Dahm, M. C. Thomas, et al. 2004. Advanced glycation end product interventions reduce diabetes-accelerated atherosclerosis. *Diabetes* 53 (7):1813–23.

Genuth, S., W. Sun, P. Cleary, X. Gao, D. R. Sell, J. Lachin, and V. M. Monnier. 2015. Skin advanced glycation end products glucosepane and methylglyoxal hydroimidazolone are independently associated with long-term microvascular complication progression of type 1 diabetes. *Diabetes* 64 (1):266–78. doi: 10.2337/db14-0215.

Hanssen, N. M., J. W. Beulens, S. van Dieren, J. L. Scheijen, A. Dl van der, A. M. Spijkerman, Y. T. van der Schouw, C. D. Stehouwer, and C. G. Schalkwijk. 2015. Plasma advanced glycation end products are associated with incident cardiovascular events in individuals with type 2 diabetes: A case-cohort study with a median follow-up of 10 years (EPIC-NL). *Diabetes* 64 (1):257–65. doi: 10.2337/db13-1864.

Hanssen, N. M., K. Wouters, M. S. Huijberts, M. J. Gijbels, J. C. Sluimer, J. L. Scheijen, S. Heeneman, et al. 2014. Higher levels of advanced glycation endproducts in human carotid atherosclerotic plaques are associated with a rupture-prone phenotype. *Eur Heart J* 35 (17):1137–46. doi: 10.1093/eurheartj/eht402.

Kilhovd, B. K., T. J. Berg, K. I. Birkeland, P. Thorsby, and K. F. Hanssen. 1999. Serum levels of advanced glycation end products are increased in patients with type 2 diabetes and coronary heart disease. *Diabetes Care* 22 (9):1543–8.

Kilhovd, B. K., A. Juutilainen, S. Lehto, T. Ronnemaa, P. A. Torjesen, K. I. Birkeland, T. J. Berg, K. F. Hanssen, and M. Laakso. 2005. High serum levels of advanced glycation end products predict increased coronary heart disease mortality in nondiabetic women but not in nondiabetic men: A population-based 18-year follow-up study. *Arterioscler Thromb Vasc Biol* 25 (4):815–20. doi: 10.1161/01.ATV.0000158380.44231.fe.

Kilhovd, B. K., A. Juutilainen, S. Lehto, T. Ronnemaa, P. A. Torjesen, K. F. Hanssen, and M. Laakso. 2007. Increased serum levels of advanced glycation endproducts predict total, cardiovascular and coronary mortality in women with type 2 diabetes: A population-based 18 year follow-up study. *Diabetologia* 50 (7):1409–17. doi: 10.1007/s00125-007-0687-z.

Kiuchi, K., J. Nejima, T. Takano, M. Ohta, and H. Hashimoto. 2001. Increased serum concentrations of advanced glycation end products: A marker of coronary artery disease activity in type 2 diabetic patients. *Heart* 85 (1):87–91.

Laakso, M. 2010. Cardiovascular disease in type 2 diabetes from population to man to mechanisms: The Kelly West Award Lecture 2008. *Diabetes Care* 33 (2):442–9. doi: 10.2337/dc09-0749.

Lind, M., M. Olsson, A. Rosengren, A. M. Svensson, I. Bounias, and S. Gudbjornsdottir. 2012. The relationship between glycaemic control and heart failure in 83,021 patients with type 2 diabetes. *Diabetologia* 55 (11):2946–53. doi: 10.1007/s00125-012-2681-3.

Lutgers, H. L., E. G. Gerrits, R. Graaff, T. P. Links, W. J. Sluiter, R. O. Gans, H. J. Bilo, and A. J. Smit. 2009. Skin autofluorescence provides additional information to the UK Prospective Diabetes Study (UKPDS) risk score for the estimation of cardiovascular prognosis in type 2 diabetes mellitus. *Diabetologia* 52 (5):789–97. doi: 10.1007/s00125-009-1308-9.

Makita, Z., H. Vlassara, A. Cerami, and R. Bucala. 1992. Immunochemical detection of advanced glycosylation end products *in vivo*. *J Biol Chem* 267 (8):5133–8.

Monnier, V. M., O. Bautista, D. Kenny, D. R. Sell, J. Fogarty, W. Dahms, P. A. Cleary, J. Lachin, and S. Genuth. 1999. Skin collagen glycation, glycoxidation, and crosslinking are lower in subjects with long-term intensive versus conventional therapy of type 1 diabetes: Relevance of glycated collagen products versus HbA1c as markers of diabetic complications. DCCT Skin Collagen Ancillary Study Group. Diabetes Control and Complications Trial. *Diabetes* 48 (4):870–80.

Monnier, V. M., W. Sun, X. Gao, D. R. Sell, P. A. Cleary, J. M. Lachin, and S. Genuth. 2015. Skin collagen advanced glycation endproducts (AGEs) and the long-term progression of sub-clinical cardiovascular disease in type 1 diabetes. *Cardiovasc Diabetol* 14 (1):118. doi: 10.1186/s12933-015-0266-4.

Mulder, D. J., P. L. van Haelst, R. Graaff, R. O. Gans, F. Zijlstra, and A. J. Smit. 2009. Skin autofluorescence is elevated in acute myocardial infarction and is associated with the one-year incidence of major adverse cardiac events. *Neth Heart J* 17 (4):162–8.

Mulder, D. J., T. V. Water, H. L. Lutgers, R. Graaff, R. O. Gans, F. Zijlstra, and A. J. Smit. 2006. Skin autofluorescence, a novel marker for glycemic and oxidative stress-derived advanced glycation endproducts: An overview of current clinical studies, evidence, and limitations. *Diabetes Technol Ther* 8 (5):523–35. doi: 10.1089/dia.2006.8.523.

Negrean, M., A. Stirban, B. Stratmann, T. Gawlowski, T. Horstmann, C. Gotting, K. Kleesiek, et al. 2007. Effects of low- and high-advanced glycation endproduct meals on macro- and microvascular endothelial function and oxidative stress in patients with type 2 diabetes mellitus. *Am J Clin Nutr* 85 (5):1236–43.

Nin, J. W., A. Jorsal, I. Ferreira, C. G. Schalkwijk, M. H. Prins, H. H. Parving, L. Tarnow, P. Rossing, and C. D. Stehouwer. 2011. Higher plasma levels of advanced glycation end products are associated with incident cardiovascular disease and all-cause mortality in type 1 diabetes: A 12-year follow-up study. *Diabetes Care* 34 (2):442–7. doi: 10.2337/dc10-1087.

Noordzij, M. J., J. D. Lefrandt, E. A. Loeffen, B. R. Saleem, R. Meerwaldt, H. L. Lutgers, A. J. Smit, and C. J. Zeebregts. 2012. Skin autofluorescence is increased in patients with carotid artery stenosis and peripheral artery disease. *Int J Cardiovasc Imaging* 28 (2):431–8. doi: 10.1007/s10554-011-9805-6.

Retnakaran, R., and B. Zinman. 2008. Type 1 diabetes, hyperglycaemia, and the heart. *Lancet* 371 (9626): 1790–9. doi: 10.1016/s0140-6736(08)60767-9.

Rosengren, A., D. Vestberg, A. M. Svensson, M. Kosiborod, M. Clements, A. Rawshani, A. Pivodic, S. Gudbjornsdottir, and M. Lind. 2015. Long-term excess risk of heart failure in people with type 1 diabetes: A prospective case-control study. *Lancet Diabetes Endocrinol.* 3(11):876–85. doi: 10.1016/s2213-8587(15)00292-2.

Sell, D.R., Sun, W., Gao, X., Strauch, C., Lachin, J.M., Cleary, P.A., Genuth, S., DCCT/EDIC Research Group, Monnier, V.M. 2016. Skin collagen fluorophore LW-1 versus skin fluorescence as markers for the long-term progression of subclinical macrovascular disease in type 1 diabetes. *Cardiovasc Diabetol* 15:30.

Stirban, A., P. Kotsi, K. Franke, U. Strijowski, W. Cai, C. Gotting, and D. Tschoepe. 2013. Acute macrovascular dysfunction in patients with type 2 diabetes induced by ingestion of advanced glycated beta-lactoglobulins. *Diabetes Care* 36 (5):1278–82. doi: 10.2337/dc12-1489.

Sveen, K. A., K. Dahl-Jorgensen, K. H. Stensaeth, K. Angel, I. Seljeflot, D. R. Sell, V. M. Monnier, and K. F. Hanssen. 2015. Glucosepane and oxidative markers in skin collagen correlate with intima media thickness and arterial stiffness in long-term type 1 diabetes. *J Diabetes Complications* 29 (3):407–12. doi: 10.1016/j.jdiacomp.2014.12.011.

Sveen, K. A., T. Nerdrum, K. F. Hanssen, M. Brekke, P. A. Torjesen, C. M. Strauch, D. R. Sell, V. M. Monnier, K. Dahl-Jorgensen, and K. Steine. 2014. Impaired left ventricular function and myocardial blood flow reserve in patients with long-term type 1 diabetes and no significant coronary artery disease: Associations with protein glycation. *Diab Vasc Dis Res* 11 (2):84–91. doi: 10.1177/1479164113518805.

Thornalley, P. J., and N. Rabbani. 2014. Detection of oxidized and glycated proteins in clinical samples using mass spectrometry—A user's perspective. *Biochim Biophys Acta* 1840 (2):818–29. doi: 10.1016/j.bbagen.2013.03.025.

21

Pathological Role of AGEs in Osteoporosis

Sho-ichi Yamagishi
Kurume University School of Medicine
Kurume, Japan

CONTENTS

KEY POINTS

- Diet has been recognized as a major environmental source of advanced glycation end products (AGEs) in humans.
- A 9-year follow-up of study revealed that baseline carboxymethyllysine levels were associated with hip fracture risk in older adults, which was independent of hip bone mineral density.
- Mechanical integrity of the collagen network in the bone might deteriorate with diabetes and/or aging due to enhanced accumulation of bone AGEs.
- AGE-RAGE interaction could not only induce apoptosis but also inhibit the proliferation and differentiation of osteoblasts.
- RAGE plays an important role in osteoclast function and differentiation.

21.1 Introduction

A nonenzymatic reaction between sugars, such as glucose and fructose, and the amino groups of proteins, lipids, and nucleic acids is known as the "Maillard reaction" [1,2]. The glycation process begins with the conversion of reversible Schiff base adducts to more stable, covalently-bound Amadori rearrangement products. Over the course of days to weeks, these Amadori products undergo further rearrangement reactions to form the irreversibly bound moieties called as advanced glycation end products (AGEs) [1,2]. The formation and accumulation of AGEs is a normal physiologic process, but increases during normal aging and markedly accelerates under hyperglycemic, inflammatory, and/or oxidative stress conditions [1,2]. AGEs could contribute to the aging of proteins and to the pathological complications of diabetes [1,2]. Indeed, cross-linking modification of the organic bone matrix proteins such as collagen and elastin by AGEs has been shown to compromise bone mechanical properties and strength and subsequently to reduce bone quality [3–5]. Moreover, there is an accumulating body of evidence that AGEs elicit oxidative stress generation and evoke proapoptotic and proinflammatory reactions in a variety of cells, including osteoblasts, osteoclasts, and osteocytes, through the interaction with a receptor for AGEs (RAGE), thereby reducing the fracture resistance of bone [6–8]. In addition, recently, diet has been recognized as a major environmental source of AGEs in humans [9]. These observations suggest that accumulation of exogenously and/or endogenously derived AGEs in the bone and resultant activation of the RAGE-downstream pathway could be involved in both reduction of bone mineral density (BMD) and impairment of bone quality, thus contributing to the development and progression of osteoporosis. Therefore, I review here the pathological role of AGEs in osteoporosis and discuss the potential therapeutic strategies that could target the AGE-RAGE axis and, therefore, prevent osteoporotic bone fractures.

21.2 Osteoporosis

Osteoporosis is a systemic skeletal disorder characterized by reduced BMD and quality, which could compromise bone strength and subsequently increase the risk of bone fractures [6]. The prevalence and cumulative incidence of osteoporosis are high in postmenopausal women and increases with age. About 40% of white postmenopausal women are suffering from osteoporosis [10]. The risk of osteoporosis-related bone fractures is also increased in both type 1 and type 2 diabetic patients [11,12]. Although increasing evidence shows that BMD is decreased in patients with type 1 diabetes, the increased risk of osteoporotic bone fractures in diabetes is not entirely explained by low BMD because BMD is increased *rather than* decreased in type 2 diabetic subjects [12,13]. Furthermore, a meta-analysis revealed that the relative risk of hip fracture in type 1 diabetic subjects was 6.9, which was much higher than that calculated based on BMD (relative risk 1.4) [12]. In addition, the Rotterdam Study showed that compared with nondiabetic individuals, bone fracture risk was higher only in already established and treated type 2 diabetic patients, but not in patients with newly diagnosed diabetes [13]. These observations suggest that the increased risk of bone fractures in diabetic subjects could be partly ascribed to the impairment of bone quality, whose deterioration was enhanced by long-term history of diabetes, thus suggesting a role of AGEs in osteoporosis.

Osteoporotic fractures, particularly vertebral and hip fractures, reduce the quality of life of patients very significantly [10]. Moreover, several papers have shown that osteoporotic bone fractures are also associated with an increased risk of morbidity and mortality [10,14,15]. Indeed, hip fracture was independently associated with a greater risk for future event of acute myocardial infarction in a large, nationwide cohort study [14]. Increased risk of all-cause mortality persisted till 5 years after hip fractures; men with hip fractures had higher risk for deaths from stroke and cancer up to 1 year post-fracture, whereas women had higher risk of coronary artery disease for 5 years after fracture [15]. Given the pathological role of AGEs in aging and/or diabetes-associated disorders, such as cardiovascular disease, cancer, and osteoporosis [6,7], AGEs might partly explain the high disability and mortality rate in osteoporotic bone fracture patients.

21.3 Food-Derived AGEs

Heat processing of food containing sugars and/or lipids and proteins stimulates the nonenzymatic browning reactions (Maillard reaction) and generates AGEs [9,16]. Nutrient composition, temperature, and method of cooking could affect the formation of AGEs in food. Food cooked at high temperature contains greater amounts of AGEs than that at lower temperature [9,16]. Under alkaline conditions, more of the hexoses are in the open chain or reducing form, whereas amino groups of proteins are in the basic form [17]. So, a higher pH condition is considered to enhance the process of AGE formation. On the contrary, excessive moisture conditions have been shown to inhibit the Maillard reactions [17].

Human studies revealed that *ca.* 10% of orally administered AGEs were absorbed, two-thirds of which remained in the body and only one-third of the absorbed AGEs was excreted into the urine within 3 days from ingestion [9,16]. Consumption of an AGE-rich meal (3-fold higher in AGE content compared with a regular diet) has been shown to increase serum AGE levels by about 1.5-fold [16]. In addition, the increase in serum AGE levels after a single AGE-rich meal is in direct proportion to the amount of AGEs consumed [18].

Hellwig et al. reported that although free Maillard reaction products, including CML, carboxyethyllysine, formyline, argpyrimidine, and pyrraline, were not substrates for the intestinal lysine transporter, dietary AGEs were absorbed into the intestinal cells as a form of dipeptides, such as alanyl-CML, alanylcarboxyethyllysine, and alanylpyrraline, by human intestinal peptide transporter hPEPT1 [19]. After hydrolysis in the intestinal cells, pyrraline, formyline, and argpyrimidine have been shown to undergo basolateral efflux by simple diffusion [19].

21.4 Association of Serum and Urinary Levels of AGEs with Osteoporosis

Serum pentosidine level was significantly increased in postmenopausal type 2 diabetic women with vertebral fractures compared with those without fractures, which was independent of BMD, risk factors for osteoporosis, diabetic status, and renal function [20]. Neumann et al. also reported that serum pentosidine levels, but not BMD or CML, were independently associated with prevalent bone fractures in type 1 diabetes [21]. These observations suggest that AGEs could impair bone quality in diabetic patients, thus increasing the risk of bone fractures in these subjects. Osteoporosis group had significantly higher serum concentrations of pentosidine and CML than healthy subjects [22]. In subgroups characterized by increased bone resorption, serum pentosidine was correlated with markers that could reflect osteoclast activity and bone resorption [22]. Furthermore, a 9-year follow-up of the Cardiovascular Health Study revealed that baseline CML levels were associated with hip fracture risk in older adults, which was independent of hip BMD [23]. Since CML is one of the major types of AGEs generated during cooking of food [9], the finding supports the concept that dietary AGEs might compromise bone biomechanical properties, thereby being involved in osteoporotic bone fractures. Yang et al. reported that serum AGE levels were negatively correlated with BMD of lumbar spine as well in menopausal women with osteoporosis [24].

Schwartz et al. have reported that elevation in urinary pentosidine levels is independently associated with both increased clinical fracture incidence and vertebral fracture prevalence in elderly patients with type 2 diabetes [25]. Moreover, Shiraki et al. showed that urinary pentosidine level was correlated with time-dependent incidence of vertebral fractures in elderly women who were not receiving any drug for the treatment of osteoporosis, which was totally independent of traditional risk factors for osteoporosis [26]. In Japanese osteoporosis patients undergoing bisphosphonate treatment, the authors also found that patients who developed incident vertebral fractures were older and had lower lumbar spine BMD, a higher prevalent vertebral fracture number, and higher urinary pentosidine levels than patients who did not develop vertebral fractures [27]. In the Cox's proportional hazard model, higher baseline urinary excretion levels of pentosidine were one of the independent predictors for incident vertebral fracture in these subjects [27].

21.5 Circulating RAGE Levels as a Biomarker of Osteoporosis

Serum levels of endogenous secretory RAGE (esRAGE)-to-pentosidine ratio in type 2 diabetic patients with vertebral fractures were significantly lower than in those without vertebral fractures [28]. Multivariate logistic regression analysis adjusted for age, serum creatinine, duration of diabetes, therapeutic agents, osteoporotic risk factors, and lumbar BMD showed that both low serum levels of esRAGE and decreased esRAGE-to-pentosidine ratio were independently associated with the prevalence of vertebral fractures in patients with type 2 diabetes as well [28]. These findings suggest that serum esRAGE level and esRAGE-to-pentosidine ratio might be more useful biomarkers than BMD for assessing the risk of vertebral fractures in type 2 diabetic patients. Bone quality is more important than BMD in defining the increased risk for osteoporotic bone fractures in type 2 diabetic patients [3–5]. Furthermore, since the AGE-RAGE system plays a role in impaired bone quality in type 2 diabetic subjects [6], the authors speculated that an insufficient amount of esRAGE to counteract AGEs could intensify the binding of AGEs to RAGE and resultantly exert harmful effects on bones, thereby being involved in the increased risk of vertebral fractures in their patients. However, soluble form of RAGE (sRAGE) can be generated both from proteolytic cleavage of cell membrane surface full-length RAGE by sheddase or novel splice variants of RAGE [29]. Circulating sRAGE in humans is mainly derived from the cleavage of membrane-bound RAGE, whereas esRAGE is one of the C-truncated splice isoforms of RAGE and only constitutes a small part of endogenous sRAGE [29]. Moreover, since interaction of RAGE with the ligands such as AGEs promotes the RAGE shedding [29], it is conceivable that sRAGE level could correlate with high levels of ongoing inflammation in diabetes. Therefore, although exogenously administered high amounts of sRAGE were shown to block the harmful effects of AGEs in animals by acting as a decoy receptor [29], it is questionable that esRAGE may also exert the same biological effects in humans, because serum concentration of esRAGE in humans is about 5000 times lower than needed for the binding to and efficiently eliminating circulating AGEs [29]. Furthermore, recently, esRAGE has been shown not to associate with prevalent bone fractures in patients with type 1 diabetes [21]. So, decreased level of esRAGE may be associated with the prevalence of vertebral fractures in only type 2 diabetic patients in unknown mechanisms other than working as a decoy RAGE. Mendelian randomization analysis revealed that single-nucleotide polymorphisms associated with lower sRAGE levels were not significantly correlated with incident death, coronary heart disease, diabetes heart failure, or chronic kidney disease in Atherosclerosis Risk in Communities Study, further supporting the concept that sRAGE, including esRAGE, may not be a causal factor in the development of AGE-related disorders, such as osteoporosis [30].

21.6 Pathological Role of AGE-RAGE Axis in Osteoporosis

1. **Effects of the AGE-RAGE axis on bone mechanical properties**

   In vitro glycation of human tibial cancellous bone cores caused microdamage and reduced bone fracture resistance [31]. AGE-modified collagen impaired lysyl oxidase enzyme–dependent physiological collagen cross-links both in primary, nondifferentiated and in differentiating mouse and rat osteoblast cells via blocking the binding of collagen to discoidin domain receptor-2 [32].

   AGE accumulation in the bone not only suppressed lysyl oxidase but also induced bone collagen degradation in a rat model of renal osteodystrophy [33]. Furthermore, despite the lack of reduction in BMD, bone mechanical properties were impaired in spontaneously diabetic WBN/Kob rats, which were coincided with decreased enzymatic cross-link formation and increased pentosidine levels in the bone collagen [34]. Accumulated uremic toxins, such as pentosidine and indoxyl sulfate, have been shown to play a role in impairing bone mechanical properties in a rat model of chronic kidney disease as well [35]. Using a high-resolution, nonlinear finite element model that incorporates cohesive elements and micro-computed tomography-based 3D meshes, Tang et al. reported that age-related increase in bone porosity and AGEs resulted in an 88% reduction in propagation toughness [36]. Trabecular pentosidine in human vertebrae was significantly associated with whole bone strength [37]. In addition, the intensity of staining of AGEs in bone specimens of osteoporotic subjects was correlated with patient age and inversely associated with the percentage of bone surface covered with osteoblasts [38]. Vitamin C transporter expression in the type 1 diabetic mouse bone and bone marrow was suppressed, which was accompanied with decreases in bone formation and lower bone quality of these animals [39]. Inclusion of tibial AGE levels significantly improved the prediction of bone strength over only tibial BMD prediction in aging female. Treatment with N-phenacylthiazolium, a cross-link breaker of AGEs significantly decreased AGE content and improved bone fragility in cancellous bone cylinders obtained from aged male [40]. Taken together, these observations suggest that mechanical integrity of the collagen network in the bone might deteriorate with diabetes and/or aging due to enhanced accumulation of bone AGEs and increased oxidative stress, being involved in osteoporosis in these subjects.

2. **Effects of the AGE-RAGE axis on osteoblasts**

AGE-modified albumin upregulated RAGE expression, increased intracellular reactive oxygen species (ROS) generation, and subsequently induced apoptotic cell death of two different osteoblast-like cell lines, rat osteosarcoma UMR 106 and mouse nontransformed MC3T3E1 cells via activation of caspase-3, a key enzyme in the execution of apoptosis [41,42]. Moreover, CML-modified collagen increased p38 and c-Jun N-terminal kinase (JNK) activity and induced apoptotic cell death of primary human cultured osteoblasts, which was blocked by anti-RAGE antibody, inhibitors of p38, or JNK [43]. Although AGEs increased activities of caspase-3, -8, and -9 in human osteoblasts, an inhibitor of caspase-8 more effectively blocked the AGE-induced caspase-3 activation and subsequent apoptotic cell death of osteoblasts than that of caspase-9, thus suggesting that cytoplasmic (caspase-8 dependent) pathway may be relatively more important than mitochondrial (caspase-9) pathway for the apoptotic signals in AGE-exposed osteoblasts [43].

Methylglyoxal is a reactive dicarbonyl compound produced by glycolytic pathway and a precursor of AGEs [44–46]. Methylglyoxal induces MC3T3E1 cell damage and impairs the osteoblastic differentiation by increasing the intracellular ROS generation via reducing mitochondrial membrane potential and intracellular ATP levels [43]. Methyglyoxal also inactivates glyoxalase I and further potentiates the formation of methyglyoxal-derived AGEs in MC3T3E1 cells [44,45]. These deleterious effects of methyglyoxal on osteoblastic MC3T3E1 cells were significantly blocked by pretreatments with aminoguanidine, an inhibitor of AGEs formation, Trolox, an antioxidant, and apocynin, an inhibitor of NADPH oxidase [44–46].

AGEs formed on type 1 collagen, a predominant matrix protein of bone could also contribute to suppressed bone formation [47,48]. Indeed, when rat osteoblastic cells were cultured on AGE-modified type 1 collagen, alkaline phosphatase (ALP) activity and osteocalcin secretion were decreased, while nodule formation was dramatically impaired [47,48]. Accelerated accumulation of AGEs was observed in the bone collagen of streptozotocin-induced diabetic rats, which was associated with reduced BMD in the diabetic animals [47]. AGE-modified type 1 collagen decreased adhesion of UMR 106 and inhibited cellular proliferation, spreading, and ALP activity through intracellular ROS production as well [49]. AGE-modification of type-I collagen may impair the integrin-mediated adhesion of osteoblastic cells to the matrix [50]. Further, the AGE-RAGE interaction has been shown to inhibit the osteoblast proliferation via suppression of Wnt-signaling in MC3T3E1 cells [51]. Pentosidine, a well-characterized glycoxidative end product also hampered the formation of bone nodules of human osteoblasts [52]. These findings suggest that the AGE-RAGE interaction could not only induce apoptosis but also inhibit the proliferation and differentiation of osteoblasts, thereby being involved in reduced BMD in diabetes.

3. **Effects of the AGE-RAGE axis on osteoclasts**

There is some controversy about the pathological role of AGEs in osteoclast function in osteoporosis. Miyata et al. reported that when mouse unfractionated bone cells containing osteoclasts were cultured on dentin slices, AGE-modified proteins increased the number of resorption pits formed by osteoclasts [53]. Moreover, bone resorption was augmented when unfractionated bone cells were cultured on AGE-modified dentin slices [53]. They also showed that AGE-modified bone particles implanted subcutaneously in rats were resorbed to a much greater extent than nonglycated control bone particles [53]. Since AGEs did not increase the number of newly formed osteoclasts, AGEs could not promote the differentiation of osteoclasts, but may activate osteoclasts or alter microenvironments favorable for bone resorption by osteoclasts. In addition, human AGE-rich cortical bone specimens were reported to increase bone resorption activities of osteoclasts [54]. These observations suggest that AGEs may activate osteoclasts, leading to the increase in bone resorption and bone loss. However, Valcourt et al. reported that when mature osteoclasts were seeded on AGE-modified bone and ivory slices, bone resorption was inhibited *rather than* increased due to decreased solubility of AGE-modified type 1 collagen molecules [55]. Moreover, they found that AGE-modified proteins inhibited osteoclastogenesis partly by blocking the differentiation of osteoblasts.

On the contrary, there is growing evidence that RAGE plays an important role in osteoclast function and differentiation [56–59]. Mice lacking RAGE had increased BMD and bone biomechanical strength and decreased number of osteoclasts and its bone resorptive activity *in vivo* [56,57]. *In vitro*-differentiated RAGE-deficient osteoclasts exhibited disrupted actin ring and sealing zone structures, impaired maturation, and reduced bone resorptive activity [56]. These findings suggest that RAGE is involved in osteoclast actin reorganization, adhesion, and activation, thereby contributing to reduced bone mass in osteoporosis. AGEs increased mRNA levels of RAGE and receptor activator of nuclear factor-κB ligand (RANKL) in osteoblasts [58]. RANKL is an essential cytokine for osteoclastogenesis, and osteoblasts express RANKL in response to bone-resorbing factors, thus further suggesting the active participation of RAGE in osteoclastogenesis [59].

4. **Effects of the AGE-RAGE axis on osteocytes**

   Mature osteocyte expresses the protein sclerostin, a negative regulator of bone mass [60]. AGEs suppressed bone formation by increasing sclerostin expression in osteocyte-like MLO-Y4-A2 cells, whereas they caused cortical bone deterioration by inducing osteocyte apoptosis [60].

5. **Effects of the AGE-RAGE axis on mesenchymal stem cells (MSCs)**

   AGE-modified albumin induced generation of ROS through the interaction with RAGE and inhibited proliferation and migration of bone marrow MSCs [61]. AGEs stimulated expression and secretion of chemokines and cytokines including CC chemokine ligand (Ccl) 2, Ccl3, Ccl4, and interleukin-1β via activation of p38, which could exert the inhibitory effects on MSCs growth and migration, thereby impairing bone repair in diabetes [61]. MSCs from rats with streptozotocin-induced diabetes were more likely to become senescent, and their ability to proliferate and differentiate to bone was reduced compared with those from control rats [62]. Glyoxal, a highly reactive dicarbonyl and one of the precursors of AGEs, which is produced by auto-oxidation of glucose, also induced senescence in bone marrow-derived telomerase-immortalized MSCs that was accompanied by increased extent of DNA breaks and AGEs accumulation [63]. Glyoxal also impaired the differentiation of MSCs, determined by decreased ALP activity and reduced mineralized matrix formation as well [63]. In addition, AGEs not only inhibited the osteoblastic differentiation and growth but also induced apoptosis of mouse stromal ST2 cells by enhancing transforming growth factor-β expression [60,64]. Furthermore, methylglyoxal suppressed the expression of osteotrophic Wnt-targeted genes, including osteoprotegerin, a decoy receptor of RANKL via oxidative stress generation, thus causing low-turnover osteoporosis in diabetes [65]. Levels of AGEs, RAGE, ROS, and apoptosis in diabetic MSCs were increased, and extensive loss of trabecular bone in the tibiae was observed in diabetic animals [62]. AGEs inhibited the proliferation, self-renewal, and osteogenic differentiation of MSCs *in vitro* [62]. We have previously reported that AGEs increase RAGE induction, ROS generation, and apoptosis and subsequently inhibit mineralization and mature bone nodule formation of MSCs [66]. Therefore, the AGE-RAGE–oxidative stress system could contribute to exhaustion of MSCs and loss of their differentiation potential to bone, thereby increasing the risk for osteoporosis.

21.7 Effects of Anti-Osteoporotic Drugs on AGE-RAGE Axis

Bisphosphonates are potent inhibitors of bone resorption and are one of the most widely used drugs for treatment of osteoporosis [67,68]. Farnesyl pyrophosphate synthase has been shown to be a molecular target of nitrogen-containing bisphosphonates, and inhibition of posttranslational prenylation of small-molecular-weight G-proteins is likely involved in their antiresorptive activity on osteoclasts [67,68]. Since AGEs exert various biological actions on a variety of cells through RAGE-mediated, NADPH oxidase-induced ROS generation and subsequent NF-κB activation via Ras-MAPK pathway [67,68], it is conceivable that nitrogen-containing bisphosphonates might have pleiotropic properties by blocking farnesylation of small G-proteins, which serve as lipid attachments for a variety of intracellular signaling molecules. Indeed, we have previously found that minodronate, a nitrogen-containing bisphosphonate, inhibits the AGE-induced vascular cell adhesion molecule-1 expression in endothelial cells by suppressing ROS generation via suppression of geranylgeranylation of Rac, a component of endothelial NADPH oxidase. Incadronate also reverted the angiogenic activity of AGEs in endothelial cells by suppressing the RAGE-downstream signaling [68]. Moreover, AGEs significantly decreased osteoblast proliferation, ALP activity, and type 1 collagen production, while increasing osteoblastic apoptosis and ROS production, all of which were completely reverted by low doses of bisphosphonates [69]. Bisphosphonates may block the deleterious actions of AGEs on osteoblastic cells via Ca(2+) influx, because an L-type calcium channel blocker, nifedipine, has been shown to inhibit the effects of bisphosphonates on AGE-exposed osteoblasts [69]. These findings could suggest a novel beneficial aspect of bisphosphonates on osteoporosis; bisphosphonates could protect against the AGE-induced bone loss partly by suppressing the RAGE-downstream signaling pathways in osteoblasts via inhibition of NADPH oxidase-mediated ROS generation.

However, it should be mentioned that 1 year of high-dose bisphosphonate therapy in dogs allowed the increased accumulation of AGEs and reduced post-yield work-to-fracture of the cortical bone matrix [70]. Furthermore, pentosidine contents were increased following 3-year treatment with incadronate in dogs [71]. Serum pentosidine levels were increased in osteoporotic females after 3 years of bisphosphonate treatment [72]. These observations suggest that long-term use of bisphosphonates might impair physiological bone remodeling, which may lead to increase in nonenzymatic cross-linking in the bone, thereby altering bone matrix quality and being involved in bisphosphonates-related atypical femoral fractures. In contrast to the observations, Hashida et al. recently reported that serum pentosidine levels in postmenopausal osteoporotic women were not changed after 3-year bisphosphonate treatment [73]. So, further clinical study is needed to test whether bisphosphonate-related AGE accumulation may impair bone quality.

Raloxifene, one of the widely used selective estrogen receptor modifiers, which has estrogen-like effects on bone and "anti-estrogen effects" on other tissues, has been developed for prevention and treatment of osteoporosis in postmenopausal women [74]. **Raloxifene ameliorates detrimental enzymatic and nonenzymatic collagen cross-links and bone strength in rabbits with hyperhomocysteinemia [74].** Pullerits et al. reported that postmenopausal rheumatoid arthritis patients receiving hormone replacement therapy (estradiol plus norethisterone acetate) displayed significantly decreased serum level of sRAGE, a marker that could reflect tissue RAGE expression, which was associated with the elevation in serum estradiol [74]. They also found that sRAGE level at baseline was correlated with bone/cartilage turnover markers. The decrease of sRAGE level after hormone replacement therapy paralleled with diminished concentration of the markers and was correlated with an increase in total BMD in these subjects [74]. These findings further support the concept that hormone replacement therapy could exert beneficial effects on bone metabolism in postmenopausal rheumatoid arthritis patients by inhibiting the AGE-RAGE-oxidative stress axis in the bone. In support of this, we have very recently found that bazedoxifene inhibits the AGE-induced ROS generation and monocyte chemoattractant protein expression in human cultured endothelial cells by suppressing RAGE expression [75].

21.8 Conclusion

We posit an overall scheme of pathological role of AGE-RAGE axis in osteoporosis (Figure 21.1). Restriction of dietary AGEs and/or blockade of the AGE-RAGE-oxidative stress system in the bone may be a novel therapeutic strategy for preventing osteoporotic bone fractures, especially in aged or diabetic subjects.

ACKNOWLEDGMENTS

This work was supported in part by Grants-in-Aid for Scientific Research (B) (grant number; 22390111) from the Ministry of Education, Culture, Sports, Science, and Technology of Japan. No potential conflicts of interest relevant to this chapter were reported.

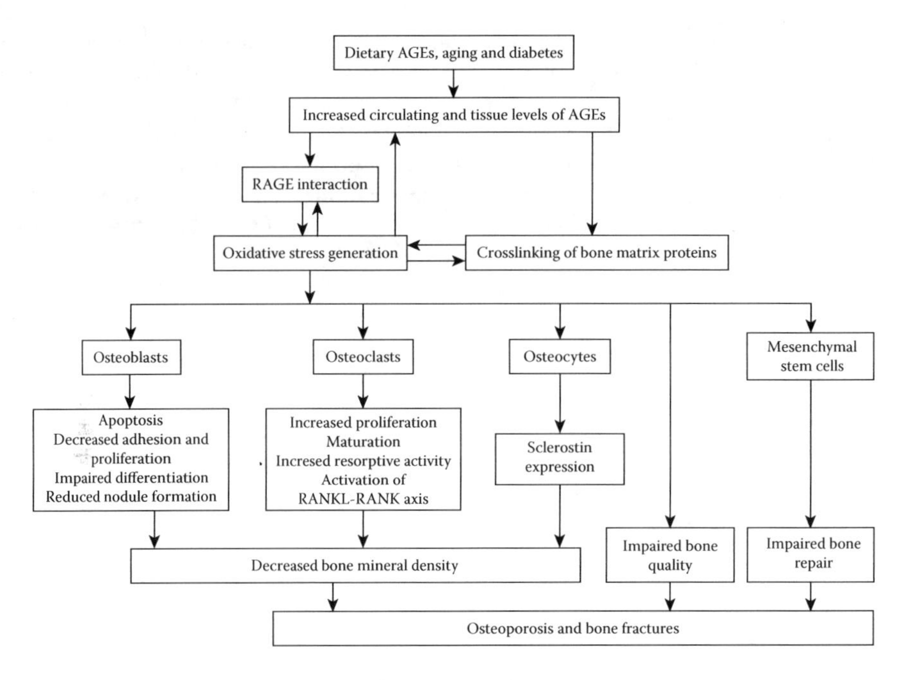

FIGURE 21.1 Pathological role of AGE-RAGE axis in osteoporosis.

REFERENCES

1. Vlassara H, Palace MR. Diabetes and advanced glycation endproducts. *J Intern Med.* 2002;251:87–101.
2. Yamagishi S, Imaizumi T. Diabetic vascular complications: Pathophysiology, biochemical basis and potential therapeutic strategy. *Curr Pharm Des.* 2005;11:2279–99.
3. Hein GE. Glycation endproducts in osteoporosis—Is there a pathophysiologic importance? *Clin Chim Acta.* 2006;371:32–6.
4. Odetti P, Rossi S, Monacelli F, Poggi A, Cirnigliaro M, Federici M, Federici A. Advanced glycation end products and bone loss during aging. *Ann N Y Acad Sci.* 2005;1043:710–17.
5. Saito M, Marumo K. Collagen cross-links as a determinant of bone quality: A possible explanation for bone fragility in aging, osteoporosis, and diabetes mellitus. *Osteoporos Int.* 2010;21:195–214.
6. Yamagishi S. Role of advanced glycation end products (AGEs) in osteoporosis in diabetes. *Curr Drug Targets.* 2011;12:2096–102.
7. Yamagishi S. Potential clinical utility of advanced glycation end product cross-link breakers in age- and diabetes-associated disorders. *Rejuvenation Res.* 2012;15:564–72.
8. Stern D, Yan SD, Yan SF, Schmidt AM. Receptor for advanced glycation endproducts: A multiligand receptor magnifying cell stress in diverse pathologic settings. *Adv Drug Deliv Rev.* 2002;54:1615–25.
9. Yamagishi S, Ueda S, Okuda S. Food-derived advanced glycation end products (AGEs): A novel therapeutic target for various disorders. *Curr Pharm Des.* 2007;13(27):2832–6.
10. Rachner TD, Khosla S, Hofbauer LC. Osteoporosis: Now and the future. *Lancet.* 2011;377:1276–87.
11. Merlotti D, Gennari L, Dotta F, Lauro D, Nuti R. Mechanisms of impaired bone strength in type 1 and 2 diabetes. *Nutr Metab Cardiovasc Dis.* 2010;20:683–90.
12. Vestergaard P. Discrepancies in bone mineral density and fracture risk in patients with type 1 and type 2 diabetes—A meta-analysis. *Osteoporos Int.* 2007;18:427–44.
13. De Liefde II, van der Klift M, de Laet CE, van Daele PL, Hofman A, Pols HA. Bone mineral density and fracture risk in type-2 diabetes mellitus: The Rotterdam Study. *Osteoporos Int.* 2005;16: 1713–20.
14. Chiang CH, Liu CJ, Chen PJ, Huang CC, Hsu CY, Chen ZY, Chan WL, et al. Hip fracture and risk of acute myocardial infarction: A nationwide study. *J Bone Miner Res.* 2013;28:404–11.

15. Koh GC, Tai BC, Ang LW, Heng D, Yuan JM, Koh WP. All-cause and cause-specific mortality after hip fracture among Chinese women and men: The Singapore Chinese Health Study. *Osteoporos Int.* 2013;24:1981–9.
16. Uribarri J, Cai W, Sandu O, Peppa M, Goldberg T, Vlassara H. Diet-derived advanced glycation end products are major contributors to the body's AGE pool and induce inflammation in healthy subjects. *Ann N Y Acad Sci.* 2005;1043:461–6.
17. Eskin NAM, Ho CT, Shahidi F. Browning reactions in foods, in N.A. Michael Eskin, Fereidoon Shahidi (Eds.), *Biochemistry of foods*, Academic Press, San Diego, CA, 2013, pp. 245–89.
18. Koschinsky T, He CJ, Mitsuhashi T, Bucala R, Liu C, Buenting C, Heitmann K, Vlassara H. Orally absorbed reactive glycation products (glycotoxins): An environmental risk factor in diabetic nephropathy. *Proc Natl Acad Sci U S A.* 1997;94:6474–9.
19. Hellwig M, Geissler S, Matthes R, Peto A, Silow C, Brandsch M, Henle T. Transport of free and peptide-bound glycated amino acids: Synthesis, transepithelial flux at Caco-2 cell monolayers, and interaction with apical membrane transport proteins. *Chembiochem.* 2011;12:1270–9.
20. Yamamoto M, Yamaguchi T, Yamauchi M, Yano S, Sugimoto T. Serum pentosidine levels are positively associated with the presence of vertebral fractures in postmenopausal women with type 2 diabetes. *J Clin Endocrinol Metab.* 2008;93:1013–19.
21. Neumann T, Lodes S, Kästner B, Franke S, Kiehntopf M, Lehmann T, Müller UA, Wolf G, Sämann A. High serum pentosidine but not esRAGE is associated with prevalent fractures in type 1 diabetes independent of bone mineral density and glycaemic control. *Osteoporos Int.* 2014;25:1527–33.
22. Hein G, Wiegand R, Lehmann G, Stein G, Franke S. Advanced glycation end-products pentosidine and N epsilon-carboxymethyllysine are elevated in serum of patients with osteoporosis. *Rheumatology (Oxford).* 2003;42:1242–6.
23. Barzilay JI, Bůžková P, Zieman SJ, Kizer JR, Djoussé L, Ix JH, Tracy RP, Siscovick DS, Cauley JA, Mukamal KJ. Circulating levels of carboxy-methyl-lysine (CML) are associated with hip fracture risk: The cardiovascular health study. *J Bone Miner Res.* 2014;29(5):1061–6.
24. Yang DH, Chiang TI, Chang IC, Lin FH, Wei CC, Cheng YW. Increased levels of circulating advanced glycation end-products in menopausal women with osteoporosis. *Int J Med Sci.* 2014;11:453–60.
25. Schwartz AV, Garnero P, Hillier TA, Sellmeyer DE, Strotmeyer ES, Feingold KR, Resnick HE, et al. Pentosidine and increased fracture risk in older adults with type 2 diabetes. *J Clin Endocrinol Metab.* 2009;94:2380–6.
26. Shiraki M, Kuroda T, Tanaka S, Saito M, Fukunaga M, Nakamura T. Nonenzymatic collagen cross-links induced by glycoxidation (pentosidine) predicts vertebral fractures. *J Bone Miner Metab.* 2008;26:93–100.
27. Shiraki M, Kuroda T, Shiraki Y, Tanaka S, Higuchi T, Saito M. Urinary pentosidine and plasma homocysteine levels at baseline predict future fractures in osteoporosis patients under bisphosphonate treatment. *J Bone Miner Metab.* 2011;29:62–70.
28. Yamamoto M, Yamaguchi T, Yamauchi M, Sugimoto T. Low serum level of the endogenous secretory receptor for advanced glycation end products (esRAGE) is a risk factor for prevalent vertebral fractures independent of bone mineral density in patients with type 2 diabetes. *Diabetes Care.* 2009;32:2263–8.
29. Yamagishi S, Matsui T. Soluble form of a receptor for advanced glycation end products (sRAGE) as a biomarker. *Front Biosci (Elite Ed).* 2010;2:1184–95.
30. Maruthur NM, Li M, Halushka MK, Astor BC, Pankow JS, Boerwinkle E, Coresh J, Selvin E, Kao WH. Genetics of plasma soluble receptor for advanced glycation end-products and cardiovascular outcomes in a community-based population: Results from the atherosclerosis risk in communities study. *PLoS One.* 2015;10:e0128452.
31. Tang SY, Vashishth D. Non-enzymatic glycation alters microdamage formation in human cancellous bone. *Bone.* 2010;46:148–54.
32. Khosravi R, Sodek KL, Faibish M, Trackman PC. Collagen advanced glycation inhibits its Discoidin Domain Receptor 2 (DDR2)-mediated induction of lysyl oxidase in osteoblasts. *Bone.* 2014;58:33–41.
33. Aoki C, Uto K, Honda K, Kato Y, Oda H. Advanced glycation end products suppress lysyl oxidase and induce bone collagen degradation in a rat model of renal osteodystrophy. *Lab Invest.* 2013;93:1170–83.
34. Saito M, Fujii K, Mori Y, Marumo K. Role of collagen enzymatic and glycation induced cross-links as a determinant of bone quality in spontaneously diabetic WBN/Kob rats. *Osteoporos Int.* 2006;17:1514–23.

35. Iwasaki Y, Kazama JJ, Yamato H, Shimoda H, Fukagawa M. Accumulated uremic toxins attenuate bone mechanical properties in rats with chronic kidney disease. *Bone.* 2013;57:477–83.
36. Tang SY, Vashishth D. The relative contributions of non-enzymatic glycation and cortical porosity on the fracture toughness of aging bone. *J Biomech.* 2011;44:330–6.
37. Viguet-Carrin S, Roux JP, Arlot ME, Merabet Z, Leeming DJ, Byrjalsen I, Delmas PD, Bouxsein ML. Contribution of the advanced glycation end product pentosidine and of maturation of type I collagen to compressive biomechanical properties of human lumbar vertebrae. *Bone.* 2006;39:1073–9.
38. Hein G, Weiss C, Lehmann G, Niwa T, Stein G, Franke S. Advanced glycation end product modification of bone proteins and bone remodelling: Hypothesis and preliminary immunohistochemical findings. *Ann Rheum Dis.* 2006;65:101–4.
39. Sangani R, Naime M, Zakhary I, Ahmad S, Chutkan N, Zhu A, Ha Y, et al. Regulation of vitamin C transporter in the type 1 diabetic mouse bone and bone marrow. *Exp Mol Pathol.* 2013;95:298–306.
40. Bradke BS, Vashishth D. N-phenacylthiazolium bromide reduces bone fragility induced by nonenzymatic glycation. *PLoS One.* 2014;9:e103199.
41. Mercer N, Ahmed H, Etcheverry SB, Vasta GR, Cortizo AM. Regulation of advanced glycation end product (AGE) receptors and apoptosis by AGEs in osteoblast-like cells. *Mol Cell Biochem.* 2007;306:87–94.
42. Schurman L, McCarthy AD, Sedlinsky C, Gangoiti MV, Arnol V, Bruzzone L, Cortizo AM. Metformin reverts deleterious effects of advanced glycation end-products (AGEs) on osteoblastic cells. *Exp Clin Endocrinol Diabetes.* 2008;116:333–40.
43. Alikhani M, Alikhani Z, Boyd C, MacLellan CM, Raptis M, Liu R, Pischon N, Trackman PC, Gerstenfeld L, Graves DT. Advanced glycation end products stimulate osteoblast apoptosis via the MAP kinase and cytosolic apoptotic pathways. *Bone.* 2007;40:345–53.
44. Suh KS, Choi EM, Rhee SY, Kim YS. Methylglyoxal induces oxidative stress and mitochondrial dysfunction in osteoblastic MC3T3-E1 cells. *Free Radic Res.* 2014;48:206–17.
45. Choi EM, Suh KS, Rhee SY, Kim YS. Sciadopitysin alleviates methylglyoxal-mediated glycation in osteoblastic MC3T3-E1 cells by enhancing glyoxalase system and mitochondrial biogenesis. *Free Radic Res.* 2014;48:729–39.
46. Suh KS, Rhee SY, Kim YS, Choi EM. Inhibitory effect of apocynin on methylglyoxal-mediated glycation in osteoblastic MC3T3-E1 cells. *J Appl Toxicol.* 2014; 35(4):350–7. doi:10.1002/jat.3016.
47. Katayama Y, Akatsu T, Yamamoto M, Kugai N, Nagata N. Role of nonenzymatic glycosylation of type I collagen in diabetic osteopenia. *J Bone Miner Res.* 1996;11:931–7.
48. Katayama Y, Celic S, Nagata N, Martin TJ, Findlay DM. Nonenzymatic glycation of type I collagen modifies interaction with UMR 201-10B preosteoblastic cells. *Bone.* 1997;21:237–42.
49. McCarthy AD, Etcheverry SB, Bruzzone L, Lettieri G, Barrio DA, Cortizo AM. Non-enzymatic glycosylation of a type I collagen matrix: Effects on osteoblastic development and oxidative stress. *BMC Cell Biol.* 2001;2:16.
50. McCarthy AD, Uemura T, Etcheverry SB, Cortizo AM. Advanced glycation endproducts interefere with integrin-mediated osteoblastic attachment to a type-I collagen matrix. *Int J Biochem Cell Biol.* 2004;36:840–8.
51. Li G, Xu J, Li Z. Receptor for advanced glycation end products inhibits proliferation in osteoblast through suppression of Wnt, PI3K and ERK signaling. *Biochem Biophys Res Commun.* 2012;423:684–9.
52. Sanguineti R, Storace D, Monacelli F, Federici A, Odetti P. Pentosidine effects on human osteoblasts *in vitro. Ann N Y Acad Sci.* 2008;1126:166–72.
53. Miyata T, Notoya K, Yoshida K, Horie K, Maeda K, Kurokawa K, Taketomi S. Advanced glycation end products enhance osteoclast-induced bone resorption in cultured mouse unfractionated bone cells and in rats implanted subcutaneously with devitalized bone particles. *J Am Soc Nephrol.* 1997;8:260–70.
54. Dong XN, Qin A, Xu J, Wang X. *In situ* accumulation of advanced glycation endproducts (AGEs) in bone matrix and its correlation with osteoclastic bone resorption. *Bone.* 2011;49:174–83.
55. Valcourt U, Merle B, Gineyts E, Viguet-Carrin S, Delmas PD, Garnero P. Non-enzymatic glycation of bone collagen modifies osteoclastic activity and differentiation. *J Biol Chem.* 2007;282:5691–703.
56. Zhou Z, Immel D, Xi CX, Bierhaus A, Feng X, Mei L, Nawroth P, Stern DM, Xiong WC. Regulation of osteoclast function and bone mass by RAGE. *J Exp Med.* 2006;203:1067–80.
57. Ding KH, Wang ZZ, Hamrick MW, Deng ZB, Zhou L, Kang B, Yan SL, et al. Disordered osteoclast formation in RAGE-deficient mouse establishes an essential role for RAGE in diabetes related bone loss. *Biochem Biophys Res Commun.* 2006;340:1091–7.

58. Franke S, Siggelkow H, Wolf G, Hein G. Advanced glycation endproducts influence the mRNA expression of RAGE, RANKL and various osteoblastic genes in human osteoblasts. *Arch Physiol Biochem.* 2007;113:154–61.
59. Kobayashi Y, Udagawa N, Takahashi N. Action of RANKL and OPG for osteoclastogenesis. *Crit Rev Eukaryot Gene Expr.* 2009;19:61–72.
60. Tanaka K, Yamaguchi T, Kanazawa I, Sugimoto T. Effects of high glucose and advanced glycation end products on the expressions of sclerostin and RANKL as well as apoptosis in osteocyte-like MLO-Y4-A2 cells. *Biochem Biophys Res Commun.* 2015;461:193–9.
61. Yang K, Wang XQ, He YS, Lu L, Chen QJ, Liu J, Shen WF. Advanced glycation end products induce chemokine/cytokine production via activation of p38 pathway and inhibit proliferation and migration of bone marrow mesenchymal stem cells. *Cardiovasc Diabetol.* 2010;9:66.
62. Stolzing A, Sellers D, Llewelyn O, Scutt A. Diabetes induced changes in rat mesenchymal stem cells. *Cells Tissues Organs.* 2010;191:453–65.
63. Larsen SA, Kassem M, Rattan SI. Glucose metabolite glyoxal induces senescence in telomerase-immortalized human mesenchymal stem cells. *Chem Cent J.* 2012;6:18.
64. Okazaki K, Yamaguchi T, Tanaka K, Notsu M, Ogawa N, Yano S, Sugimoto T. Advanced glycation end products (AGEs), but not high glucose, inhibit the osteoblastic differentiation of mouse stromal ST2 cells through the suppression of osterix expression, and inhibit cell growth and increasing cell apoptosis. *Calcif Tissue Int.* 2012;91:286–96.
65. Mori K, Kitazawa R, Kondo T, Mori M, Hamada Y, Nishida M, Minami Y, Haraguchi R, Takahashi Y, Kitazawa S. Diabetic osteopenia by decreased β-Catenin signaling is partly induced by epigenetic derepression of sFRP-4 gene. *PLoS One.* 2014;9:e102797.
66. Kume S, Kato S, Yamagishi S, Inagaki Y, Ueda S, Arima N, Okawa T, Kojiro M, Nagata K. Advanced glycation end-products attenuate human mesenchymal stem cells and prevent cognate differentiation into adipose tissue, cartilage, and bone. *J Bone Miner Res.* 2005;20:1647–58.
67. Okamoto T, Yamagishi S, Inagaki Y, Amano S, Koga K, Abe R, Takeuchi M, Ohno S, Yoshimura A, Makita Z. Angiogenesis induced by advanced glycation end products and its prevention by cerivastatin. *FASEB J.* 2002;16:1928–30.
68. Okamoto T, Yamagishi S, Inagaki Y, Amano S, Takeuchi M, Kikuchi S, Ohno S, Yoshimura A. Incadronate disodium inhibits advanced glycation end products-induced angiogenesis *in vitro*. *Biochem Biophys Res Commun.* 2002;297:419–24.
69. Gangoiti MV, Cortizo AM, Arnol V, Felice JI, McCarthy AD. Opposing effects of bisphosphonates and advanced glycation end-products on osteoblastic cells. *Eur J Pharmacol.* 2008;600:140–7.
70. Tang SY, Allen MR, Phipps R, Burr DB, Vashishth D. Changes in non-enzymatic glycation and its association with altered mechanical properties following 1-year treatment with risedronate or alendronate. *Osteoporos Int.* 2009;20:887–94.
71. Saito M, Mori S, Mashiba T, Komatsubara S, Marumo K. Collagen maturity, glycation induced-pentosidine, and mineralization are increased following 3-year treatment with incadronate in dogs. *Osteoporos Int.* 2008;19:1343–54.
72. Uchiyama S, Ikegami S, Kamimura M, Mukaiyama K, Nakamura Y, Nonaka K, Kato H. The skeletal muscle cross sectional area in long-term bisphosphonate users is smaller than that of bone mineral density-matched controls with increased serum pentosidine concentrations. *Bone.* 2015;75:84–7.
73. Hashidate H, Kamimura M, Ikegami S, Mukaiyama K, Uchiyama S, Nakamura Y, Kato H. Serum pentosidine levels after 3 years of bisphosphonate treatment in post-menopausal osteoporotic women. *Endocr Res.* 2014:1–5.
74. Pullerits R, d'Elia HF, Tarkowski A, Carlsten H. The decrease of soluble RAGE levels in rheumatoid arthritis patients following hormone replacement therapy is associated with increased bone mineral density and diminished bone/cartilage turnover: A randomized controlled trial. *Rheumatology (Oxford).* 2009;48:785–90.
75. Ishibashi Y, Matsui T, Ueda S, Fukami K, Okuda S, Ohta H, Yamagishi S. Bazedoxifene blocks AGEs-RAGE-induced superoxide generation and MCP-1 level in endothelial cells. *Climacteric.* 2015;18:426–30.

22

Is There a Relationship between Dietary AGEs and Food Allergies?

Masako Toda
Paul-Ehrlich-Institut
Langen, Germany

CONTENTS

KEY POINTS

- AGEs of food allergens are produced during thermal processing of food products.
- The formation of AGEs may enhance T-cell immunogenicity of food allergens, since AGEs are efficiently endocytosed by antigen-presenting cells (APCs) via interaction with receptor binding to AGE such as scavenger receptor type A, thus increasing antigen presentation to $CD4^+$ T-cells.
- Depending on the type of allergens contained in allergic foods, the type and concentration of reducing-sugars, and food-processing conditions (e.g., temperature, moisture, and treatment time), the formation of AGEs alter IgE reactivity of food allergens.
- AGEs of food allergens are, therefore, involved in the pathological mechanisms of food allergy.
- AGE masking of IgE epitopes in food allergens may lead to the development of food products with reduced allergenicity.

22.1 Introduction

The prevalence of food allergies has increased worldwide over the past decades [1,2]. Food allergies are caused by various types of food products such as hen's eggs, cow's milk, soy, peanuts, tree nuts, wheat, fish, shellfish, vegetables, and fruits [1,2]. Naturally occurring proteins in these foods act as allergens. When allergenic foods are subjected to thermal processing, conformational changes of food allergens and interactions with other food components such as carbohydrates, lipids, and food matrix are induced. The Maillard reaction is one of the most common chemical reactions between reducing-sugars and free amino groups in proteins. Via formation of Amadori products, the Maillard reaction modifies lysine and arginine residues with various types of glycation structures, including N^{ε}-carboxymethyl-lysine (CML), pyrraline, pyridine, and methylglyoxal-H1 [3]. Products formed at the late stage of the Maillard reaction are collectively called advanced glycation end products (AGEs). Accumulating evidence suggests that AGEs of food allergens may influence type I hypersensitivity, an allergic reaction characteristic for food products, via glycation structures.

22.2 Basic Mechanism of Food Allergies

Type I hypersensitivity reaction consists of sensitization and elicitation phases. In the sensitization phase, an allergen is captured and endocytosed by antigen-presenting cells (APCs) such as dendritic cells (DCs) and macrophages (Figure 22.1a). APC-captured allergens are processed into short peptides, loaded onto major histocompatibility complex (MHC) class II molecules, and presented to $CD4^+$ T-cells. Upon recognition of the antigenic peptide-MHC class II complex by the surface T-cell receptor (TCR), $CD4^+$ T-cells are activated and differentiated into several subsets: T helper type 1 (Th1) cells producing interferon-γ (IFN-γ) and tumor necrosis factor (TNF)-α; Th2 cells producing IL-4, IL-5, and IL-13; Th9 cells producing IL-9; Th17 cells producing IL-17A, and regulatory T-cells producing transforming growth factor (TGF)-β and/or IL-10. Among these subsets, Th2 cells play an essential role in the development of food allergies. Cytokines produced by Th2 cells induce IgE production by B-cells and maturation of other immune cells such as mast cells and eosinophils.

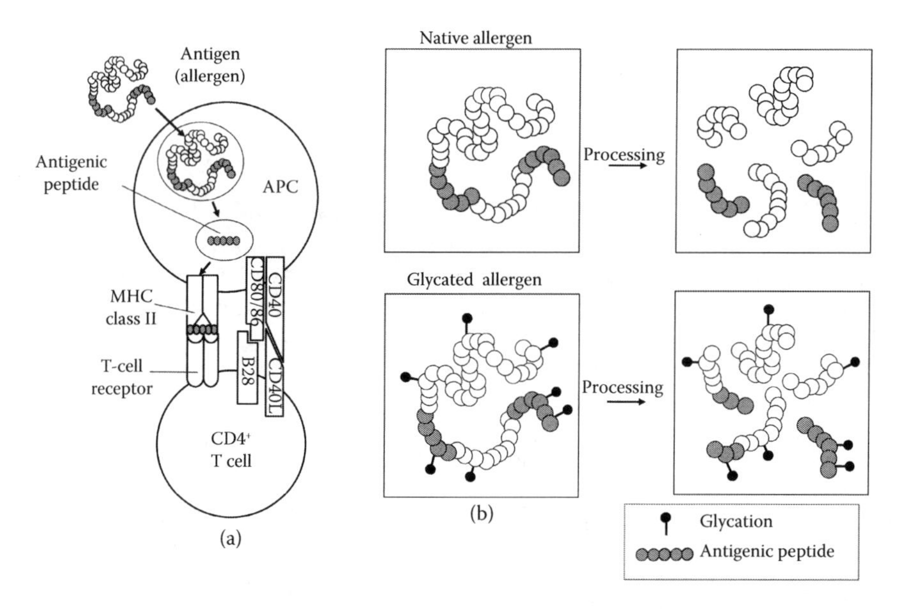

FIGURE 22.1 Influence of glycation on processing pattern of allergen in APC. (a) Allergen capture, processing, and presentation to CD4+ T-cells by antigen-presenting cell (APC). (b) A comparison in processing of native and glycated allergens by APC.

Mast cells and basophils play a critical role in the elicitation phase. The complex of allergens with IgE antibodies captured by FcεRI (the high affinity IgE receptor) on the cell surface of mast cells and basophils induces the release of a wide variety of anaphylactic mediators such as histamine, resulting in immediate allergic symptoms. Activated mast cells via FcεRI engagement also produce various cytokines and chemokines that drive maturation and migration of inflammatory eosinophils and neutrophils, leading to inflammation in local tissues.

22.3 AGE Involvement in the Sensitization Phase of Food Allergies

22.3.1 AGE Uptake by APCs

AGEs of food allergens appear to be involved in the sensitization phase of food allergies via interaction with APCs. DCs and macrophages express several receptors that could bind AGEs such as macrophage scavenger receptor class A (SR-A) [4], scavenger receptor class B (SR-B) [5], CD36 [6], galectin-3 [7], and RAGE [8,9]. The majority of putative AGE-binding receptors are known to endocytose their ligands. Recent studies have shown that [1) DCs take up more AGE-OVA, which is a crude product of the Maillard reaction between ovalbumin (OVA, egg white allergen) and glucose in phosphate-buffered saline (PBS) at 50°C for 6 weeks, compared to native OVA, and 2) SR-A mediates the uptake of AGE-OVA via interaction with glycation structures [10,11]. In a murine model of food allergy, AGE-OVA induced higher levels of OVA-specific CD4$^+$ T-cell activation and IgE production than native OVA [12]. Burgdorf et al. have reported that SR-A delivers its ligand to MHC class II loading compartments in APCs for better antigen presentation to CD4$^+$ T-cells [13]. These results suggest that AGEs of food allergens possess higher T-cell immunogenicity than native forms of allergens. Since Th2 cells, a subset of CD4$^+$ T-cells, play a critical role in inducing IgE production by B-cells, AGE-OVA could potentially exhibit higher allergenicity than native OVA.

AGEs are crude products modified with many glycation structures. There has been debate whether specific glycation structure(s) is responsible for interaction of AGEs with immune cells. To address this question, Heilmann et al. used selectively modified OVA with representative glycation structures (i.e., N$^\varepsilon$-carboxymethyl lysine, N$^\varepsilon$-carboxyethyl lysine, pyrraline, or methylglyoxal-derived arginine derivative) [12]. Interestingly, only pyrraline-modified OVA appeared to interact with SR-A expressed in DCs, and induced higher OVA-specific T-cell responses and IgE production than native OVA. The results have suggested that pyrraline potentially enhances the allergenicity of food allergens. High amounts of pyrraline have been detected in roasted peanuts, an allergenic food [14]. However, information about the profile of glycation structures in thermally processed or stored allergenic foods is still limited. Identifying glycation structures in such foods and investigating its interaction with receptors expressed in immune cells should provide further insights into the allergenicity of food allergens.

It should also be noticed that the observed effect of AGE-OVA would not be directly translatable to AGEs of all other allergens. CD4$^+$ T-cells are activated when TCR recognize the antigenic peptide/MHC class II complex presented by APCs. If the peptide contains a T-cell epitope (i.e., the amino acid sequence recognized by specific T-cells) with glycated lysine and/or arginine, it may not be able to bind to MHC class II molecules, or be recognized by TCRs, because of conformational or electric changes. Glycation may also alter the processing pattern of food allergens in APCs, and antigenic peptides may not be generated (Figure 22.1b). In this case, AGEs of food allergens would exhibit lower T-cell immunogenicity than native allergens. Therefore, the influence of glycation on T-cell immunogenicity of food allergens would depend on the allergen type.

22.3.2 APC Maturation by AGEs

In addition to antigen uptake, maturation is required for APCs to induce optimal T-cell activation. Mature APCs increase the surface expression of MHC class II and co-stimulatory molecules such as CD80, CD86, and CD40, which are crucial for naive T-cell activation and subsequent differentiation. Several studies have shown diverse effects of AGEs on APC maturation. AGEs derived from bovine serum albumin augmented maturation of human DCs and increased their capacity to stimulate allogeneic T-cell activation [15]. AGEs of plasma β2-glycoprotein I (β2GPI) induced maturation of human monocyte-derived DCs via interaction of AGEs with RAGE followed by the activation of the nuclear factor-κB signaling pathway [16]. AGE-β2GPI also exhibited capacity inducing Th2 polarization. In contrast, adrenocorticotropic hormone-derived AGEs inhibited maturation and T-cell stimulatory capacity of human DCs [17]. The difference in these findings may be attributed to the variations in RAGE expression on APCs, the amount and type of AGE modifications, or the presence of endotoxin in the samples. RAGE is known to stimulate proinflammatory responses in leukocytes and endothelial cells [18,19]. If AGEs of food allergens induce APC maturation, it would subsequently enhance T-cell responses to the allergens. Muller et al. have shown that roasted peanuts contain AGE-modified Ara h 1 that can bind to RAGE [20]. However, there is no direct evidence showing the effect of AGEs of food allergens on APC maturation via interaction with RAGE. Further studies are necessary to determine whether AGEs of food allergens trigger APC maturation and promote allergen-specific immune responses in the allergic state.

22.4 AGE Involvement in the Elicitation Phase of Food Allergies

IgE is the immunoglobulin that elicits allergic responses by triggering degranulation (i.e., mediator release) of mast cells and basophils. IgE recognizes protein conformation (conformational epitopes) or peptide sequences (sequential epitopes) of allergens, and glycation of food allergens by the Maillard reaction may alter their IgE reactivity. Therefore, AGE-modified and native food allergens may be involved in the elicitation phase of food allergies at different levels [21]. It has been assumed that AGEs of food allergens have higher IgE reactivity compared to unmodified allergens, which is based on the observation that some patients were allergic only to cooked products [22,23]. However, recent studies have shown that the glycation effects on allergenicity of food allergens depend on type and concentration of allergens, or reducing sugar, and treatment conditions (e.g., temperature, duration, and moisture) (Figure 22.2).

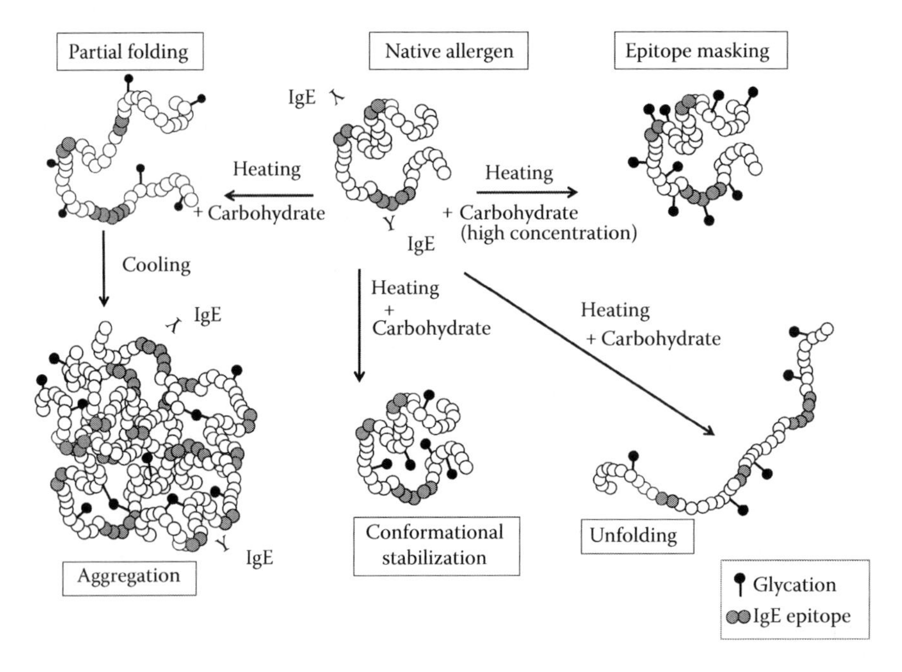

FIGURE 22.2 Influence of glycation on IgE reactivity of allergen. Depending on the type of food allergen, the type and concentration of reducing-sugar, and heating condition, glycation influences structure and electric charge of proteins and thereby changes IgE reactivity of food allergens.

22.4.1 Peanuts

Peanuts are one of the highly allergenic foods inducing severe allergic reactions. It has been suggested that roasting enhances allergenicity of peanuts, because IgE antibodies from peanut allergic patients exhibited stronger reactivities to the extracts from roasted peanuts compared with raw peanuts [24]. The presence of AGEs in roasted peanut extracts supported a role of glycation in the enhanced IgE reactivity of peanut allergens [25]. Therefore, glycation effects on IgE reactivity of the major peanut allergens Ara h 1 and Ara h 2 have been extensively investigated using peanut-isolated allergens or their recombinant forms.

Ara h 1 is 7/8 S globulin (vicilin) of seed storage proteins, which belong to the cupin superfamily. The 7/8 S globulins are major food allergens in legumes, nuts, and seeds. This type of allergens often aggregate by heat treatment, that is, unfolding by heating partially, and subsequent refolding, oligomerization, and aggregation by cooling. Blanc et al. have shown that Ara h 1 subjected to heating at 100°C in PBS without reducing sugar for 15 minutes aggregates and thereby reduces IgE reactivity and capacity to stimulate mediator release from basophils: incubation of Ara h 1 with glucose in the same conditions did not change these effects [26]. The same research group has shown that Ara h 1 aggregates by heating at 145°C for 20 minutes in dry conditions, and exhibits significantly enhanced mediator release capacity [27]. In this case, the presence of glucose reduced the IgE reactivity of Ara h 1 but did not change the effect on the mediator release capacity. The capacity to induce mediator release from basophils is a more reliable measure in the assessment of the potential allergenicity of allergens, compared to the IgE reactivity. Therefore, the results suggest that heat treatment can affect the allergenicity of Ara h 1 with or without glycation.

Ara h 2 belongs to 2S albumins of the prolamin superfamily, and is known as a thermostable allergen. Ara h 2 incubated at 100°C–110°C for 15 minutes in PBS, showed partial aggregation, which reduced its IgE reactivity and capacity to induce mediator release by basophils [28]; the incubation of Ara h 2 with glucose in the same conditions did not produce any additional effects. If dry Ara h 2 was heated with glucose at 145°C for 20 minutes, glycation counteracted the loss of mediator release capacity caused by heating [27]. However, Muller et al. have shown that in roasted peanuts, the most of Ara h 2 molecules may not be modified with AGEs, possibly because of a limited number of lysine residues [20]. Therefore, glycated products of Ara h 2 are not likely to be involved in the elicitation phase of peanut allergy.

22.4.2 Hazelnuts

Hazelnuts are one of the most common tree nuts that cause allergic reactions in European countries. Cucu et al. have shown that the capacity of crude hazelnut proteins to induce mediator release by basophils was reduced by incubation in PBS with glucose at 70°C for 48 hours [29]. It has been suggested that the reduction was due to glycation of hazelnut allergens Cor a 1 and Cor a 2, which resulted in the modification of nucleophilic amino acids and changes in protein tertiary structures. Cor a 1 and Cor a 2 belong to the pathogenesis-related protein Bet v I family and profilin protein family, respectively, which comprise heat-liable proteins. Another study has shown that the capacity of the major hazelnut allergen Cor a 11 (a vicilin-like protein) to induce mediator release by basophils was enhanced by heating at 145°C for 20 minutes in dry conditions [30], while glucose counteracted the heat-induced effect. This finding indicates that the presence of carbohydrates attenuates the enhanced allergenicity of hazelnuts induced by thermal treatment, suggesting that food-processing conditions of potentially allergenic foods should be carefully selected.

22.4.3 Buckwheat

Buckwheat is one of the common allergic diets in Asian countries. It often induces severe allergic reaction. Fag t 3 is a major allergenic protein, and 11S globulin seed storage protein belonging to cupin superfamily. Glycation of Fag t 3 by crude polysaccharides, which was isolated from buckwheat, in PBS at 70°C for 3 days reduced its IgE reactivity, while heating without crude polysaccharides did not change it [31]. The effect of glycation was correlated with disruption of protein structure of Fag t 3, suggesting that conformational IgE epitope(s) was destroyed by incubation with polysaccharides.

22.4.4 Fruit

Birch pollen–induced oral allergy syndrome is one of the most common causes of IgE-mediated food allergy in northern and central Europe, and North America [2]. This allergy mainly results from IgE cross-reactivity between the major birch pollen allergen Bet v 1 and homologous allergens contained in stone fruits, hazelnuts, certain vegetables, and legumes. Pru av 1 is an allergenic homologue of Bet v 1 found in cherry. Glycation of Pru av 1 by fructose or ribose in PBS at 100°C for 90 minutes significantly reduced its IgE reactivity [32]. It is well-known that Bet v 1 homologues easily lose their IgE reactivity after heat treatment because of the loss of conformational epitopes.

Nonspecific lipid transfer proteins (nsLTPs) are the major food allergens found in plants of the Mediterranean region; they have high thermostability and often trigger severe allergic reactions [2]. Sancho et al. have shown that glycation of Mal d 3, an LTP allergen present in apple, in harsh thermal treatment at 100°C in PBS with glucose for 2 hours protected loss of the IgE reactivity and mediator release capacity of the allergen by heating [33].

22.4.5 Hen's Eggs

Ovomucoid (OVM) is the most clinically relevant egg white allergen. OVA is another egg white allergen, but its allergenic activity and thermal stability is weaker than that of OVM and heat-liable. Thermal treatment at 50°C for 96 hours under dry conditions reduced the IgE reactivity of both OVM and OVA [34]. However, while glucose in the same conditions did not affect the IgE reactivity of OVA, it increased that of OVM, suggesting that glycation may enhance thermal stability of OVM structure.

22.4.6 Cow's Milk

Beta-lactoglobulin (β-LG) is one of the major allergens found in cow's milk. Glycation of β-LG by incubation with high concentration of ribose in PBS at 60°C for 72 hours had a "masking" effect on IgE epitopes, and reduced IgE reactivity [35]. However, this masking effect was not observed when β-LG was incubated with high concentration of lactose, galactose, or lactose in the same heating conditions.

22.4.7 Seafood

Tropomyosin is one of the major allergens found in many shellfish: crustaceans and mollusks; it is a thermostable cytoskeletal protein highly expressed in muscle tissue. The IgE reactivity and mediator release capacity of shellfish tropomyosin were enhanced after 3 hours' incubation with glucose and ribose at 60°C under dry conditions [36]. In contrast, the IgE reactivity of squid tropomyosin decreased because of structural changes induced by heat treatment rather than blockage of lysine residues in incubation at 60°C and relative humidity of 35% for 180 minutes [37].

In summary, glycation influences IgE reactivity of food allergens diversely (Figure 22.2) [21] (1) Some allergens could lose their allergenicity after heat treatment because of the loss of conformational IgE epitopes and/or masking of sequential epitopes for IgE antibodies by denaturation, or aggregation. (2) In contrast, allergenicity of some allergens may be enhanced after heat treatment if IgE epitope(s) is exposed. (3) AGE formation may either enhance heating effects or protect from them by promoting denaturation, or aggregation of allergens. (4) Glycation may stabilize protein conformation of some allergens, and protect from the loss of conformational IgE epitopes by heat treatment. (5) AGE formation may reduce or enhance the affinity and/or accessibility of allergens to specific IgE antibodies by causing changes not only in protein structure but also in electric charge, and/or hydrophobicity. (6) High levels of AGE formation achieved by incubation with high concentrations of carbohydrates may mask IgE epitopes and reduce allergenicity of food allergens.

22.5 Potential AGE Involvement in the Inflammatory Phase of Food Allergies

Food allergies cause inflammation and clinical symptoms systemically and/or locally in gastrointestinal, respiratory, and cutaneous tissues. Tessier et al. have shown that mice accumulate CML a component of dietary AGE, in many organs, in particular, kidneys, intestines, and lungs after feeding CML-BSA [38]. Although the study protocols and processes cannot be directly transferred, dietary AGEs may accumulate in humans similarly. Several studies have shown that RAGE expression is upregulated in chronic tissue inflammation including allergic asthma [39,40]. It would be important to investigate whether accumulated dietary AGEs including AGEs of food allergens interact with RAGE, and thereby enhance proinflammatory cascades in inflamed tissues of food allergic patients.

22.6 Conclusions

AGEs of food allergens could interact with immune mechanisms in both sensitization and elicitation phases of allergic diseases. AGEs of some allergens may have higher immunogenicity and allergenicity than unmodified native forms. However, if thermal conditions were adjusted to mask epitopes of food allergens by AGE formation, it would be possible to develop food products with reduced allergenicity. So far, the effects of AGE formation on immunogenicity and allergenicity of food allergens have been assessed using isolated or recombinant form of allergens that were subjected to *in vitro* thermal incubation with a limited number of reducing-sugars. Comprehensive investigation in biochemical, immunological, and allergic properties of AGEs of allergens contained in thermally processed foods would further elucidate the role of AGEs in the pathogenic mechanisms underlying food allergy, and promote the development of food products with low allergenicity.

REFERENCES

1. Sicherer, S. H., and H. A. Sampson. 2010. Food allergy. *J. Allergy Clin. Immunol.* 125:S116–25.
2. Nwaru, B. I., L. Hickstein, S. S. Panesar, G. Roberts, and A. Muraro, A. Sheikh, EAACI Food Allergy and Anaphylaxis Guidelines Group. 2014. Prevalence of common food allergies in Europe: A systematic review and meta-analysis. *Allergy.* 69:992–1007.
3. Henle, T. 2005. Protein-bound advanced glycation endproducts (AGEs) as bioactive amino acid derivatives in foods. *Amino Acids.* 29:313–22.
4. Suzuki, H., Y. Kurihara, M. Takeya, N. Kamada, M. Kataoka, K. Jishage, et al. 1997. A role for macrophage scavenger receptors in atherosclerosis and susceptibility to infection. *Nature.* 386:292–6.
5. Ohgami, N., R. Nagai, A. Miyazaki, M. Ikemoto, H. Arai, S. Horiuchi, et al. 2001. Scavenger receptor class B type I-mediated reverse cholesterol transport is inhibited by advanced glycation end products. *J. Biol. Chem.* 276:13348–55.
6. Ohgami, N., R. Nagai, M. Ikemoto, H. Arai, A. Kuniyasu, S. Horiuchi, et al. 2001. CD36, a member of the class b scavenger receptor family, as a receptor for advanced glycation end products. *J. Biol. Chem.* 276:3195–202.
7. Vlassara, H., Y. M. Li, F. Imani, D. Wojciechowicz, Z. Yang, F. T. Liu, et al. 1995. Identification of galectin-3 as a high-affinity binding protein for advanced glycation end products (AGE): A new member of the AGE-receptor complex. *Mol. Med.* 1:634–46.
8. Neeper, M., A. M. Schmidt, J. Brett, S. D. Yan, F. Wang, Y. C. Pan, et al. Cloning and expression of a cell surface receptor for advanced glycosylation end products of proteins. 1992. *J. Biol. Chem.* 267:14998–5004.
9. Schmidt, A. M., M. Vianna, M. Gerlach, J. Brett, J. Ryan, J. Kao, et al. 1992. Isolation and characterization of two binding proteins for advanced glycosylation end products from bovine lung which are present on the endothelial cell surface. *J. Biol. Chem.* 267:14987–97.

10. Ilchmann, A., S. Burgdorf, S. Scheurer, Z, Waibler, R. Nagai, A. Wellner, et al. 2010. Glycation of a food allergen by the Maillard reaction enhances its T-cell immunogenicity: Role of macrophage scavenger receptor class A type I and II. *J. Allergy Clin. Immunol.* 125:175–83.
11. Hilmenyuk, T., I. Bellinghausen, B. Heydenreich, A. Ilchmann, M. Toda, S. Grabbe, et al. 2010. Effects of glycation of the model food allergen ovalbumin on antigen uptake and presentation by human dendritic cells. *Immunology.* 129:437–45.
12. Heilmann, M., A. Wellner, G. Gadermaier, A. Ilchmann, P. Briza, M. Krause, et al. 2014. Ovalbumin modified with pyrraline, a Maillard reaction product, shows enhanced T-cell immunogenicity. *J. Biol. Chem.* 289:7919–28.
13. Burgdorf, S., and C. Kurts. 2008. Endocytosis mechanisms and the cell biology of antigen presentation. *Curr. Opin. Immunol.* 20:89–95.
14. Wellner, A., L. Nusspickel, and T. Henle. 2012. Glycation compounds in peanuts. *Eur. Food Res. Technol.* 234:423–9.
15. Ge, J., Q. Jia, C. Liang, Y. Luo, D. Huang, A. Sun, et al. 2005. Advanced glycosylation end products might promote atherosclerosis through inducing the immune maturation of dendritic cells. *Arterioscler. Thromb. Vasc. Biol.* 25:2157–63.
16. Buttari, B., E. Profumo, A. Capozzi, F. Facchiano, L. Saso, M. Sorice, et al. 2011. Advanced glycation end products of human β2 glycoprotein I modulate the maturation and function of DCs. *Blood.* 117:6152–61.
17. Price, C. L., P. S. Sharp, M. E. North, S. J. Rainbow, and S. C. Knight. 2004. Advanced glycation end products modulate the maturation and function of peripheral blood dendritic cells. *Diabetes.* 53:1452–8.
18. Litwinoff, E., C. Hurtado Del Pozo, R. Ramasamy, and A. M. Schmidt. 2015. Emerging targets for therapeutic development in diabetes and its complications: The RAGE signaling pathway. *Clin. Pharmacol. Ther.* 98:135–44.
19. Chuah, Y. K., R, Basir, H. Talib, T. H. Tie, and N. Nordin. 2013. Receptor for advanced glycation end products and its involvement in inflammatory diseases. *Int. J. Inflam.* 2013:403460.
20. Mueller, G. A., S. J. Maleki, K. Johnson, B. K. Hurlburt, H. Cheng, S. Ruan, et al. 2013. Identification of Maillard reaction products on peanut allergens that influence binding to the receptor for advanced glycation end products. *Allergy.* 68:1546–54.
21. Toda, M., M. Heilmann, A. Ilchmann, and S. Vieths. 2014. The Maillard reaction and food allergies: Is there a link? *Clin. Chem. Lab. Med.* 52:61–7.
22. Berrens, L. 1996. Neoallergens in heated pecan nut: Products of Maillard-type degradation? *Allergy.* 51:277–8.
23. Simonato, B., G. Pasini, M. Giannattasio, A. D. Peruffo, F. De Lazzari, and A. Curioni. 2001. Food allergy to wheat products: The effect of bread baking and *in vitro* digestion on wheat allergenic proteins. A study with bread dough, crumb, and crust. *J. Agric. Food Chem.* 49:5668–73.
24. Maleki, S. J., S. Y. Chung, E. T. Champagne, and J. P. Raufman. 2000. The effects of roasting on the allergenic properties of peanut proteins. *J. Allergy Clin. Immunol.* 106:763–8.
25. Chung, S. Y., and E. T. Champagne. 2001. Association of end-product adducts with increased IgE binding of roasted peanuts. *J. Agric. Food Chem.* 49:3911–16.
26. Blanc, F., Y. M. Vissers, K. Adel-Patient., N. M. Rigby, A. R. Mackie, A. P. Gunning, et al. 2011. Boiling peanut Ara h 1 results in the formation of aggregates with reduced allergenicity. *Mol. Nutr. Food Res.* 55:1887–94.
27. Vissers, Y. M., M. Iwan, K. Adel-Patient, P. Stahl Skov, N. M. Rigby, P. E. Johnson, et al. 2011. Effect of roasting on the allergenicity of major peanut allergens Ara h 1 and Ara h 2/6: The necessity of degranulation assays. *Clin. Exp. Allergy.* 41:1631–42.
28. Vissers, Y. M., F. Blanc, P. S. Skov, P. E. Johnson, N. M. Rigby, L. Przybylski-Nicaise, et al. 2011. Effect of heating and glycation on the allergenicity of 2S Albumins (Ara h 2/6) from peanut. *PLoS One.* 6:e23998.
29. Cucu, T., B. De Meulenaer, C. Bridts, B. Devreese, and D. Ebo. 2012. Impact of thermal processing and the Maillard reaction on the basophil activation of hazelnut allergic patients. *Food Chem. Toxicol.* 50:1722–8.
30. Iwan, M., Y. M. Vissers, E. Fiedorowicz, H. Kostyra, E. Kostyra, H. F. Savelkoul, et al. 2011. Impact of Maillard reaction on immunoreactivity and allergenicity of the hazelnut allergen Cor a 11. *J. Agric. Food Chem.* 59:7163–71.

31. Yang, Z. H., C. Li, Y. Y. Li, and Z. H. Wang. 2013. Effects of Maillard reaction on allergenicity of buckwheat allergen Fag t 3 during thermal processing. *J. Sci. Food Agric.* 93:1510–15.
32. Gruber, P., S. Vieths, A. Wangorsch, J. Nerkamp, and T. Hofmann. 2004. Maillard reaction and enzymatic browning affect the allergenicity of Pru av 1, the major allergen from cherry (Prunus avium). *J. Agric. Food Chem.* 52:4002–7.
33. Sancho, A. I., N. M. Rigby, L. Zuidmeer, R. Asero, G. Mistrello, S. Amato, et al. The effect of thermal processing on the IgE reactivity of the non-specific lipid transfer protein from apple, Mal d 3. *Allergy.* 2005;60:1262–68.
34. Jimenez-Saiz, R., J. Belloque, E. Molina, and R. Lopez-Fandino. 2011. Human immunoglobulin E (IgE) binding to heated and glycated ovalbumin and ovomucoid before and after *in vitro* digestion. *J. Agric. Food Chem.* 59:10044–51.
35. Taheri-Kafrani, A., J. C. Gaudin, H. Rabesona, C. Nioi, D. Agarwal, M. Drouet, et al. 2009. Effects of heating and glycation of beta-lactoglobulin on its recognition by IgE of sera from cow milk allergy patients. *J. Agric. Food Chem.* 57:4974–82.
36. Nakamura, A., K. Watanabe, T. Ojima, D. H. Ahn, and H. Saeki. 2005. Effect of Maillard reaction on allergenicity of scallop tropomyosin. *J. Agric. Food Chem.* 53:7559–64.
37. Nakamura, A., F. Sasaki, K. Watanabe, T. Ojima, D. H. Ahn, and H. Saeki. 2006. Changes in allergenicity and digestibility of squid tropomyosin during the Maillard reaction with ribose. *J. Agric. Food Chem.* 54:9529–34.
38. Tessier, F. J., C. Niquet-Léridon, P. Jacolot, C. Jouquand, M. Genin, A. M. Schmidt, et al. 2016. Quantitative assessment of organ distribution of dietary protein-bound 13 C-labeled Nε-carboxymethyllysine after a chronic oral exposure in mice. *Mol. Nutr. Food. Res.* 60:2446–56.
39. Ramasamy, R., S. F. Yan, and A. M. Schmidt. 2012. Advanced glycation endproducts: From precursors to RAGE: Round and round we go. *Amino Acids.* 42:1151–61.
40. Sukkar, M. B., M. A. Ullah, W. J. Gan, P. A. Wark, K. F. Chung, J. M. Hughes, et al. 2012. RAGE: A new frontier in chronic airways disease. *Br. J. Pharmacol.* 167:1161–76.

23

Quantitation and Potential Health Effects of Advanced Glycation End Products in Pet Foods

Guido Bosch
Wageningen University
Wageningen, The Netherlands

Wouter Hendriks
Utrecht University
Utrecht, The Netherlands

CONTENTS

KEY POINTS

- Commercial pet foods and their ingredients are produced using processing techniques that favor the Maillard reaction and formation of advanced glycation end products (AGEs).
- Quantitative data on AGEs in pet foods are highly limited. Considerable variation is found in AGE contents of dry extruded and wet retorted pet foods.
- Estimated intake of studied AGEs is similar or higher in adult dogs and cats than that in humans.
- The contribution of the AGE load to the pathogenesis of diseases in pet dogs and cats is unknown and is an important area for future (fundamental) studies.

23.1 Introduction

Pet dogs (*Canis familiaris*) and cats (*Felis silvestris catus*) play an important role in many people's lives. Over 140 million dogs and 160 million cats live in households in Europe and the United States (FEDIAF 2012a; Pet Food Institute 2014) and their numbers are increasing, particularly in Asia and Latin America. In time, our relationship with dogs and cats has intensified and many of us now consider them "family members." Where their ancestors, the wolves (*C. lupus*) and wildcats (*F. s.* spp), were carnivores that had to hunt for prey and struggled for survival, most of our modern pet dogs and cats have a relatively sedentary lifestyle and are cared for throughout their lives. Although pets have been considered as social parasites (Archer 1997), pet ownership has been associated with increased social engagement and cohesion in communities, and with psychological, physiological, and physical health benefits (McNicholas et al. 2005). The affection for our pets has fueled the development of industries targeting pet care. The pet food industry is a prime example and offers owners a plethora of nutritious products to support specific pet breeds and sizes, particular life stages, and disease predispositions, in various formats and packaging styles, and at different prices (Aldrich 2006). The pet food industry thrives to provide optimal and safe nutrition for health and longevity. Considering the potential impact of advanced glycation end products (AGEs) on health, as indicated in previous chapters, this chapter aims to present an overview of our current knowledge on the levels of AGEs in commercial pet foods and their potential role in health and disease in pet dogs and cats. As readers may lack some background information on the pet food manufacturing process that underlies the potential formation and presence of AGEs, the production of pet food is first described.

23.2 Pet Food Production

Of the different formats, the dry extruded and moist retorted foods are the most popular among pet owners in Western countries (Laflamme et al. 2008). During the manufacturing of these types of pet foods, thermal treatments are used to not only improve the safety and nutritive properties of the foods but also to create the optimal texture and shape of the product (Hendriks et al. 1999). In addition, many of the ingredients used for the formulation of pet foods have already undergone processing including extensive thermal treatment. Meat and by-product meals of poultry, beef, pig, lamb, and/or fish are produced by a rendering-process, which applies extensive cooking (130°C for several hours), drying, and grinding. The plant-derived ingredients like cereal grains and their by-products are often ground and dried. Furthermore, palatability enhancers are created for mostly dry pet foods by digesting animal tissues. The resulting amino acids and fatty acids are highly palatable to cats and dogs, which is further increased by heating the hydrolysates with sugars promoting the formation of aromatic compounds generated during the Maillard reaction.

23.2.1 Dry Extruded Pet Foods

Dry extruded pet foods are produced in several processing steps. The ingredient mixture is first precooked in a preconditioner in which water and/or steam are uniformly applied to achieve a moisture content of 10% to 25% and mixture temperature of 70°C to 90°C at the discharge of the preconditioner (Rokey et al. 2010). The mixture is retained for about 45 seconds in the preconditioner (Crane et al. 2010). Other liquid ingredients like fresh meat, oil, flavors, and coloring agents may also be introduced in the preconditioner. The material flows from the preconditioner into the extruder barrel, which contains one or two screws to transport the material from the inlet zone to the die. In the barrel, the material is kneaded into an amorphous dough, compressed and forced through the die of the extruder. Due to the mechanical energy dissipated through the rotating screw(s) and possibly assisted by direct steam injection or from external thermal energy sources, the temperature of the dough rises. Furthermore, the die restricts the product flow causing increased pressure and shear. The final temperature prior to the die is 125°C to 150°C, the moisture content is 23% to 28%, and the pressure rises to between 34 and 37 atmospheres (Rokey et al. 2010). When the dough is pressed through the orifice of the die plate, it encounters ambient pressure and temperature, resulting in rapid evaporation of moisture and expansion of the product. The expansion is at least 50% greater than the die diameter and results in the characteristic porous texture of dry pet food, which is retained by the loss of between 3% and 5% moisture (Colonna et al. 1989). The size and shape of the food are determined by the orifice shape and the knife located directly behind the die that cuts the expanded product exiting the die. Most extruded foods are dried in about 15 minutes to a moisture content of less than 10% on a horizontal conveyor dryer where heated air (90°C to 180°C) is passed through the bed of product (Colonna et al. 1989; Rokey et al. 2010). The product is coated with fat, palatability enhancers, and potentially heat-labile additives (e.g., probiotics) to enhance the acceptance and functionality of the pet food. The coated kibbles are cooled, packaged, and prepared for transport.

23.2.2 Wet Retorted Foods

Wet pet foods in airtight cans, containers, or flexible pouches are also produced in multiple processing steps. The basic ingredients for wet food recipes are fresh and/or frozen meats and other animal tissues, mash grains, or other ground starch sources, vitamin and mineral premixes, and water (Crane et al. 2010). The animal tissues are ground and combined with the other ingredients to a homogenous mixture, which is heated (25°C to 85°C) to gelatinize starches and denature proteins and to promote the texture and flavor of the product (Crane et al. 2010). The cans, containers, or flexible pouches are filled with the product and prepared for the sterilization in a retort or pressure cooker. The process of retorting is continuous or via a batch system and both follow the three phases. In the first phase, the temperature of the food is gradually increased to 80°C to 100°C. Then, the sterilization phase starts during which the temperature is further increased and maintained above 116°C for a period long enough to kill all pathogenic bacteria (Crane et al. 2010). The sterilization in a retort is a temperature/time-dependent process for which the lethality of the heat employed on the product is expressed using an F0-value (Hendriks et al. 1999). The F0-value represents the time equivalent in minutes of a heating process to destroy microorganisms at the reference temperature of 121.1°C. Generally, the minimal time to kill pathogenic bacteria is 3 minutes at 121.1°C (F0-value of 3) (Crane et al. 2010) but in practice F0-values of more than 10 are used (Hendriks et al. 1999). After sterilization, the product is cooled to 32°C and 40°C after which the dried packages are labeled and prepared for maturing and transport.

23.3 AGEs in Pet Foods

Considering the composition and the processing techniques applied to produce pet foods and palatability enhancers, it would be expected that the Maillard reaction is promoted during processing, and its products are present in the finished pet foods. Indeed, in 1983, it was reported that dry dog food contained 0.910 g/kg furosine (Chiang 1983), which would equal 3.45 g/kg fructoselysine using 32% as a correction factor (mole-by-mole basis) (Krause et al. 2003) (Table 23.1). Most studies, however, focused on the impact of the Maillard reaction on the nutritional value of pet foods based on the quantification of the nonglycated (reactive) as well as total lysine and using *in vitro* and *in vivo* assays. The ratio of reactive to total lysine is highly variable in pet foods with values as low as 0.38 (Rutherfurd et al. 2007; Van Rooijen et al. 2014b; Williams et al. 2006), which is caused by the Maillard reaction during processing of the ingredients and the pet foods (for a review, see Van Rooijen et al. 2013). To compensate for the amino acid degradation and modifications, pet foods are commonly formulated to contain considerably more protein.

The study of the AGEs in pet foods is, however, still in its infancy with only six studies focusing on the quantification of six AGEs (Table 23.1, Figure 23.1). Acrylamide was quantified in dry extruded foods for dogs ($n = 5$) and cats ($n = 3$), with values ranging between 66 and 358 μg/kg (Veselá and Šucman 2013). The energy contents of these foods were not reported, which hampers accurate estimation of the daily intake of acrylamide. Assuming an average metabolizable energy content of 3.57 and 3.55 kcal/g for grocery dog and cat food brands (Hand et al. 2000) and a daily metabolizable energy requirement of 130×kg $BW^{0.75}$ for adult dogs and 100×kg $BW^{0.67}$ for adult cats (NRC 2006), a 20 kg adult dog and a 4 kg adult cat would have a daily intake between 3.86 and 13.04 μg/kg $BW^{0.75}$ and between 1.66 and 6.79 μg/kg $BW^{0.75}$, respectively. These intake levels are higher than that in adult humans, with mean intake ranges between 1.16 and 2.60 μg/kg $BW^{0.75}$ and 95th percentile estimates between 1.74 and 5.79 μg/kg $BW^{0.75}$ (EFSA 2015). The heterocyclic amines MeIQx (2-amino-3,8-dimethylimidazo[4,5-*f*]quinoxaline) and PhIP (2-amino-1-methyl-6-phenylimidazo[4,5-*b*]pyridine) have been, respectively, found in 13 and 10 of the 14 evaluated commercial foods for growing and adult dogs and cats (Knize et al. 2003). The compound 2-amino-(1,6-dimethylfuro[3,2-*e*]imidazo[4,5-b])pyridine (IFP), which is found in well-done meat (Pais et al. 2000), was not detected in the samples. Knize et al. (2003) estimated that the daily intake of the heterocyclic amines in pets would be 5-fold higher than that in humans. Details regarding food format and the energy contents were not reported, which hampers verification of this estimate. Recently, Van Rooijen et al. (2014a) reported the content of the fructoselysine (analyzed as furosine), 5-hydroxymethylfurfural, and N^{ε}-carboxymethyllysine in 57 commercial dry extruded and wet retorted foods for growing and adult

TABLE 23.1
Advanced Glycation End Products in Pet Foods

Ref[a]	Component[b]	Species	Life Stage	n	Unit[c]	Amount	
						Mean ± SD	**Range**
I	Fructoselysine[d]	Dog	NS[e]	1	μg/kg	2844	
II	Acrylamide	Dog	Growing	1	μg/kg	214	
			Adult	4	μg/kg	201 ± 117	106–358
		Cat	Adult	3	μg/kg	146 ± 108	66–269
III	MeIQx	Dog	Growing	2	ng/g	1.00 ± 0.14	0.90–1.10
			Adult	10	ng/g	0.86 ± 1.00	0.04–3.30
		Cat	Growing	1	ng/g	0.57	
			Adult	1	ng/g	0.53	
III	PhIP	Dog	Growing	2	ng/g	2.00 ± 0.57	1.60–2.40
			Adult	10	ng/g	13.80 ± 21.48	0.05–70.00
		Cat	Growing	1	ng/g	3.50	
			Adult	1	ng/g	1.70	

[a] I, Chiang (1983); II, Veselá and Šucman (2013); III, Knize et al. (2003).
[b] MeIQx, 2-amino-3,8-dimethylimidazo[4,5-*f*]quinoxaline; PhIP, 2-amino-1-methyl-6-phenylimidazo [4,5-*b*]pyridine.
[c] Presumably on as is basis (authors did not specify).
[d] Calculated as analyzed furosine/(32/100) (Krause et al. 2003).
[e] NS, not specified.

dogs and cats (Figure 23.1). For dry extruded dog and cat foods, fructoselysine contents were lower than previously reported (Chiang 1983) and considerably lower than those in wet retorted dog and cat foods. Similarly, wet retorted dog and cat foods contained more N^{ε}-carboxymethyllysine on a dry matter basis. The 5-hydroxymethylfurfural contents in pet foods seem slightly higher in retorted formats although considerable variation was noted. With daily 5-hydroxymethylfurfural intakes between 2.17 and 23.17 mg for a Spanish diet (Rufián-Henares and de la Cueva 2008) and a median intake of 3.04 mg and a maximum intake of 32.6 mg for a Norwegian diet (Husøy et al. 2008), the intake for adult humans (70 kg) would have ranged between 0.09 and 1.35 mg/kg $BW^{0.75}$. These daily intakes for adult pets are considerably higher and highly variable. For adult dogs, the estimated 5-hydroxymethylfurfural intake ranged between 8.1 and 55.1 mg/kg $BW^{0.75}$ for dry extruded foods and 36.9 and 94.4 mg/kg $BW^{0.75}$ for wet retorted foods and for adult cats this was, respectively, between 4.7 and 18.6 mg/kg $BW^{0.75}$ and 15.3 and 33.0 mg/kg $BW^{0.75}$ (Van Rooijen et al. 2014a). The intake of N^{ε}-carboxymethyllysine in adult dogs and cats is high when fed wet retorted foods (0.60 to 1.52 and 0.51 to 1.17 mg/kg $BW^{0.75}$, respectively) but in the ranges observed for human infants. For a 6-month-old infant, the average daily N^{ε}-carboxymethyllysine intake from infant formulas was estimated to be 4.6 mg (Šebeková et al. 2008), which equals 0.97 mg/kg $BW^{0.75}$ assuming a body weight of 8 kg. Hydrolyzed infant formulas contain more N^{ε}-carboxymethyllysine than regular formulas (Dittrich et al. 2006; Šebeková et al. 2008). For example, the maximum N^{ε}-carboxymethyllysine content in hydrolyzed formula is six times higher than that in regular formula with intake levels of, respectively, 2.97 and 0.52 mg/kg $BW^{0.75}$ for a 6 kg infant consuming 1 L of milk (Dittrich et al. 2006). Daily N^{ε}-carboxymethyllysine intake estimates for Spanish adolescent males for a low and high AGE diet were, respectively, 0.26 and 0.54 mg/kg $BW^{0.75}$ (Delgado-Andrade et al. 2012) and French adults (18–24 years old) on a low and high AGE diet had N^{ε}-carboxymethyllysine intakes of, respectively, 2.2 and 5.4 mg (Birlouez-Aragon et al. 2010) or 0.09 and 0.22 mg/kg $BW^{0.75}$ assuming a body weight of 70 kg. The daily intake of fructoselysine is particularly high, with values between 14.8 and 58.1 mg/kg $BW^{0.75}$ for dry extruded foods and 95.4 and 273.6 mg/kg $BW^{0.75}$ for wet retorted foods for adult dogs and 9.5 and 31.0 mg/kg $BW^{0.75}$ for dry extruded foods and 83.1 and 120.6 mg/kg $BW^{0.75}$ for wet retorted foods for adult cats (based on Van Rooijen et al. 2014a). Based on the current knowledge, it can be concluded that dry and moist pet foods contain multiple AGEs to variable levels. The origin and control of

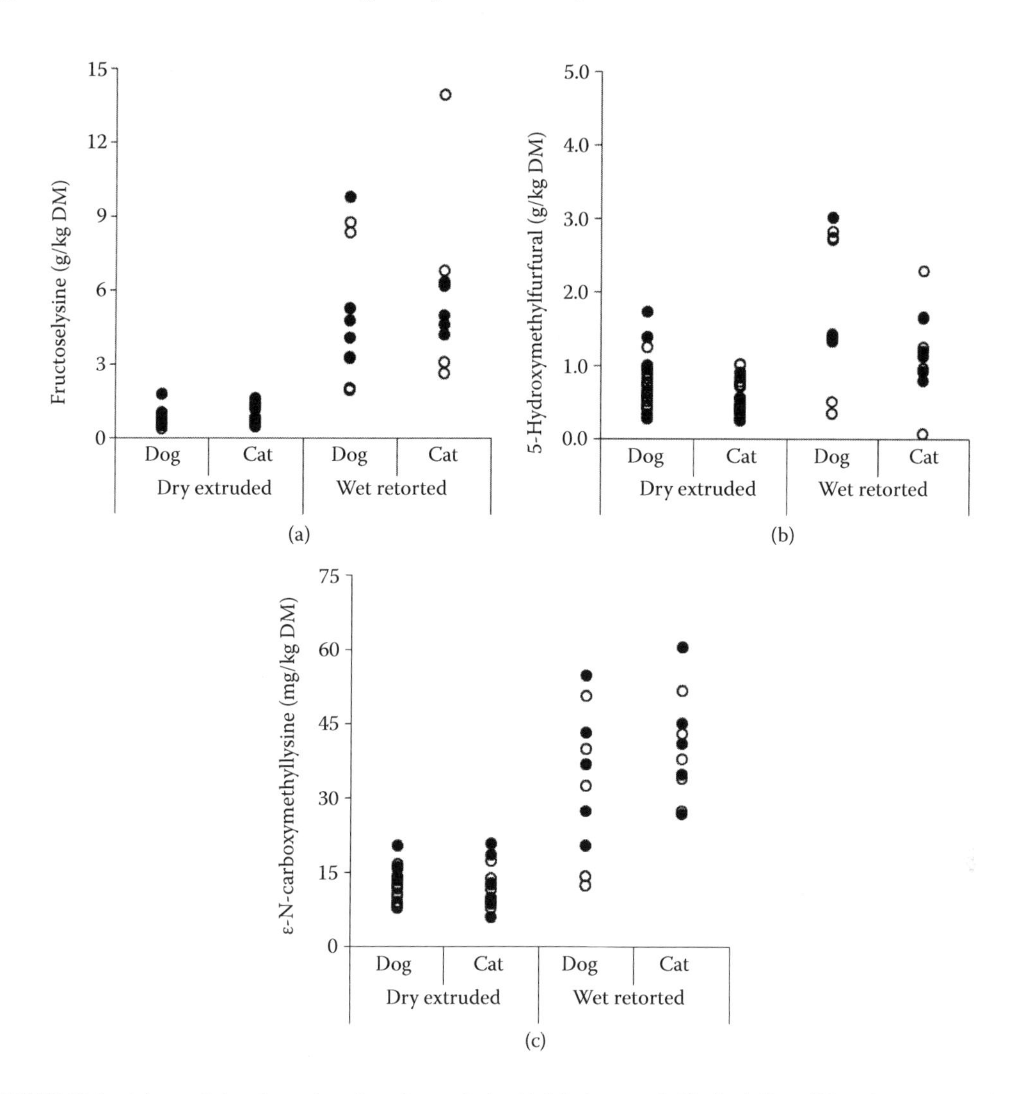

FIGURE 23.1 Advanced glycation end products fructoselysine (a), 5-hydroxymethylfurfural (b), and Nε-carboxymethyllysine (c) in pet foods categorized by pet species (dog, cat), processing type (dry extruded, wet retorted), and life stage (adult, growing). (From Van Rooijen, C., et al., *J. Agric. Food Chem.*, 62, 8883–8891, 2014a.) The symbol ● refers to with $n = 5$ dry extruded foods for adult dogs and cats and ○ refers to $n = 16$ dry extruded foods for growing dogs and $n = 11$ dry extruded foods for growing cats, $n = 5$ wet retorted foods for growing dogs and cats.

this variation, for example, via modification of ingredient or pet food-processing conditions, warrants further study. The estimates for intake of AGEs in evaluated pet foods in the literature suggest similar (N^{ε}-carboxymethyllysine) to higher (other AGEs) intake in adult dogs and cats compared to humans. Further work is required to quantify other AGEs potentially present in pet foods and to understand the key processes of pet food manufacturing that underlie the formation of AGEs.

23.4 AGEs Products and Pet Health

The impact of consumption of processed pet foods containing AGEs on the health of dogs and cats is under debate (Freeman et al. 2013; Knueven 2014). This debate is in line with that in human food research where AGEs are associated with pathologies of organs and tissues, including cardiovascular, renal, orthopedic, periodontal, ocular, and nervous tissues (Henle 2005; Smit and Lutgers 2004). Next to dietary AGEs, the endogenously formed AGEs contribute the AGE load in dogs and cats as it does in humans. In particular, dry extruded pet foods can contain up to 60% digestible carbohydrates, which provides a glycemic load that can result in increased endogenous glycation of proteins and formation of AGEs. There are indications that AGEs can impact functionality of, and accumulate in, tissues in dogs. For example, injections of ribose in the knee joint resulted in increased pentosidine levels in the femoral cartilage, which predisposed dogs to develop osteoarthritis (DeGroot et al. 2004). In aging dogs, AGEs were found to accumulate in the brain, predominantly in the cytoplasm of neurons of cerebellum and brainstem (AGE types not defined) (Weber et al. 1998) and in the aorta but not in the left ventricle of the heart (N^{ε}-carboxymethyllysine) (Shapiro et al. 2008). Furthermore, three cases of spontaneously arising atherosclerosis in dogs were associated with AGE accumulation (Chiers et al. 2010). There is no evidence that dietary and/or endogenously formed AGEs truly contribute to the pathogenesis of these diseases in dogs and cats. Also in humans, it has been indicated that unambiguous defined toxicological effects of individual AGEs are lacking and even positive aspects are noted including antioxidative properties and inhibition of tumor cell growth (see Henle 2005).

A potential contribution of dietary AGEs to the pathogenesis of diseases in pet dog and cats would depend on the absorption, metabolism, detoxification, elimination, and the sensitivity to AGEs. For each of these factors, there are virtually no studies performed in dogs or cats indicating there is a lack of fundamental knowledge to assess the health risks of the types and amounts of AGEs consumed via dry extruded and wet retorted pet foods. Absorption and build up in tissues of acrylamide, which may be consumed by dogs and cats in relatively high quantities, has been studied in dogs. Oral administration of large amounts of acrylamide (1 mg/kg BW) to an adult dog showed that after 14 hours, 59% was excreted via the urine and 7% via the feces, and acrylamide was mostly present in muscle, liver, and blood, and little in brain, testis, lung, kidney, spleen, heart, bile, and fat (Ikeda et al. 1987). Intravenously administered acrylamide (5 mg/kg BW) to dogs in late gestation is also passed on to fetuses (Ikeda et al. 1983). For adult humans, the intake of acrylamide is not of concern as it is well below the benchmark dose lower confidence limit of 10% of the effect level for neurotoxicity and carcinogenicity, that is, a factor of >125 (EFSA 2015). To assess the risk of acrylamide intake in dogs and cats, more studies are required regarding the quantity and bioavailability of acrylamide in the pet food matrix as well as its potency to cause or contribute to the pathogenesis of diseases in pet dogs and cats. Bioavailability of other AGEs in dogs and cats are not described in literature, although a recent cat trial in our group indicated that both fructoselysine and N^{ε}-carboxymethyllysine are excreted via the urine and at least are partially bioavailable (Van Rooijen et al. 2016). Next to the content and absorption of dietary AGEs, post-absorptive metabolism may impact bioactivity of AGEs. For example, fructoselysine can be oxidized to N^{ε}-carboxymethyllysine (Ahmed et al. 1986), which can interact with the receptor for AGE (RAGE) accelerating oxidative stress and inflammation. Considering the high levels of fructoselysine in commercial pet foods fed to dogs and cats, the N^{ε}-carboxymethyllysine load may, therefore, be higher than expected based on its content in food. Effects of AGE are avoided or regulated by renal AGE elimination and detoxification, antioxidant systems, and suppression of signaling via the AGE receptor AGER1 (Vlassara and Striker 2011). The detoxification and elimination efficiency and sensitivity to specific dietary or endogenously formed AGEs in dogs and cats may be different than in other species including humans, rats, and mice. Examples of common human food sources being toxic to dogs are grapes and raisins (caused by unknown compounds), chocolate (methylxanthine alkaloids), and onions and garlic (organo-sulfoxides) (FEDIAF 2012b). Such differences in sensitivity to compounds originate from differences in the evolutionary background of animal species. Dogs and cats are domesticated carnivores and during evolution their digestive physiology and metabolism has been geared toward an animal-based diet consisting mainly of protein and fat, with little digestible carbohydrates (Bosch et al. 2015; Plantinga et al. 2011). Although wolves also consumed ungulate livers containing glycogen and occasionally some fruits, strong fluctuations in blood glucose (i.e., high glycemic loads) would have been rare (Bosch et al. 2015). For the omnivorous humans, digestible carbohydrate consumption would have been more common, resulting in stronger fluctuations in blood sugar levels promoting endogenous formation of AGEs, potentially a more efficient elimination and detoxification of these AGEs. This may have resulted in an increased capacity to lower the load of specific AGEs in humans as opposed to dogs and cats. Specificity of RAGEs to AGEs like N^{ε}-carboxymethyllysine and downstream processes after RAGE-binding in dogs and cats are also currently unknown. Fundamental understanding on these aspects would significantly improve our insight on the role of AGEs in pathogenesis of diseases.

23.5 Conclusions

Limited information is available on AGEs quantities in commercial pet foods. The data suggest that variable contents and estimated daily intakes of adult dogs and cats can be considerably higher than that in adult humans. Whether this high load of AGEs results in the pathogenesis of diseases is unknown and would depend on numerous factors including absorption, metabolism, detoxification, and elimination of AGEs as well as the sensitivity to AGEs via binding to RAGEs. The carnivorous evolutionary background, characterized by low levels of endogenous AGE formation, might have resulted in sensitivity to AGEs being different from that of more well-studied omnivorous species like humans and rats. Considering the daily intake of AGEs throughout the life of pet dogs and cats, the potential species-specific capacities to cope with these AGEs and sensitivity to AGEs as well as the role of AGEs in the pathogenesis of diseases warrants further study.

REFERENCES

Ahmed, M. U., S. R. Thorpe, and J. W. Baynes. 1986. Identification of n^{ε}-carboxymethyllysine as a degradation product of fructoselysine in glycated protein. *Journal of Biological Chemistry* 261: 4889–4894.

Aldrich, G. 2006. Rendered products in pet food. In: D. L. Meeker (ed.), *Essential rendering.* pp. 159–178. Kirby Lithographic Company, Arlington, VA.

Archer, J. 1997. Why do people love their pets? *Evolution and Human Behavior* 18: 237–259.

Birlouez-Aragon, I. 2010. A diet based on high-heat-treated foods promotes risk factors for diabetes mellitus and cardiovascular diseases. *American Journal of Clinical Nutrition* 91: 1220–1226.

Bosch, G., E. A. Hagen-Plantinga, and W. H. Hendriks. 2015. Dietary nutrient profiles of wild wolves: Insights for optimal dog nutrition? *British Journal of Nutrition* 113: S40–S54.

Chiang, G. H. 1983. A simple and rapid high-performance liquid chromatographic procedure for determination of furosine, lysine-reducing sugar derivative. *Journal of Agricultural and Food Chemistry* 31: 1373–1374.

Chiers, K., V. Vandenberge, and R. Ducatelle. 2010. Accumulation of advanced glycation end products in canine atherosclerosis. *Journal of Comparative Pathology* 143: 65–69.

Colonna, P., J. Tayeb, and C. Mercier. 1989. Extrusion cooking of starch and starchy products. In: C. Mercier, P. Linko and J. M. Harper (eds.) *Extrusion cooking.* pp. 247–319. American Association of Starch Chemists, St. Paul, MN.

Crane, S. W. 2010. Commercial pet foods. In: M. S. Hand, C. D. Thatcher, R. L. Remillard, P. Roudebush and B. J. Novotny (eds.), *Small animal clinical nutrition.* pp. 157–190. Mark Morris Institute, Topeka, KS.

DeGroot, J. 2004. Accumulation of advanced glycation end products as a molecular mechanism for aging as a risk factor in osteoarthritis. *Arthritis and Rheumatism* 50: 1207–1215.

Delgado-Andrade, C., F. Tessier, C. Niquet-Leridon, I. Seiquer, and M. Pilar Navarro. 2012. Study of the urinary and faecal excretion of n^{ε}-carboxymethyllysine in young human volunteers. *Amino Acids* 43: 595–602.

Dittrich, R. 2006. Concentrations of n^{ε}-carboxymethyllysine in human breast milk, infant formulas, and urine of infants. *Journal of Agricultural and Food Chemistry* 54: 6924–6928.

EFSA. 2015. Scientific opinion on acrylamide in food. *EFSA Journal* 13: 4104.

FEDIAF. 2012a. *Facts & figures No. 2014.* The European Pet Food Industry Federation, Bruxelles, Belgium.

FEDIAF. 2012b. *Nutritional guidelines for complete and complementary pet food for cats and dogs.* FEDIAF—European Pet Food Industry Federation, Bruxelles, Belgium.

Freeman, L. M., M. L. Chandler, B. A. Hamper, and L. P. Weeth. 2013. Current knowledge about the risks and benefits of raw meat-based diets for dogs and cats. *Journal of the American Veterinary Medical Association* 243: 1549–1558.

Hand, M. S., C. D. Thatcher, R. L. Remillard, and P. Roudebush (Editors). 2000. *Small animal clinical nutrition.* Mark Morris Institute, Topeka, KS, 1192 p.

Hendriks, W. H., M. M. A. Emmens, B. Trass, and J. R. Pluske. 1999. Heat processing changes the protein quality of canned cat foods as measured with a rat bioassay. *Journal of Animal Science* 77: 669–676.

Henle, T. 2005. Protein-bound advanced glycation endproducts (ages) as bioactive amino acid derivatives in foods. *Amino Acids* 29: 313–322.

Husøy, T. 2008. Dietary exposure to 5-hydroxymethylfurfural from Norwegian food and correlations with urine metabolites of short-term exposure. *Food and Chemical Toxicology* 46: 3697–3702.

Ikeda, G. J., E. Miller, P. P. Sapienza, T. C. Michel, and P. B. Inskeep. 1987. Comparative tissue distribution and excretion of [1-^{14}c]acrylamide in beagle dogs and miniature pigs. *Food and Chemical Toxicology* 25: 871–875.

Ikeda, G. J. 1983. Distribution of ^{14}c-labelled acrylamide and betaine in foetuses of rats, rabbits, beagle dogs and miniature pigs. *Food and Chemical Toxicology* 21: 49–58.

Knize, M. G., C. P. Salmon, and J. S. Felton. 2003. Mutagenic activity and heterocyclic amine carcinogens in commercial pet foods. *Mutation Research* 539: 195–201.

Knueven, D. 2014. Processed pet foods. *Journal of the American Veterinary Medical Association* 244: 405.

Krause, R., K. Knoll, and T. Henle. 2003. Studies on the formation of furosine and pyridosine during acid hydrolysis of different amadori products of lysine. *European Food Research and Technology* 216: 277–283.

Laflamme, D. P. 2008. Pet feeding practices of dog and cat owners in the United States and Australia. *Journal of the American Veterinary Medical Association* 232: 687–694.

McNicholas, J. 2005. Pet ownership and human health: A brief review of evidence and issues. *British Medical Journal* 331: 1252–1254.

NRC. 2006. *Nutrient requirements of dogs and cats.* National Academies Press, Washington, DC.

Pais, P., M. J. Tanga, C. P. Salmon, and M. G. Knize. 2000. Formation of the mutagen IFP in model systems and detection in restaurant meats. *Journal of Agricultural and Food Chemistry* 48: 1721–1726.

Pet Food Institute. 2014. *Pet dog and cat population No. 2014* http://www.petfoodinstitute.org/?page=PetPopulation. (Accessed December 12, 2014).

Plantinga, E. A., G. Bosch, and W. H. Hendriks. 2011. Estimation of the dietary nutrient profile of free-roaming feral cats: Possible implications for nutrition of domestic cats. *British Journal of Nutrition* 106: S35–S48.

Rokey, G. J., B. Plattner, and E. M. De Souza. 2010. Feed extrusion process description. *Revista Brasileira de Zootecnia* 39: 510–518.

Rufián-Henares, J.A., and S. P. de la Cueva. 2008. Assessment of hydroxymethylfurfural intake in the Spanish diet. *Food Additives and Contaminants—Part A Chemistry, Analysis, Control, Exposure and Risk Assessment* 25: 1306–1312.

Rutherfurd, S. M., K. J. Rutherfurd-Markwick, and P. J. Moughan. 2007. Available (ileal digestible reactive) lysine in selected pet foods. *Journal of Agricultural and Food Chemistry* 55: 3517–3522.

Šebeková, K. 2008. Plasma concentration and urinary excretion of n^{ε}-(carboxymethyl)lysine in breast milk- and formula-fed infants. *Annals of the New York Academy of Sciences* 1126: 177–180.

Shapiro, B. P. 2008. Advanced glycation end products accumulate in vascular smooth muscle and modify vascular but not ventricular properties in elderly hypertensive canines. *Circulation* 118: 1002–1010.

Smit, A. J., and H. L. Lutgers. 2004. The clinical relevance of advanced glycation endproducts (age) and recent developments in pharmaceutics to reduce age accumulation. *Current Medicinal Chemistry* 11: 2767–2784.

Van Rooijen, C. 2013. The maillard reaction and pet food processing: Effects on nutritive value and pet health. *Nutrition Research Reviews* 26: 130–148.

Van Rooijen, C. 2014a. Quantitation of maillard reaction products in commercially available pet foods. *Journal of Agricultural and Food Chemistry* 62: 8883–8891.

Van Rooijen, C. 2014b. Reactive lysine content in commercially available pet foods. *Journal of Nutritional Science* 3: e35.

Van Rooijen, C., G. Bosch, C. I. Butré, A. F. B. Van der Poel, P. A. Wierenga, L. Alexander, and W. H. Hendriks. 2016. Urinary excretion of dietary Maillard reaction products in healthy adult female cats. *Journal of Animal Science* 94: 185–195. doi:10.2527/jas.2015–9550

Veselá, H., and E. Šucman. 2013. Determination of acrylamide in dry feedstuff for dogs and cats. *Acta Veterinaria Brno* 82: 203–208.

Vlassara, H., and G. E. Striker. 2011. Age restriction in diabetes mellitus: A paradigm shift. *Nature Reviews Endocrinology* 7: 526–539.

Weber, K., W. Schmahl, and G. Münch. 1998. Distribution of advanced glycation end products in the cerebellar neurons of dogs. *Brain Research* 791: 11–17.

Williams, P. A., S. M. Hodgkinson, S. M. Rutherfurd, and W. H. Hendriks. 2006. Lysine content in canine diets can be severely heat damaged. *Journal of Nutrition* 136: 1998S–2000S.

24

The Role of AGEs in the Pathogenesis of Macrovascular Complications in Diabetes Mellitus

Marisa Passarelli
University of Sao Paulo Medical School
Sao Paulo, Brazil

CONTENTS

KEY POINTS

- AGEs are increased in diabetes mellitus and are related to the development of micro- and macrovascular complications in this condition.
- AGEs are recognized by the receptor for AGEs (RAGE) leading to intracellular reactive oxygen species generation and transactivation of inflammatory genes.
- AGEs damages insulin sensitivity and disturbs lipid and lipoprotein metabolism.
- AGEs reduce the amount of high-density lipoprotein receptor, ABCA-1, diminishing the exportation of excess cholesterol from these cells.
- The reduction in cholesterol exportation causes cholesterol accumulation in macrophages contributing to atherogenesis.

24.1 Introduction

Advanced glycation end products (AGEs) are prevalent in diabetes mellitus (DM) mainly due to hyperglycemia but also as consequence of kidney function impairment and consumption of high AGE-containing diets. By interacting with the receptor for AGEs (RAGE), they elicit reactive oxygen species (ROS) generation triggering NF-κB activation and the transactivation of inflammatory genes, *Rage*, and other components related to the development of DM long-term complications (Wendt et al. 2006; Ott et al. 2014) (Figure 24.1). Signal transduction triggered by RAGE ligands requires the interaction of its cytoplasmic domain with the formin, DIAPH1 (Shekhtman et al. 2017).

The oxidative stress elicited by AGEs leads to the activation of poly ADP ribose polymerase (PARP) that not only protects DNA structure but also leads to the modification of the glycolytic enzyme, glyceraldehyde 3-phosphate dehydrogenase (G3PD). This impairs the flow along the glycolysis shifting upstream substrates to the formation of methylglyoxal (MGO), leading to further generation of AGEs and ROS (Pacher et al. 2005). Methylglyoxal is a very reactive oxoaldehyde that reacts with lysine and arginine residues in the polypeptide chain leading to the irreversible formation of AGEs (Brownlee 2001). Other carbonyl

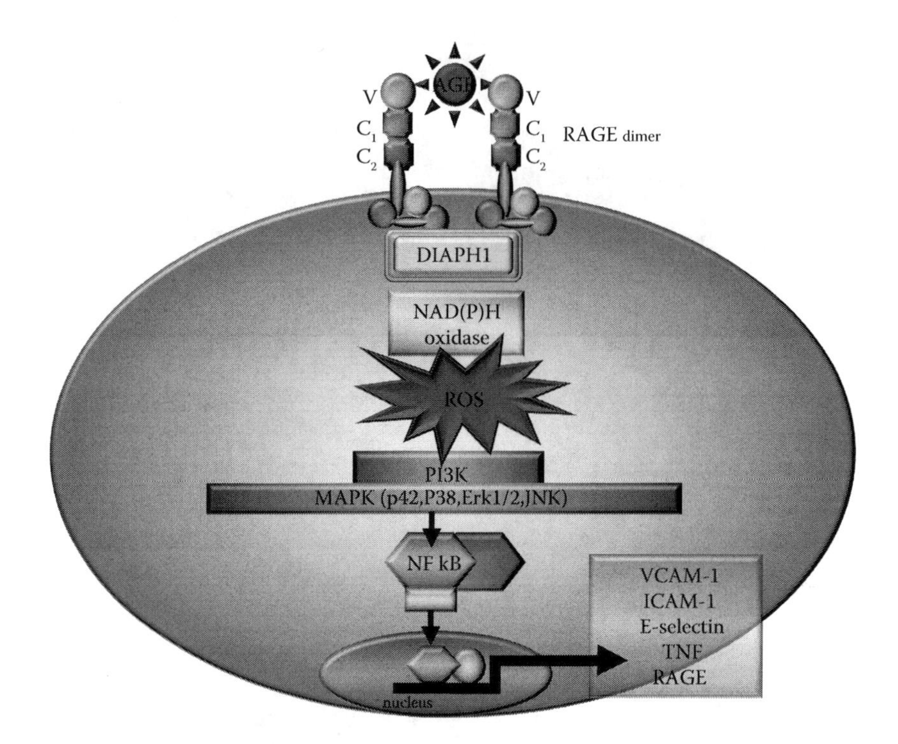

FIGURE 24.1 AGE-RAGE signaling. Advanced glycation end products (AGEs) interact with the receptor for AGEs (RAGE), leading to the generation of reactive oxygen species (ROS) by the NADPH system. Signal transduction triggered by RAGE ligands requires the interaction of its cytoplasmic domain with the formin, DIAPH1. This signaling pathway culminates in the activation NF-κB and transactivation of inflammatory genes, Rage and other components related to the development of DM long-term complications. (Adapted from Ramasamy, R., et al., *Vascul. Pharmacol.*, 57, 160–167, 2012; Shekhtman, A., et al., *Expert Rev. Proteomics.*, 14, 147–156, 2017.)

compounds, such as glyoxal, glycolaldehyde, and 3-deoxyglucosone, can be generated due to Schiff Base and Amadori Product rearrangements in many cases involving oxidative reactions. In addition, the myeloperoxidase reaction, the oxidation of polyunsaturated fatty acids, some aminoacids, and ketone bodies may also lead to oxoaldehyde formation changing macromolecules by AGEs (Henning et al. 2016).

The role of AGEs in the pathophysiology of micro- and macrovascular complications of DM has been extensively demonstrated as well as the implication of growing strategies to limit AGE generation and/or signaling through RAGE (Moriya et al. 2014; Kajikawa et al. 2015; Shah et al. 2016; Shekhtman et al. 2017).

24.2 Role of AGEs in Macrovascular Complications of DM

Levels of glycated hemoglobin (HbA1c) predict the development of micro- and macrovascular complications as demonstrated by many epidemiological diabetes clinical trials. In this sense, an intensive glycemic control established early confers benefits in comparison to subjects maintained in conventional treatment even after a subsequent period of bad glycemic control (Stratton et al. 2000; Nathan et al. 2014). This observation from different clinical trials raised a concept of metabolic memory or legacy effect that lies on the chemical and functional changes imposed by AGEs and oxidative stress in cellular biomolecules (Yamagishi et al. 2017). In additional, epigenetic modulation can also alter long-term gene transcription, contributing to DM complications after a period of diabetic decompensation (Yamagishi et al. 2017).

Skin biopsies from DM patients show different AGE structures whose levels relate to the incidence of DM complications. In addition, the measurement of skin auto fluorescence positively correlated with tissue and circulating AGEs allowing prediction of DM complications with a noninvasive clinical tool (Genuth et al. 2015; Sveen KA et al. 2015; Monnier et al. 2016; Fokkens et al. 2016; Sell et al. 2016).

AGEs predict cardiovascular and total mortality; their plasma concentrations relate to the number of vessels compromised by obstructive coronary disease (Kiuchi et al. 2001). The highest concentration of carboxymethyllysine (CML)—the major AGE structure found *in vivo*—positively correlates with cardiovascular and all-cause mortality (Semba et al. 2009).

Mechanistic studies reveal that endogenous as well as exogenous AGEs alter endothelial function, disrupt nitric oxide synthesis and action, favor endothelin 1–mediated vasoconstriction, and trigger local and systemic inflammation (Brownlee 2001).

Even in the absence of a diabetic milieu, AGEs induce systemic effects that compromise body glycemic homeostasis. In pancreatic islets, AGEs—intraperitoneally administered or from diet source—induced cytoarchitecture damage and compromised insulin secretion (Coughlan et al. 2011). More recent evidence shows that in soleus muscle from healthy rats AGEs induce endoplasmic reticulum stress markers and activate inflammation, leading to a repression of *Slc2a4*/GLUT4 expression and ultimately impaired glucose uptake. In healthy rats chronically administered with AGE-albumin, a worsening in insulin tolerance test was observed reflecting an induced whole-body insulin resistance. This was accompanied by a reduction in *Slc2a4* mRNA and GLUT4 protein and increased nuclear content of NF-κB p105 subunit (Pinto et al. 2016). In adipose tissue, an enhancement in macrophage infiltration is observed, setting the adipocyte to an inflammatory state that may also aggravate insulin resistance (Silva et al. 2016).

By altering insulin sensitivity, AGEs favor alterations in plasma lipid concentration since lipoprotein metabolism is intimately regulated in many steps by insulin (Filippatos et al. 2017). In addition, AGEs increase plasma triglycerides by diminishing the catabolism of chylomicrons and very low-density lipoproteins (VLDL) by the lipoprotein lipase (Mamo et al. 1990). Glycated VLDL and low-density lipoprotein (LDL) are not recognized by the B-E receptor but are recognized by macrophage receptors. AGEs increase the risk of atherosclerosis and cardiovascular mortality (Younis et al. 2008; Soran et al. 2011).

Atherosclerosis is initiated by the formation of foam cell due to the uptake of modified LDL by arterial macrophages. The enhanced half-life of glycated LDL in circulation favors its access to the arterial wall compartment and the uptake by monocyte-derived macrophages (Horiuchi et al. 2003). The intracellular accumulation of cholesterol and inflammation may be counteracted by the excess cholesterol exportation to high-density lipoprotein (HDL). Nonetheless, due to glycation, HDL is removed faster from plasma reducing the availability of cholesterol acceptors that may hamper the reverse cholesterol transport system (RCT) whereby excess of cholesterol is removed from macrophages and transported back to the liver for secretion in bile. Alterations in RCT are well described in DM and genetic diseases favoring atherosclerosis (Yamamoto et al. 2016).

Lipid poor apo A-I (the main apolipoprotein of HDL) and nascent discoidal HDL (named pre beta HDL) interact with the ATP-binding cassette transporter A1 (ABCA-1) in cell membrane. The hydrolysis of two molecules of ATP linked to the nucleotide-binding domain of ABCA-1 promotes cholesterol transfer to the outer membrane leaflet allowing its uptake by apo A-I or pre beta HDL. After cholesterol esterification by the lecithin cholesterol acyltransferase (LCAT), larger HDL particles (HDL_2) are formed with a hydrophobic core filled with esterified cholesterol. These particles remove cell cholesterol and toxic oxysterols by interacting with ABCG-1 transporter. The scavenger receptor class B type 1 (SR-BI) also contributes to cholesterol removal from macrophages, creating a hydrophobic channel by which cholesterol is transferred to HDL. Cholesteryl ester transfer protein (CETP) transfers esterified cholesterol from HDL to apo B-containing lipoproteins (chylomicrons, very low-density lipoprotein, VLDL, and LDL) that are taken up by the B-E receptors in the liver. In addition, esterified cholesterol can be selectively removed by the hepatic SR-BI. Then, cholesterol is converted into bile acids and excreted in feces (Yamamoto et al. 2016).

Lipoprotein glycation alters LCAT, CETP, and SR-BI activity disrupting the cholesterol flow along the RCT (Ohgami et al. 2003; Low et al. 2012; Filippatos et al. 2017). In addition, HDL advanced glycation impairs its ability to remove cell cholesterol and its anti-inflammatory and antioxidant properties (Tan 2009) (Figure 24.2). In mice with alloxan-induced DM type 1, the *in vivo* macrophage-to-feces RCT was 20% lower than in control animals, which was attributed to a decrease in hepatic lipid uptake (de Boer et al. 2012).

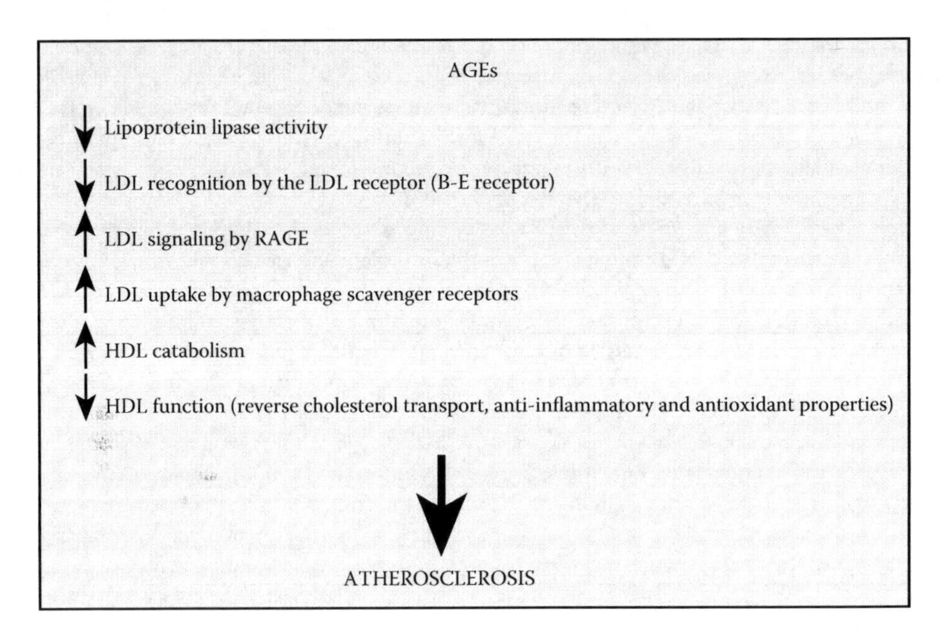

FIGURE 24.2 AGEs adversely affect lipoprotein metabolism favoring atherosclerosis development.

Human skin fibroblasts and macrophages treated with the oxoaldehydes, glycolaldehyde, or glyoxal presented a dose-dependent reduction in ABCA-1 protein content without changes in its mRNA. Consequently, cholesterol efflux to apo A-I is dramatically reduced (Passarelli et al. 2005). Metformin that reduces AGE formation and helps in oxoaldehyde detoxification *in vivo* and the antioxidant and antiglycation drug aminoguanidine were able to prevent alterations in cholesterol efflux in macrophages (Machado et al. 2006).

Oxysterols that derivate from cholesterol oxidation are also enhanced in cells treated with AGEs, especially 7-ketocholesterol (Iborra et al. 2011) that is related to inflammation and apoptosis in atherosclerotic lesion areas favoring plaque rupture.

Albumin is the major serum protein modified by glycation due to its elevated concentration in serum, long half-life, as well as great amount of lysine and arginine residues in its primary structure (Dozio et al. 2017). An enhanced flow of albumin to the interstitial compartment is reported in endothelial dysfunction and atherosclerosis enhancing the susceptibility of albumin to the modification by AGEs generated by local inflammation and oxidative stress (Nerlich et al. 1999; Baidoshvili et al. 2004). Levels of glycated albumin are clinical parameters of glycemic control together with HbA1c (Dozio et al. 2017).

In nondiabetic apo E-KO mice, 1-month intraperitoneal administration of AGE-albumin increased lipid infiltration in aortic arch, as compared to animals that received control albumin. A higher amount of CML, RAGE, 4-hydroxynonenal (a marker of lipid peroxidation), and interleukin 6 (IL-6) were also observed in AGE-albumin-treated mice. These findings reinforce that independent of hyperglycemia, AGEs trigger lipid accumulation in the arterial wall compartment (Gomes et al. 2016).

Advanced glycated albumin reduces ABCA-1 protein levels in macrophages lowering the cholesterol efflux and inducing intracellular accumulation of lipids. The reduction of ABCA-1 was related to the oxidative stress and endoplasmic reticulum stress elicited in those cells by AGEs. Interestingly, the use of aminoguanidine that reduced ROS generation was able to recover ABCA-1 levels (de Souza Pinto et al. 2012). Similarly, cell treatment with a chemical chaperone (4-phenylbutiric acid) that alleviates ER stress restored ABCA-1 and cholesterol efflux to apo A-I (Castilho et al. 2012).

There are data in the literature on the inflammatory role of AGEs, although results from cell cultures may have been biased by endotoxin contamination in AGE-protein samples utilized. Macrophages treated with endotoxin free-AGE-albumin do not increase the secretion of inflammatory markers. On the contrary, AGE-albumin primes macrophages to inflammation elicited by lipopolysaccharides (LPS) or S100B calgranulin. The conditioned medium from cells incubated with AGE-albumin and further with LPS or calgranulin—enriched in IL-6, tumor necrosis factor (TNF), monocyte chemoattractant protein 1 (MCP-1), and vascular cell adhesion molecule 1 (VCAM-1)—reduced cholesterol efflux and ABCA-1 content in naive macrophages (Okuda et al. 2012). In poorly controlled DM, total AGE and CML in albumin purified from serum (corrected per milligram of albumin) are higher when compared to albumin isolated from nondiabetic individuals. In agreement with results observed with *in vitro* glycated albumin, AGE-albumin from DM1 and DM2 patients impaired macrophage cholesterol efflux and selectively altered gene expression. Among genes involved in cell lipid flow, a significant increment was observed in the expression of *Nadphoxidase* (NADPH oxidase) and *Scd1* (stearoyl-CoA desaturase-1). The first is linked to oxidative stress induced by AGE-albumin while the second may confer ABCA-1 mRNA instability due to the action of polyunsaturated fatty acid on the ABCA1 message. On the contrary, the expression of janus kinase (janus kinase 2) was reduced. Janus kinase 2 improves ABCA-1 binding to apo A-I that increases cholesterol efflux and prevents ABCA-1 degradation in the cell surface. Although no changes were observed in *Abca1* gene expression, it is well known that ABCA-1 is mainly regulated by post-transcriptional mechanisms (Machado-Lima et al. 2013; Machado-Lima et al. 2015). In fact, the reduction in ABCA-1 protein levels in macrophages treated with AGE-albumin is consequent to a faster decay rate of the protein due to the ubiquitin/proteasome and lysosomal systems-mediated degradation (Iborra et al. 2014) (Figure 24.3).

Rosuvastatin, a cholesterol-lowering medication that inhibits the activity of HMG CoA reductase, is demonstrated as able to improve cholesterol efflux from macrophage foam cells by blocking the harmful effects of AGEs, namely by suppressing NADPH oxidase activity (Ishibashi et al. 2011).

In streptozotocin-induced DM pigs, the amount of ABCA-1 in the aorta was greatly reduced as compared to nondiabetic animals, pointing the role of hyperglycemia in the down regulation of ABCA-1 increasing atherosclerosis *in vivo* (Passarelli et al. 2005).

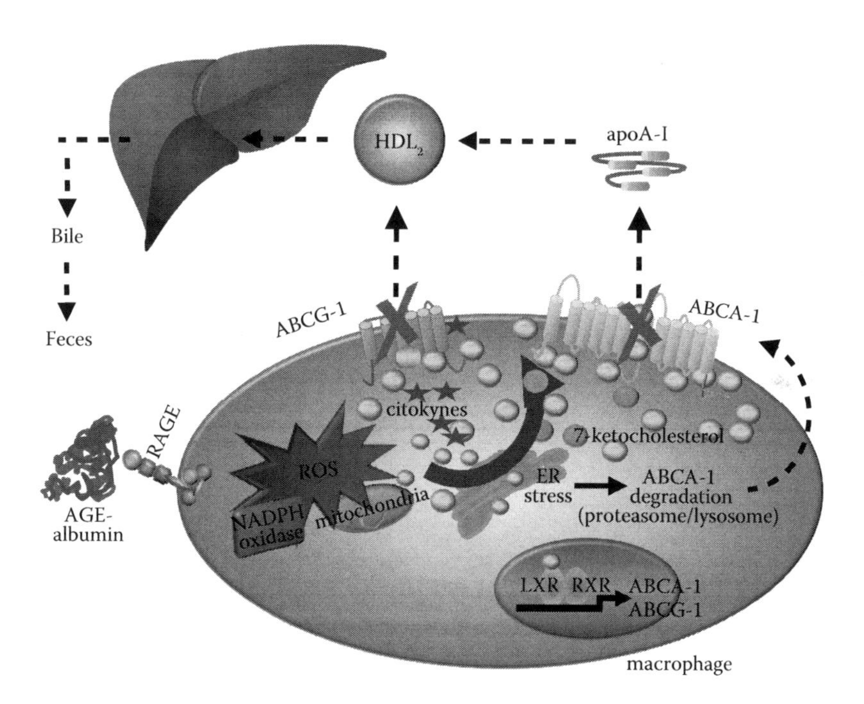

FIGURE 24.3 AGE-albumin impairs macrophage reverse cholesterol transport. In macrophages, AGE-albumin induces ROS generation by the mitochondrial and NADPH oxidase systems, endoplasmic reticulum stress, and inflammatory stress that are related to the reduction of HDL receptors (ABCA-1 and ABCG-1), independent of changes in ABCA-1 mRNA. ABCA-1 protein is faster degradated by the proteasomal and lysosomal systems. The reduction in the exportation of excess cholesterol to apo A-I and large HDL compromises the reverse cholesterol transport, a system that drives cholesterol back to the liver allowing its excretion into bile and feces. This favors intracellular accumulation of cholesterol and toxic oxysterols, such as 7-ketocholesterol, leading to inflammation and atherogenesis.

Serum albumin was isolated prior to and after adequate glycemic control in human DM subjects. Interestingly, the reduction in cholesterol efflux from macrophages elicited by AGE-albumin isolated during the inadequate glycemic control was no longer observed in cells incubated with albumin drawn after adjusted glycemic control, represented by lower levels of fructosamine, glycated albumin, HbA1c, and CML-albumin. In addition, the effect of AGE-albumin on cell lipid homeostasis was abrogated by RAGE-silencing or by utilizing macrophages from RAGE-KO mice (Machado-Lima et al. 2016).

RAGE is highly expressed in atherosclerotic lesions, particularly in macrophages. In those cells, cholesterol efflux to apolipoprotein A-I and HDL and reverse cholesterol transport to plasma, liver, and feces were reduced in diabetic macrophages through RAGE (Daffu et al. 2015), which mediates lipid accumulation in macrophages (Xu et al. 2016). In fact, RAGE deletion or antagonism by soluble RAGE reduces neointima formation and diminishes the atherosclerotic lesion development in diabetic apo E-KO mice which is attributed to reduction in macrophages and vascular inflammation (Park et al. 1998; Bu et al. 2010; Morris-Rosenfeld et al. 2011).

In chronic kidney disease, atherosclerosis is not only prevalent in and related to the presence of traditional risk factors but also to nontraditional risk factors such as AGEs. Independent of hyperglycemia, AGE formation in CKD is accelerated due to failure in detoxification of intermediate products of the glycation reaction as well as due to the increased oxidative stress (Stinghen et al. 2016). Circulating AGEs and lipid peroxidation products (TBARS) are elevated in CKD rats as compared to healthy control animals. In addition, and in resemblance of DM-albumin, serum albumin from CDK-rats impairs macrophage cholesterol efflux and elicits endoplasmic reticulum stress in macrophages. Interestingly, N-acetylcysteine, a potent antioxidant, reduces plasma AGEs and TBARS and ameliorates the cholesterol efflux by diminishing endoplasmic reticulum stress (Machado et al. 2014). On the contrary, no changes in the *in vivo* RCT were found in uremic mice despite elevated AGEs (Low et al. 2012).

24.3 Conclusion

In summary, AGEs directly influence atherogenesis by inducing oxidative stress, endoplasmic reticulum stress, and inflammation, leading to intracellular lipid accumulation. Also, by considering its role in metabolic memory and epigenetics, AGEs seem to contribute to the association observed between hyperglycemia and cardiovascular risk in DM as shown by epidemiological studies such as UKPS and DCCT/EDIC.

Considering the high amount of AGEs in processed foods and high-fat diets and the fast generation of AGEs independently of hyperglycemia, recent evidence indicates an important role of AGEs in the pathophysiology of DM. In this regard, strategies to improve glycemic control, to reduce exogenous AGEs, inducing AGE intermediates detoxification and/or blocking AGE signaling may be useful to prevent derangements in glucose and lipid homeostasis and to avoid the deleterious effects of AGEs on the development of atherosclerosis and other chronic complications of DM.

REFERENCES

Baidoshvili A, Niessen HW, Stooker W, Huybregts RA, Hack CE, Rauwerda JA, Meijer CJ, et al. 2004. N(omega)-(carboxymethyl)lysine depositions in human aortic heart valves: Similarities with atherosclerotic blood vessels. *Atherosclerosis.* 174:287–92.

Brownlee M. 2001. Biochemistry and molecular cell biology of diabetic complications. *Nature* 414:813–20.

Bu DX, Rai V, Shen X, Rosario R, Lu Y, D'Agati V, Yan SF, et al. 2010. Activation of the ROCK1 branch of the transforming growth factor-beta pathway contributes to RAGE-dependent acceleration of atherosclerosis in diabetic apoE-null mice. *Circ Res* 106:1040–51.

Castilho G, Okuda LS, Pinto RS, Iborra RT, Nakandakare ER, Santos CX, Laurindo FR, et al. 2012. ER stress is associated with reduced ABCA-1 protein levels in macrophages treated with advanced glycated albumin—Reversal by a chemical chaperone. *Int J Biochem Cell Biol.* 44:1078–86.

Coughlan MT, Yap FY, Tong DC, Andrikopoulos S, Gasser A, Thallas-Bonke V, Webster DE, et al. 2011. Advanced glycation end products are direct modulators of β-cell function. *Diabetes* 60:2523–32.

Daffu G, Shen X, Senatus L, Thiagarajan D, Abedini A, Hurtado Del Pozo C, Rosario R, et al. 2015. RAGE suppresses ABCG1-Mediated macrophage cholesterol efflux in diabetes. *Diabetes* 64:4046–60.

de Boer JF, Annema W, Schreurs M, van der Veen JN, van der Giet M, Nijstad N, Kuipers F, et al. 2012. Type I diabetes mellitus decreases *in vivo* macrophage-to-feces reverse cholesterol transport despite increased biliary sterol secretion in mice. *J Lipid Res.* 53:348–57.

de Souza Pinto R, Castilho G, Paim BA, Machado-Lima A, Inada NM, Nakandakare ER, Vercesi AE, et al. Inhibition of macrophage oxidative stress prevents the reduction of ABCA-1 transporter induced by advanced glycated albumin. 2012. Inhibition of macrophage oxidative stress prevents the reduction of ABCA-1 transporter induced by advanced glycated albumin. *Lipids* 47:443–50.

Dozio E, Di Gaetano N, Findeisen P, Corsi Romanelli MM. 2017. Glycated albumIn: From biochemistry and laboratory medicine to clinical practice. *Endocrine* 55:682–90.

Filippatos T, Tsimihodimos V, Pappa E, Elisaf M. 2017. Pathophysiology of diabetic dyslipidaemia. *Curr Vasc Pharmacol.* 31. doi: 10.2174/1570 161115666170201105425.

Fokkens BT, Smit AJ. 2016. Skin fluorescence as a clinical tool for non-invasive assessment of advanced glycation and long-term complications of diabetes. *Glycoconj J.* 33:527–35.

Genuth S, Sun W, Cleary P, Gao X, Sell DR, Lachin J; DCCT/EDIC Research Group, Monnier VM. 2015. Skin advanced glycation end products glucosepane and methylglyoxal hydroimidazolone are independently associated with long-term microvascular complication progression of type 1 diabetes. *Diabetes* 64:266–78.

Gomes DJ, Velosa AP, Okuda LS, Fusco FB, da Silva KS, Pinto PR, Nakandakare ER, et al. 2016. Glycated albumin induces lipid infiltration in mice aorta independently of DM and RAS local modulation by inducing lipid peroxidation and inflammation. *J Diabetes Complications* 30:1614–21.

Henning C, Glomb MA. 2016. Pathways of the Maillard reaction under physiological conditions. *Glycoconj J.* 33:499–512.

Horiuchi S, Sakamoto Y, Sakai M. 2003. Scavenger receptors for oxidized and glycated proteins. *Amino Acids* 25:283–92.

Iborra, R.T. 2011. Advanced glycation in macrophages induces intracellular accumulation of 7-ketocholesterol and total sterols by decreasing the expression of ABCA-1 and ABCG-1. *Lipids Health Dis.* 10:172.

Iborra RT, Machado-Lima A, Castilho G, Nunes VS, Abdalla DS, Nakandakare ER, Passarelli M. 2014. Selective inhibition of proteasomal and lysosomal degradation pathways partially prevent abca-1 reduction in macrophages induced by advanced glycated albumin. *Atherosclerosis* 235(2):e97–8.

Ishibashi Y, Matsui T, Takeuchi M, Yamagishi S. 2011. Rosuvastatin blocks advanced glycation end products-elicited reduction of macrophage cholesterol efflux by suppressing NADPH oxidase activity via inhibition of geranylgeranylation of Rac-1. *Horm Metab Res.* 43:619–24.

Kajikawa M, Nakashima A, Fujimura N, Maruhashi T, Iwamoto Y, Iwamoto A, Matsumoto T, et al. 2015. Ratio of serum levels of AGEs to soluble form of RAGE is a predictor of endotelial function. *Diabetes Care* 38:119–25.

Kiuchi K, Nejima J, Takano T, Ohta M, Hashimoto H. 2001. Increased serum concentrations of advanced glycation end products: A marker of coronary artery disease activity in type 2 diabetic patients. *Heart.* 85:87–91.

Low H, Hoang A, Forbes J, Thomas M, Lyons JG, Nestel P, Bach LA, et al. 2012. Advanced glycation end-products (AGEs) and functionality of reverse cholesterol transport in patients with type 2 diabetes and in mouse models. *Diabetologia* 55:2513–21.

Machado AP, Pinto RS, Moysés ZP, Nakandakare ER, Quintão EC, Passarelli M. 2006. Aminoguanidine and metformin prevent the reduced rate of HDL-mediated cell cholesterol efflux induced by formation of advanced glycation end products. *Int J Biochem Cell Biol.* 38:392–403.

Machado JT, Iborra RT, Fusco FB, Castilho G, Pinto RS, Machado-Lima A, Nakandakare ER, et al. 2014. N-acetylcysteine prevents endoplasmic reticulum stress elicited in macrophages by sérum albumin drawn from chronic kidney disease rats and selectively affects lipid transporters, ABCA-1 and ABCG-1. *Atherosclerosis.* 237:343–52.

Machado JT, Iborra RT, Fusco FB, Castilho G, Pinto RS, Machado-Lima A, Nakandakare ER, et al. 2013. Advanced glycated albumin isolated from poorly controlled type 1 diabetes mellitus patients alters macrophage gene expression impairing ABCA-1-mediated reverse cholesterol transport. *Diabetes Metab Res Rev.* 29:66–76.

Machado-Lima A, Iborra RT, Pinto RS, Castilho G, Sartori CH, Oliveira ER, Okuda LS, et al. 2015. In type 2 diabetes mellitus glycated albumin alters macrophage gene expression. impairing ABCA1-mediated cholesterol efflux. *J. Cell Physiol.* 230:1250–7.

Machado-Lima, A, Torres R, Mello M, Bonavolonta SAR, Machado UF, Correa-Giannella MLC, Nakandakare ER, et al. 2016. Mejora del control glucémico incrementa el ABCA-1 en macrófagos incubados com albumina aislada de diabéticos. Paper presented at the 2nd Simposio Iberoamericano AGEs. Santiago, Universidade de Chile.

Mamo JC, Szeto L, Steiner G. 1990. Glycation of very low density lipoprotein from rat plasma impairs its catabolism. *Diabetologia.* 33:339–45.

Monnier VM, Genuth S, Sell DR. 2016. The pecking order of skin Advanced Glycation Endproducts (AGEs) as long-term markers of glycemic damage and risk factors for micro- and subclinical macrovascular disease progression in Type 1 diabetes. *Glycoconj J.* 33:569–79.

Moriya S, Yamazaki M, Murakami H, Maruyama K, Uchiyama S. Two soluble isoforms of receptors for advanced glycation end products (RAGE) in carotid atherosclerosis: the difference of soluble and endogenous secretory RAGE. 2014. *J Stroke Cerebrovasc Dis.* 23:2540–6.

Morris-Rosenfeld S, Blessing E, Preusch MR, Albrecht C, Bierhaus A, Andrassy M, Nawroth PP, et al. 2011. Deletion of bone marrow-derived receptor for advanced glycation end products inhibits atherosclerotic plaque progression. *Eur J Clin Invest* 41:1164–71.

Nathan DM; DCCT/EDIC Research Group. 2014. The diabetes control and complications trial/epidemiology of diabetes interventions and complications study at 30 years: Overview. *Diabetes Care* 37:9–16.

Nerlich AG, Schleicher ED. 1999. N(epsilon)-(carboxymethyl)lysine in atherosclerotic vascular lesions as a marker for local oxidative stress. *Atherosclerosis* 144(1):41–7.

Ohgami, N. 2003. Advanced glycation end products (AGE) inhibit scavenger receptor class B type I-mediated reverse cholesterol transport: A new crossroad of AGE to cholesterol metabolism. *J Atheroscler Thromb.* 10:1–6.

Okuda LS, Castilho G, Rocco DD, Nakandakare ER, Catanozi S, Passarelli M. 2012. Advanced glycated albumin impairs HDL anti-inflammatory activity and primes macrophages for inflammatory response that reduces reverse cholesterol transport. *Biochim Biophys Acta.* 1821:1485–92.

Ott C, Jacobs K, Haucke E, Navarrete Santos A, Grune T, Simm A. 2014. Role of advanced glycation end products in cellular signaling. *Redox Biol.* 2:411–29.

Pacher P, Szabó C. 2005. Role of poly(ADP-ribose) polymerase-1 activation in the pathogenesis of diabetic complications: Endothelial dysfunction, as a common underlying theme. *Antioxid Redox Signal.* 7:1568–80.

Park L, Raman KG, Lee KJ, Lu Y, Ferran LJ Jr, Chow WS, Stern D, et al. 1998. Suppression of accelerated diabetic atherosclerosis by the soluble receptor for advanced glycation endproducts. *Nat Med* 4:1025–31.

Passarelli M, Tang C, McDonald TO, O'Brien KD, Gerrity RG, Heinecke JW, Oram JF. 2005. Advanced glycation end product precursors impair ABCA1-dependent cholesterol removal from cells. *Diabetes* 54:2198–205.

Pinto Jr DC, Silva KS, Passarelli M, Machado UF. 2016. Advanced glycation end products-induced insulin resistance involvement of skeletal muscle GLUT4 repression. *Paper presented at the 2nd Simposio Iberoamericano AGEs.* Santiago, Universidade de Chile.

Ramasamy R, Yan SF, Schmidt AM. 2012. The diverse ligand repertoire of the receptor for advanced glycation endproducts and pathways to the complications of diabetes. *Vascul Pharmacol.* 57:160–7.

Sell DR, Sun W, Gao X, Strauch C, Lachin JM, Cleary PA, Genuth S; DCCT/EDIC Research Group, Monnier VM. 2016. Skin collagen fluorophore LW-1 versus skin fluorescence as markers for the long-term progression of subclinical macrovascular disease in type 1 diabetes. *Cardiovasc Diabetol.* 15:30. doi: 10.1186/s12933-016-0343-3.

Semba RD, Bandinelli S, Sun K, Guralnik JM, Ferrucci L. 2009. Plasma carboxymethyl-lysine, an advanced glycation end product, and all-cause and cardiovascular disease mortality in older community-dwelling adults. *J Am Geriatr Soc.* 57:1874–80.

Shah MS, Brownlee M. 2016. Molecular and cellular mechanisms of cardiovascular disorders in diabetes. *Circ Res.*118:1808–29.

Shekhtman A, Ramasamy R, Schmidt AM. 2017. Glycation & the RAGE axis: Targeting signal transduction through DIAPH1. *Expert Ver Proteomics.* 14:147–56.

Silva, KS, Pinto PR, Gomes DJ, Fabre NT, Thieme K, Shimizu MHM, Okamoto M, et al. 2016. N-acetylcysteine prevents lipid peroxidation, inflammation and insulin resistance induced by advanced glycated albumin in Wistar rats. *Paper presented at the 2nd Simposio Iberoamericano AGEs*. Santiago, Universidade de Chile.

Soran H, Durrington PN. 2011. Susceptibility of LDL and its subfractions to glycation. *Curr Opin Lipidol.* 22:254–61.

Stinghen, A.E., Massy, Z.A., Vlassara, H., Striker, G.E., Boullier, A. 2016. Uremic toxicity of advanced glycation end products in CKD. *J Am Soc Nephrol.* 27(2):354–70.

Stratton IM, Adler AI, Neil HA, Matthews DR, Manley SE, Cull CA, Hadden D, et al. 2000. Association of glycaemia with macrovascular and microvascular complications of type 2 diabetes (UKPDS 35): Prospective observational study. *BMJ.* 321:405–12.

Sveen KA, Dahl-Jørgensen K, Stensaeth KH, Angel K, Seljeflot I, Sell DR, Monnier VM, et al. 2015. Glucosepane and oxidative markers in skin collagen correlate with intima media thickness and arterial stiffness in long-term type 1 diabetes. *J Diabetes Complications* 29:407–12.

Tan, K.C. 2009. Reverse cholesterol transport in type 2 diabetes mellitus. *Diabetes Obes Metab* 11:534–43.

Wendt T, Harja E, Bucciarelli L, Qu W, Lu Y, Rong LL, Jenkins DG, et al. 2006. RAGE modulates vascular inflammation and atherosclerosis in a murine model of type 2 diabetes. *Atherosclerosis* 185:70–7.

Xu L, Wang YR, Li PC, Feng B. 2016. Advanced glycation end products increase lipids accumulation in macrophages through upregulation of receptor of advanced glycation end products: Increasing uptake, esterification and decreasing efflux of cholesterol. *Lipids Health Dis.* 15:161–73.

Yamagishi SI, Nakamura N, Matsui T. 2017. Glycation and cardiovascular disease in diabetes: A perspective on the concept of metabolic memory. *J Diabetes.* 9:141–8.

Yamamoto S, Narita I, Kotani K. 2016. The macrophage and its related cholesterol efflux as a HDL function index in atherosclerosis. *Clin Chim Acta.* 457:117–22.

Younis N, Sharma R, Soran H, Charlton-Menys V, Elseweidy M, Durrington PN. 2008. Glycation as an atherogenic modification of LDL. *Curr Opin Lipidol.* 19:378–84.

Section IV

Therapeutic Alternatives to Deal with Dietary AGEs

25

Plant-Derived Products with Antiglycation Activity

Laura C. Cogoi
Universidad de Buenos Aires
Buenos Aires, Argentina

Rosana Filip
CONICET-Universidad de Buenos Aires
Instituto de Química y Metabolismo del Fármaco (IQUIMEFA)
Buenos Aires, Argentina

CONTENTS

KEY POINTS

- Plant extracts and phytochemicals evidenced the capacity to prevent some diseases associated with oxidative stress and advanced glycation end product (AGE) formation.
- Polyphenols are the main group of compounds with anti-AGE activities and the published scientific evidence is presented.
- The ability of polyphenols to prevent AGE formation depends on their structure (phenolic acids, flavonoids, and stilbenes).
- Terpenoids (terpenes and carotenoids) have gained relevance as potential anti-AGE agents in recent times.
- This review focuses on the potential of plant-derived products to develop medicines for treating diseases at a lower cost and toxicity than synthetic antiglycant pharmaceutical agents.

25.1 Introduction

Nonenzymatic glycation involves a series of chemical reactions that occur between the carbonyl group of reducing sugars and the amino group of proteins, lipids, and nucleic acids [1,2]. After a series of reactions, a complex family of stable covalent adducts called advanced glycation end products (AGEs) is formed [3]. AGEs can be derived from diet or from endogenous generation. The nonenzymatic reaction between the free amino groups of proteins and carbonyl groups of reducing sugars or other carbonyl compounds is known as Maillard reaction. In the human body, the process of forming AGEs can be considered as having three stages: early, intermediate, and late. At the early stage, the amino groups of biological amines react with the carbonyl groups of glucose or other reducing sugars to form the Schiff bases, which further undergo arrangements to form Amadori adducts. In the secondary stage, α-dicarbonyls and highly reactive compounds such as glyoxal (GO), methylglyoxal (MGO), and 3-deoxyglucosone (3-DG) are formed (from oxidation or hydrolysis of the Amadori adducts), which react with proteins to form AGEs. In the last stage, most AGEs form intermolecular or intramolecular cross-links on long-lived proteins. AGE-modified proteins lose their specific functions and undergo accelerated degradation to form free AGEs such as 2-(2-furoyl)-4(5)-furanyl-1H-imidazole, imidazolone, N-ε-carboxymethyllysine (CML), N-ε-carboxyethyllysine, glyoxal-lysine dimer, and methylglyoxal-lysine dimer, among others [4–6].

Other pathways involved in AGE generation include autoxidation of glucose, or ascorbate and lipid peroxidation. Dicarbonyl intermediates, for example, MGO, GO, 3-DG glycolaldehyde, 1-DG [7], and free radicals [8] have been shown to have a strong relationship with AGE formation.

Cross-linking of extracellular matrix proteins leads to increased vascular stiffness and diminished vascular compliance [9]. AGEs contribute to the development of a proinflammatory and proliferative state with increased oxidative stress, resulting in endothelial dysfunction, the common underlying mechanism leading to organ damage [10]. On the contrary, AGEs interact with the receptor for AGEs (RAGE) to initiate intracellular signaling that disturbs cellular function, with the triggering of inflammatory response and oxidative stress. AGEs are known to have a pathogenic significance in diabetes, nephropathy, retinopathy, neuropathy, atherosclerosis, Alzheimer's disease, and arthritis, among several other chronic diseases [11]. In addition to AGEs that form within the body, AGEs also exist in processed foods, and several strategies to limit their formation have been reported [12]. Recent studies demonstrated the potential use of extracts of *Ilex paraguariensis* for the prevention of AGE formation and lipoperoxidation during the process of frying eggs [13].

The discovery of compounds that could act as endogenous AGE inhibitors would offer a potential preventive tool and therapeutic approach for lowering the risks of pathogenic complications caused by AGE formation in the body.

Synthetic compounds have been evaluated as inhibitors against the formation of AGEs, however, they were withdrawn from clinical trials due to relatively low efficacy and unsatisfactory safety [14,15]. Natural products have been proven to be relatively safe for human consumption when compared with synthetic compounds. Medicines of natural origin appear to offer the possibility of treating diseases at a lower cost and with low toxicity. Recent studies have highlighted the benefits of using plants with antiglycation properties in diabetic patients [16]. Some plant extracts and compounds derived from them have been examined for their activities to inhibit AGE formation. As oxidative stress accompanies and accelerates the formation of AGEs, there is an increasing interest in the antioxidant effects of compounds derived from plants that could be relevant in relation to their role in the disease state. Many plant extracts and natural substances isolated from them have been tested for their ability to prevent AGE formation [17].

Some polyphenols [18,19], triterpenes and saponins [20–22], and carotenoids [23] were shown to decrease AGE formation.

Polyphenols constitute the major group of plant-derived compounds with anti-AGE activities, mainly due to the ability to decrease AGE formation [18,19]; however, other phytochemicals like terpenoids have gained relevance in this area in recent times [20–28].

This report focuses on the scientific evidence on the anti-AGE activities of the main polyphenols and terpenoids present in plants.

25.2 Polyphenols

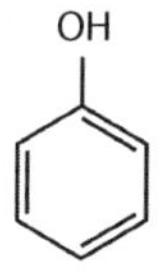

The basic structural feature of phenolic compounds is an aromatic ring bearing one or more hydroxyl groups (Figure 25.1). Plant phenolic compounds are classified as simple phenols or polyphenols based on the number of phenol units in the molecule. Thus, plant phenolics comprise simple phenols, phenolic acids, flavonoids coumarins, lignins, lignans, and condensed and hydrolysable tannins [29].

FIGURE 25.1 Basic structure of phenol.

Polyphenols present in dietary and medicinal plant species are the most abundant antioxidants. On a molecular level, all of these compounds "absorb" harmful free radicals and chelate prooxidant metal ions. Most of them also modulate cellular biochemical reactions and the expression of genes and proteins associated with oxidative stress. They have been shown to have many health benefits, such as preventing heart disease [30,31], reducing inflammation [32,33], lowering the incidence of cancers [34–37] and diabetes [38,39], as well as reducing the rates of mutagenesis in human cells [34,40].

Polyphenols have been classified by the source of origin, biological function, and chemical structure. The majority of polyphenols in plants exist as glycosides with different sugar units and with sugars acylated at different positions of the polyphenol skeletons [41]. Chemically, this group is highly diverse and can be divided into different classes according to the structures of aglycones that determine their bioactivity [42–45].

25.2.1 Phenolic Acids

Phenolic acids have two parent structures: hydroxycinnamic and hydroxybenzoic acid. Hydroxybenzoic acids contain a C6-C1 aromatic ring with one or more hydroxyl groups and hydroxycinnamic acids, a C6-C3 skeleton with one or more hydroxyl groups (Figure 25.2). The effect of phenolic acids derivatives on inhibition of protein glycation has been determined by several groups. Hydroxybenzoic acids (gallic acid and vanillic acid) and hydroxycinnamic acids (ferulic acid and chlorogenic acid) showed inhibitory activity of glycation of bovine serum albumin (BSA) [46].

Gallic acid derivatives isolated from *Rhus verniciflua* extracts have been shown to inhibit recombinant human aldose reductase as well as the accumulation of AGEs in BSA-glucose model system [47].

Cyperus rotundus extracts showed a potent inhibitory activity on AGEs formation and protein oxidation due to gallic acid and *p*-coumaric acid [48]. A new gallic acid derivative, 7-*O*-galloyl-D-sedoheptulose, isolated from *Cornus officinalis* reduced renal damage, AGE formation, and oxidative stress in diabetic rats. Moreover, this compound reduced Maillard reaction–induced CML formation *via* the marked inhibition of mitochondrial lipid peroxidation. It also effectively ameliorates the increases in serum creatinine and urinary protein to nearly normal levels [49].

(a)

Cinnamic acid ($R_1 = R_2 = R_3 = R_4 = H$)
Caffeic acid ($R_2 = R_3 = OH; R_1 = R_4 = H$)
Ferulic acid ($R_2 = OMe; R_3 = OH; R_1 = R_4 = H$)
o-Coumaric acid ($R_1 = OH; R_2 = R_3 = R_4 = H$)
m-Coumaric acid ($R_2 = OH; R_1 = R_3 = R_4 = H$)
p-Coumaric acid ($R_3 = OH; R_1 = R_2 = R_4 = H$)

(b)

Benzoic acid ($R_1 = R_2 = R_3 = R_4 = H$)
p-Hydroxibenzoic acid ($R_2 = OH; R_1 = R_3 = R_4 = H$)
Vanillic acid ($R_1 = OMe; R_2 = OH; R_3 = R_4 = H$)
Gallic acid ($R_1 = R_2 = R_3 = OH; R_4 = H$)
Protocacheuic acid ($R_1 = R_2 = OH; R_3 = R_4 = H$)

FIGURE 25.2 Basic structures of phenolic acids. (a) Cinnamic acid derivatives. (b) Benzoic acid derivatives.

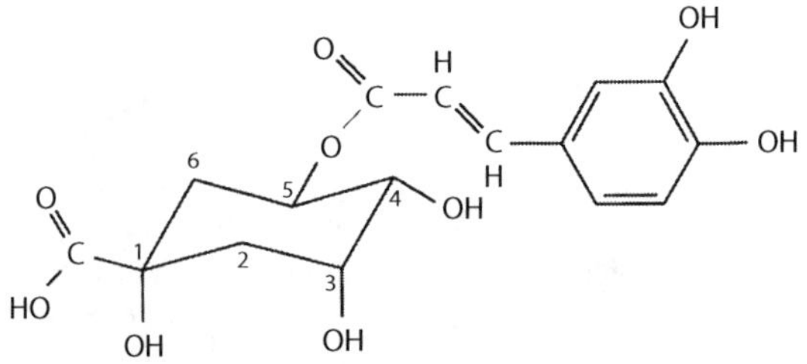

FIGURE 25.3 Structure of 5-caffeoylquinic acid (chlorogenic acid) which shows the IUPAC (International Union of Pure Applied Chemistry) numbering for the quinic acid residue.

I. paraguariensis and *Chrysanthemum* spp. extracts demonstrated marked inhibition of the formation of AGEs and CML in *in vitro* model systems associated with the presence of caffeic acid and chlorogenic acid (5-caffeoylquinic acid) [15] (Figures 25.2 and 25.3). Moreover, chlorogenic acid may interfere with intestinal glucose absorption and has been shown to modulate gene expression of antioxidant enzymes [50]. In coffee extracts, chlorogenic acid together with polyphenols such as caffeoylquinic, *p*-coumaroylquinic, feruloylquinic, and dicaffeoylquinic acids contributed to about 70% of the antioxidant capacity of the coffee fractions [51]. Caffeoylquinic acid derivatives isolated from ethyl acetate soluble extract of the leaves and stems of *Erigeron annuus* exhibited potent inhibitory activity against AGE formation; inhibition of RLAR (rat lens aldose reductase), AGE-BSA cross-linking, and cataractogenesis were also observed [52].

Ferulic acid, another cinnamic acid, which occurs naturally in some fruits and vegetables possesses free radical–scavenging properties toward hydroxyl radicals, peroxynitrite, and oxidized low-density lipoprotein (LDL) *in vitro* [53]. It has also been shown that ferulic acid can bind human serum albumin to form complexes, providing unusual protective effects against protein oxidation. It was also reported that ferulic acid reduces the formation of CML and fluorescent AGEs *in vitro* [54].

Miroliaei et al. [55] reported the presence of rosmarinic acid, a dimer of caffeic acid, in *Melissa officinalis* L. (balm) extract. The chaperone-like activity of this compound would afford a protective effect against AGE-induced toxicity by suppression of receptor signaling pathways, for example, RAGE antagonists.

Comparing the structures of the phenolic acids with their anti-AGE activities, some authors concluded that the hydroxyls in positions 3, 4, and 5 are positive to the activities, while the methoxylation of these positions is negative. In addition, the hydrogenation of the unsaturated bonds of the substituents enhances the anti-AGE activities of phenolic acids. In caffeoylquinic acids, caffeoyl groups contributed to the activity of quinic acid derivatives on inhibiting AGE formation. Caffeoyl group at position 4 showed much stronger activity than that with the one at position 3 [9].

25.2.2 Flavonoids

Flavonoids have the C6–C3–C6 general structural backbone in which the two C6 units (ring A and ring B) are of phenolic nature. General structure and numbering pattern for common flavonoids are shown in Figure 25.4. Due to the hydroxylation pattern and variations in the structure of ring C, flavonoids may be divided into six different major classes (flavones, flavonols, flavanones, flavanols [flavan-3-ol], isoflavones, and anthocyanins) [56,57]. While the vast majority of the flavonoids have their ring B attached to the C2 position of ring C, in some flavonoids such as isoflavones, ring B is connected at the C3 of ring C. Linkages, unsaturation positions, and functional groups of each flavonoid subclass are summarized in Table 25.1.

Numerous flavonoids are well-known antioxidants due to the ability to scavenge free radicals, chelation of transition metal ions, sparing of LDL-associated antioxidants, and binding to macromolecules or interaction with other kinds of antioxidants [58]. The antioxidant capacity of flavonoids depends on both their structure and their glycosylation pattern.

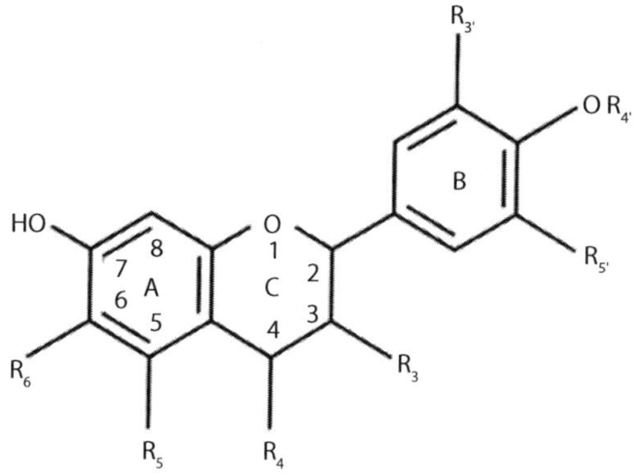

FIGURE 25.4 General structure and numbering pattern for common flavonoids. For most flavonoids, $R_{4'}$ = H, R_5 = OH, and R_6 = H.

TABLE 25.1

Flavonoid Subclasses, Their Chemical Characteristics and Name of Prominent Flavonoids

Flavonoid Subclass	C Ring Unsaturation	C Ring Functional Group	Prominent Flavonoid
Flavonol	2-3 Double bond	3-hydroxy4-Oxo	Isorhamnetin Kaempferol Myricetin Quercetin
Flavones	2-3 Double bond	4-Oxo	Apigenin Luteolin
Flavanone	None	4-Oxo	Naringenin Hesperitin
Flavanol	None	3-hydroxy3-O-gallate	(+)-Catechin (-)-Epicatechin (+)-Gallocatechin (-)-Epicatechin-3-gallate
Isoflavones	2-3 Double bond	4-Oxo	Daidzein Genistein
Anthocyanidins	1-2, 3-4 Double bonds	3-hydroxy	Cyanidin Delphinidin Petunidin

Source: Adapted from Patel, J.M., *Lethbridge Undergrad. Res J.*, 3, 2008.

25.2.2.1 *Flavones, Flavonols, and Flavanones*

Flavones and their 3-hydroxy derivatives, flavonols, including their glycosides, methoxides, and other acylated products, make the largest subgroup among all polyphenols [41].

Kaempferol is a well-known antioxidant flavonol aglycone that possesses anti-inflammatory activity. This compound showed the ability to diminish the formation of reactive species, inhibition of the inducible nitric oxide (NO) synthase and cyclooxygenase-2, and the downregulation of NF-κB pathway [59]. It was demonstrated that the short-term feeding of aged rats with kaempferol modulated both AGE accumulation and RAGE expression. Furthermore, kaempferol suppressed age-related NF-κB activation and its proinflammatory genes through the suppression of AGE-induced NADPH oxidase activation [60].

Quercetin is another example of flavonol. Plant extracts containing quercetin and quercetin-derived glycosides, as well as gallic acid and ferulic acid, significantly decreased fasting blood glucose levels in streptozotocin-induced diabetic rats, decreased glycation products and lipid peroxidation, and improved the antioxidant status in a dose-dependent manner [61].

The flavonoid glycosides isoquercitrin (quercetin-3-β-glucopyranoside) and hyperin (quercetin-3-D-galactoside) showed outstanding antioxidant activity in yeast cells by increasing the activity of superoxide dismutase. Inhibition of the hydroxyl radical, superoxide anion generation, and lipopolysaccharide-induced NO production were also reported for these compounds [62].

Rutin (quercetin-3-O-rutinoside) showed potent antioxidant capacities in different *in vitro* antioxidant models and remarkable inhibitory activities on RLAR and AGE formation [63]. Rutin was also found to be an effective inhibitor of lipoprotein glycation by increasing the resistance of LDL to HG/Cu (II)-mediated oxidation [64].

Apigenin (4',5,7-trihydroxyflavone) and luteolin (2-(3,4-dihydroxyphenyl)-5,7-dihydroxy-4-chromenone) demonstrated their role in inhibiting AGE formation *in vitro* [24]. Vitexin (apigenin-8-C-glucoside) and isovitexin (apigenin-6-C-glucoside) are flavone C-glucosides with anti-inflammatory, antirheumatic, and antimicrobial activities. Their antiglycation activity could be attributed to their free radical–scavenging and/or metal ion–trapping activities, as they failed to directly trap reactive carbonyl species, such as MGO [65].

The number of flavanones and their 3-hydroxy derivatives (flavanols) identified in the last 15 years has significantly increased. Flavanones isolated from *Viscum album* (European mistletoe) showed a potent antiglycation activity, as well as superoxide anion scavenging capacity. The antioxidant potential of 4′,5-dimethoxy-7-hydroxy flavanone was determined to be greater than that of rutin used as a standard [16].

25.2.2.2 Flavanols

Flavanols or flavan-3-ols are often called catechins. They differ from most flavonoids in that they do not have a double bond between C2 and C3, and there is no C4 carbonyl group in ring C (Table 25.1). The presence of catechins was reported in green tea, which is an excellent source of many polyphenol antioxidants. Catechins have been investigated broadly on their bioactive properties such as anti-inflammation, anticancer, and antiobesity [66]. The most important catechins of green tea are: (-)-epicatechin, (-) epicatechin-3-gallate, (-)- epigallocatechin, and (-) epigallocatechin-3-gallate (EGCG) [67]. Green tea also significantly reduced advanced glycation, accumulation of AGEs, and cross-linking of tail tendon collagen in diabetes [66]. This antihyperglycemic effect may be linked to enhanced basal and insulin-stimulated glucose uptake in rat adipocytes, inhibition of the intestinal glucose transporter, and decreased expression of genes that control gluconeogenesis [68,69].

One of the major polyphenolic constituents in green tea is EGCG, which demonstrated to be responsible for decreased AGE-stimulated gene expression and production of tumor necrosis factor-α and matrix metalloproteinase-13 in human chondrocytes [70]. EGCG has also been shown to prevent intracellular AGE formation, trapping reactive dicarbonyl species, such as MGO and GO, and enhancing the production of proinflammatory cytokines in monocytes under hyperglycemic conditions. EGCG was also able to bind lipoproteins and to enhance the antioxidant and antiglycation properties of LDL [71,72].

Flavanones and flavanol with hydroxyl groups at the 3'-, 4'-, 5'-, and 7-positions have shown a significant inhibitory activity against AGEs in *in vitro* experiments [62].

25.2.2.3 Isoflavones

Isoflavones have their ring B attached to the C3 position of ring C (Figure 25.4, Table 25.1) [73]. They are mostly found in the Leguminosae family of plants [41]. Soybean isoflavones showed both antioxidant and phytoesterogenic activities that may contribute to their potential anticarcinogenic and cardioprotective effects. Genistein and daidzein are the two main isoflavones in soy along with glycetein, biochanin A, and formononetin [74]. Soy isoflavones supplementation significantly decreased the concentration of protein carbonyls in the liver, kidney, and brain in D-galactose-treated mice in a dose-dependent manner. The mechanism of isoflavones inhibiting the formation of AGEs has been ascribed to their abilities to trap reactive dicarbonyl species such as MGO. Positions 6 and 8 of the A-ring were believed to be the major active sites. A 5,7-dihydroxy structure was favorable to the activity of isoflavones [75].

25.2.2.4 Anthocyanins

Anthocyanins are water-soluble glycosides and acyl glycosides of anthocyanidins. Proanthocyanidins are the oligomeric and polymeric forms of flavan-3-ols and traditionally considered to be condensed tannins. Biologically, they are regarded as molecules with chemopreventive activities in chronic diseases such as cancer and diabetes mellitus. Proanthocyanidins from grape seeds extracts were investigated on their therapy efficacies on diabetic complications. They also exerted various protective effects on glucose consumption impaired by high MGO concentrations through potential interaction with proteins involved in insulin signaling pathways [71].

The relationship between the AGE formation inhibitory activities and flavonoids chemical structure has been reported [9]. The hydroxylation on both A-ring and B-ring improved the inhibitory activity on AGE formation, while hydroxylation on C ring decreased the activity. On the contrary, methylation generally reduced the anti-AGE activity except for the 3-O-methylation of flavonols. Glycosylation of hydroxyl groups usually but not always decreases inhibitory activities on AGE formation. Hydrogenation of the C2=C3 double bond of flavones slightly weakened their activities.

The phenolic acids with multiple hydroxyls showed strong inhibition against AGE formation, and an *ortho-* or *meta-*dihydroxyl structure on the benzene ring was essential to the anti-AGE activity. The presence of galloyl groups was important for the activity of catechins, and α-hydroxyl group at C-3 was much more effective than β-hydroxyl group at C-3.

Proanthocyanidins dimer or trimers showed a stronger inhibitory activity than catechins.

25.2.3 Stilbenes

Stilbenes chemically belong to the family of phenylpropanoids showing antioxidative and anti-inflammatory properties [76]. Stilbenes efficiently inhibit the formation of AGEs in a dose-dependent manner by trapping reactive MGO under physiological conditions [77].

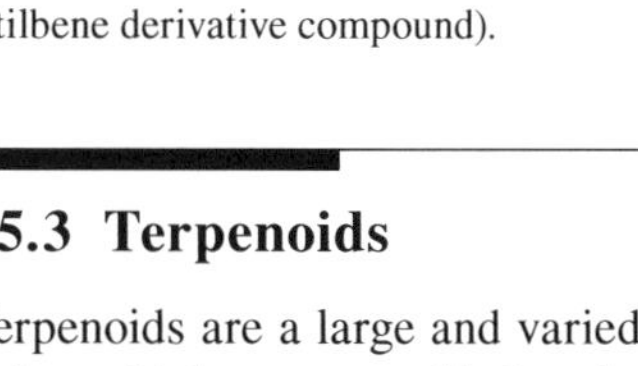

Resveratrol (Figure 25.5), a natural stilbene present in grape skin and red wine, is a well-known antioxidant, which attenuates complications derived from hyperglycemia. It was reported that this compound attenuates vasculopathy and renal damage through inhibiting RAGE, AGE-induced proliferation, and collagen synthesis activity, as well as reducing oxidative stress [78,79].

The hydroxylation on B ring and the methylation of stilbenes decreased their inhibitory activity.

OH
HO
OH
OH

FIGURE 25.5 Structure of resveratrol (stilbene derivative compound).

25.3 Terpenoids

Terpenoids are a large and varied class of organic compounds derived from five carbon isoprene (C5) units, which are assembled and modified in thousands of different ways. These C5 units are linked together in a head-to-tail manner. Based on the number of the isoprene units, terpenoids are classified as monoterpenes (C10), sesquiterpenes (C15), diterpenes (C20), sesterpenes (C25), triterpenes (C30), tetraterpenes (C40), and polyterpenes [80]. Monoterpenes and sesquiterpenes are the main constituents of the essential oils. However, di- and triterpenoids, which are not volatile compounds, are generally found in gums and resins. Tetraterpenoids constitute a group of terpenoids called carotenoids. This group includes carotenes, xanthophylls, and carotenoic acids [81].

The main terpenoid structures with antiglycation activity are shown in Figure 25.6.

Chloroform extracts from *Aegle marmelos* leaves showed inhibition of protein glycation, pentosidine formation, and protein carbonyl formation, with the monoterpene Limonene

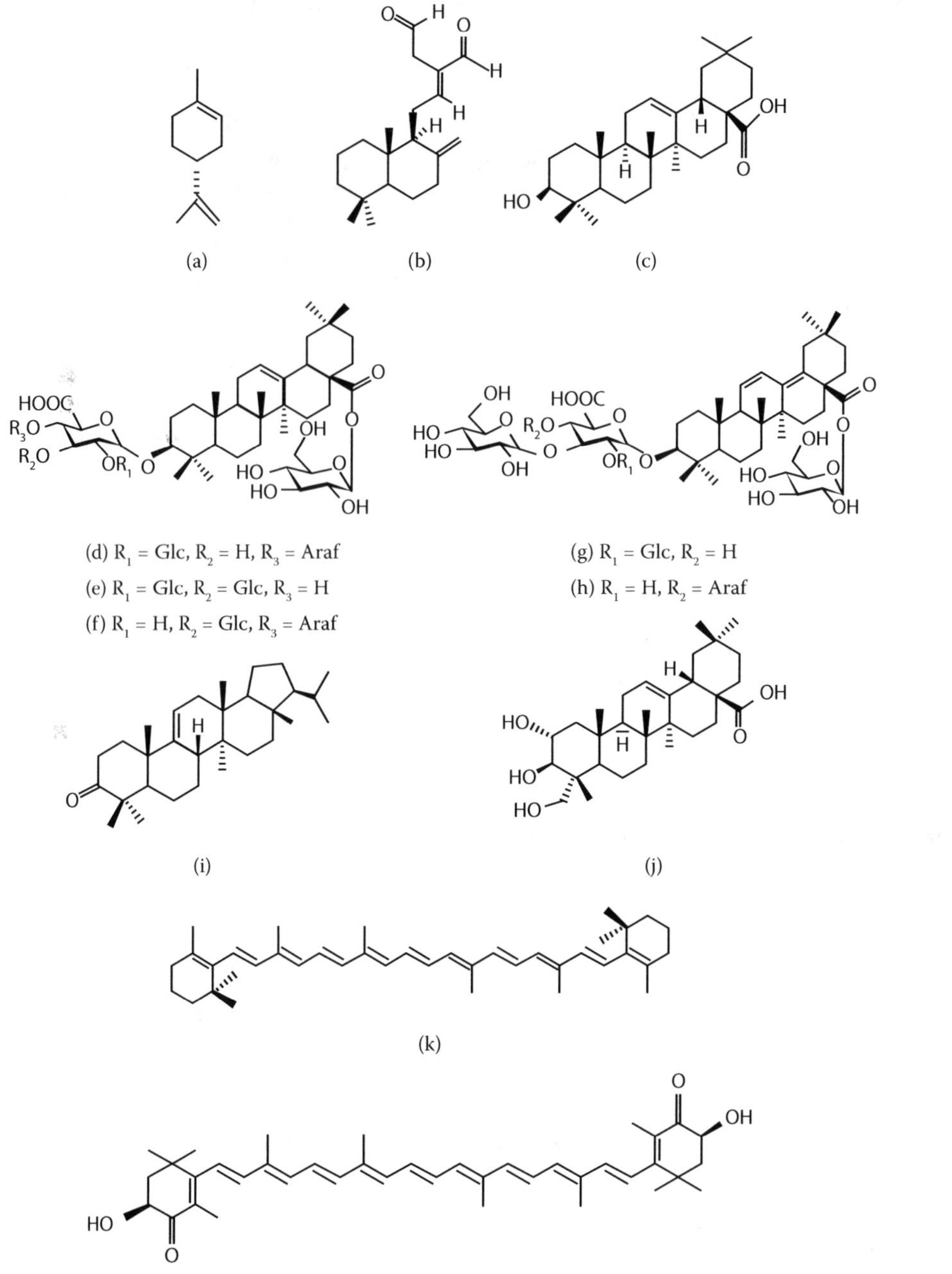

(a) (b) (c)

(d) R_1 = Glc, R_2 = H, R_3 = Araf

(e) R_1 = Glc, R_2 = Glc, R_3 = H

(f) R_1 = H, R_2 = Glc, R_3 = Araf

(g) R_1 = Glc, R_2 = H

(h) R_1 = H, R_2 = Araf

(i) (j)

(k)

(l)

FIGURE 25.6 Terpenoid compounds with antiglycation activity. (Adapted from Ashish, A., et al., *Roy. Soc Chem Adv.*, 5, 31113, 2015.) (a) Limonene, (b) Labdadiene, (c) Oleanolic acid, (d) 3-O-{b-D-glucopyranosyl-(1/2)-[a-D-arabinofuranosyl-(1/4)]-b-D-glucuronopyranosyl}-oleanolic acid 28-O-b-D-glucopyranosyl ester; (e) 3-O-{b-D-glucopyranosyl-(1/2)-[b-D-glucopyran osyl-(1/3)]-b-D-glucuronopyranosyl}-oleanolic acid 28-O-b-D-glucopyranosyl ester; (f) 3-O- {b-D-glucopyranosyl-(1/3)-[a-D-arabinofuranosyl-(1/4)]-b-D-glucuronopyranosyl}-oleanolic acid 28-O-b-D-glucopyranosylester; (g) 3-O-{b-D-glucopyranosyl-(1/2)-[b-Dglucopyranosyl-(1/3)]-b-D-glucuronopyranosyl}-olean-11,13-(18)-diene-28-oic acid 28-O-b-D-glucopyranosyl ester; (h) 3-O-{b-D-glucopyranosyl-(1/3)-[a-D-arabinofuranosyl-(1/4)]-b-Dglucuronopyranosyl}-olean-11,13(18)-diene-28-oic acid 28-O-b-D-glucopyranosyl ester; (i) Arborinone; (j) Arjunolic acid, (k) β-carotene; (l) Astaxanthin.

(Figure 25.6a) identified as responsible for the antiglycation activity. Labdane diterpene, labdadiene (Figure 25.6b), isolated from the rhizomes of *Alpinia zerumbet* exhibited inhibitory activities on the formation of fructosamine adducts and alpha-dicarbonyl compounds and could be used to prevent glycation-associated complications in diabetes.

Oleanolic acid (Figure 25.6c), a pentacyclic triterpene, has been found to exhibit an antiglycation effect in the kidneys of diabetic mice [41]. This compound along with two phenolic acids, caffeic acid, and chlorogenic acid from *I. paraguariensis* extracts, also showed antiglycation activity [35].

Glycoside esters of oleanolic acid (Figure 25.6d through f) isolated from the root bark of *Aralia taibaiensis*, as well as two oleanolic acid–derived saponins with an 11,13-diene system (Figure 25.6g and h), have been found to exhibit moderate antiglycation and antioxidant activities.

The pentacyclic triterpenoid arborinone (Figure 25.6i), along with a 5,7-dihydroxyisofavone derivative compound present in *Iris loczyi* extract, inhibited the activity of α-glucosidase and had antiglycation potential. Arjunolic acid (Figure 25.6j), a pentacyclic triterpenic acid present in *Terminalia arjuna*, has been found to be effective in preventing the formation of HbA1c, reactive oxygen species, AGEs, and oxidative stress signaling, and protecting from DNA fragmentation. The tetraterpenoid β-carotene (Figure 25.6k) has been found to exhibit an inhibitory effect on the formation of AGEs [82].

The green microalga *Chlorella zofingiensis* is known as a natural source of astaxanthin (l), a red ketocarotenoid that is a potent antioxidant. The astaxanthin diester was found to have antiglycative properties.

25.4 Conclusions

Plant-derived extracts and compounds isolated from them could be considered a promising alternative for the development of natural medicines with antiglycation activity, lowering the incidence of adverse 3.

ACKNOWLEDGMENT

This work was supported by UBACYT 20020130100686BA from the Buenos Aires University.

REFERENCES

1. Ahmed N. Advanced glycation end products-role in pathology of diabetic complications. *Diabetes Res Clin Pract*. **2005**, *67*, 3–21.
2. Rahman A, Choudhary MI, Basha FZ, Abbas G, Khan SN, Shah SA. Science at the interface of chemistry and biology: Discoveries of a-glucosidase inhibitors and antiglycation agents. *Pure Appl Chem Lett*. **2007**, *79* (12), 2263–2268.
3. Gutiérrez RMP, Diaz SL, Reyes IC, Gonzalez AMN. Antiglycation effect of spices and chilies used in traditional Mexican cuisine. *J Nat Prod*. **2010**, *3*, 95–102.
4. Kikuchi S, Shinpo K, Takeuchi M, Yamagishi S, Makita Z, Sasaki N, Tashiro K. Glycation: A sweet temper for neuronal death. *Brain Res Rev*. **2003**, *41*, 306–323.
5. Sell DR, Biemel KM, Reihl O, Lederer MO, Strauch CM, Monnier VM. Glucosepane is a major protein cross-link of the senescent human extracellular matrix. Relationship with diabetes. *J Biol Chem*. **2005**, *280* (13), 12310–12315.
6. Liu LH, Xie YX, Song ZQ, Shang SB, Chen XQ. Influence of dietary flavonoids on the glycation of plasma proteins. *Mol Biosyst*. **2012**, *8*, 2183–2187.
7. Zhang Q, Ames JM, Smith RD, Baynes JW, Metz TO. A perspective on the Maillard reaction and the analysis of protein glycation by mass spectrometry: Probing the pathogenesis of chronic disease. *J Proteome Res*. **2009**, *8*, 754–769.
8. Elosta A, Ghous T, Ahmed N. Natural products as anti-glycation agents: Possible therapeutic potential for diabetic complications. *Curr Diabetes Rev*. **2012**, *8*, 92–108.
9. Shikata K, Makino H, Sugimoto H, Kushiro M, Ota K, Akiyama K, et al. Localization of advanced glycation endproducts in the kidney of experimental diabetic rats. *J Diabetes Complications*. **1995**, *9*, 269–271.

10. Nishino T, Horii Y, Shiiki H, Yamamoto H, Makita Z, Bucala R, et al. Immunohistochemical detection of advanced glycosylation end products within the vascular lesions and glomeruli in diabetic nephropathy. *Hum Pathol.* **1995**, *26*, 308–313.
11. Xie Y, Chen X. Structures required of polyphenols for inhibiting advanced glycation end products formation. *Curr Drug Metabol.* **2013**, *14*, 414–431.
12. Uribarri J, Woodruff S, Goodman S, Cai W, Chen X, Pyzik R, Yong A, Striker GE, Vlassara H. Advanced glycation end products in foods and a practical guide to their reduction in the diet. *J Am Diet Assoc.* **2010**, *110* (6), 911–916. doi: 10.1016/j.jada.2010.03.018.
13. Peralta I, Filip R, Anesini C. Antioxidant and antiglycant activity of Ilex paraguariensis. Poster presentation 2°. Simposio Iberoamericano sobre AGEs y la Salud. Santiago de Chile, Setiembre **2016**. Available from: https://www.researchgate.net/publication/309785811_ANTIOXIDANT_AND_ANTIGLYCANT_ACTIVITY_OF_ILEX_PARAGUARIENSIS (Accessed July 24, 2017).
14. Kawanishi K, Ueda H, Moriyasu M. Aldose reductase inhibitors from the nature. *Curr Med Chem.* **2003**, *10* (15), 1353–1374.
15. Manzanaro S, Salva J, de la Fuente JA. Phenolic marine natural products as aldose reductase inhibitors. *J Nat Prod.* **2006**, *69* (10), 1485–1487.
16. Wu C, Huang S, Lin J, Yen G. Inhibition of advanced glycation end product formation by foodstuffs. *Food Funct.* **2011**, *2*, 224–234.
17. Lee GY, Jang DS, Lee YM, Kim JM, Kim JS. Naphthopyrone glucosides from the seeds of Cassia tora with inhibitory activity on advanced glycation end products (AGEs) formation. *Arch Pharm Res.* **2006**, *29* (7), 587–590.
18. Tsuji-Naito K, Saeki H, Hamano M. Inhibitory effects of Chrysanthemum species extracts on formation of advaced glycation end products. *Food Chem.* **2009**, *116* (4), 854–859.
19. Choudhary MI, Maher S, Begum A, Abbaskhan A, Ali S, Khan A, Shafique-ur-Rehman, Atta-ur-Rahman. Characterization and antiglycation activity of phenolic constituents from Viscum album (European Mistletoe). *Chem Pharm Bull (Tokyo)* **2010**, *58* (7), 980–982.
20. Manna P, Das J, Ghosh J, Sil PC. Contribution of type 1 diabetes to rat liver dysfunction and cellular damage via activation of NOS, PARP, IkappaBalpha/NFkappaB, MAPKs, and mitochondria-dependent pathways: Prophylactic role of arjunolic acid. *Free Radic Biol Med.* **2010**, *48* (11), 1465–1484.
21. Wang ZH, Hsu CC, Huang CN, Yin MC. Anti-glycative effect of oleanolic acid and ursolic acid in kidney of diabetic mice. *Eur J Pharmacol.* **2010**, *628* (1–3), 255–260.
22. Mosihuzzman M, Naheed S, Hareem S, Talib S, Abbas G, Khan SN, Choudhary MI, Sener B, Tareen RB, Israr M. *Life Sci.* **2013**, *92*, 187.
23. Sun Z, Liu J, Zeng X, Huangfu J, Jiang Y, Wang M, Chen F. Astaxanthin is responsible for antiglycoxidative properties of microalga Chlorell zofingiensis. *Food Chem.* **2011**, *126* (4), 1629–1635.
24. Farsi DA, Harris CS, Reid L, Bennett SAL, Haddad PS, Martineau LC, Arnason JT. Inhibition of non-enzymatic glycation by silk extracts from a Mexican land race and modern inbred lines of maize (Zea mays). *Phytother. Res.* **2008**, *22*, 108–112.
25. Harris CS, Beaulieu LP, Fraser MH, McIntyre KL, Owen PL, Martineau LC, et al. Inhibition of advanced glycation end product formation by medicinal plant extracts correlates with phenolic metabolites and antioxidant activity. *Planta Med.* **2011**, *77*, 196–204.
26. Ferchichi L, Derbre S, Mahmood K, Toure K, Guilet D, Litaudon M, Awang K, Hadi A. Le Ray AM, Richomme P. Bioguided fractionation and isolation of natural inhibitors of advanced glycation end-products (AGEs) from Calophyllum flavoramulum. *Phytochemistry.* **2012**, *78*, 98.
27. Sun C, McIntyre K, Saleem A, Haddad PS, Arnason JT. The relationship between antiglycation activity and procyanidin and phenolic content in commercial grape seed products. *Can. J Physiol Pharmacol.* **2012**, *90*, 167–174.
28. Yao Y, Cheng XZ, Wang LX, Wang SH, Ren GX. Major phenolic compounds, antioxidant capacity and antidiabetic potential of Rice Bean (Vigna umbellata L.) in China. *Int J Mol Sci.* **2012**, *13*, 2707–2716.
29. Chirinos R, Betalleluz-Pallardel I, Huamán A, Arbizu C, Pedreschi R, Campos D. HPLC-DAD characterisation of phenolic compounds from Andean oca (Oxalis tuberosa Mol.) tubers and their contribution to the antioxidant capacity. *Food Chem.* **2009**, *113*, 1243–1251.
30. Wijngaard HH, Rößle C, Brunton N. A survey of Irish fruit and vegetable waste and byproducts as a source of polyphenolic antioxidants. *Food Chem.* **2009**, *116*, 202–207.

31. Jin D, Mumper RJ. Plant phenolics: Extraction, analysis and their antioxidant and anticancer properties. Review. *Molecules*. **2010**, *15*, 7313–7352.
32. Zhang L, Ravipati AS, Koyyalamudi SR, Jeong S, Reddy N, Smith PT, Bartlett J, Shanmugam K, Münch G, Wu MJ. Antioxidant and anti-inflammatory activities of selected medicinal plants containing phenolic and flavonoid compounds. *J Agric Food Chem*. **2011**, *59*, 12361–12367.
33. Mohanlal S, Parvathy R, Shalini V, Mohanan R, Helen A, Jayalekshmy A. Chemical indices, Antioxidant activity and anti-inflammatory effect of extracts of the medicinal rice "Njavara" and staple varieties. *J Food Biochem*. **2012**, *36*, 1–12.
34. Sawadogo WR, Maciuk A, Banzouzi JT, Champy P, Figadere B, Guissou IP, Nacoulma OG. Mutagenic effect, Antioxidant and anticancer activities of six medicinal plants from Burkina Faso. *Nat Prod Res*. **2012**, *26*, 575–579.
35. Pieme CA, Penlap VN, Ngogang J, Costache M. *In vitro* cytotoxicity and antioxidant activities of five medicinal plants of Malvaceae family from Cameroon. *Environ Toxicol Pharmacol*. **2010**, *29*, 223–228.
36. Ramos S. Cancer chemoprevention and chemotherapy: Dietary polyphenols and signaling pathways. *Mol Nutr Food Res*. 2008, *52*, 507–526.
37. Slivova V, Zaloga G, DeMichele SJ, Mukerji P, Huang YS, Siddiqui R, Harvey K, Valachovicova T, Sliva D. Green tea polyphenols modulate secretion of urokinase plasminogen activator (uPA) and inhibit invasive behavior of breast cancer cells. *Nutr Cancer*. **2005**, *52*, 66–73.
38. Kusirisin W, Srichairatanakool S, Lerttrakarnnon P, Lailerd N, Suttajit M, Jaikang C, Chaiyasut C. Antioxidative activity, Polyphenolic content and anti-glycation effect of some Thai medicinal plants traditionally used in diabetic patients. *Med. Chem*. **2009**, *5*, 139–147.
39. Scalbert A, Manach C, Remesy C, Morand C. Dietary polyphenols and the prevention of diseases. *Crit Rev Food Sci Nutr*. **2005**, *45*, 287–306.
40. Pedreschi R, Cisneros-Zevallos L. Antimutagenic and antioxidant properties of phenolic fractions from Andean purple corn (*Zea mays* L.). *J Agric Food Chem*. **2006**, *54*, 4557–4567.
41. Tsao R. Chemistry and biochemistry of dietary polyphenols. *Nutrients*. **2010**, *2*, 1231–1246.
42. Xiao J, Kai G. A review of dietary polyphenol-plasma protein interactions: Characterization, influence on the bioactivity, and structure-affinity relationship. *Crit Rev Food Sci Nutr*. **2012**, *52*, 85–101.
43. Heim KE, Tagliaferro AR, Bobilya DJ. Flavonoid antioxidants: Chemistry, metabolism and structure-activity relationships. *J Nutr Biochem*. **2002**, *13*, 572–584.
44. Cao G, Sofic E, Prior RL. Antioxidant and prooxidant behavior of flavonoids: Structure-activity relationships. *Free Rad Biol Med*. **1997**, *22*, 749–760.
45. Rice-Evans CA, Miller NJ, Paganga G. Structure-antioxidant activity relationships of flavonoids and phenolic acids. *Free Rad Biol Med*. **1996**, *20*, 933–956.
46. Wu CH, Yeh CT, Shih PH, Yen GC. Dietary phenolic acids attenuate multiple stages of protein glycation and high glucose-stimulated proinflammatory IL-1 activation by interfering with chromatin remodeling and transcription in monocytes. *Mol Nutr Food Res*. **2010**, *54*, S127–S140.
47. Lee EH, Song DG, Lee JY, Pan CH, Um BH, Jung SH. Inhibitory effect of the compounds isolated from *Rhus verniciflua* on aldose reductase and advanced glycation endproduct. *Biol Pharm Bull*. **2008**, *31* (8), 1626–1630.
48. Yazdanparast R, Ardestani A, Jamshidi S. Experimental diabetes treated with Achillea santolina: Effect on pancreatic oxidative parameters. *J Ethnopharmacol*. **2007**, *112* (1), 13–18.
49. Yamabe N, Kang KS, Park CH, Tanaka H, Yokozawa T. 7-O-Galloyl D-sedoheptulose is a novel therapeutic agent against oxidative stress and advanced glycation endproducts in the diabetic kidney. *Biol Pharm Bull*. **2009**, *32* (4), 657–664.
50. Fiuza SM, Gomes C, Teixeira LJ, Gir o da Cruz MT, Cordeiro MN, Milhazes N, Borges F, Marques MP. Phenolic acid derivatives with potential anticancer properties—A structure-activity relationship study. Part 1: Methyl, propyl and octyl esters of caffeic and gallic acids. *Bioorgan Med Chem*. **2004**, *12* (13), 3581–3589.
51. Verzelloni E, Tagliazucchi D, Rio D, Calani L, Conte A. Antiglycative and antioxidative properties of coffee fractions. *Food Chem*. **2011**, *124* (4), 1430–1435.
52. Jang DS, Yoo NH, Kim NH, Lee YM, Kim CS, Kim J, Kim JH, Kim JS. 3,5-Di-O-caffeoyl-epi-quinic Acid from the leaves and stems of erigeron annuus inhibits protein glycation, aldose reductase, and cataractogenesis. *Biol Pharm Bull*. **2010**, *33*, 329–333.
53. Kikuzaki H, Hisamoto M, Hirose K, Akiyama K, Taniguchi H. Antioxidant properties of ferulic acid and its related compounds. *J Agric Food Chem*. **2002**, *50* (7), 2161–2168.

54. Silván JM, Assar SH, Srey C, Dolores del Castillo M, Ames JM. Control of the Maillard reaction by ferulic acid. *Food Chem.* **2011**, *128* (1), 208–213.
55. Miroliaei M, Khazaei S, Moshkelgosha S, Shirvani M. Inhibitory effects of Lemon balm (Melissa officinalis, L.) extract on the formation of advanced glycation end products. *Food Chem.* **2011**, *129* (2), 267–271.
56. Harborne JB, Mabry TJ, Mabry H. *The Flavonoids*, Chapman and Hall, London, **1974**.
57. Beecher GR. Overview of dietary flavonoids: Nomenclature, occurrence and intake. *J Nutr.* **2003**, *133*, 3248–3254.
58. Fraga CG. Plant polyphenols: How to translate their *in vitro* antioxidant actions to *in vivo* conditions. *IUBMB Life.* **2007**, *59* (4–5), 308–315.
59. García-Mediavilla V, Crespo I, Collado PS, Esteller A, Sánchez-Campos S, Tuñón MJ, González-Gallego J. The anti-inflammatory flavones quercetin and kaempferol cause inhibition of inducible nitric oxide synthase, cyclooxygenase-2 and reactive C protein, and down-regulation of the nuclear factor kappaB pathway in Chang Liver cells. *Eur J Pharmacol.* **2007**, *557* (2–3), 221–229.
60. Kim JM, Lee EK, Kim DH, Yu BP, Chung HY. Kaempferol modulates proinflammatory NF-κB activation by suppressing advanced glycation end products induced NADPH oxidase. *Am Aging Assoc.* **2010**, *32* (2), 197–208.
61. Soman S, Rauf AA, Indira M, Rajamanickam C. Antioxidant and antiglycative potential of ethyl acetate fraction of *Psidium guajava* leaf extract in steptozotocin-induced diabetic rats. *Plant Foods Hum Nutr.* **2010**, *65* (4), 386–391.
62. Lee S, Park HS, Notsu Y, Ban HS, Kim YP, Ishihara K, Hirasawa N, et al. Effects of hyperin, isoquercitrin and quercetin on lipopolysaccharide-induced nitrite production in rat peritoneal macrophages. *Phytother Res.* **2008**, *22* (11), 1552–1556.
63. Jung HA, Jung YJ, Yoon NY, Jeong da M, Bae HJ, Kim DW, Na DH, Choi JS. Inhibitory effects of Nelumbo nucifera leaves on rat lens aldose reductase, advanced glycation end products formation, and oxidative stress. *Food Chem Toxicol.* **2008**, *46* (12), 3818–3826.
64. Wu CH, Lin JA, Hsieh WC, Yen GC. Low-Density-Lipoprotein (LDL)-Bound flavonoids increase the resistance of LDL to oxidation and glycation under pathophysiological concentrations of glucose *in vitro*. *J Agric Food Chem.* **2009**, *57* (11), 5058–5064.
65. Peng X, Zheng Z, Cheung KW, Shan F, Ren GX, Chen SF, Wang M. Inhibitory effect of mung bean extract and its constituents vitexin and isovitexin on the formation of advanced glycation endproducts. *Food Chem.* **2008**, *106* (2), 457–481.
66. Babu PV, Sabitha KE, Shyamaladevi CS. Effect of green tea extract on advanced glycation and cross-linking of tail tendon collagen in streptozotocin induced diabetic rats. *Food Chem Toxicol.* **2008**, *46* (1), 280–285.
67. McKay DL, Blumberg JB. The role of tea in human health: An update. *J Am Coll Nutr.* **2002**, *21* (1), 1–13.
68. Kobayashi Y, Suzuki M, Satsu H, Arai S, Hara Y, Suzuki K, Miyamaoto Y, Shimizu, M. Green tea polyphenols inhibit the sodium dependent glucose transporter of intestinal epithelial cells by a competitive mechanism. *J Agric Food Chem.* **2000**, *48* (11), 5618–5623.
69. Wu LY, Juan CC, Ho LT, Hsu YP, Hwang LS. Effect of green tea supplementation on insulin sensitivity in Sprague-Dawley rats. *J. Agric Food Chem.* **2004**, *52* (3), 643–648.
70. Rasheed Z, Anbazhagan AN, Akhtar N, Ramamurthy S, Voss FR, Haqqi TM. Green tea polyphenol epigallocatechin-3-gallate inhibits advanced glycation end product-induced expression of tumor necrosis factor-alpha and matrix metalloproteinase-13 in human chondrocytes. *Arthritis Res Ther.* **2009**, *11* (3), R71.
71. Peng X, Ma J, Chao J, Sun Z, Chang RCC, Tse I, Li ETS, Chen F, Wang M. Beneficial Effects of cinnamon proanthocyanidins on the formation of specific advanced glycation endproducts and methylglyoxal-induced impairment on glucose consumption. *J Agric Food Chem.* **2010**, *58*, 6692–6696.
72. Wu CH, Yeh CT, Yen GC. Epigallocatechin gallate (EGCG) binds to low-density lipoproteins (LDL) and protects them from oxidation and glycation under high-glucose conditions mimicking diabetes. *Food Chem.* **2010**, *121* (3), 639–644.
73. Patel JM. A review of potential health benefits of flavonoids. *Lethbridge Undergrad Res J.* **2008**, *3*. Available from: http://www.lurj.org/issues/volume-3-number-2/flavonoids (accessed December 29, 2014).

74. Rimbach G, Boesh-Saadatmandi C, Frank J, Fuchs D, Wenzel U, Daniel H, Hall WL, Weinberg PD. Dietary isoflavones in the prevention of cardiovascular disease. A molecular perspective. *Food Chem Toxicol.* **2008**, *46* (4), 1308–1319.
75. Lv LS, Shao X, Chen HD, Ho CT, Sang SM. Genistein inhibits advanced glycation end product formation by trapping methylglyoxal. *Chem Res Toxicol.* **2011**, *24*, 579–586.
76. Lv L, Gu X, Tang J, Ho CT. Antioxidant activity of stilbene glycoside from Polygonum multiflorum Thunb *in vivo*. *Food Chem.* **2007**, *104* (4), 1678–1681.
77. Lv L, Shao X, Wang L, Huang D, Ho CT, Sang S. Stilbene glucoside from polygonum multiflorum thunb: A novel natural inhibitor of advanced glycation end product formation by trapping of methylglyoxal. *J Agric Food Chem.* **2010**, *58* (4), 2239–2245.
78. Liu FC, Hung LF, Wu WL, Chang DM, Huang CY, Lai JH, Ho LJ. Chondroprotective effects and mechanisms of resveratrol in advanced glycation end products-stimulated chondrocytes. *Arthritis Res Ther.* **2010**, *12*. R167.
79. Palsamy P, Subramanian S. Resveratrol protects diabetic kidney by attenuating hyperglycemia-mediated oxidative stress and renal inflammatory cytokines via Nrf2-Keap1 signaling. *BBA-Mol Basis Dis.* **2011**, *1812*, 719–731.
80. Wang G, Tang W, Bidigare RR. Terpenoids As Therapeutic Drugs and Pharmaceutical Agents. In Zhang, L. & Demain, A.L., (Eds.), *Natural products drug discovery and therapeutic medicine terpenoids as therapeutic drugs as pharmaceutical agents*. Humana Press, Totowa, NJ, **2005**, 197–237.
81. Sameeno B. *Chemistry of natural compounds.* **2007**. Available from: http://nsdl.niscair.res.in/bitstream/123456789/700/1/revised+terpenoids.pdf (October 9, 2011).
82. Ashish A, Chinchansure A, Arvind M, Korwar B, Mahesh JK, Swati PJ. Recent development of plant products with antiglycation activity: A review. *Roy. Soc Chem Adv.* **2015**, *5*, 31113. doi: 10.1039/C4RA14211J.

26

Dietary Intake of AGEs and ALEs and Inflammation: Nutritional Aspects

Stig Bengmark
University College London
London, United Kingdom

CONTENTS

KEY POINTS

- Chronic, silent, often low-grade, inflammation is associated with almost all lifestyle-associated chronic diseases.
- The degree of inflammation is enforced by postprandial inflammation induced by certain foods.

- Among factors documented to enhance chronic and postprandial inflammation are exposure to glycated, lipoxidated products; proteins such as gluten and casein; long-chain fatty acids, and lack of anti-inflammatory factors such as vitamin D and omega fatty acids.
- Chronic and postprandial inflammation is strongly associated with impaired and poorly functioning gut microbiota and impaired innate immune functions.
- Gut reconditioning—supply of bioactive lactic acid bacteria, bioactive plant fibers, and plant antioxidants by plant foods such as cloves, turmeric, Ceylon cinnamon, chili pepper, black pepper, wild caraway, and many other plants may have the ability to reduce chronic and postprandial inflammation.

26.1 Western Life Style and Food Habits—A Real Threat to Health

Most Western diseases are strongly associated with physical and mental stress, lack of exercise, and overconsumption of processed Western-type foods—often leading to metabolic syndrome and manifested in, what has been called the "deadly quartet": excessive body weight, hypertension, impaired glucose homeostasis, and atherogenic dyslipidemia (changes in serum cholesterol, increased triglycerides, decreased high density lipoprotein [HDL] cholesterol, and an increase of low-density lipoprotein [LDL] particles)—manifestations, which often lead to severe acute and chronic diseases such as diabetes mellitus type 2, cardiovascular disease (CVD), cancers (breast, colorectal, and pancreas), neurodegenerative diseases (e.g., Alzheimer's disease), pregnancy complications (gestational diabetes and preeclampsia), fertility problems (polycystic ovarian syndrome), and many more [1–4].

The development of metabolic syndrome with its components of abdominal obesity, high blood pressure, elevated blood sugar, elevated blood triglycerides, low HDL cholesterol, and high uric acid in blood is often, if not always, a result of malfunctioning gut flora (dysbiosis), induced endotoxemia, low-grade systemic inflammation, and malfunctioning immune system [1,2]—all constituting, what I call a "mother of disease" [3]. This chapter focuses only on the effects of Western food habits and its association to dysbiosis, in particular with the inflammation and immune dysfunctions induced by intake of glycated and lipoxidated molecules, often combined with lack of organ rest, recuperation, regeneration, and detoxification.

26.2 Inflammation—Early Warnings

Dysbiosis, which always induces a low-grade, often silent, inflammation and a malfunctioning immune system, leads early on to a series of various, seemingly benign manifestations in the body, for which the sufferers often seek medical advice at their local general practitioner, and often receive symptomatic treatment. However, these benign but irritating symptoms should nevertheless be taken seriously as they may be signs of ongoing low-grade inflammation, which with time might bring a series of consequences—severe diseases and eventually death. Such signals should be regarded as "early warnings" and encourage radical changes in lifestyle, especially in food habits.

Among these "early warnings" are manifestations such as acne, dandruff, unexplained fatigue, sleep problems, frequent headache, hair loss, gray hair, skin rashes, dry eyes, frail nails, dry mouth or increased salivation, reduced sex functions, irregular menstruations, obstipation or diarrhea, osteoporosis, overweight, frequent infections, mental depression, breathlessness, sweaty feet and palms, vaginal flour, and several more. If ignored—worse is to come. To treat these manifestations with lifestyle changes is more important than using drugs.

26.3 Without Lifestyle Changes—Worse Is to Come

A series of well-done published studies suggest that the incidence of most of the endemic chronic diseases from Attention Deficit/Hyperactivity Disorders (ADHD), Alzheimer, and diabetes, to prostatic and other cancers will in average triple by the year 2050. Incidence of diabetes will double [5] and that of ADHD, Alzheimer disease [6], and cancer [7] will triple or more. No health insurance system, governmental or private, will have a chance to survive under such conditions. Even in times of low inflation, health care costs seem to double in each 10-year period [8], and this has been happening for several decades. It is expected that in the United States, the country with the highest health care costs in the world, by the year 2020 the costs of health care will correspond to half (>$15,000) of the average family income (about $46,000) after tax (app 30,000)—sales taxes excluded.

A rather recent and most interesting study looked at the prospective landscape of health and disease up to the year 2030 in the United States and the United Kingdom [9], two countries already with the highest rates of obesity and chronic diseases in the world and representing approximately 5% of the world's population. The study suggests that these countries combined will by the year of 2030 have another 76 million obese adults, and have an additional 6–8.5 million cases of diabetes, 6–7 million cases of cardiovascular disease, 492,000–669,000 additional cases of cancer, which will result in another loss of between 26 and 55 million quality-adjusted life years and a dramatic increase in costs of care (the authors calculated to be $50–$68 billion per year) [9].

26.4 Easy Access of Food and High Consumption of Processed Foods Is the Problem

For some decades, the epidemic of obesity and chronic diseases has mainly been a problem for the Western world. Modern agricultural techniques, techniques for mass production, and easy access to cheap foods has led to a much too large consumption of agricultural foods, frequently and increasingly industrially manipulated and rich in processed and easy digestible products such as meat, dairy, and wheat, and foods that are often also rich in advanced glycation and lipoxidated end products—AGEs and ALEs (10–12). Similar developments are now observed in other parts of the world, largely in parallel to the adoption of "modern"/Western food habits.

Presently, the epidemic of obesity and associated diseases seems to have its epicenter in the Southern United States [13]; states like Alabama, Louisiana, and Mississippi having the highest incidence of obesity and chronic diseases in the United States and the world. These diseases are spreading around the world much like a tsunami; to the West to New Zeeland and Australia, to the North to Canada, to both Eastern and Western Europe, and now also to the Arab world and Asia, and to the South, particularly to Mexico and Brazil, most often in the footprints of the development of modern agriculture.

26.5 Developing Countries Soon to Take Over the "Yellow Jersey"

Japan was the first country outside the Western hemisphere to adapt a Western lifestyle and it suffers now the burden of Western diseases— to an extent not seen before. The island of Okinawa, once said to have the healthiest populace and the greatest numbers of centenarians in the world, has lost its leading position of having the lowest incidence of obesity and chronic diseases, and the highest number of centenarians in the world. This occurred after the United States built military bases on the island, thereby westernizing the island—today, the island ranks among the lowest from the perspective of health when the 50 Japanese states (prefectures) are studied.

The mortality rate of prostatic cancer increased 25-fold and almost linearly between the years 1948 and 1998, when Japan after the Second Word War, at least to some extent, adopted its food habits to

Western agriculture-based foods, which happened in parallel to the increase in the consumption of eggs (7-fold), meat (9-fold), and milk products (20-fold) [14,15]. Now, the same development is seen not only in China, India, and other Asian countries but also to a great extent in African countries. China, for example, once known for its extremely good lifestyle and food habits, especially in rural areas, and low incidence of obesity as well as chronic diseases with high numbers of centenarians [16] is today badly affected by obesity and chronic diseases, much in parallel to the introduction of western-type agriculture and especially in parallel to the increased production and consumption of dairy products. I have had difficulties in accessing official information, but my colleagues in China tell me that the incidence of chronic diseases such as coronary heart diseases, diabetes, and cancers such as breast cancer and prostatic cancer seem to double every 10 years, especially in the large cities.

26.6 Incidence of Obesity and Chronic Disease Increases with Unprecedented Speed

It has been recently reported that the incidence of metabolic syndrome and cardiovascular risk rose dramatically in the Chinese population in the 8 years between 2002 and 2010 [17]. A 4-fold increase in the incidence of metabolic syndrome was observed, affecting only 5.4% of the population in 2002 and rising to as much as 21.3% in 2010. The situation seems even more worrisome considering that the rate of hyperglycemia rose five times from 9.1% in 2002 to 53.1% in 2010. Furthermore, the age-standardized prevalence of obesity did double during the same period, from 13.5% to 25.4%, much in parallel to the increased incidence in hypertension (from 23.6% to 40.8%), hypertriglyceridemia (from 12.1% to 17.4%), and an alarming rise of low-density cholesterol LDL (from 32.1% to 71.1%).

It is also reported that the gap in the incidence of metabolic syndrome and its serious consequences, previously much in favor of rural compared to urban populations, decreased significantly during the 8 years, from 2002 to 2010 [17]. A just published study reports much similar development in cancer disease in Southeast Asia—exemplified by fast increasing instances of prostatic cancer, already high in Japan, Taiwan, Hong Kong, and Korea, with Shanghai and most likely also Beijing—and the whole of urban China—fast following in the footprints of the most affected large cities [18]. Furthermore, Western food habits are increasingly being adopted by the Chinese youth, which is even more worrisome. Metabolic syndrome and obesity are increasing faster in younger age groups and the prevalence of juvenile type 2 diabetes is reported to have doubled within the recent 5-year period.

26.7 The Interval between Change of Lifestyle and Signs of Ill Health Is Shorter Than Ever Before

It is of great interest to observe that the interval between change of lifestyle and altered pattern of disease is much shorter than previously ever believed. What took about 100 years to occur in the Western world is happening in Southeast Asia in less than 10 years. The large increase in dairy production and consumption, which exploded after the shift of the millennium, was seemingly followed almost immediately by a typhoon of obesity and chronic diseases.

Feeding large populations with cheap, calorie-condensed foods are seemingly one of the greatest political priorities, and a favored political task in almost all countries. Western politicians know well the negative health consequences of such policies and have done so for decades, but they seem unwilling to make any serious attempt to stop the epidemic of obesity and chronic diseases that follows. Both in Europe and in the United States, governments continue to subsidize mass agriculture with large sums of money in order to produce even more of such disease-promoting foods and are obviously prepared to pay for subsequent attempts to try to cure those who have been affected by disease due to overconsumption of cheap, calorie-condensed agricultural foods.

Consumption of refined sugar, strongly associated with obesity and Western diseases, has sky-rocketed in the last 150 years from a decent half a kg in 1,850 to presently about 50 kg/person/year in Western and even more in South American countries. The consumption of sugar is still comparatively low in Asian countries—usually below 10 kg/person/year, but is growing fast. Asian countries, in addition to having a considerable internal and fast-growing production, are big importers of sugar. For example, India and China are the largest importers of sugar in the world—China is expected to be by far the largest importer in the year 2020. One can only speculate about the damaging effects on public health that such a development will lead to. Africa is now following in the same path—a recent study reports a fast increasing public health problem with obesity in Tanzanian women with damaging physical and social consequences—the prevalence of overweight reported as considerable for the continent: 16% overweight and 6% obese [19].

Behind dysbiosis, the 10 most important factors contributing to chronic inflammation and subsequent chronic diseases are the following:

- Very high intake of insulinogenic foods such as refined carbohydrates; cereals, bread, sweets, cookies, rice, pasta, cooked tubers, including potatoes, and foods that are highly absorbed in the small intestine and are of no or minimal benefit to microbiota.
- Too high intake of fructose, above 25 g a day, particularly of high fructose corn syrup.
- High intake of dairy products, especially butter, cheese, and milk powder, rich in long-chain fatty acids, absorbed via the thoracic duct and remaining for hours in general circulation, contributing to postprandial endotoxemia and postprandial inflammation.
- High intake of foods rich in hormones and growth factors such as IGF1.
- High intake of meat, especially inflammation-inducing processed and cured meat, such as bacon and sausages, meatballs, which also are detrimental to microbiota and induce dysbiosis.
- High intake of foods exposed to industrial processes and heated in temperatures above 80°C/175F° known to induce synthesis of molecules such as AGEs and ALEs.
- Exposure to microbe-derived highly inflammation-inducing endotoxin, especially rich in meat hung for several days, hard cheeses, pork, and ice creams.
- Intake of foods rich in proteotoxin pesticides such as casein, gluten, and zein (maize).
- Intake of chemicals of all kinds, also including alcohol, nicotine, most pharmaceutical drugs, even pain relievers, sedatives, sleeping pills, proton pump inhibitors, all detrimental to microbiota.
- Too small intake of plant fibers, fresh and raw greens, fresh spices, and vegetables, and too little intake of antioxidants, minerals (especially magnesium-rich), and other anti-inflammatory nutrients.

26.8 Postprandial Inflammation: A "Deadly" Threat to Long-Term Health

The factors mentioned above do, more or less all, contribute to severe postprandial inflammation, especially when consuming a meal rich in long-chain fatty acids, sugars, and AGEs and ALEs. Frequent episodes of postprandial inflammation has for years been recognized as a key factor behind the development of arteriosclerosis [20] and various other chronic diseases, especially metabolic syndrome [21], diabetes [22], and hepatosteatosis [23]. Every meal rich in fat is associated with significant derangement of microbiota [24], cascades of markers of inflammatory and oxidative stress [25], particularly tumor necrosis factor-α (TNF-α) [26] and significant endothelial dysfunction [27].

Plasma endotoxin levels were studied in 12 healthy men (20–58 years, mean age: 32 years) after exposure to no meal, three cigarettes, and a high-fat meal, or a high-fat meal with three cigarettes [26]. The high-fat meal with or without cigarettes, but not the no meal or smoking alone, reduced significantly ($P < 0.05$) endotoxin neutralization capacity of plasma, an indirect measure of endotoxin exposure. The levels of endotoxin/plasma increased with a mean of 50% ($P < 0.05$) and remained significantly elevated for about 1.5 hours, while the triacylglycerol concentrations remained statistically significantly elevated as long as 4 hours after the meal [26]. This study provides strong support to the hypothesis of food/dysbiosis/endotoxemia-induced postprandial inflammation as a major contributor to endothelial activation and development of atherosclerosis. It is also observed that simultaneous intake of sugars significantly potentiates the postprandial inflammation induced by a high-fat meal [27]. The inflammatory response in vascular endothelial cells varies directly with the subject's postprandial serum triglyceride level and waist circumference [28].

26.9 Abdominal/Visceral Obesity Enhances Postprandial Inflammation

Visceral obesity was extremely rare among our forefathers and remained so until only a few decades ago. A recent study that measured anthropometric parameters using nuclear magnetic resonance was performed in 54 otherwise healthy volunteers with BMI ranging from 19 to 57 kg/m^2 and demonstrated that visceral obesity can vary from only a few milliliters in lean individuals to over 6 L in morbidly obese individuals [24]. Furthermore, a strong correlation was observed between visceral amount of fat, waist circumference, and waist-to-hip ratio [29]. It is of the greatest interest that visceral adipocytes exposed to stress secrete significantly more free fatty acids and also approximately three times as much proinflammatory factors such as IL-6 and PAI-1 per gram tissue compared with subcutaneous fat cells. These observations might well explain the high risk of acute and also chronic diseases in individuals with visceral obesity [29]. As a matter of fact, the stress-induced load on the vascular endothelium and particularly those of the brain, the heart, and the lungs can be extreme as the proinflammatory and procoagulant molecules can vary up to 1,000 times. These observations provide strong support to what has been called the "portal theory", which proposes that the liver when exposed to larger amounts of free fatty acids and proinflammatory factors, released from visceral depots of fat into the portal vein, especially in obese individuals, will promote development of liver steatosis and hepatic insulin resistance, and enhance the development of metabolic syndrome, particularly type 2 diabetes [30]. Dysbiosis with metabolic endotoxemia is strongly associated with general obesity and insulin resistance both in mice and humans, supporting a strong linkage between gut microbes, gut barrier function, acute and chronic inflammation, adipose tissue inflammation, endothelial inflammation and dysfunction, obesity, chronic inflammation and insulin resistance, and various chronic diseases.

26.10 Postprandial Inflammation Induced by Long-Chain but Not Medium-Chain Fatty Acids

The metabolism of consumed medium-chain fatty acids (MCFAs, C6-C12) in the body is fundamentally different from long-chain fatty acids (C12 – C21). This is an observation which is receiving increasing interest. Medium-chain triglycerides (MCT) are among the most readily hydrolyzed nutritional fats, much in contrast to long-chain triglycerides (LCT). MCFAs are known to be absorbed from the small intestine by a pathway, which is more direct and much more rapid than that of long-chain fatty acids (LCFAs), for example, via the portal vein to the liver. Since several decades ago, it is known that MCTs undergo a rapid hydrolysis by the gastric, salivary, or pancreatic lipases, most likely due to much better solubility and motility of the MCT lipid droplet. MCFAs are rapidly transported as nonesterified fatty acids into the portal blood stream to reach the liver, while LCFAs are transported as chylomicrons into the thoracic duct and after remaining up to several hours in the general circulation are redistributed as LCTs by hepatic lipoproteins to nonhepatic tissues [31,32].

The effects of fatty acid chain length were tested on male Wistar rats which were fed iso-caloric high-fat diets containing triacylglycerols composed of either MCFAs or LCFA. After 4 weeks, insulin sensitivity was reduced by 30% in the LCFA group, while it remained nonaffected in the MCFA group [33]. Triacylglycerol concentrations in muscle were higher in both high-fat groups compared to controls. No diet-induced changes were found in acyl-CoA oxidase (ACO) activity (liver and muscle) in the MCFA group, while feeding significantly raised carnitine palmitoyltransferase activity in the LCFA group. It was concluded that the chain length of saturated fatty acids clearly affects whole-body insulin sensitivity and mitochondrial fatty acid uptake, even in the absence of obesity. It was also observed that MCT compared to LCT feeding resulted in significantly lowered fasted and postprandial triglyceride concentrations [33]. Feeding sows with diets containing 15% MCTs resulted in a significantly lower mortality of newborns and promoted development, particularly of underweight piglets [33,34].

26.11 Reduced Intake of LCFAs and Increased Intake of MCFAs Are Good for Microbiota and Health

Numerous studies have demonstrated significant beneficial impacts of feeding MCFAs on both composition of the intestinal microbiota and inhibitory effects on bacterial concentrations in the digesta, mainly on Salmonella and coliforms. Apart from the specific nutritional and metabolic effects of MCTs and MCFA, especially their rapid digestion, passive absorption, and obligatory oxidation, they also possess immunomodulatory effects. While LCTs and LCFAs have meat and dairy as their dominating food source, MCTs and MCFAs typically come from plant fats. The MCT content is especially high in coconut oil: caprylic acid (C8), 3.2%–15% of capric acid (C1), and 41%–56% of lauric acid (C12). High contents of caprylic (2.4%–6.2%), capric (2.6%–7.0%), and lauric acid (41%–55%) can also be found in palm kernel oil. Cuphea seeds (family of loosestrife) have a broad species-dependent diversity in MCFA. Oil from Cuphea seeds has an extraordinarily high content of MCFA; Cuphea lanceolata and Cuphea ignea oils containing over 80 % capric acid have been used particularly as sources of MCTs in piglets [35].

Too few studies have been performed in humans. Some studies, however, report positive clinical effects of increased consumption of MCTs or MCFAs. One study reported that plasma triglycerides decreased from a mean of 1,601 to 554 mg/dL ($p < 0.05$), total cholesterol levels were reduced from 417 to 287 mg/dL ($p < 0.001$), and slight decreases in fasting glucose (–8%) and uric acid levels (–12%) when patients with severe hypertriglyceridemia were treated for 7 days with a formula diet rich in omega-3 fatty acids and MCT [36]. Positive effects of supplementation with MCFAs are also reported in conditions such as obesity (reduced body weight, waist line, and insulin resistance) [37,38], mild-to-moderate dementia in Alzheimer (improved cognition) [39], in type 1 diabetic subjects [40], on aging and arteriosclerosis [41], inherited cardiomyopathy [42,43], and chronic pancreatitis [44].

26.12 Intake of Animal-Based Foods Induces Dysbiosis and Inflammation within 24 Hours

As discussed above, the gut microbiota over the years has decreased in size and diversity. As a matter of fact, recent studies suggest a decrease of up to 40% [45] when compared to the Paleolithic microbiota, and evidence suggests that it will continue to do so [46]. Furthermore, recent studies demonstrate that such changes occur within 24 hours as immediate reaction to the content of our daily food [47]. Consumption of a diet high in saturated (milk- or meat-derived) fats (MF), but not consumption of polyunsaturated (safflower oil) fat (PUFA), changes the conditions for microbial assemblage and promotes expansion of the sulfite-reducing pathobiont, *Bilophila wadsworthia*, which induces a shift in hepatic conjugation of bile acids, from glycocholic to taurocholic acid that is especially important for solubilizing a hydrophobic diet such as milk. These changes are strongly associated with a strong proinflammatory TH1 immune response and increased incidence of inflammatory conditions such as colitis [48,49].

Numerous environmental and other toxins have AGE- ALE-like effects on the microbiota, immune system, and disease development, including uremic toxins. About 100 such toxins have been identified today, but most likely there exists many more, yet unidentified, with profound negative effects on health [50]. Several identified and unidentified uremic toxins are badly removed by renal dialysis, particularly those, which much like AGEs, are bound to proteins, such as p-cresyl sulfate (PCS) [50].

High intake, especially of meat, but also to some extent milk, and to a large extent powdered milk and a large majority of processed foods [51], is strongly associated with high intake of AGEs and ALEs, factors that in turn further support the development of inflammatory conditions. A recent review addressed the role of saturated fatty acid, sodium, advanced glycation end products (AGEs), nitrates/nitrites, heme iron, trimethylamine N-oxide (TMAO), branched amino acids (BCAAs), and endocrine disruptor chemicals (EDCs)—all more or less strong inducers of inflammation—in the development of type 2 diabetes [52].

26.13 No AGE-Preventing Drug Available—But Lifestyle Changes Are Very Effective

There are currently no drugs available that are effective and nontoxic at preventing AGE formation, and/or target preformed AGEs. Both aminoguanidine (AG) and the thiazolium-derived compound algebrium showed potential, but studies with both were discontinued due to safety and/or efficacy concerns. The fact that several second-generation compounds in experimental studies exhibit increased AGE inhibition and ability to breaking activity compared to the first-generation compounds including aminoguanidine gives some hope [53], but it will most likely take many years, if ever to happen, for such a "magic pill" to be available. It is, however, clear that significant benefits will be obtained by reducing the intake of cheese, meats, powdered milk, and other processed foods such as heated oils, and also of bread, and instead increase the consumption of vegetables and fruits, especially when raw. These recommendations are in line with the policy of various expert organizations with the aim to reduce chronic diseases such as cancer, heart diseases, and hypertension: American Cancer Society [54], American Heart Association Nutrition Committee [55], and the US Department of Health and Human Services [56].

26.14 AGE-Reducing Eating Habits

Eating foods preferably raw or at least prepared at a low temperature (below 80°C), steam-cooked or boiled, with minimal cooking time are much healthier than eating foods prepared by frying, grilling, microwaving, and roasting but also salting. Recent information warns against microwaving food that may dramatically accelerate the rate of AGE formation [57]. A randomized cross-over trial compared the metabolic effects of two different diets, one based on mild steam cooking while the other was based on high-temperature cooking in 62 volunteers (university students) during a period of 4 weeks [58]. Consuming the steamed-cooked food for 1 month induced significantly improved insulin sensitivity and increased plasma levels of omega-3 fatty acids (217%, $p = 0.002$), vitamin C (213%, $p = 0.0001$), and vitamin E (28%, $p = 0.01$) in comparison to the high temperature–exposed diet. Furthermore, significant reductions in concentrations of plasma cholesterol (5%, $p = 0.01$) and triglycerides (9%, $p = 0.01$) were also reported in the steamed-cooked foods group.

A great challenge for the future, and especially for the Western world, is to find techniques to produce bread at or below 100°C/215°F as the Chinese have done for centuries and continue to do. The synthesis of the toxic/inflammation-inducing substance acrylamide, normally not detected in unheated control or boiled foods (<5 µg/kg), increases when temperatures exceed 120°C/250°F and is found to be increased manifold at temperatures usually used for baking bread in Western Societies, often as high as 275°C/530° F [59,60]. High levels of acrylamide (up to 4,000 µg/kg) are observed in conventionally baked bread, being the highest in crispbreads, and also high in high temperature oven–baked or grilled vegetables, especially when vegetables are rich in carbohydrates, such as potatoes, carrots, beetroots, parsnips, and even more so in most commercially heated products such as potato chips, French fries, and toasted bread [61,62].

26.15 Reduction in Intake of Protein, Especially Sulfur-Containing, Is Also of Importance for Health

Some prevention is offered by marinating the foods for some hours at room temperature with ingredients such as antioxidant-rich herbs, garlic, tea, red wine, onions, olive oil, and beers, which significantly, but not totally, reduces the development of AGEs/ALEs [63]. Reduction in total intake of proteins [64], and most likely a particular reduction in methionine and other sulfur-containing amino acids, is an additional issue of relevance [65]. Significant reduction in body content of AGEs/ALEs in comparison to controls (eating standard Western food) is observed in individuals, who for >2 years practiced what is called caloric restriction (CR)—eating only two-thirds of what they would like to. This practice was accompanied by significant health advantages compared to the matched controls: lower blood pressure (102/61 ± 7 vs. 131/83 mm Hg) and lower levels of markers of inflammation such as CRP (0.3 vs. 1.9 mg /L), TNF-α (0.8 vs. 1.5 pg/ mL^{-1}), and TGF-β (29.4 vs. 35.4 ng/mL^{-1}) [66].

Elevated RAGE and low sRAGE is frequently seen in patients with active rheumatoid arthritis [67]. Thirty-seven obese individuals (mean BMI 28.3 ± 3.2) with rheumatoid arthritis were treated with calorie restriction, and after 8 weeks demonstrated not only significantly lower levels of pentosidine (an often-measured AGE) in urine, and reduction in BMI (6.3%, $p < 0.001$), waist circumference (5.7%, $p < 0.002$), triglycerides (11.9 % $p < 0.002$), and AGEs (7.21%, $p < 0.001$) but also much lower disease activity [68]. As an example, forced expiratory volume (FEV1), an expression of lung function, almost doubled.

26.16 Antioxidants and Vitamins

Provision of vitamins such as A, various B (especially B6 and B12), C, D, E, and K, as well as glutathione and folic acid, is often recommended for the prevention of accumulation in the body of AGEs/ALEs. Many plant antioxidants, particularly those collectively defined as polyphenols, are claimed to have oxidation-quenching properties, some say up to 10 times more powerful than conventional vitamins. They are also claimed to have great chemo-preventive properties, marked ability to prevent accumulation of AGEs/ALEs in the body, and significant capacity to reduce inflammation and to prevent impaired organ function and premature aging [69–72]. It is regrettable, as emphasized in a recent systematic review of the literature regarding antioxidant intake and protein glycation in normoglycemic individuals, that human trials with polyphenol-rich supplements are not only few but also characterized by high heterogeneity, poor design, and small sample size [73]. During the last 20 years, only 14 trials have tried polyphenols as a means to reduce glycation in nondiabetic individuals [73,74].

Plant antioxidants exist in nature in many thousands—most probably hundreds of thousands of different compounds. More than 4,000 have been identified only among flavonoids, and almost 1,000 among carotenoids. Most investigated antioxidants have been isothiocyanates in cruciferous vegetables; anthocyanins and hydroxycinnamic acids in cherries; epigallo-catechin-3-gallate (EGCG) in green tea; chlorogenic acid and caffeic acid in fresh coffee beans and also in fresh tobacco leaves; capsaicin in hot chili peppers; chalcones in apples; eugenol in cloves; gallic acid in rhubarb; hesperidin and naringin in citrus fruits; kaempferol in white cabbage; myricetin in berries; rutin and quercetin in apples and onions; resveratrol and other procyanidin dimers in red wine and virgin peanuts; various curcumenoids, the main yellow pigments in turmeric curry foods; and daidzein and genistein from the soy bean [10–12]. Most of these substances/foods are not yet tried in experimental or clinical studies, which is discouraging. It is clear that antioxidant molecules in food have a wide range of functions, but many of these seem unrelated to the ability to absorb free radicals.

A recent study looked at the anti-AGE effects of nine different plants. Three spices, namely seeds from *Coriandrum sativum* (cilantro or Chinese parsley), bark from *Cinnamomum zeylanicum* (Ceylon cinnamon) bark, and flower buds from *Syzygium aromaticum* (clove tree)—all well-known and common spices among the 20 spices with the highest antioxidant capacity, demonstrated a high ability to inhibit *in vitro* cross-linking [75].

26.17 Turmeric with Its Curcumenoids: Strong Inhibitors of Inflammatory Genes Such as COX-2—"The World's Healthiest Food"

Central to inflammation is the expression of numerous inflammation-inducing genes such as COX-2, matrix metalloproteinase-9 (MMP-9), inducible nitric oxide synthase (iNOS), TNF, IL-8, eotaxin, various cell surface adhesion molecules, and antiapoptotic proteins, regulated by NF-κB. COX-2 is inducible and barely detectable under normal physiological conditions, but is rapidly, but transiently, induced as an early response to proinflammatory mediators and mitogenic stimuli.

Curcuminoids, important bioactive ingredient of turmeric, are not only inexpensive atoxic and potent inflammation inhibitors (COX-2 and iNOS) but also potent inducers of heat shock proteins (HSPs) and other cytoprotecting factors. The most important chemical components of turmeric are a family of compounds called curcuminoids, which include several important anti-inflammatory substances, which seemingly interact, and should be used in combination, among them curcumin (diferuloylmethane), demethoxycurcumin, and bisdemethoxycurcumin. At least 5% of turmeric consists in curcumenoids of which curcumin is about 3% of the powdered turmeric. In addition, other important health-promoting ingredients are volatile oils such as turmerone, atlantone, and zingiberene. Half of the turmeric contains important fibers in addition to the several important vitamins as well as some well-defined sugars, proteins, and resins—all good reasons why this food often has been called "the world's healthiest food" (76–78). The curcumenoids inhibit not only COX-2 but also LOXs and leukotrienes, such as LBT4 and 5HETE, especially when bound to phosphatidylcholine micelles and are suggested to be especially effective in Th1-mediated immune conditions [79]. A recent publication suggests, based on *in vitro* studies, that curcuminoid effect reducing AGEs is achieved by interrupting leptin signaling [80].

26.18 Curcuminoid Treatment—Strong Clinical Effects

Although no human studies, known to me, have dealt with the specific effects of curcuminoids on AGE/ALE-induced chronic inflammation, numerous clinical studies support strong positive effects induced by numerous other similar lifestyle-associated factors. Here are some recent examples:

To prevent release of proinflammatory cytokines. Thirty obese individuals were randomized to receive pure curcumin 1 g/day or matched placebo for 4 weeks. Following a 2-week washout period, each group was assigned to the alternate treatment regimen for another 4 weeks. Serum samples were collected at the start and end of each study period. Serum levels of IL-1α, IL-1β, IL-2, IL-4, IL-6, IL-8, IL-10, VEGF, IFNγ, EGF, MCP-1, and TNF α were measured using a multiplex Biochip Array Technology–based method. Only, but importantly, mean serum IL-1β ($P = 0.042$), IL-4 ($P = 0.008$), and VEGF ($P = 0.01$) were significantly reduced by 4 weeks of curcumin therapy [81].

To reduce metabolic syndrome. A total of 50 patients diagnosed with metabolic syndrome (MS) according to the NCEP-ATPIII criteria, who were receiving standard of care, were assigned for 8 weeks to curcuminoids (1,000 mg/day) while another 50 MS patients received placebo. In order to improve the oral bioavailability, curcuminoids were coadministered with piperine in a ratio of 100:1 [82]. Significant positive impacts of curcuminoid supplementation were observed on triglycerides ($p = 0.003$), total cholesterol ($p = 0.042$), Lp(a) ($p < 0.001$), and non-HDL-C ($p = 0.009$), but not HDL-C ($p = 0.235$) or LDL-C ($p = 0.833$); all changes remained statistically significant after adjustment for baseline BMI [82]. In another study, overweight/obese type 2 diabetic patients (BMI ≥ 24.0; fasting blood glucose ≥7.0 mmol/L or postprandial blood glucose ≥11.1 mmol/L) were randomly assigned to curcuminoids (300 mg/day) or placebo for 3 months [83]. A total of 100 patients (curcuminoids, $n = 50$; placebo, $n = 50$) completed the trial. Curcuminoid supplementation significantly decreased fasting blood glucose ($p < 0.01$), HbA1c ($p = 0.031$), and insulin resistance index (HOMA-IR) ($p < 0.01$). In addition, curcuminoids also induced a significant decrease in serum total FFAs ($p < 0.01$), triglycerides ($P = 0.018$), and an increase in LPL activity ($p < 0.01$) [83].

To improve lung function, especially in smokers. Curry intake (at least once monthly) was significantly associated with better forced expiratory volume (FEV1) ($b = 0.045 \pm 0.018$, $p = 0.011$) and FEV1/FVC ($b = 1.14 \pm 0.52$, $p = 0.029$) in multivariate analyses that controlled simultaneously for gender, age, height, height-squared, smoking, occupational exposure and asthma/COPD history, and other dietary or supplementary intakes. Increasing levels of curry intake ("never or rarely," "occasional," "often," and "very often") were associated with higher mean adjusted FEV1 (p for linear trend = 0.001) and FEV1/FVC% (p for linear trend = 0.048). Significant effect modifications were observed for FEV1 (curry* smoking interaction, $p = 0.028$) and FEV1/FVC ($p = 0.05$). There were significantly larger differences in FEV1 and FEV1/FVC% between curry intake and noncurry intake among current and past smokers—the mean adjusted FEV1 associated with curry intake being 9.2% higher among current smokers, 10.3% higher among past smokers, and 1.5% higher among nonsmokers [84].

To reduce risk of arteriosclerosis in diabetes. The effects of curcumin on risk factors for atherosclerosis in individuals with diabetes were investigated during a 6-month period in a randomized, double-blinded, and placebo-controlled clinical trial, in which 107 individuals were treated with 1.5 g curcumin and 106 with placebo. Curcumin intervention significantly reduced pulse wave velocity ($P < 0.001$) and decreased level of leptin ($P < 0.001$) but increased level of serum adiponectin ($P < 0.001$). These results were associated with reduced levels of homeostasis model assessment-insulin resistance (HOMA) ($P < 0.001$), triglycerides ($P < 0.001$), uric acid ($P < 0.001$), visceral fat ($P < 0.001$), and total body fat ($P < 0.001$) [85].

To improve mood in mental depression. A total of 56 individuals with a major depressive disorder were treated with curcumin (500 mg twice daily) or placebo for 8 weeks. From Weeks 4 to 8, curcumin was significantly more effective than placebo in improving several mood-related symptoms, demonstrated by significant differences in both IDS-SR30 total score ($p = 0.045$) and IDS-SR30 mood score ($p = 0.014$), in addition to a nonsignificant trend for STAI trait score ($p = 0.097$). Greater efficacy from curcumin treatment was identified in a subgroup of individuals with atypical depression [86].

To reduce osteoarthritis. A total of 185 and 182 patients with knee osteoarthritis were randomly assigned into curcumin *(C. domestica)* extracts and ibuprofen groups, respectively. All WOMAC showed significant improvement scores at Weeks 0, 2, and 4 when compared to the baseline in both groups. All scores, WOMAC total, WOMAC pain, and WOMAC function scores showed no difference between the groups at Week 4. The number of patients complaining of abdominal pain/discomfort was significantly higher in the ibuprofen group ($P = 0.046$). Most subjects (96%–97%) were satisfied with the treatment, and two-thirds rated themselves as improved in a global assessment [87]. Others have observed similar effects [88].

To reduce disease activity in rheumatoid arthritis. Forty-five patients diagnosed with rheumatoid arthritis were randomized into three groups to receive daily curcumin (500 mg), and diclofenac sodium (50 mg) alone or in combination for 8 weeks [89]. The primary endpoints were reduction in Disease Activity Score (DAS). The secondary endpoints included American College of Rheumatology (ACR) criteria for reduction in tenderness and swelling of joint scores. Patients in all three treatment groups showed statistically significant changes in their DAS scores. It is of special interest that the curcumin group showed the highest percentage of improvement in overall DAS and ACR scores (ACR 20, 50, and 70) and these scores were significantly better than the patients in the diclofenac sodium group. It is important to note that curcumin treatment was found to be safe and no adverse events were reported [89].

To reduce inflammation in dialysis patients and reduce pruritus. A total of 100 HD patients with end-stage renal disease (ESRD) and suffering from severe pruritus were randomized into two groups: turmeric and placebo. The pruritus score and biochemical determinants including high-sensitivity C-reactive protein (hs-CRP) were compared before and at the end of the study between the two groups. A significant reduction of pruritus scores accompanied by a significant decrease in inflammation (hs-CRP) was observed in the turmeric group ($p = 0.012$) compared to the placebo group ($p = 0.001$) [90]. Other authors have observed similar effects [91].

To maintain remission in ulcerative colitis. A total of 45 patients were randomized for 6 months to curcumin treatment (2 g/day) and 44 patients to placebo. All patients received in parallel treatment with sulfasalazine or mesalamine. Four percent of patients in the curcumin group relapsed at 6 months compared to 18% of patients in the placebo group ($P = 0.06$). Twenty-two percent of the curcumin-treated patients had relapsed at 12 months compared to 32% of placebo patients ($P = 0.31$). A total of nine adverse events were reported in seven patients. Both clinical activity index (CAI) and endoscopic index were significantly lower in the curcumin-treated group than in the placebo group after 6 months [92]. Others have also obtained similar results [93].

26.19 Probiotics, Especially When Combined with Plant Fibers (Synbiotics), Are Effective to Eliminate Poisonous Substances

Some specific lactobacilli might well have the ability to eliminate AGEs/ALEs from foods, in a way that is very similar to that demonstrated for gluten [94] and also for heterocyclic amines [95]. *In vitro* studies have shown that fructoselysine, the dominating AGE in heated milk, can be effectively eliminated when incubated with fresh intestinal flora [96]. It is a weakness that no study up to this point seems to have investigated the possibilities to eliminate AGEs and ALEs through gut reconditioning, for example, achieved by supplementation of live lactobacilli with or without simultaneous supply of plant fibers. Significant detoxification and clinical improvements are, however, reported when applied to reduce other noxious substances—here follows some examples, which gives strong support to the assumption that supply of probiotics or better synbiotics might have strong positive clinical effects in individuals exposed to larger amounts of AGEs and ALEs.

To prevent effects of local toxic metal exposure. A study in Mwanza, Tanzania, investigated the efficacy of probiotic foods, nutritious and affordable means to prevent consequences of high local toxic metal exposures. A group of 44 school-aged children was followed over 25 days, and 60 pregnant women were followed over their last two trimesters until birth [97]. A yogurt containing 10^{10} colony-forming units (CFU) *Lactobacillus rhamnosus* GR-1 per 250 g was administered, while control groups received either whole milk or no intervention. Changes in blood metal levels were assessed, and the gut microbiomes of the children were profiled by analyzing 16S rRNA sequencing via the Ion Torrent platform. The children and pregnant women in the study were found to have elevated blood levels of lead and mercury compared to age- and sex-matched Canadians. Consumption of probiotic yogurt had a statistically significant protective effect against further increases in mercury (3.2 nmol/L; $p = 0.035$) and arsenic (2.3 nmol/L; $p = 0.011$) blood levels in the pregnant women, but this trend was not statistically significant in the children [97].

To improve intestinal barrier function and prevent leakage. Twenty-five healthy subjects were randomized into two groups: Group A (13 subjects) was given an active formulation containing 250 mg of tara gum, a plant fiber, and 1 billion viable cells of a potential probiotic, *Streptococcus thermophilus* ST10, whereas 12 subjects were given a placebo formulation, one dose per day for 30 consecutive days [98]. The presence and concentration of exopolysaccharides (EPSs) in the feces was determined at Time 0, after 30 days of treatment, and at the end of a 2-week follow-up period. The monosaccharide composition of EPSs was used to quantify the possible contribution of tara gum (a substance similar to guar gum) to the amount of polysaccharides detected in the fecal material. Intestinal permeability was evaluated at the same time by means of the lactitol/mannitol ratio (LM ration expresses small intestine permeability) and sucralose concentration (expression of colonic permeability) in urine specimens sampled after specified times. Supplementation with *S. thermophilus* ST10 and tara gum increased significantly the fecal EPSs concentration compared with placebo ($P < 0.001$) in parallel to induce significant decreases in intestinal permeability, both of the small bowel and colon. The L/M ratio diminished from 0.021 in the active group to 0.014 and 0.015 after 30 and 45 days, respectively ($P = 0.045$ and $P = 0.033$ compared with placebo). The sucralose concentration decreased from 35.8 to 27.9 mg and 29.1 mg ($P = 0.038$ and $P = 0.026$ compared with placebo) at the end of the supplementation period and after the follow-up, respectively. No significant differences were recorded in the placebo after 30 days or at the end of the follow-up [98].

To reduce exposure to hepatotoxins and carcinogens. Both *in vitro* and *in vivo* studies suggest that selected strains of probiotic bacteria can form tight complexes with aflatoxin B1 and other carcinogens and eliminate them. Ninety healthy young men from Guangzhou, China, were enrolled in a study aimed to determine whether administration of probiotic bacteria could block the intestinal absorption of aflatoxin B1 and thereby lead to reduced urinary excretion of aflatoxin B1-N(7)-guanine (AFB-N(7)-guanine), a marker for a biologically effective dose of aflatoxin exposure [99]. They were randomly assigned into two groups; one group received a mixture of *Lactobacillus rhamnosus* LC705 and *Propionibacterium freudenreichii* subsp. shermanii strains two times per day for 5 weeks, and the other group received a placebo preparation. The percentage of samples with negative AFB-N(7)-guanine values were higher in the probiotic group than in the placebo group after the 5-week intervention period ($p = 0.052$), and the decrease in urinary AFB-N(7)-guanine was statistically significant in the probiotic group ($p < 0.05$). The observed reduction was 36% after 3 weeks and 55% after 5 weeks. The geometric means for the probiotic and placebo groups during the intervention period were 0.24 and 0.49 ng AFB-N(7)-guanine/mL, respectively ($p = 0.005$) [99].

To reduce the accumulation of urea in chronic kidney disease. Patients with chronic kidney disease (CKD) show an increase in bowel aerobic bacteria that produce uremic toxins and decreased anaerobic bacteria as bifidobacteria and lactobacillus [100]. Different strains of *Lactobacillus casei* Shirota (LcS) were tried for 8 weeks in CKD patients in a randomized, controlled clinical trial in two doses: Group A: 8×10^9 CFU and Group B: 16×10^9 CFU. The larger dose induced a statistically significant reduction in blood urea concentrations [100].

To reduce inflammation in dialysis patients. Peritoneal dialysis patients received one capsule of a probiotic containing 10^9 cfu *Bi-fidobacterium bifidum* A218, 10^9 cfu *Bifidobacterium catenulatum* A302, 10^9 cfu *Bifidobacterium longum* A101, and 10^9 cfu *Lactobacillus plantarum* A87 daily for 6 months, and a placebo group received maltodextrin for the same duration [101]. A total of 39 patients completed the study (21 in the probiotics group and 18 in the placebo group). The serum levels of proinflammatory cytokines TNF-α, IL-5, IL-6, and endotoxin were significantly decreased after 6 months of treatment, while serum levels of anti-inflammatory cytokine IL-10 were significantly increased in the active group. In contrast, no significant changes in levels of serum cytokines and endotoxin occur in the placebo group after 6 months. Importantly, the residual renal function was well preserved in patients receiving probiotics [101].

To reduce uremic waste products in patients with CKD. In a 6-month cross-over trial, 46 outpatients were supplemented with a probiotic formulation consisting of a gel capsule containing a mix of *Lactobacillus acidophilus* KB27, *B. longum* KB31, and *S. thermophilus* KB19, totaling 1.5×1010 CFU/day [102]. Significant improvements were observed in terms of enhanced well-being (quality of life—QLT), absence of serious adverse effects, and impressive reductions in blood urea nitrogen (BUN)—the improvement in QOL as well as in BUN being statistically significant ($P < 0.05$). BUN levels decreased by 63% ($P < 0.05$), serum creatinine levels by 43%, and uric acid levels by 33%. The improvement in QOL was estimated to be 86% ($p < 0.05$) [102].

26.20 First Ever Trial with Synbiotic Treatment in Chronic Renal Disease Published in 2011

The first study ever undertaken to investigate the effects of combined fiber/probiotic (synbiotic treatment) was recently published [103]. This study demonstrated that fecal flora before supplementation with probiotics contained not only a significantly greater proportion of aerobic bacteria (specifically *Escherichia coli*)—100 times higher than that in healthy matched controls—but also significantly lower levels of the beneficial bifidobacteria. A significant decrease in both pathogenic Enterobacteria and in serum indoxyl sulfate levels was observed in dialysis patients receiving a supplement with a combination of 10^8 *Lactobacillus casei* strain Shirota, 10^8 *Bifidobacterium breve* (Yakult), and 4 g of the plant fibregalacto-oligosaccharides, three times a day for 2 weeks—a well-known prebiotic. The serum p-cresol level, poorly removed by dialysis, was significantly decreased during the treatment. Patients with a high serum p-cresol level tend to have often hard, but sometimes muddy, stools, and difficulty with defecation—a problem, which was eliminated by synbiotic treatment—replaced by normal ones [103]. However, the effects are not long-lasting, both protein-bound uremic toxins, PCS and IS, do return to pre-intervention levels 2 weeks after conclusion of the studies [104]. Most likely future should aim to, in addition to radical diet changes, supply pre-, pro-, and synbiotics on a regular basis as the disease remains, and most likely also provide both pre- and probiotics (synbiotics) in significantly larger doses.

A recent meta-analysis at the effectiveness of pre-, pro-, and synbiotics on reducing two protein-bound uremic toxins, PCS and IS, summarizes all studies published before 2012 [104]. Eight studies were found to have investigated prebiotics, six probiotics, one synbiotics, one both pre- and probiotics. The quality of the studies ranged from *moderate* to *very low*. Twelve studies were included in the meta-analyses, which reported statistically significant reductions in both IS and PCS. Their conclusion was that "there is a limited but supportive evidence for the effectiveness of pre- and probiotics on reducing PCS and IS in the CKD population," but that "further studies are needed to provide more definitive findings before routine clinical use can be recommended" [104].

26.21 Rest, Recuperation, Cleansing, Detoxification—Important to Reduce Poisonous Substances and Maintain Health

Daily nocturnal fasting is important in order to reduce/eliminate poisonous substances from blood and tissues, particularly from the liver, kidneys, skeletal muscles, and brain. Disturbed function of the diurnal clocks is strongly associated with impaired glucose tolerance in diseases such as Alzheimer's disease, type 2 diabetes, Parkinson's disease, multiple sclerosis, epilepsy, other seizure disorders, amyotrophic lateral sclerosis, Huntington's disease, restless legs, obstructive sleep apnea, and other chronic disorders [1]. Significant positive physiological consequences of time-restricted feeding are observed in experimental animals (mice). In an experimental study, two groups of animals receive exactly the same food and the same amounts of calories; the only difference was that one group was allowed to consume freely day and night, while the other had its food intake restricted to only half of the 24-hour day. Dramatic positive differences in body weight, glucose intolerance (insulin resistance), leptin resistance, liver pathology (fatty infiltration), degree of inflammation, and motor coordination were observed in the group with time-restricted food intake [105].

26.22 Paleolithic Lifestyle Stimulates a Robust Circadian Rhythm and a Healthy and Long-Lasting Life

Observations that our forefathers might have eaten only twice a day are supported by studies in people with similar lifestyle. One such group is the Hunzas in Northern Pakistan, today known for their good health and high number of centenarians. The adult Hunzas are reported to live on a daily 1,800-calorie 99% plant-based diet, consisting of 73% of mostly unrefined/unprocessed carbohydrates, 17% fat, and 10% protein (http://thepdi.com/hunza_health_secrets.htm). They go out to work in the fields around 5 o'clock in the morning on an empty stomach, and eat their main meal of the day at noon, and a lighter meal just before going to bed around dusk (http://projectavalon.net/forum4/showthread.php?48210HUNZAS-a-people-who-live-to-age-145-)— allowing the organs 15–18 hours daily for rest, cleansing, and detoxification.

REFERENCES

1. Bengmark, S. 2015. Obesity, the deadly quartet and the contribution of the neglected daily organ rest—A new dimension of un-health and its prevention. *HepatoBiliary Surg Nutr.* 4:278–288. doi: 10.3978/j.issn.2304-3881.2015.07.02
2. Bengmark, S. 2013. Gut microbiota, immune development and function. *Pharmacol Res.* 69:87–113.
3. Bengmark, S. 2004. Acute and "chronic" phase reaction—A mother of disease. *Clin Nutr.* 23:1256–1266.
4. Danaei G, Ding EL, Mozaffarian D, et al. 2009. The preventable causes of death in the United States: Comparative risk assessment of dietary, lifestyle, and metabolic risk factors. *PLoS Med.* 6(4):e1000058.
5. Boyle JP, Thompson TJ, Gregg EW, et al. 2010. Projection of the year 2050 burden of diabetes in the US adult population: Dynamic modeling of incidence, mortality, and prediabetes prevalence. *Popul Health Metr.* 8:29.
6. Hebert LE, Scherr PA, Bienias JL, et al. 2003. Alzheimer disease in the US population: Prevalence estimates using the 2000 census. *Arch Neurol.* 60:1119–1112.
7. Bray F, Møller B. 2006. Predicting the future burden of cancer. *Nat Rev Cancer.* 6:63–74.

8. Heffler S, Smith S, Keehan S, et al. 2005. U.S. health spending projections for 2004–2014. *Health Aff (Millwood).* W5-74-W5-85.
9. Wang YC, McPherson K, Marsh T, et al. 2011. Health and economic burden of the projected obesity trends in the USA and the UK. *Lancet.* 378:815–825.
10. Bengmark, S. 2007. Advanced glycation and lipoxidation end products—Amplifiers of inflammation: The role of food. *JPEN.* 31:430–440.
11. Bengmark, S. 2010. AGE, ALE RAGE and disease—A foods perspective. In *Handbook of Prebiotic and Probiotic Ingredients: Health Benefits and Food Applications*, Edited by Cho SS, Finocchiaro T. CRC Press, Taylor and Francis Group, Boca Raton, FL, pp. 139–162.
12. Bengmark, S. 2011. Modified amino acid-based molecules: Accumulation and health implications. In *Amino Acids in Human Nutrition and Health*, Edited by Mello JFD. CABI, Wallingford, UK, pp. 382–405.
13. http://www.cdc.gov/obesity/data/trends.html and http://www.cdc.gov/diabetes /data/trends.html
14. Li XM, Ganmaa D, Sato A. 2003. The experience of Japan as a clue to the etiology of breast and ovarian cancers: Relationship between death from both malignancies and dietary practices. *Med Hypotheses.* 60:268–275.
15. Ganmaa D, Li XM, Wang J, et al. 2002. Incidence and mortality of testicular and prostatic cancers in relation to world dietary practices. *Int J Cancer.* 98:262–267.
16. Campbell T, Campbell TC. 2006. *The China Study: The Most Comprehensive Study of Nutrition Ever Conducted and the Startling Implications for Diet, Weight Loss, and Long-term Health.* Ben Bella Books, Dallas, TX.
17. Lao XQ, Ma WJ, Sobko T, et al. 2014. Dramatic escalation in metabolic syndrome and cardiovascular risk in a Chinese population experiencing rapid economic development. *BMC Public Health.* 14:983.
18. Zhu Y, Wang HK, Qu YY, et al. 2015. Prostate cancer in East Asia: Evolving trend over the last decade. *Asian J Androl.* 17:48–57.
19. Keding GB, Msuya JM, Maass BL, et al. 2013. Obesity as a public health problem among adult women in rural Tanzania. *Glob Health Sci Pract.* 1:359–371.
20. Ebenbichler CF, Kirchmair R, Egger C, et al. Postprandial state and atherosclerosis. *Curr Opin Lipidol.* 6:286–290.
21. Meneses ME, Camargo A, Perez-Martinez P, et al. 2011. Postprandial inflammatory response in adipose tissue of patients with metabolic syndrome after the intake of different dietary models. *Mol Nutr Food Res.* 55:1759–1770.
22. Sottero B, Gargiulo S, Russo I. 2015. Postprandial dysmetabolism and oxidative stress in type 2 diabetes: Pathogenetic mechanisms and therapeutic strategies. *Med Res Rev.* 35(5):968–1031.
23. Mager DR, Mazurak V, Rodriguez-Dimitrescu C, et al. 2013. A meal high in saturated fat evokes postprandial dyslipemia, hyperinsulinemia, and altered lipoprotein expression in obese children with and without nonalcoholic fatty liver disease. *J Parenter Enteral Nutr.* 37:517–528.
24. Thomas EL, Saeed N, Hajnal JV, et al. 1998. Magnetic resonance imaging of total body fat. *J Appl Physiol.* 85:1778–1785.
25. Ceriello A, Quagliaro L, Piconi L, et al. 2004. Effect of postprandial hypertriglyceridemia and hyperglycemia on circulating adhesion molecules and oxidative stress generation and the possible role of simvastatin treatment. *Diabetes.* 53:701–710.
26. Erridge C, Attina T, Spickett CM, et al. 2007. A high-fat meal induces low-grade endotoxemia: Evidence of a novel mechanism of postprandial inflammation. *Am J Clin Nutr.* 86:1286–1292.
27. Ceriello A, Cavarape A, Martinelli L, et al. 2004. The post-prandial state in Type 2diabetesand endothelial dysfunction: Effects of insulin aspart. *Diabet Med.* 21:171–175.
28. Wang YI, Schulze J, Raymond N, et al. 2011. Endothelial inflammation correlates with subject triglycerides and waist size after a high-fat meal. *Am J Physiol Heart Circ Physiol.* 300:H784–H791.
29. Alessi MC, Peiretti F, Morange P, et al. 1997. Production of plasminogen activator inhibitor 1 by human adipose tissue: Possible link between visceral fat accumulation and vascular disease. *Diabetes.* 46:860–867.
30. Item F, Konrad D. 2012. Visceral fat and metabolic inflammation: The portal theory revisited. *Obes Rev.* 13 Suppl 2:30–39.
31. Guillot E, Vaugelade P, Lemarchal P, et al. 1993. Intestinal absorption and liver uptake of medium-chain fatty acids in non-anaesthetized pigs. *Br J Nutr.* 69:431–442.

32. Buttet M, Traynard V, Tran TT, et al. 2014. From fatty-acid sensing to chylomicron synthesis: Role of intestinal lipid-binding proteins. *Biochimie*. 96:37–47.
33. Wein S, Wolffram S, Schrezenmeir J, et al. 2009. Medium-chain fatty acids ameliorate insulin resistance caused by high-fat diets in rats. *Diabetes Metab Res Rev*. 25:185–194.
34. Zentek J, Buchheit-Renko S, Ferrara F, et al. 2011. Nutritional and physiological role of medium-chain triglycerides and medium-chain fatty acids in piglets. *Anim Health Res Rev*. 12:83–93.
35. Dierick NA, Decuypere JA, Degeyter I. The combined use of whole Cuphea seeds containing medium chain fatty acids and an exogenous lipase in piglet nutrition. *Arch Tierernahr*. 57:49–63.
36. Hauenschild A, Bretzel RG, Schnell-Kretschmer H, et al. 2010. Successful treatment of severe hypertriglyceridemia with a formula diet rich in omega-3 fatty acids and medium-chain triglycerides. *Ann Nutr Metab*. 56:170–175.
37. Han JR, Deng B, Sun J, et al. 2007. Effects of dietary medium-chain triglyceride on weight loss and insulin sensitivity in a group of moderately overweight free-living type 2 diabetic Chinese subjects. *Metabolism*. 56:985–991.
38. Siener R, Ehrhardt C, Bitterlich N, et al. 2011. Effect of a fat spread enriched with medium-chain triacylglycerols and a special fatty acid-micronutrient combination on cardiometabolic risk factors in overweight patients with diabetes. *Nutr Metab*. 8:21.
39. Sharma A, Bemis M, Desilets AR. 2014. Role of medium chain triglycerides (Axona(R)) in the treatment of mild to moderate Alzheimer's disease. *Am J Alzheimers Dis Other Demen*. 29:409–414.
40. Page KA, Williamson A, Yu N, et al. 2009. Medium-chain fatty acids improve cognitive function in intensively treated type 1 diabetic patients and support *in vitro* synaptic transmission during acute hypoglycemia. *Diabetes*. 58:1237–1244.
41. Kaunitz H. 1986. Medium chain triglycerides (MCT) in aging and arteriosclerosis. *J Environ Pathol Toxicol Oncol*. 6:115–121.
42. Iemitsu M, Shimojo N, Maeda S, et al. 2008. The benefit of medium-chain triglyceride therapy on the cardiac function of SHRs is associated with a reversal of metabolic and signaling alterations. *Am J Physiol Heart Circ Physiol*. 295:H136–H144.
43. Footitt EJ, Stafford J, Dixon M, et al. 2010. Use of a long-chaintriglyceride-restricted/medium-chaintriglyceride-supplemented diet in a case of malonyl-CoA decarboxylase deficiency with cardiomyopathy. *J Inherit Metab Dis*. 33:S253–S256.
44. Shea JC, Bishop MD, Parker EM, et al. An enteral therapy containing medium-chain triglycerides and hydrolyzed peptides reduces postprandial pain associated with chronic pancreatitis. *Pancreatology*. 3:36–40.
45. Clemente JC, Pehrsson EC, Blaser MJ, et al. 2015. The microbiome of uncontacted Amerindians. *Sci Adv*. 1(3):e1500183.
46. Walter J, Ley R. 2011. The human gut microbiome: Ecology and recent evolutionary changes. *Annu Rev Microbiol*. 65:411–429.
47. David LA, Maurice CF, Carmody RN, et al. 2014. Diet rapidly and reproducibly alters the human gut microbiome. *Nature*. 505:559–563.
48. Devkota S, Wang Y, Musch MW, et al. 2012. Dietary-fat-induced taurocholic acid promotes pathobiont expansion and colitis in Il10-/- mice. *Nature*. 487:104–108.
49. Devkota S, Chang EB. 2015. Interactions between diet, bile acid metabolism, gut microbiota, and inflammatory bowel diseases. *Dig Dis*. 33:351–356.
50. Sirich TL. 2015. Dietary protein and fiber in end stage renal disease. *Semin Dial*. 28:75–80.
51. Baptista JAB, Carvalho RCB. 2004. Indirect determination of Amadori compounds in milk-based products by HPLC/ELSD/UV as an index of protein deterioration. *Food Res Int*. 37:739–747.
52. Kim Y, Keogh J, Clifton P. 2015. A review of potential metabolic etiologies of the observed association between red meat consumption and development of type 2diabetes mellitus. *Metabolism*. 64:768–779.
53. Furlani RE, Richardson MA, Podell BK, et al. 2015. Second generation 2-aminoimidazole based advanced glycation end product inhibitors and breakers. *Bioorg Med Chem Lett* 25(21):4820–4823.
54. American Cancer Society. 2006. Choices for good health: American Cancer Society guidelines for nutrition and physical activity for cancer prevention. *CA – A Cancer J Clin*. 56:310–312.
55. Lichtenstein AH, Brands M, Franch HA, et al. 2006. Diet and lifestyle recommendations revision 2006. A scientific statement from the American Heart Association Nutrition Committee. *Circulation*. 114:82–96.

56. US Department of Health and Human Services, National Institutes of Health, and National Heart, Lung, and Blood Institute. 2006. *Your Guide to Lowering Your Blood Pressure with Dietary Approach to Stop Hypertension (DASH)*. NIH Publication 06-4082.
57. Visentin S, Medana C, Barge A, et al. 2010. Microwave-assisted Maillard reactions for the preparation of advanced glycation end products (AGEs). *Organ Biomol Chem.* 21:2473–2477.
58. Birlouez-Aragon I, Saavedra G, Tessier FJ, et al. 2010. A diet based on high-heat-treated foods promotes risk factors for diabetes mellitus and cardiovascular diseases. *Am J Clin Nutr.* 91:1220–1226.
59. Tareke E, Rydberg P, Karlsson P, et al. 2002. Analysis of acrylamide, a carcinogen formed in heated foodstuffs. *J Agric Food Chem.* 50:4998–5006.
60. Tareke E, Heinze TM, Gamboa da Costa G, et al. 2009. Acrylamide formed at physiological temperature as a result of asparagine oxidation. *J Agric Food Chem.* 57:9730–9733.
61. Granby K, Nielsen NJ, Hedegaard RV, et al. 2008. Acrylamide-asparagine relationship in baked/toasted wheat and rye breads. *Food Addit Contam, Part A. Chem Anal Control Expo Risk Assess.* 25:921–929.
62. Pedreschi F, Mariotti MS, Granby K. 2014. Current issues in dietary acrylamide: Formation, mitigation and risk assessment. *J Sci Food Agric.* 94:9–20.
63. Melo A, Viegas O, Petisca C, et al. 2008. Effect of beer/red wine marinades on the formation of heterocyclic aromatic amines in pan-fried beef. *J Agric Food Chem.* 56:10625–10632.
64. Uribarri J, Tuttle KR. 2006. Advanced glycation end products and nephrotoxicity of high-protein diets. *Clin J Am Soc Nephrol.* 1:1293–1299.
65. McCarty MF, Barroso-Aranda J, Contreras F. 2009. The low-methionine content of vegan diets may make methionine restriction feasible as a life extension strategy. *Med Hypotheses.* 72:125–128.
66. Meyer TE, Kovacs SJ, Ehsani AA, et al. 2006. Long-term caloric restriction ameliorates the decline in diastolic function in humans. *J Am Coll Cardio.* 47:398–402.
67. Iwashige K, Kouda K, Kouda M, et al. 2004. Calorie restricted diet and urinary pentosidine in patients with rheumatoid arthritis. *J Physiol Anthropol Appl Human Sci.* 23:19–24.
68. Gugliucci A, Kotani K, Taing J, et al. 2009. Short-term low calorie diet intervention reduces serum advanced glycation end products in healthy overweight or obese adults. *Ann Nutr Metab.* 54:197–201.
69. Delmas D, Jannin B, Latruffe N. 2005. Resveratrol: Preventing properties against vascular alterations and ageing. *Mol Nutr Food Res.* 49:377–395.
70. Rahman I, Biswas SK, Kode A. 2006. Oxidant and antioxidant balance in the airways and airway diseases. *Eur J Pharmacol.* 533:222–239.
71. Rahman I, Biswas SK, Kirkham PA. 2006. Regulation of inflammation and redox signalling by dietary polyphenols. *Biochem Pharmacol.* 72:1439–1452.
72. Sun AY, Wang Q, Simonyi A, et al. 2010. Resveratrol as a therapeutic agent for neurodegenerative diseases. *Mol Neurobiol.* 41:375–383.
73. Vlassopoulos A, Lean ME, Combet E. 2014. Oxidative stress, protein glycation and nutrition—Interactions relevant to health and disease throughout the lifecycle. *Proc Nutr Soc.* 73:430–438.
74. Oxygen Radical Absorbance Capacity (ORAC) of Selected Foods, Release 2. 2010. http://www.ars.usda.gov/services/docs.htm?docid=15866
75. Perera HK, Handuwalage CS. 2015. Analysis of glycation induced protein cross-linking inhibitory effects of some antidiabetic plants and spices. *BMC Complement Altern Med.* 15:175.
76. Bengmark S. 2006. Curcumin: An atoxic antioxidant and natural NF-κB, COX-2, LOX and iNOS inhibitor—A shield against acute and chronic diseases. *JPEN J Parenter Enteral Nutr.* 30:45–51.
77. Bengmark S. 2006. Plant-derived health-effects of turmeric and Curcumenoids. *Kuwait Med J.* 38:267–275.
78. Bengmark S. 2009. Control of systemic inflammation and chronic disease—The use of turmeric and curcumenoids. In *Nutrigenomics and proteonomics in health and disease. Food factors and gene interaction.* Edited by Mine Y, Miyashita K, Shahidi F. Wiley-Blackwell, Chichester, pp. 161–180.
79. Castro CN, Barcala TAE, Winnewisser J, et al. 2014. Curcumin ameliorates autoimmune diabetes. Evidence in accelerated murine models of type 1 diabetes. *Clin Exp Immunol.* 177:149–160.
80. Tang Y, Chen A. 2014. Curcumin eliminates the effect of advanced glycation end-products (AGEs) on the divergent regulation of gene expression of receptors of AGEs by interrupting leptin signalling. *Lab Invest.* 94:503–516.
81. Ganjali S, Sahebkar A, Mahdipour E, et al. 2014. Investigation of the effects of curcumin on serum cytokines in obese individuals: A randomized controlled trial. *Scientific World J.* 2014:898361.

82. Panahi Y, Khalili N, Hosseini MS, et al. 2014. Lipid-modifying effects of adjunctive therapy with curcuminoids-piperine combination in patients with metabolic syndrome: Results of a randomized controlled trial. *Complement Ther Med.* 22:851–857.
83. Na LX, Li Y, Pan HZ, et al. 2013. Curcuminoids exert glucose-lowering effect in type 2 diabetes by decreasing serum free fatty acids: A double-blind, placebo-controlled trial. *Mol Nutr Food Res.* 57:1569–1577.
84. Ng TP, Niti M, Yap KB, et al. 2014. Dietary and supplemental antioxidant and anti-inflammatory nutrient intakes and pulmonary function. *Public Health Nutr.* 17:2081–2086.
85. Chuengsamarn S, Rattanamongkolgul S, Phonrat B, et al. 2014. Reduction of atherogenic risk in patients with type 2diabetesby curcuminoid extract: A randomized controlled trial. *J Nutr Biochem.* 25:144–150.
86. Lopresti AL, Maes M, Maker GL, et al. 2014. Curcumin for the treatment of major depression: A randomised, double-blind, placebo controlled study. *J Affect Disord.* 67:368–375.
87. Kuptniratsaikul V, Dajpratham P, Taechaarpornkul W, et al. 2014. Efficacy and safety of Curcuma domestica extracts compared with ibuprofen in patients with knee osteoarthritis: A multicenter study. *Clin Interv Aging.* 9:451–458.
88. Madhu K, Chanda K, Saji MJ. 2013. Safety and efficacy of Curcuma longa extract in the treatment of painful knee osteoarthritis: A randomized placebo-controlled trial. *Inflammopharmacology.* 21:129–136.
89. Chandran B, Goel A. 2012. A randomized, pilot study to assess the efficacy and safety of curcuminin patients with active rheumatoid arthritis. *Phytother Res.* 26:1719–1725.
90. Pakfetrat M, Basiri F, Malekmakan L, et al. 2014. Effects of turmeric on uremic pruritus in end stage renal disease patients: A double-blind randomized clinical trial. *J Nephrol.* 27:203–207.
91. Sanmukhani J, Satodia V, Trivedi J, et al. 2014. Efficacy and safety of curcumin in major depressive disorder: A randomized controlled trial. *Phytother Res.* 28:579–585.
92. Kumar S, Ahuja V, Sankar MJ, et al. 2012. Curcumin for maintenance of remission in ulcerative colitis. *Cochrane Database Syst Rev.* 10:CD008424.
93. Hanai H, Iida T, Takeuchi K, et al. 2006. Curcumin maintenance therapy for ulcerative colitis: Randomized, multicenter, double-blind, placebo-controlled trial. *Clin Gastroenterol Hepatol.* 4:1502–1506.
94. di Cagno R, de Angelis M, Alfonsi G. et al. 2005. Pasta made from durum wheat semolina fermented with selected lactobacilli as a tool for a potential decrease of the gluten intolerance. *J Agric Food Chem.* 53;4393–4402.
95. Takada M, Hirata K, Ajiki T, et al. 2004. Expression of receptor for advanced glycation end products (RAGE) and MMP-9 in human pancreatic cancer cells. *Hepatogastroenterol* 51:928–930.
96. Erbersdobler H, Gunsser I, Weber G. 1970. Abbau von Fructoselysine durch die Darmflora. *Zentralblatt für Veterinärmedizin* A17:573–575. (in German).
97. Bisanz JE, Enos MK, Mwanga JR, et al. 2014. Randomized open-label pilot study of the influence of probiotics and the gut microbiome on toxic metal levels in Tanzanian pregnant women and school children. *MBio.* 5:e01580-14.
98. Del Piano M, Balzarini M, Carmagnola S, et al. 2014. Assessment of the capability of a gelling complex made of tara gum and the exopolysaccharides produced by the microorganism Streptococcus thermophilus ST10 to prospectively restore the gut physiological barrier: A pilot study. *J Clin Gastroenterol.* 48 Suppl 1:S56–S61.
99. El-Nezami HS, Polychronaki NN, Ma J, et al. 2006. Probiotic supplementation reduces a biomarker for increased risk of liver cancer in young men from Southern China. *Am J Clin Nutr.* 83:1199–1203.
100. Miranda Alatriste PV, Urbina Arronte R, Gómez Espinosa CO, et al. 2014. Effect of probiotics on human blood urea levels in patients with chronic renal failure. *Nutr Hosp.* 29:582–590.
101. Wang IK, Wu YY, Yang YF, et al. 2015. The effect of probiotics on serum levels of cytokine and endotoxin in peritoneal dialysis patients: A randomised, double-blind, placebo-controlled trial. *Benef Microbes.* 6:423–430.

102. Ranganathan N, Ranganathan P, Friedman EA, et al. 2010. Pilot study of probiotic dietary supplementation for promoting healthy kidney function in patients with chronic kidney disease. *Adv Ther.* 27:634–647.
103. Nakabayashi I, Nakamura M, Kawakami K, et al. 2011. Effects of synbiotic treatment on serum level of p-cresol in haemodialysis patients: A preliminary study. *Nephrol Dial Transplant* 26:1094–1098.
104. Rossi M, Klein K, Johnson DW, Campbell KL. 2012. Pre-, pro-, and synbiotics: Do they have a role in reducing uremic toxins? A systematic review and meta-analysis. *Int J Nephrol* 2012:673631
105. Chaix A, Zarrinpar A, Miu P, et al. 2014. Time-restricted feeding is a preventative and therapeutic intervention against diverse nutritional challenges. *Cell Metab* 20:991–1005.

27

Effects of a Low-AGE Diet on Insulin Sensitivity

Barbora de Courten and Estifanos Baye
Monash University
Clayton, VIC, Australia

CONTENTS

KEY POINTS

- Diets high in advanced glycation end products (AGEs) have been suggested to increase insulin resistance in humans.
- Reduction in dietary AGEs can be effectively achieved by cooking at low temperatures for a short time and by using acidic marinades.
- Recent clinical studies have shown that consumption of low-AGE diets improved insulin sensitivity in nondiabetic individuals.
- Only one trial used gold standard measure of insulin sensitivity.
- Long-term, high-quality clinical trials with larger sample sizes using gold standard measurements for insulin sensitivity are warranted.

27.1 Introduction

Advanced glycation end products (AGEs) are formed endogenously from the nonenzymatic reaction of the carbonyl group of sugars with a nucleophilic amino group of amino acids. This forms intermediate Amadori products via the Maillard reaction or methylglyoxal-derived AGEs such as methylglyoxal derived–hydroimidazolones (MG-H1). Oxidation of Amadori products leads to stable irreversible formation of N^{ε}-(carboxymethyl) lysine (CML) on lysine residues.

Apart from endogenous AGE formation, AGEs are also absorbed through ingestion of highly heated processed foods typical of Western diets. Browning of foods during cooking generates large amounts of AGEs (Maillard reaction). This contributes some desirable culinary properties such as flavor, color and aroma and prolongs the shelf-life of foods [1]. The rate of the Maillard reaction depends on the reaction time, processing temperature, concentrations of reactants, availability of water, pH level, and

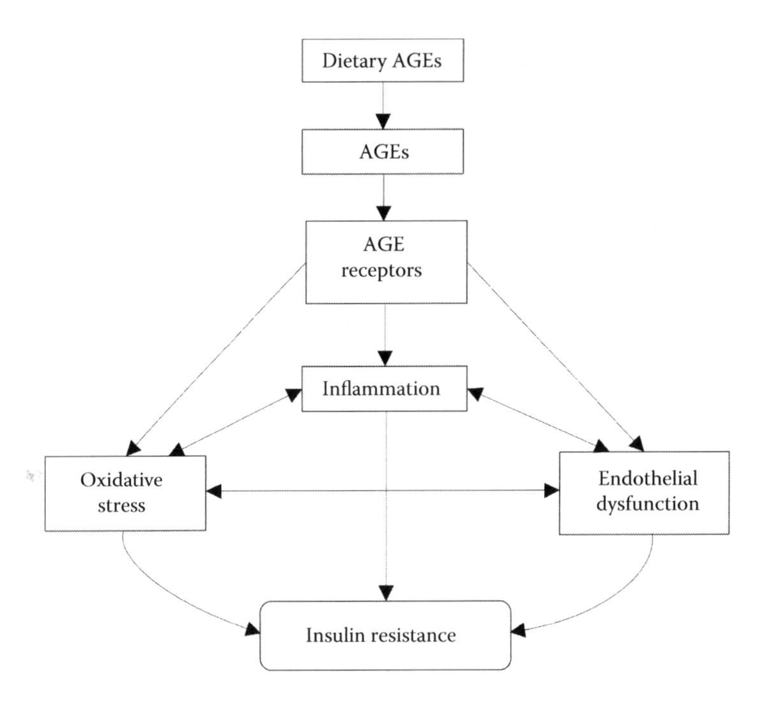

FIGURE 27.1 Relationship between dietary advanced glycation end products (AGEs) and circulating AGEs, inflammation, oxidative stress, endothelial dysfunction, and insulin resistance.

pro- and antioxidants. Higher dietary AGEs are generated in foods rich in lipid and protein content that are exposed to dry heat compared to foods cooked at lower temperatures for longer time periods in the presence of water content and an acidic environment [2–4]. Consistent with this, increased consumption of fish, legumes, vegetables, whole grains, and low-fat foods significantly reduces levels of dietary AGEs [5,6].

In humans, about 10%–30% of diet-derived AGEs are absorbed, and only one-third of the absorbed AGEs are excreted into the urine and feces within 3 days of ingestion [7]. The remaining two-thirds of dietary AGEs are retained and added to the body's total AGE load [1]. CML and MG-H1 are the most common AGEs and also the most commonly investigated in foods and human research. Both MG-H1 and CML have been previously used in clinical studies as indicators of dietary AGE intake [3]. In the tissues, CML binds to the receptor for AGEs. Interaction of AGEs with the AGE receptor (RAGE) triggers oxidative stress and inflammation (Figure 27.1). AGEs can directly cross-link with proteins, thereby alter their function [8–13]. In this chapter, we summarize current evidence regarding the effects of dietary AGE modulation in the pathophysiology of insulin resistance in humans.

27.2 Relationship between Dietary AGEs, Circulating AGEs, and Insulin Resistance

27.2.1 Evidence from Cross-Sectional Studies

There is contradictory evidence regarding the relationships between dietary AGE intake and serum AGEs as well as between dietary AGEs and insulin resistance, inflammation, endothelial dysfunction, and oxidative stress from cross-sectional studies.

Dietary AGE intake correlates well with both serum CML and MG levels in infants [14], healthy middle age and older individuals [15–17], as well as in patients with type 2 diabetes [18,19] and patients on dialysis [9]. Some studies reviewed in this chapter measured dietary AGE intake, while others measured circulating or urinary AGEs or both.

A cross-sectional study in 172 clinically healthy individuals demonstrated that dietary AGE intake was positively associated with serum levels of high-sensitivity C-reactive protein (hsCRP), CML and MG-H1 even after adjustment for age, gender, body mass index (BMI), and caloric intake [16]. Serum CML was positively related to insulin resistance as measured by homeostatic model assessment (HOMA-IR) [16]. Similarly, cross-sectional data obtained from 166 healthy term infants (aged 3–14 months) of Central European descent showed that high dietary AGE intake ingested through infant formulas significantly increased circulating CML levels and AGE-associated skin fluorescence [14]. However, there was no change in HOMA-IR oxidative stress or concentrations of plasma leptin, adhesion molecules, and markers of inflammation. Of note, HOMA-IR is not validated as a measure of insulin sensitivity in infants. In 322 older nondiabetic Japanese individuals, serum AGEs were independently correlated with HOMA-IR after adjustment for metabolic and anthropometric variables [20]. Another cross-sectional study conducted in 207 (97 male and 110 female) healthy nonobese Chinese individuals also supported these findings [21]. This study found that serum AGEs were independent determinants of insulin resistance in both males and females.

Similarly, a study in 273 elderly individuals (88 healthy controls, 90 individuals with impaired fasting glucose, and 95 patients with type 2 diabetes) found a positive correlation between serum AGE levels and fasting glucose, and advanced oxidation protein products and HOMA-IR in those with type 2 diabetes [22]. In addition, lower plasma soluble RAGE (sRAGE) levels and higher CML levels were found in patients with type 2 diabetes compared to healthy controls. In this study, sRAGE was independently associated with HOMA-IR, hemoglobin A1c, and circulating CRP levels [23]. Another study in healthy individuals found that levels of serum AGEs or sRAGE concentrations were not associated with insulin sensitivity measured by euglycemic hyperinsulinemic glucose clamp, the gold standard measure of insulin sensitivity. However, there was an association between serum AGEs with early phase insulin secretion, independent of age, sex, BMI, and waist circumference [24]. Moreover, circulating AGEs, sRAGE, and endogenous secretory receptor for AGEs (esRAGE) concentrations were inversely related to 2-hour plasma glucose concentrations [24].

Interestingly, a cross-sectional study conducted in 139 male nondiabetic patients with obstructive sleep apnea showed that serum AGEs were independently associated with insulin resistance (HOMA-IR) as well as apnea–hypopnea index, duration of SaO_2 <90%, minimum SaO_2, and plasma hsCRP levels. These relationships were independent of obesity, suggesting that chronic inflammation and oxidative stress in patients with obstructive sleep apnea may increase AGEs [25]. Another cross-sectional study investigated 325 healthy young (18–45 years) and older (>60 years) adults and 66 chronic kidney disease (CKD) patients [17]. Dietary AGE intake was independently associated with 8-isoprostane, vascular cell adhesion molecule-1 (VCAM-1), and RAGE and $p66^{shc}$ mRNAs. Subgroup analyses revealed that in healthy subjects only, both serum CML and MG levels were correlated with AGE receptor-1 (AGER1) mRNA expression [17]. Another study in 93 older (>60 years old) healthy individuals showed that dietary AGEs were correlated with serum MG levels and both were positively correlated with serum CML, plasma 8-isoprostanes, leptin, tumor necrosis factor alpha protein (TNFα) in peripheral blood mononuclear cells (PBMCs), and RAGE mRNA, but inversely with adiponectin levels which has been shown to be associated with insulin sensitivity [15].

A cross-sectional study by Chao et al. [18] included 74 healthy controls, 50 patients with type 2 diabetes and low AGE intake (≤300 μg), and 68 with high AGE intake (>300 μg). All participants completed a 7-day dietary record. Comparison of patients with type 2 diabetes who had high AGE intake showed significantly higher frequency in consuming soybean sauce and frying oil, as well as using deep frying process for food preparation. They also had higher plasma AGE concentrations compared to patients with type 2 diabetes with low AGE intake as well as healthy controls [18]. These findings suggest a significant contribution of dietary AGE intake to the endogenous AGE pool. Furthermore, patients with type 2 diabetes who had high AGE intake showed positive associations between concentrations of plasma AGEs and markers of inflammation such as interleukin-1α (IL-1α), TNF-α, and monocyte chemoattractant protein-1 (MCP-1) levels and plasma markers of oxidative stress such as 8-isoprostane levels, superoxide dismutase (SOD) activity, and glutathione. Therefore, increased dietary AGE intake may result in insulin resistance through the prooxidative and proinflammatory effects of AGEs.

27.2.2 Evidence from Longitudinal Studies

Only three longitudinal studies investigated a role of AGEs in the development of insulin resistance. In 93 older healthy adults, baseline dietary AGE intake was associated with circulating AGEs and markers of oxidative stress at follow-up. High baseline serum MG levels were independent predictors of cognitive decline over 9 months, and changes in serum MG levels correlated with changes in HOMA-IR as well as with serum CML levels [15]. In a study by Vlassara et al. [17], 49 healthy participants were followed for 2 years. Changes in dietary AGE intake were strongly correlated with changes in serum CML and MG levels. In addition, serum CML levels were significantly related to changes in markers of inflammation, endothelial dysfunction, and oxidative stress [17]. In pregnant women with pre-eclampsia, esRAGE levels were threefold higher in patients who developed pre-eclampsia (200 ng/L) compared to controls (63 ng/L). In addition, esRAGE levels were correlated with insulin resistance, CRP and adiponectin levels as well as with systolic and diastolic blood pressure and renal function [26]. The positive association between esRAGE and CRP and the negative correlation between esRAGE and HOMA-IR persisted after adjustment for age, creatinine, systolic blood pressure, and adiponectin [26]. Interestingly, median esRAGE concentrations 6 months after the delivery were significantly lower in patients with existing preeclampsia (270 ng/L) than in controls (342 ng/L) in contrast to the results obtained during pregnancy.

In summary, observational studies indicate that circulating AGEs relate well to dietary AGE intake in different AGE groups as well as in healthy and diseased states. Several studies show relationship between dietary AGEs and/or circulating AGEs and the indirect measure of insulin resistance, HOMA-IR. HOMA-IR cannot differentiate between insulin sensitivity and secretion, which is the main limitation of the studies. Only one study measured insulin resistance by hyperinsulinemic euglycemic glucose clamp, a direct measure of insulin sensitivity, and found no correlation between AGE concentrations and insulin resistance but found a correlation with insulin secretion measured by intravenous glucose tolerance test. Current observational evidence supports a role for dietary AGEs in increasing proinflammatory and prooxidative states, which seems to be more prominent in diseases associated with proinflammatory and prooxidative profiles. A small amount of evidence also supports temporal effects of dietary AGE on insulin sensitivity.

27.2.3 Evidence from Clinical Trials

There is some evidence from clinical trials that changes in dietary AGE consumption result in changes in circulating [27], urinary, and fecal concentrations of AGEs [27,28].

Previous studies have suggested that a single meal challenge high in dietary AGE content can alter glucose homeostasis [29,30]. One study administered modified wheat flakes to healthy participants where addition of a fermentation step and suppression of high temperature cooking improved satiety as well as insulin index - a surrogate measure of insulin secretory response to various foods [29]. Another study in patients with type 2 diabetes found that varieties of French bread with similar ingredients have different insulin indices during a meal challenge, which is likely due to differences in bread processing [31].

Birlouez-Aragon et al. [28] compared two 4-week-long diets in a randomized crossover trial with 10-day washout—one with predominantly steamed foods (low-AGE diet) and the other with high heat-treated foods (high-AGE diet) in 62 healthy student volunteers (age >18 years and BMI <25 kg/m^2) [28]. All meals were provided on campus. Although the diets were designed to contain comparable amounts of energy and nutrients, the high-AGE diet was significantly more energy dense (10% in higher caloric intake) and had a greater content of fat and carbohydrates and lower vitamin C. However, changes in macronutrient and vitamin C intakes were not associated with metabolic changes. Both plasma protein CML content and urinary CML concentrations (but not fecal concentrations) were increased during consumption of the high-AGE diet [28]. The low-AGE diet resulted in lower fasting plasma insulin levels and HOMA-IR as well as favorable lipid profiles with lower cholesterol and triglyceride levels [28].

Mark et al. [27] performed a randomized controlled trial investigating if consumption of a diet low in AGEs for 4 weeks improved insulin sensitivity (HOMA-IR and insulin sensitivity index) in healthy overweight women [27]. Seventy-four women were randomized to a diet high or low in AGEs, together with fructose or glucose supplements. Baseline anthropometric and metabolic characteristics of the two intervention groups were well matched. Change in dietary AGEs was achieved by providing cooking instructions. Diets were matched for energy content but not macronutrient content. The low-AGE diet was lower in fat content. Percentage of energy derived from fat and carbohydrate was higher (22% and 10%, respectively) and protein was lower (15%) in the high-AGE group compared to the low-AGE group. This was likely a reason for the significant reduction observed in all anthropometric parameters including weight, BMI, and waist circumference in the low-AGE group. The low-AGE diet resulted in decreased urinary CML and MG-H1 levels and improved insulin resistance, which was significant after adjustment for age, and change in weight and waist circumference. Plasma glucose did not change in either group. Supplementation with sugar did not affect the outcome measures [27].

Another parallel trial investigated 18 healthy individuals aged above 60 years who were randomized to a high-AGE (>15 AGE Eq/day) or low-AGE diet (<10 AGE Eq/day) for 4 months [32]. Change in dietary AGEs was achieved by providing instructions for cooking and resulted in 50% lower dietary AGE content in the low-AGE group (without caloric restriction). No information was available about differences in macronutrient content in the study or whether the two groups changed their body weight during the intervention. Dietary restriction of AGE intake significantly decreased serum AGEs (both CML and MG) as well as 8-isoprostanes, TNFa protein in PBMCs, full length RAGE, and AGER1 mRNA.

In the parallel clinical trial by Vlassara and colleagues [17], 40 healthy volunteers were randomized to either a low-AGE or high-AGE diet (dietary AGE intake >13 AGE Eq/day) for 4 months. Similarly, nine patients with CKD were also randomly assigned to these diets for 4 weeks. In healthy subjects, the low-AGE diet significantly reduced the levels of serum CML and MG as well as AGER1, RAGE, and $p66^{shc}$mRNA. In addition, the low-AGE diet reduced 8-isoprostanes, VCAM-1, and TNF-α protein in PBMCs. In patients with CKD, the low-AGE diet showed a similar reduction in all parameters, except AGER1. AGER1 was increased by 60%, which was similar to the values seen in healthy young subjects.

Tantalaki et al. [33] conducted a clinical trial (nonrandomized) in 34 women with polycystic ovary syndrome. Polycystic ovary syndrome is the most common endocrine condition in women and is underpinned by hormonal disturbances including insulin resistance and hyperandrogenism (high testosterone levels) [34]. They studied women during three 2-month dietary interventions—a hypocaloric diet with ad libitum AGEs (energy deficit of 500 kcals was assigned) followed by an isocaloric diet with high-AGE content for another 2 months and afterward an isocaloric diet with low-AGE content for the following 2 months [33]. The dietary intervention was delivered by providing cooking instructions with weekly support by a dietician. The low-AGE diet consisted of 50% less dietary AGEs and the high-AGE diet consisted of 50% more dietary AGEs compared to baseline, and these two diets had a similar caloric content. Macronutrient content was not assessed. The low-AGE diet resulted in improved HOMA-IR and lower fasting insulin levels, oxidative stress markers, and testosterone levels compared to the high-AGE diet and was superior with regard to its metabolic impact compared to the hypocaloric diet with ad libitum AGEs. During the low-AGE dietary period, dietary AGE intake correlated with insulin levels, and serum AGE levels correlated with both plasma insulin levels and HOMA-IR [33]. Results from this study suggest that low-AGE diets may be metabolically more beneficial in preventing and treating insulin resistance than hypocaloric ad libitum AGE diets.

Uribarri et al. [35] conducted a randomized controlled clinical trial in 18 healthy controls and 18 patients with type 2 diabetes. Participants were randomly assigned to an isocaloric high-AGE diet (their usual diet, >20 AGE Eq/day) or a low-AGE diet (<10 AGE Eq/day) for 4 months. Twenty percent of patients with type 2 diabetes were on diet only, and 80% were on oral medical therapy, including insulin sensitizers such as metformin and pioglitazone, as well as other drugs which influence glucose metabolism and markers of inflammation such as aspirin, angiotensin-converting enzyme inhibitors, and statins. The intervention was delivered by provision of cooking instructions with weekly support from a dietician. Caloric and macronutrient content of the diets was not reported. There was no significant change in body weight from baseline to follow-up but data in each intervention group were not reported. Low-AGE intake significantly reduced serum CML and MG levels in both healthy controls and patients with type 2 diabetes. In patients with type 2 diabetes, a low-AGE diet reduced HOMA-IR, fasting insulin, 8-isoprostanes, RAGE, TNF-α and leptin levels. It also reduced nuclear factor kappa beta and increased expression of AGER1 in PBMCs and levels of adiponectin [35]. In healthy subjects, there was no change in HOMA-IR, but there was a decrease in RAGE, 8-isoprostanes, and TNF-α [35].

Vlassara et al. [11] conducted two intervention studies in 24 patients with type 2 diabetes. Eleven patients were randomized to a 2-week crossover trial and 13 patients to a 6-week parallel design trial. Four patients from the second study were treated with statins (Lipitor) and two with aspirin. In the crossover trial, patients were randomized to a 2 week high- or low-AGE diet with 1–2 weeks washout. Dietary intervention included providing packaged meals for breakfast, lunch, dinner, and snacks and in addition, patients received cooking instructions. Diets resulted in significant changes in both serum and urinary AGEs. Investigators attempted to match isocaloric and macronutrient content of the diets; however, there was a small but significant difference in body weight between the interventions. In the 6-week parallel design trial, there was a significant decrease in plasma glucose which was at normal range by the end of the study. None of the metabolic and cardiovascular parameters changed in the 2-week crossover trial. In both trials, consumption of a low-AGE diet significantly reduced markers of inflammation and endothelial function [11].

In another parallel design trial conducted by Vlassara and colleagues [36], 138 obese individuals with metabolic syndrome were randomly assigned to consume either low-AGE or high-AGE (regular) diets for 1 year. Similar baseline characteristics were reported in both groups, except for a relatively lower BMI, VCAM-1 levels, and glyoxalase I in the low-AGE groups. Circulating AGEs, markers of inflammation, and oxidative stress, as well as body weight, were significantly reduced after consumption of low-AGE diets. On the contrary, high-AGE diets increased AGE levels, inflammation, and oxidative stress. Compared to the high-AGE diets, HOMA-IR was markedly improved after low-AGE diets. Importantly, this effect remained significant after adjusting for baseline BMI and intake of calories and macronutrients as well as age, sex, and race. Even in those participants on low-AGE diets who did not lose body weight, significant reductions in serum AGEs, inflammatory markers, oxidative stress, and insulin resistance was observed. There were no adverse events reported in this trial. These findings clearly suggest that long-term intake of low-AGE diets can help to delay or prevent the development of chronic diseases such as type 2 diabetes and cardiovascular diseases without any side effects of the intervention.

De Courten et al. [37] performed a randomized, double-blind, crossover trial in 20 overweight and obese otherwise healthy adults. In this study, participants alternately consumed low- and high-AGE diets matched in both energy and macronutrient contents for 2 weeks each and separated by a 4-week washout period. Baseline values for insulin sensitivity and secretion, circulating AGEs, and anthropometric variables did not differ between groups before each test diet. Insulin sensitivity measured by hyperinsulinemic euglycemic clamp was improved after consumption of low-AGE diets compared to high-AGE diets.

Serum and urinary CML, MG-H1, and Nε-(carboxyethyl) lysine (CEL) levels, however, did not change between the two diets. No differences in body weight and insulin secretion were reported and no side effects associated with the intervention were observed. The findings of this study further support the positive effects of low-AGE diets in reducing the risk of developing type 2 diabetes in high-risk groups and suggest that the effect of AGEs on glucose metabolism is primarily mediated via insulin sensitivity.

In summary, the data from clinical trials suggest that low-AGE diets are beneficial for improving insulin sensitivity in nondiabetic individuals including healthy and overweight adults, obese people with metabolic syndrome, and women with polycystic ovary syndrome as well as glucose metabolism in patients with type 2 diabetes. The limitations of current trials are that the majority of trials published thus far did not match both energy and macronutrient content, which often resulted in changes in body weight. This suggests that low-AGE diets that the low-AGE diet improved glucose metabolism due to changes in body weight and/or macronutrient intake. In addition, HOMA-IR, an indirect measure of insulin sensitivity, was used in all trials except one study by de Courten et al. [37] that used the gold standard measurements for insulin sensitivity—hyperinsulinemic euglycemic glucose clamps. As mentioned previously, HOMA-IR cannot differentiate between insulin sensitivity and secretion and is also not validated in children and patients with type 2 diabetes. Furthermore, the crossover trials [11,28] had only 1–2 weeks washout which might not have been sufficient and did not assess for carry-over effects of the previous diet.

27.2.4 Evidence from Systematic Reviews

In 2013, a systematic review was conducted with a focus on dietary AGE restriction for attenuation of insulin resistance, oxidative stress, and endothelial dysfunction and identified 12 clinical trials. It concluded that a low-AGE diet reduced serum CML levels in healthy individuals but not in patients with renal failure. Low-quality evidence was also observed for the effects of long-term low-AGE diet markers of inflammation, oxidative stress, and endothelial dysfunction in healthy individuals. There was contradictory evidence on the effects of a low-AGE diet on insulin resistance in healthy individuals and very low-quality evidence was found for patients with type 2 diabetes. The authors were unable to draw conclusions regarding the effects of dietary AGE restriction on insulin resistance, markers of inflammation and oxidative stress in patients with type 2 diabetes or kidney disease because of the poor methodological quality of the clinical trials reviewed [2].

Clarke and colleagues [38] conducted another systematic review with the aim of examining the effect of consumption of a high-AGE diet on biomarkers of chronic disease, including CKD. In this systematic review, 12 randomized controlled trials were included with a total of 293 participants. High-AGE diets increased circulating TNFα and AGEs levels in all populations, 8-isoprostanes in healthy adults, and VCAM-1 in patients with diabetes. It was concluded that dietary AGEs may play an important role in the promotion of chronic conditions such as type 2 diabetes, cardiovascular diseases, and CKD through increasing inflammation, oxidative stress, and advanced glycation. As pointed out by the authors, the generalizability of the findings from this review may be limited due to the low quality of included trials.

27.3 Conclusions and Recommendations

Modern food processing due to globalization and utilization of industrialized methods has dramatically altered our diets. These highly processed foods, which are replete with appetite-enhancing AGEs, have been suggested to promote inflammation and oxidative stress, and thereby increase insulin resistance and contribute to the development of type 2 diabetes. Low-AGE diets are a relatively simple, noninvasive, and well-tolerated approach that can be achieved in three different ways: (1) daily choice of foods with low-AGE content, (2) healthier cooking methods (such as lower heat food preparation, use of water and acidic marinades) to minimize the production of AGEs, and (3) high antioxidant intake that prevents AGE formation [39]. Current evidence from both observational and intervention studies is supportive of dietary restriction of our usual high-AGE diet, without altering nutrient or caloric intake to reduce markers of oxidative stress, inflammation, and endothelial dysfunction and improve insulin sensitivity in healthy individuals and patients with type 2 diabetes. However, these studies suggest that the effect of dietary AGEs on insulin resistance may depend on the health status of the individual. The main limitations of current trials include the methods used for measurement of insulin sensitivity, as well as not accounting for the effect of weight loss and change in energy and macronutrient intake. Thus, long-term, multi-center, high-quality clinical trials with large sample sizes and hard clinical outcomes such as development of type 2 diabetes are needed. Trials should include both healthy individuals and patients with type 2 diabetes to clarify the effects of low-AGE diets in the prevention and treatment of insulin resistance and type 2 diabetes.

REFERENCES

1. Ottum M, Mistry A. Advanced glycation end products: Modifiable environmental factors profoundly mediate insulin resistance. *J Clin Biochem Nutr.* 2015;57(1):1–12.
2. Kellow NJ, Savige GS. Dietary advanced glycation end-product restriction for the attenuation of insulin resistance, oxidative stress and endothelial dysfunction: A systematic review. *Eur J Clin Nutr.* 2013;67(3):239–48.
3. Poulsen MW, Hedegaard RV, Andersen JM, de Courten B, Bugel S, Nielsen J, et al. Advanced glycation endproducts in food and their effects on health. *Food Chem Toxicol.* 2013;60:10–37.

4. Vlassara H, Uribarri J. Glycoxidation and diabetic complications: Modern lessons and a warning? *Rev Endocr Metabol Disord.* 2004;5(3):181–8.
5. Goldberg T, Cai W, Peppa M, Dardaine V, Baliga BS, Uribarri J, et al. Advanced glycoxidation end products in commonly consumed foods. *J Am Diet Assoc.* 2004;104(8):1287–91.
6. Uribarri J, Woodruff S, Goodman S, Cai W, Chen X, Pyzik R, et al. Advanced glycation end products in foods and a practical guide to their reduction in the diet. *J Am Diet Assoc.* 2010;110(6):911–16.e12.
7. Semba RD, Nicklett EJ, Ferrucci L. Does accumulation of advanced glycation end products contribute to the aging phenotype? *J Gerontol Series A, Biol Sci Med Sci.* 2010;65(9):963–75.
8. Cai W, Gao QD, Zhu L, Peppa M, He C, Vlassara H. Oxidative stress-inducing carbonyl compounds from common foods: Novel mediators of cellular dysfunction. *Mol Med.* 2002;8(7):337–46.
9. Uribarri J, Peppa M, Cai W, Goldberg T, Lu M, Baliga S, et al. Dietary glycotoxins correlate with circulating advanced glycation end product levels in renal failure patients. *Am J Kidney Dis.* 2003;42(3):532–8.
10. Vlassara H. The AGE-receptor in the pathogenesis of diabetic complications. *Diabetes/Metabol Res Rev.* 2001;17(6):436–43.
11. Vlassara H, Cai W, Crandall J, Goldberg T, Oberstein R, Dardaine V, et al. Inflammatory mediators are induced by dietary glycotoxins, a major risk factor for diabetic angiopathy. *Proc Natl Acad Sci U S A.* 2002;99(24):15596–601.
12. Vlassara H, Striker GE. AGE restriction in diabetes mellitus: A paradigm shift. *Nat Rev Endocrinol.* 2011;7(9):526–39.
13. Yamagishi S, Ueda S, Okuda S. Food-derived advanced glycation end products (AGEs): A novel therapeutic target for various disorders. *Curr Pharmaceut Design.* 2007;13(27):2832–6.
14. Klenovics KS, Boor P, Somoza V, Celec P, Fogliano V, Sebekova K. Advanced glycation end products in infant formulas do not contribute to insulin resistance associated with their consumption. *PLoS One [Electronic Resource].* 2013;8(1):e53056.
15. Cai W, Uribarri J, Zhu L, Chen X, Swamy S, Zhao Z, et al. Oral glycotoxins are a modifiable cause of dementia and the metabolic syndrome in mice and humans. *Proc Natl Acad Sci U S A.* 2014;111(13):4940–5.
16. Uribarri J, Cai W, Peppa M, Goodman S, Ferrucci L, Striker G, et al. Circulating glycotoxins and dietary advanced glycation endproducts: Two links to inflammatory response, oxidative stress, and aging. *J Gerontol Series A-Biol Sci Med Sci.* 2007;62(4):427–33.
17. Vlassara H, Cai W, Goodman S, Pyzik R, Yong A, Chen X, et al. Protection against loss of innate defenses in adulthood by low advanced glycation end products (AGE) intake: Role of the antiinflammatory AGE receptor-1. *J Clin Endocrinol Metabol.* 2009;94(11):4483–91.
18. Chao PC, Huang CN, Hsu CC, Yin MC, Guo YR. Association of dietary AGEs with circulating AGEs, glycated LDL, IL-1alpha and MCP-1 levels in type 2 diabetic patients. *Eur J Nutr.* 2010;49(7):429–34.
19. Luevano-Contreras C, Garay-Sevilla ME, Preciado-Puga M, Chapman-Novakofski KM. The relationship between dietary advanced glycation end products and indicators of diabetes severity in Mexicans and non-Hispanic whites: A pilot study. *Int J Food Sci Nutr.* 2013;64(1):16–20.
20. Tahara N, Yamagishi S, Matsui T, Takeuchi M, Nitta Y, Kodama N, et al. Serum levels of advanced glycation end products (AGEs) are independent correlates of insulin resistance in nondiabetic subjects. *Cardiovasc Therapeut.* 2012;30(1):42–8.
21. Tan KC, Shiu SW, Wong Y, Tam X. Serum advanced glycation end products (AGEs) are associated with insulin resistance. *Diabetes/Metabol Res Rev.* 2011;27(5):488–92.
22. Gradinaru D, Borsa C, Ionescu C, Margina D. Advanced oxidative and glycoxidative protein damage markers in the elderly with type 2 diabetes. *J Proteomics.* 2013;92:313–22.
23. Basta G, Sironi AM, Lazzerini G, Del Turco S, Buzzigoli E, Casolaro A, et al. Circulating soluble receptor for advanced glycation end products is inversely associated with glycemic control and S100A12 protein. *J Clin Endocrinol Metabol.* 2006;91(11):4628–34.
24. Forbes JM, Sourris KC, de Courten MP, Dougherty SL, Chand V, Lyons JG, et al. Advanced glycation end products (AGEs) are cross-sectionally associated with insulin secretion in healthy subjects. *Amino Acids.* 2014;46(2):321–6.
25. Xu JX, Cai W, Sun JF, Liao WJ, Liu Y, Xiao JR, et al. Serum advanced glycation end products are associated with insulin resistance in male nondiabetic patients with obstructive sleep apnea. *Sleep Breath.* 2015;19(3):827–33.

26. Fasshauer M, Seeger J, Waldeyer T, Schrey S, Ebert T, Lossner U, et al. Endogenous soluble receptor for advanced glycation endproducts is increased in preeclampsia. *J Hypertens.* 2008;26(9):1824–8.
27. Mark AB, Poulsen MW, Andersen S, Andersen JM, Bak MJ, Ritz C, et al. Consumption of a diet low in advanced glycation end products for 4 weeks improves insulin sensitivity in overweight women. *Diabetes Care.* 2014;37(1):88–95.
28. Birlouez-Aragon I, Saavedra G, Tessier FJ, Galinier A, Ait-Ameur L, Lacoste F, et al. A diet based on high-heat-treated foods promotes risk factors for diabetes mellitus and cardiovascular diseases. *Am J Clin Nutr.* 2010;91(5):1220–6.
29. Lioger D, Fardet A, Foassert P, Davicco MJ, Mardon J, Gaillard-Martinie B, et al. Influence of sourdough prefermentation, of steam cooking suppression and of decreased sucrose content during wheat flakes processing on the plasma glucose and insulin responses and satiety of healthy subjects. *J Am Coll Nutr.* 2009;28(1):30–6.
30. Vaaler S, Hanssen KF, Aagenaes O. The effect of cooking upon the blood glucose response to ingested carrots and potatoes. *Diabetes Care.* 1984;7(3):221–3.
31. Rizkalla SW, Laromiguiere M, Champ M, Bruzzo F, Boillot J, Slama G. Effect of baking process on postprandial metabolic consequences: Randomized trials in normal and type 2 diabetic subjects. *Eur J Clin Nutr.* 2007;61(2):175–83.
32. Uribarri J, Cai W, Pyzik R, Goodman S, Chen X, Zhu L, et al. Suppression of native defense mechanisms, SIRT1 and PPARgamma, by dietary glycoxidants precedes disease in adult humans; relevance to lifestyle-engendered chronic diseases. *Amino Acids.* 2014;46(2):301–9.
33. Tantalaki E, Piperi C, Livadas S, Kollias A, Adamopoulos C, Koulouri A, et al. Impact of dietary modification of advanced glycation end products (AGEs) on the hormonal and metabolic profile of women with polycystic ovary syndrome (PCOS). *Hormones.* 2014;13(1):65–73.
34. Legro RS, Kunselman AR, Dodson WC, Dunaif A. Prevalence and predictors of risk for type 2 diabetes mellitus and impaired glucose tolerance in polycystic ovary syndrome: A prospective, controlled study in 254 affected women. *J Clin Endocrinol Metabol.* 1999;84(1):165–9.
35. Uribarri J, Cai W, Ramdas M, Goodman S, Pyzik R, Chen X, et al. Restriction of advanced glycation end products improves insulin resistance in human type 2 diabetes: Potential role of AGER1 and SIRT1. *Diabetes Care.* 2011;34(7):1610–16.
36. Vlassara H, Cai W, Tripp E, Pyzik R, Yee K, Goldberg L, et al. Oral AGE restriction ameliorates insulin resistance in obese individuals with the metabolic syndrome: A randomised controlled trial. *Diabetologia.* 2016;59(10):2181–92.
37. de Courten B, de Courten MP, Soldatos G, Dougherty SL, Straznicky N, Schlaich M, et al. Diet low in advanced glycation end products increases insulin sensitivity in healthy overweight individuals: A double-blind, randomized, crossover trial. *Am J Clin Nutr.* 2016;103(6):1426–33.
38. Clarke RE, Dordevic AL, Tan SM, Ryan L, Coughlan MT. Dietary advanced glycation end products and risk factors for chronic disease: A systematic review of randomised controlled trials. *Nutrients.* 2016;8(3):125.
39. Xanthis A, Hatzitolios A, Koliakos G, Tatola V. Advanced glycosylation end products and nutrition—A possible relation with diabetic atherosclerosis and how to prevent it. *J Food Sci.* 2007;72(8):R125–9.

28

Clinical Trials with an AGE-Restricted Diet

Jaime Uribarri
Icahn School of Medicine at Mount Sinai
New York, NY

CONTENTS

KEY POINTS

- Intervention trials with low dietary advanced glycation end products (AGE) intake demonstrate that dietary AGEs are significant contributors to the body AGE pool both in health and in disease.
- Restriction of dietary AGEs reduces serum levels of AGEs as well as markers of inflammation and oxidative stress in healthy subjects and in subjects with the metabolic syndrome, diabetes, or chronic kidney disease.
- Restriction of dietary AGE intake improves insulin resistance in people with the metabolic syndrome and diabetes.
- Application of a low-AGE diet is a safe and practical intervention that can be easily performed mainly by changing cooking methods.
- A restricted AGE diet agrees with the dietary recommendations of most health organizations.

28.1 Introduction

Advanced glycation end products (AGEs) represent a large and heterogeneous group of compounds that are formed by the nonenzymatic reaction of sugars with free amino groups on proteins, peptides, or amino acids. This is the Maillard reaction, which is also called browning reaction because of the formation of dark colored compounds. AGEs, however, may also form through many other biochemical pathways.

AGEs form endogenously as part of the normal metabolism at a constant physiologic rate, which is known to increase in the presence of hyperglycemia and high oxidative stress. We now know, however, that AGEs are also introduced into the body from exogenous sources, mostly tobacco and food (Uribarri et al. 2016). Tobacco curing in the presence of reducing sugars generates AGEs. Smokers have increased circulating and tissue AGE levels compared to nonsmokers (Cerami et al. 1997). Nowadays, diet is recognized as an important exogenous source of AGEs; these AGEs generate during cooking of food under dry-heat conditions and can be partially absorbed by the gastrointestinal system, contributing significantly to the total AGE body burden (Goldberg et al. 2004; Uribarri et al. 2010).

AGEs, endogenous and exogenous, share the same pathogenetic mechanisms and lead to tissue damage by two main pathways. They can covalently cross-link proteins, producing direct modification of their structure and therefore function. AGEs can also increase intracellular generation of reactive oxygen species and inflammatory cytokines, acting through both receptor-dependent and receptor-independent pathways. For example, AGE interaction with the receptor for AGEs (RAGE) initiates a cascade of intracellular events leading to inflammation and oxidative stress (Yan et al. 2010).

In mice, an increased dietary AGE intake is accompanied by significant increase in circulating AGE levels as well as increased diseases related to inflammation and oxidative stress, such as atherosclerosis, diabetes, and chronic kidney disease (CKD), while dietary AGE restriction does exactly the opposite (see Chapter 5).

Over the past two decades, a large amount of human data have been reported on the role for food-derived AGEs in causing chronic human disease. This chapter will deal with the results of clinical trials testing the effect of dietary AGE restriction in different populations.

28.2 Restricted AGE Diet Intervention in Healthy Subjects

Our team took a group of healthy subjects, equally divided among young and older ages, and randomly assigned them to follow either their own regular diet or a low-AGE diet (AGE levels 50% below the amount consumed normally) for the next 4 months (Vlassara et al. 2009). Participants were selected only if they had a habitually high-normal dAGE intake, defined as >15 AGE Eq/day. Therefore, their baseline levels of sAGEs and related markers were also at the upper end of the normal range. They met with a research dietitian and received detailed instructions on how to prepare the assigned diet at home. A great effort was placed in keeping the diets of equal calorie, nutrient, and micronutrient content as baseline. After 4 months, significant reductions in serum levels of two AGEs (carboxymethyllysine [CML] and methylglyoxal [MG] derivatives) were noted, with parallel reductions in plasma levels of 8-isoprostanes, vascular cell adhesion molecule-1 (VCAM-1), and mononuclear cells–derived TNFα below baseline "normal" values. There was no change in total calorie or nutrient consumption by this group, ruling out effects due to energy intake changes; in support of this fact, participants did not lose weight during the study period. The effects were not different between younger and older participants (Vlassara et al. 2009).

Another randomized, crossover study with 62 healthy volunteers in France compared the effect of two diets, one based on mild steam cooking (low AGE) and the other one based on high-temperature cooking (high AGE), each one followed for 1 month. The low-AGE diet significantly decreased circulating CML levels and improved insulin sensitivity, as assessed by the HOMA index (Birlouez et al. 2010).

Different results were obtained in another study with 24 healthy adults, aged 50–69 years, who were randomized to either low- or high-AGE dietary intervention for 6 weeks. In this study, the low-AGE diet decreased serum and urinary CML levels significantly, but it had no significant impact on peripheral arterial tonometry or levels of any inflammatory mediators (Semba et al. 2014).

28.3 Restricted AGE Diet Intervention in Diabetic Patients

Our team tested the effect of the low dietary AGE intervention in two groups of diabetic patients. The first trial studied a group of diabetic patients who followed both a low- and a regular-AGE diet in a crossover design. All foods were prepared at the Mount Sinai School of Medicine Clinical Research Center kitchen, and patients picked them up twice a week during the duration of the study. The low-AGE diet subjects showed falling levels of circulating AGEs (both CML and MG), VCAM-1, hsCRP, and TNFα, while the high-AGE group showed exactly the opposite changes (Vlassara et al. 2002).

The second study included a group of type 2 diabetes patients with insulin resistance who were randomized to follow either their regular-AGE diet or a low-AGE diet for 4 months (Uribarri et al. 2011). The main difference with the previous study is that participants prepared their own food at home under detailed instructions from the research dietitian who followed them closely. At the end of the study, patients in the low-AGE diet showed not only decreased circulating levels of AGEs, 8-isoprostane, RAGE, and TNFα but also decreased HOMA (an index of insulin resistance) and increased AGER1 and SIRT1 compared with those in the regular-AGE diet.

In another study of 26 diabetic patients randomized to either a high- (n = 13) or a low-AGE (n = 13) for 6 weeks, the low-AGE diet decreased markers of inflammation (TNFα) and oxidative stress (malondialdehyde) significantly, but did not affect marker of insulin resistance (HOMA) (Luevano-Contreras et al. 2013).

28.4 Restricted AGE Diet Intervention in Overweight or Obese Subjects and in Subjects with the Metabolic Syndrome

A group in Denmark randomized 74 overweight women to follow either a high- or a low-AGE diet for 4 weeks. The low-AGE diet decreased urinary AGEs, fasting insulin concentrations, and HOMA compared with the high-AGE diet (Mark et al. 2014).

In Mexico, 43 overweight or obese men (BMI > 25), aged 30–55 years, participated in a 12-week study in which they were randomly assigned to one of three groups: low-AGE diet, exercise with habitual food intake, or exercise plus low-AGE diet. Exercise was for 45 minutes at 65% to 75% of their maximum heart rate three times a week. Exercise alone was associated with only decreased somatometric variables; the low-AGE diet had the same effects, but also decreased serum CML and MG and when combined with exercise reproduced all these effects, but also decreased triacylglycerols and increased high-density lipoprotein (Macias-Cervantes et al. 2015).

Another study looked at whether a low-AGE diet could modulate insulin sensitivity and secretion in healthy, overweight individuals. For this, they performed a double-blind, randomized, crossover trial of diets in 20 participants (6 women and 14 men; mean ± SD BMI = 29.8 ± 3.7). Isocaloric- and macronutrient-matched diets that were high or low in AGE content were alternately consumed for 2 weeks and separated by a 4-week washout period. Insulin sensitivity increased after the low-AGE diet (P = 0.004), whereas it showed a tendency to decrease after the high-AGE diet (P = 0.086). There was no difference in body weight or insulin secretion between the diets (De Courten et al. 2016).

We have tested the effects of the low dietary AGE intervention for 1 year in a group of subjects with two or more features of the metabolic syndrome (Vlassara et al. 2016). Subjects were chosen from a pool of otherwise healthy subjects whose habitual dietary AGE intake was greater than 12 AGE Eq/day and randomized into two parallel groups either following a baseline high-AGE diet or a low-AGE diet. The low-AGE diet produced a significant decrease in serum, cellular, and urinary AGEs, TNFα, and 8-isoprostane as well as an improvement in insulin resistance as assessed by HOMA (Vlassara et al. 2016).

28.5 Restricted AGE Diet Intervention in CKD Patients Not on Dialysis

To determine the relative impact of the low-AGE diet intervention on subjects with different renal abilities to handle oxidants, a group of subjects with established and characterized CKD not requiring dialysis and without diabetes was included in a randomized parallel study comparing regular versus low-AGE diet for 4 months (Vlassara et al. 2009). At the end of the intervention, the effects of the low-AGE diet in these CKD patients mimicked those in healthy participants and in diabetic patients (40%–60% reduction in inflammation).

28.6 Restricted AGE Diet Intervention in ESRD Patients on Peritoneal Dialysis

The low-AGE diet intervention was also done for 4 weeks in a group of nondiabetic, end-stage renal disease (ESRD) patients maintained on chronic peritoneal dialysis. There was a significant fall of circulating AGEs and hsCRP in these patients compared with similar cohort maintained on a regular-AGE diet. This was a randomized trial (Uribarri et al. 2003).

28.7 CKD Subjects on a Regular Diet Exposed to Agents That Bind AGEs in the Gastrointestinal Tract

A Japanese group demonstrated that the oral administration of AST-120 (6 g/day for 3 months; Kremezin™) decreased significantly the serum levels of AGEs in a small group of CKD patients. *In vitro* studies showed that this compound could adsorb CML (Ueda et al. 2006).

We recently studied a group of 20 CKD patients with diabetes type 2 in a crossover study, with one period of sevelamer carbonate (1,600 mg TID with meals) and another one of calcium carbonate (1,200 mg TID with meals) for 8 weeks each. Sevelamer therapy, in contrast to calcium carbonate, reproduced all the previous findings observed on the low dietary AGE intervention, namely reduced circulating levels of AGEs, 8-isoprostane, TNFα, and RAGE and increased SIRT1. Of interest, sevelamer also decreased HbA1c significantly. *In vitro* studies documented that sevelamer, not calcium carbonate, binds AGEs quite effectively (Vlassara et al. 2012).

More recently, a similar study was performed in a larger group of CKD patients with type 2 diabetes, exposed to the low-AGE diet for a more prolonged periods of time. In this randomized study, 117 CKD diabetic patients were randomized into two parallel groups of either sevelamer or calcium carbonate for 6 months without changing their usual diet at any time. As in the previous study, the sevelamer group showed significant decrease in circulating and cellular AGEs as well as markers of oxidative stress and inflammation compared with the calcium carbonate group (Yubero-Serrano et al. 2015).

The latter three studies mentioned above do not represent trials testing the effect of a low-AGE diet in a strict sense, but they are discussed here because their results mimic those of a restricted dietary AGE intake most likely reflecting the effect of these medications in binding dietary AGEs within the gastrointestinal lumen.

28.8 Conclusions

These data (Table 28.1) highlight the following points: (1) dietary AGEs are significant contributors to the AGE pool both in health and disease; (2) the chronic intake of these exogenous prooxidant substances gradually erodes native defenses, setting the stage for abnormally high oxidative stress and inflammation, by themselves precursors of chronic illnesses; (3) these abnormalities may be present not only in patients with established elevated oxidative stress such as diabetes or CKD but also in healthy subjects, prior to onset of overt disease; (4) since this dietary intervention effectively decreased oxidative stress, one may conclude that increased oxidative stress, whether in healthy aging or in diseases, may be reversible; and (5) the introduction of a low-AGE diet is a feasible, safe, and practical intervention that can be easily performed mainly by learning how to change cooking methods as we have widely described in other publications (ref).

TABLE 28.1

Clinical Trials with an AGE-Restricted Diet

Author/Year	Population	Dietary Study Design	Outcome
Vlassara et al. 2002	Diabetics (USA)	Crossover	↓ Circulating AGEs and OS/ inflammation markers
Uribarri et al. 2003	Nondiabetic ESRD (USA)	Two parallel groups (high and low AGE)	↓ Circulating AGEs and inflammation markers
Vlassara et al. 2009	Healthy and nondiabetic CKD (USA)	Two parallel groups (high and low AGE)	↓ Circulating AGEs and OS/ inflammation markers
Uribarri et al. 2010	Type II diabetics with insulin resistance (USA)	Two parallel groups (high and low AGE)	↓ Circulating AGEs and OS/ inflammation markers and HOMA
Birlouez et al. 2010	Healthy (France)	Two parallel groups (high and low AGE)	↓ Circulating AGEs and HOMA
Luevano-Contreras et al. 2013	Type II diabetics (Mexico)	Two parallel groups (high and low AGE)	↓ Circulating OS/inflammation markers
Mark et al. 2014	Overweight women (Denmark)	Two parallel groups (high and low AGE)	↓ Urinary AGEs and HOMA
Semba et al. 2014	Healthy (USA)	Two parallel groups (high and low AGE)	↓ Circulating AGEs but no effect on inflammation markers
Macias-Cervantes et al. 2015	Overweight or obese men (Mexico)	Three parallel groups (diet + exercise)	↓ Circulating AGEs and weight
De Courten et al. 2016	Overweight healthy men and women (Australia)	Two parallel groups (high and low AGE)	↓ Circulating AGEs and IR
Vlassara et al. 2016	Metabolic syndrome (USA)	Two parallel groups (high and low AGE)	↓ Circulating AGEs and IR

Note: AGEs, advanced glycation end products; CKD, chronic kidney disease; ESRD, end-stage renal disease; HOMA, homeostatic model assessment; IR, insulin resistance; OS, oxidative stress.

REFERENCES

Birlouez-Aragon I, Saaveda G, Tessier FJ, Galinier A, Ait-Ameur L, Lacoste F, Niamba CN, Alt N, Somoza V, Lecerf JM. A diet based on high-heat-treated foods promotes risk factors for diabetes mellitus and cardiovascular disease. *Am J Clin Nutr* 2010; 91: 1220–6.

Cerami C. Tobacco smoke is a source of toxic reactive glycation products. *Proc Natl Acad Sci U S A* 1997; 94: 13915–20.

De Courten B. Diet low in advanced glycation end products increases insulin sensitivity in healthy overweight individuals: A double-blind, randomized, crossover trial. *Am J Clin Nutr* 2016; 103: 1426–33.

Goldberg T. Advanced glycoxidation end products in commonly consumed foods. *JADA* 2004; 104: 1287–91.

Luevano-Contreras C. 2013. Dietary advanced glycation end products restriction diminishes inflammation markers and oxidative stress in patients with type 2 diabetes mellitus. *J Clin Biochem Nutr* 2013; 52: 22–6.

Macias-Cervantes MH. Effect of an advanced glycation end product-restricted diet and exercise on metabolic parameters in adult overweight men. *Nutrition* 2015; 31: 446–51.

Mark AB. Consumption of a diet low in advanced glycation end products for 4 weeks improves insulin sensitivity in overweight women. *Diabetes Care* 2014; 37: 88–95.

Semba RD. Dietary intake of advanced glycation end products did not affect endothelial function and inflammation in healthy adults in a randomized controlled trial. *J Nutr* 2014; 144: 1037–42.

Ueda S, Yamagishi S, Takeuchi M, Kohno K, Shibata R, Matsumoto Y, Kaneyuki U, Fujimura T, Hayashida A, Okuda S. Oral adsorbent AST-120 decreases serum levels of AGEs in patients with chronic renal failure. *Mol Med* 2006; 12: 180–84.

Uribarri J, Peppa M, Cai W, Goldberg T, Lu M, He C, Vlassara H. Restriction of dietary glycotoxins reduces excessive advanced glycation end products in renal failure patients. *J Am Soc Nephrol* 2003; 14: 728–31.

Uribarri J. Advanced glycation end products in foods and a practical guide to their reduction in the diet. *JADA* 2010; 110: 911–16.

Uribarri J. Restriction of advanced glycation end products improves insulin resistance in human type 2 diabetes: Potential role of AGER1 and SIRT1. *Diabetes Care* 2011; 34(7): 1610–16.

Uribarri J. Dietary advanced glycation end products and their role in health and disease. *Adv Nutr* 2015; 6: 461–73.

Vlassara H, Cai W, Crandall J, Goldberg T, Oberstein R, Dardaine V, Peppa M, Rayfield EJ. Inflammatory mediators are induced by dietary glycotoxins, a major risk factor for diabetic angiopathy. *Proc Natl Acad Sci U S A* 2002; 99: 15596–155601.

Vlassara H. Protection against loss of innate defenses in adulthood by low advanced glycation end products (AGE) intake: Role of the antiinflammatory AGE receptor-1. *J Clin Endocrinol Metab* 2009; 94: 4483–91.

Vlassara H. Effects of sevelamer on HbA1c, inflammation, and advanced glycation end products in diabetic kidney disease. *Clin J Am Soc Nephrol* 2012; 7: 934–42.

Vlassara H. Oral AGE restriction ameliorates insulin resistance in obese individuals with the metabolic syndrome: A randomised controlled trial. *Diabetologia* 2016; 59: 2181–92.

Yan SF. The RAGE axis: A fundamental mechanism signaling danger to the vulnerable vasculature. *Circ Res* 2010; 106: 842–53.

Yubero-Serrano EM. Effects of sevelamer carbonate on advanced glycation end products and antioxidant/pro-oxidant status in patients with diabetic kidney disease. *Clin J Am Soc Nephrol* 2015; 10: 759–66.

29

Blocking Gastrointestinal Absorption of AGEs

Rabi Yacoub
University at Buffalo
Buffalo, NY

CONTENTS

KEY POINTS

- Advanced glycation end products (AGEs) have been shown to have a detrimental effect on health and are linked to the progression of different diseases.
- Intestinal AGE absorption is variable and depends on different intra-intestinal factors such as the gut microbiota and intestinal enzymes.
- To date, and due to the diversity of AGEs, the exact intestinal absorption mechanism for AGEs is not fully elucidated.
- No selective and specific intervention to block or decrease AGE gastrointestinal absorption is available.
- To date, such intervention is limited to general resins that are nonselective and might have undesirable effects beyond scavenging AGEs.

29.1 Introduction

Advanced glycation end products (AGEs) are a heterogeneous group of compounds that are formed nonenzymatically by the reaction of reducing sugars or α-carbonylic compounds with free amino groups. AGEs are normally formed endogenously and a significant amount is being incorporated with food. Different approaches to decrease the amount of absorbed AGEs have been studied and proposed. Although the most commonly recommended method is change of dietary habits and food preparation, this is generally not well adhered to and patients usually return back to their usual dietary habits. Other theoretical methods of decreasing AGEs include prevention of AGEs formation, AGE breakers, AGE signaling blockers, anti-RAGE antibodies and RAGE antagonists, antioxidants, and blocking AGE absorption.

It is generally accepted that AGEs correlate and are directly associated with increased cardiovascular risk, diabetes, aging, and renal dysfunction [1]. AGE accumulation can be harmful through different mechanisms including forming cross-links with proteins affecting the structure and function of these proteins, increasing stiffness of the protein matrix resulting in increased resistance to removal by proteolytic measures, and affecting tissue remodeling. These changes are accelerated in diabetes and aging, leading to stiffness of the aorta [2]. AGEs formed in the vessel matrix causes lipoproteins trapping and impaired cholesterol efflux, leading to increased atherosclerosis and cardiovascular events [3,4]. AGEs are also are involved in the activation of receptors such as RAGE, resulting in the production of reactive oxygen species (ROS) [5] and several transcription factors including nuclear factor kappa-B (NF-κB) [6], and subsequent upregulation of chemokines, such as Monocyte Chemoattractant Protein-1 (MCP-1), and profibrogenic mediators, such as Transforming growth factor beta (TGFβ) in addition to proinflammatory cytokines, which are known to be involved in thrombogenesis, vascular inflammation, and pathological angiogenesis. These AGE receptors–mediated events contribute to many of the long-term complications of diabetes and other diseases [7].

29.2 AGE Intestinal Absorption

With high temperatures, as used in the deep-frying process with red meat, starch, and carbohydrate-rich diet, Western modern diets contain large amounts of AGEs [8,9], and the estimated amount supplied ranges from 25 to 75 mg of mainly pyrraline and carboxymethyllysine (CML) [10]. Intestinal AGE absorption is variable for different AGEs from minimal intestinal absorption (10%–30%) and up to 70% for certain products, which might have substantial biological and health effects when excretion is limited, especially in patients with impaired renal function [10–12]. At the same time, studies have shown conflicting results even when evaluating the same product. In a crossover study including 20 healthy adolescent males, the fecal excretion, not the urinary excretion of CML, was greater when a high-CML diet was consumed [13]. In another study, the biodistribution and elimination of AGEs in ICR mice were studied *in vivo* following tail vein injection and intragastric administration of ^{18}F-CML [14]. Twenty minutes after tail injection, ^{18}F-CML was quickly distributed via the blood, and it was rapidly excreted through the kidneys. However, after intragastric administration, ^{18}F-CML was only slightly absorbed and intense accumulation of radioactivity in the intestines was still observed at 150 minutes post intragastric administration. All of above suggest that the intestinal absorption of these compounds is highly variable and might be affected by digestive enzymes and also by the bacteria of the gut [15].

Blocking AGE absorption is still under intense investigation, and several approaches including dietary modification to decrease its intestinal transport and increase its fecal elimination, blocking its receptor using different therapeutic agents and modifying the gut microbiota have been studied. Since the mechanisms of intestinal AGE transport have not been fully elucidated, it is hard to efficiently and effectively design a therapeutic intervention. Therefore, delineation of the exact mechanisms by which AGEs are absorbed and transported in the intestinal lumen is of crucial importance. Some evidence suggests that AGEs are transported by diffusion, and others suggest that glycation-modified lysine is transported neither by the major peptide carrier (PEPT-1) nor by carriers for neutral amino acids [16]. At the same time, another study found that pyrraline-containing peptides are transported by H^+-coupled peptide transporter 1 (hPEPT1) in an electronic manner into intestinal cells [17]. All the above evidence confirms that different AGEs seem to be absorbed though different mechanisms.

29.3 Therapies to Decrease AGE Absorption by Enhancing Fecal Elimination

29.3.1 Sevelamer

Sevelamer is a nonabsorbable calcium-free phosphate binder, used in patients with advanced chronic kidney disease (CKD) and those with end-stage renal disease (ESRD) on dialysis. It has been shown in previous studies to decelerate the progression of coronary artery disease and decrease mortality when compared with calcium-based phosphate binders [18–21]. Randomized controlled trials have found that sevelamer decreases AGE blood levels and suggested that this compound might act as a nonabsorbable resin sequestering AGEs in the intestinal lumen and eliminating them in the stool [22–24]. *In vitro* analysis showed that sevelamer binds to AGE-modified bovine serum albumin (BSA) in a pH-dependent and reversible fashion [24]. Less than 5% of ^{125}I-AGE-BSA bound to sevelamer carbonate at pH 1 (the approximate stomach pH). Whereas more than 80% of ^{125}I-AGE-BSA bound to sevelamer carbonate at pH 7, and lowering the pH from 7 to 1 resulted in release of ^{125}I-AGE-BSA, which was later bound to sevelamer again once the pH returned to 7. The mechanism of binding the negatively charged AGEs to sevelamer was proposed to be due to formation of imidazolium adduct between amino groups and methylglyoxal (MG) [24]. However, these clinical human studies [22–24] were limited by the dietary details, and though a strong body of evidence suggests that sevelamer binds AGEs and thus decreases their absorption, it is also plausible to assume that sevelamer-induced loss of appetite might have influenced the dietary intake and overall AGE consumption. It was also shown in another study involving patients with diabetic nephropathy that the usual daily dose of 2.4 g sevelamer did not change the serum concentration of CML and MG compared to placebo, while higher doses showed significant reduction in AGE levels, indicating the need for higher doses in clinical conditions [25]. At the same time, the most commonly studied *in vitro* model of high AGEs is based on BSA incubated with glucose in order to become a glycated "AGE-BSA." This high-AGE model does not seem to be a good one for studying real structure–function relationships on a cellular level, as incubation of BSA in the presence of glucose predominantly forms early reaction products, "Amadori products." Only a small amount of AGEs is formed in glucose-modified BSA in contrast to fructoselysine, which accounts for about 90% of the detectable lysine derivatization [10]. Therefore, it is questionable whether the biological effects seen in these studies are due to AGEs or other modification products [26].

29.3.2 Orlistat

Foods of the fat group showed the highest amounts of AGEs [9,11]; thus, it is conceivable to assume that decreasing fat absorption would result in decreased AGE intestinal absorption. Orlistat is a pancreatic lipase inhibitor that blocks the absorption of 30% of ingested fat, and it has been shown to decrease the serum AGE levels when given either as a single dose post high-AGE meal [27], or for a 6-months period coupled with diet restriction in patients with polycystic ovarian disease [28]. Same results were found when orlistat was given with high-AGE meals for 2 days [29]. Unfortunately, these studies did not have a placebo arm and the effects found, though significant, need further confirmations. These studies postulated that AGEs are absorbed from exogenous sources and that fat influences the absorption of these food glycotoxins more than proteins and carbohydrates.

29.3.3 AST-120 (Kremezin)

The oral charcoal adsorbent AST-120 has been shown to decrease the serum levels of many uremic toxins (indoxyl sulfate, p-cresyl sulfate, phenyl sulfate) in patients with ESRD [30], and moderate to severe CKD [31]. It was also shown to reduce carotid intima media thickness and arterial stiffness in pre-dialysis CKD patients. These observations led researchers to speculate that beneficial effects of AST-120 could be due its ability to adsorb diet-derived AGEs and subsequently decrease serum AGE levels. In a small study [32], 3 months treatment with daily 6 g AST-120 orally significantly decreased serum CML levels. To further confirm these findings and to study the effects of AST-120 on atherosclerosis and endothelial dysfunction, the authors incubated human umbilical vein endothelial cells with serum from participants who received AST-120 before and after treatment (before treatment used as control), and found a significant decrease in mRNA levels of receptor for AGEs, monocyte chemoattractant protein–1, and vascular adhesion molecule–1 when incubated with after treatment serum compared to pretreatment. AST-120 was also found to adsorb CML in *in vitro* studies [31]. Recently, a large randomized controlled trial of AST-120 including 579 patients with advanced CKD (stages III–IV) was published [33]. After 36 months, both treatment and control arms showed similar results. Indoxyl sulfate and β2-microglobulin, mortality, hospitalization, estimated glomerular filtration rate (eGFR), and change in proteinuria were not significantly different between the two groups. At the same time, a recent 5-year retrospective analysis of 278 CKD stage III–IV patients, 128 of whom received AST-120 (6 g/day orally) showed significant results [34]. The prevalence of dialysis induction, mortality, and cardiac and stroke events in patients treated with AST-120 was significantly lower after 3 and 5 years ($p < 0.0001$) compared with the prevalence observed in the untreated patients. Findings of this retrospective study were confirmed in animal models [35]. It remains to be determined whether this beneficial effect of AST-120 therapy resulted from reduction of AGE levels or other mechanisms such as sequestering uremic toxins. Treating spontaneous hypertensive rats with AST-120 post experimental myocardial infarction was associated not only with lower blood pressure and better cardiac function tests but also with decreased indoxyl sulfate levels and urinary biomarkers of kidney injury (KIM-1, NGAL, L-FABP), suggesting an antioxidant role of AST-120 probably through its chelating properties. Though these epidemiological studies have shown conflicting results and the most recent randomized trial failed to show any significant reduction in hard outcomes, it is important to mention that in one randomized control trial [33], there was a trend toward less eGFR decline in the AST-120 group. At the same time, a significant number of participants in the AST-120 dropped out (mostly due to AST-related GI side effects), and lastly, authors could not determine compliance rate that might have played a major role in these negative results. It is also important to mention that the side effects were higher in the AST-120 participants compared with control (constipation, nausea, vomiting, and decreased appetite). No significant difference was found between the groups with regard to major side effects.

29.3.4 Carnosine

Reactive carbonyl species (RCS) react with amino acid residues on proteins to generate stable adducts or cross-links (AGEs) [35–39], and thus, sequestering RCS in the gastrointestinal (GI) tract would result in decreased AGE availability in the gut and decreased absorption. Carnosine is a selective RCS-sequestering agent, but is rapidly hydrolyzed by serum carnosinase, and extensive drug studies have been conducted to develop carnosine products that are stable in both GI tract and patients' serum. L-carnosine (L-CAR, beta-alanyl-L-histidine) was initially developed as such a drug, but was later found to be rapidly hydrolyzed in human serum by carnosinase. Later, D-carnosine (D-CAR, β-alanyl-D-histidine), which maintains the same quenching activity of L-CAR, was developed by isomerization of the histidine residue [40]. D-CAR is poorly absorbed in the GI tract but when given as an octylester, it was found to have a 2.6-fold increase in its bioavailability [41]. Studies [42,43] evaluating apolipoprotein E (APOE)-null mice fed with high-AGE diets and D-CAR showed promising results. D-CAR-treated mice showed reduced atherosclerosis lesion area and a more stable plaque phenotype compared with untreated animals, with reduced foam cell accumulation, inflammation, and apoptosis and increased clearance of apoptotic bodies and collagen deposition, resulting in decreased necrotic core formation. It also showed decreased renal lesions and lower inflammation, apoptosis, and fibrosis in the kidneys. A significant body of evidence is available confirming the beneficial effects of carnosine in ameliorating AGE-related diseases such as diabetic kidney disease, diabetic retinopathy, and vascular diseases along with endothelial cell and podocytes dysfunction in animal models [44–48]. However, unlike humans, rodents lack carnosinase, and to date, no human study evaluating carnosine effects is available. With the development of the stable form (D-CAR) and the observation of its poor GI tract absorption, D-CAR might be after all a suitable therapeutic agent to sequester AGEs in the GI tract preventing their absorption.

29.4 Carbonyl Traps and AGE Cross-Link Breakers

In the absence of effective therapeutic agents to selectively prevent the absorption of AGEs in the GI tract, scientists have studied different treatments aiming at decreasing AGE blood levels and found that many drugs including renin angiotensin system blockers [49–52], diabetes medications such as metformin, lipid-lowering agents such as statins [53–55], and vitamin B6 [56] are associated with decreased serum levels of AGEs through either scavenging effects or breaking AGE cross-links. However, there is no available study evaluating the effects of these agents on the exogenous AGEs inside the GI tract, and whether the decreased serum AGE levels are in part due to increased AGE cross-link breakage or sequestering in the GI tract is not clear.

29.4.1 Alagebrium

Alagebrium (ALT-711, 3-phenyacyl-4,5-dimethylthiazolium chloride), a thiazolium derivative, which catalytically breaks established AGE cross-links between proteins, has been extensively studied and found to result in increased vascular compliance, decreased arterial stiffness [57], and decreased ventricular mass and diastolic filling in patients with diastolic dysfunction [58]. However, recent long-term and larger studies failed to replicate these results and showed no significant differences in AGE serum levels, endothelial dysfunction, and vascular compliance [59,60]. Alagebrium has been extensively studied in multiple clinical trials sponsored by Synvista Therapeutics from 2002 to 2010 (oral administration). However, whether alagebrium interacts with AGEs in the GI system resulting in decreased intestinal AGE absorption is an interesting yet to be studied mechanism.

29.4.2 Metformin

There is evidence suggesting that metformin therapy decreases AGE serum level in humans and animal models [61–64]. These decreased serum AGE levels were independent of glucose control, suggesting a direct interaction between certain AGEs and metformin. *In vitro* studies have shown that metformin reacts chemically with MG and forms a metformin–MG adduct characterized as a triazepinone (2-amino-4-(dimethyl-amino)-7-methyl-5,7-dihydro-6H-[1,3,5]triazepin+ ++-6-one). This interaction most likely occurs *in vivo*, but as mentioned above, no study has evaluated or confirmed whether metformin interacts with MG in the GI tract.

29.5 Conclusions

AGEs are a group of heterogeneous products with different chemical properties that seem to affect our health. Though many therapeutic agents and interventions beyond dietary restriction have been proposed, clinical studies have shown limited and conflicting results on the efficacy of these therapies on hard outcomes. The relatively low GI absorption of these products has suggested for a long time that exogenous AGEs are probably harmless, but recent studies have revealed a direct and close correlation between dietary AGEs and their serum levels, supporting the need for selective and specific intervention to block or decrease their GI absorption. To date, such intervention is limited to general resins that are nonselective and might have undesirable effects beyond scavenging AGEs.

REFERENCES

1. Ross R. The pathogenesis of atherosclerosis: A perspective for the 1990s. *Nature* 1993;362:801–809.
2. McCance DR, Dyer DG, Dunn JA, Bailie KE, Thorpe SR, Baynes JW, Lyons TJ. Maillard reaction products and their relation to complications in insulin-dependent diabetes mellitus. *J Clin Invest* 1993;91:2470–2478.
3. Bierhaus A, Hofmann MA, Ziegler R, Nawroth PP. AGEs and their interaction with AGE-receptors in vascular disease and diabetes mellitus. I. The AGE concept. *Cardiovasc Res* 1998;37:586–600.
4. Chappey O, Dosquet C, Wautier MP, Wautier JL. Advanced glycation end products, oxidant stress and vascular lesions. *Eur J Clin Invest* 1997;27:97–108.
5. Rosca MG, Mustata TG, Kinter MT, Ozdemir AM, Kern TS, Szweda LI, Brownlee M, Monnier VM, Weiss MF. Glycation of mitochondrial proteins from diabetic rat kidney is associated with excess superoxide formation. *Am J Physiol Renal Physiol* 2005;289:F420–F430.
6. Morita M, Yano S, Yamaguchi T, Sugimoto T. Advanced glycation end products-induced reactive oxygen species generation is partly through NF-kappa B activation in human aortic endothelial cells. *J Diabetes Complications* 2013;27:11–15.

7. Schmidt AM, Hori O, Chen JX, Li JF, Crandall J, Zhang J, Cao R, Yan SD, Brett J, Stern D. Advanced glycation endproducts interacting with their endothelial receptor induce expression of vascular cell adhesion molecule-1 (VCAM-1) in cultured human endothelial cells and in mice. A potential mechanism for the accelerated vasculopathy of diabetes. *J Clin Invest* 1995;96:1395–1403.
8. Vlassara H, Uribarri J. Glycoxidation and diabetic complications: Modern lessons and a warning? *Rev Endocr Metab Disord* 2004;5:181–188.
9. Goldberg T, Cai W, Peppa M, Dardaine V, Baliga BS, Uribarri J, Vlassara H. Advanced glycoxidation end products in commonly consumed foods. *J Am Diet Assoc* 2004;104:1287–1291.
10. Henle T. AGEs in foods: Do they play a role in uremia? *Kidney Int Suppl* 2003:S145–S147.
11. Koschinsky T, He CJ, Mitsuhashi T, Bucala R, Liu C, Buenting C, Heitmann K, Vlassara H. Orally absorbed reactive glycation products (glycotoxins): An environmental risk factor in diabetic nephropathy. *Proc Natl Acad Sci U S A* 1997;94:6474–6479.
12. Foerster A, Henle T. Glycation in food and metabolic transit of dietary AGEs (advanced glycation end-products): Studies on the urinary excretion of pyrraline. *Biochem Soc Trans* 2003;31:1383–1385.
13. Delgado-Andrade C, Tessier FJ, Niquet-Leridon C, Seiquer I, Pilar Navarro M. Study of the urinary and faecal excretion of Nepsilon-carboxymethyllysine in young human volunteers. *Amino Acids* 2012;43:595–602.
14. Xu H, Wang Z, Wang Y, Hu S, Liu N. Biodistribution and elimination study of fluorine-18 labeled Nepsilon-carboxymethyl-lysine following intragastric and intravenous administration. *PLoS One* 2013;8:e57897.
15. Ames JM, Wynne A, Hofmann A, Plos S, Gibson GR. The effect of a model melanoidin mixture on faecal bacterial populations *in vitro*. *Br J Nutr* 1999, 82:489–495.
16. Grunwald S, Krause R, Bruch M, Henle T, Brandsch M. Transepithelial flux of early and advanced glycation compounds across Caco-2 cell monolayers and their interaction with intestinal amino acid and peptide transport systems. *Br J Nutr* 2006;95:1221–1228.
17. Geissler S, Hellwig M, Zwarg M, Markwardt F, Henle T, Brandsch M. Transport of the advanced glycation end products alanylpyrraline and pyrralylalanine by the human proton-coupled peptide transporter hPEPT1. *J Agric Food Chem* 2010;58:2543–2547.
18. Chertow GM, Burke SK, Raggi P, Treat to Goal Working Group. Sevelamer attenuates the progression of coronary and aortic calcification in hemodialysis patients. *Kidney Int* 2002;62:245–252.
19. Chertow GM, Burke SK, Dillon MA, Slatopolsky E. Long-term effects of sevelamer hydrochloride on the calcium x phosphate product and lipid profile of haemodialysis patients. *Nephrol Dial Transplant* 1999;14:2907–2914.
20. Chertow GM, Raggi P, McCarthy JT, Schulman G, Silberzweig J, Kuhlik A, Goodman WG, Boulay A, Burke SK, Toto RD. The effects of sevelamer and calcium acetate on proxies of atherosclerotic and arteriosclerotic vascular disease in hemodialysis patients. *Am J Nephrol* 2003;23:307–314.
21. Jamal SA, Vandermeer B, Raggi P, Mendelssohn DC, Chatterley T, Dorgan M, Lok CE, Fitchett D, Tsuyuki RT. Effect of calcium-based versus non-calcium-based phosphate binders on mortality in patients with chronic kidney disease: An updated systematic review and meta-analysis. *Lancet* 2013;382:1268–1277.
22. Kakuta T, Tanaka R, Hyodo T, Suzuki H, Kanai G, Nagaoka M, Takahashi H, Hirawa N, Oogushi Y, Miyata T, et al. Effect of sevelamer and calcium-based phosphate binders on coronary artery calcification and accumulation of circulating advanced glycation end products in hemodialysis patients. *Am J Kidney Dis* 2011;57:422–431.
23. Yubero-Serrano EM, Woodward M, Poretsky L, Vlassara H, Striker GE, Group AG-IS. Effects of sevelamer carbonate on advanced glycation end products and antioxidant/pro-oxidant status in patients with diabetic kidney disease. *Clin J Am Soc Nephrol* 2015;10:759–766.
24. Vlassara H, Uribarri J, Cai W, Goodman S, Pyzik R, Post J, Grosjean F, Woodward M, Striker GE. Effects of sevelamer on HbA1c, inflammation, and advanced glycation end products in diabetic kidney disease. *Clin J Am Soc Nephrol* 2012;7:934–942.
25. Vlassara H, Cai W, Chen X, Serrano EJ, Shobha MS, Uribarri J, Woodward M, Striker GE. Managing chronic inflammation in the aging diabetic patient with CKD by diet or sevelamer carbonate: A modern paradigm shift. *J Gerontol A Biol Sci Med Sci* 2012;67:1410–1416.
26. Nowotny K, Jung T, Hohn A, Weber D, Grune T. Advanced glycation end products and oxidative stress in type 2 diabetes mellitus. *Biomolecules* 2015;5:194–222.

27. Diamanti-Kandarakis E, Piperi C, Alexandraki K, Katsilambros N, Kouroupi E, Papailiou J, Lazaridis S, et al. Short-term effect of orlistat on dietary glycotoxins in healthy women and women with polycystic ovary syndrome. *Metabolism* 2006;55:494–500.
28. Diamanti-Kandarakis E, Katsikis I, Piperi C, Alexandraki K, Panidis D. Effect of long-term orlistat treatment on serum levels of advanced glycation end-products in women with polycystic ovary syndrome. *Clin Endocrinol (Oxford)* 2007;66:103–109.
29. Diamanti-Kandarakis E, Piperi C, Alexandraki KI, Papailiou J, Ekonomou F, Koulouri E, Kandarakis H, Creatsas G. The acute effect of Orlistat on dietary glycotoxins in diabetics and healthy women. *Minerva Endocrinol* 2009;34:97–104.
30. Yamamoto S, Kazama JJ, Omori K, Matsuo K, Takahashi Y, Kawamura K, Matsuto T, Watanabe H, Maruyama T, Narita I. Continuous reduction of protein-bound uraemic toxins with improved oxidative stress by using the Oral Charcoal Adsorbent AST-120 in haemodialysis patients. *Sci Rep* 2015;5:14381.
31. Schulman G, Agarwal R, Acharya M, Berl T, Blumenthal S, Kopyt N. A multicenter, randomized, double-blind, placebo-controlled, dose-ranging study of AST-120 (Kremezin) in patients with moderate to severe CKD. *Am J Kidney Dis* 2006;47:565–577.
32. Ueda S, Yamagishi S, Takeuchi M, Kohno K, Shibata R, Matsumoto Y, Kaneyuki U, Fujimura T, Hayashida A, Okuda S. Oral adsorbent AST-120 decreases serum levels of AGEs in patients with chronic renal failure. *Mol Med* 2006;12:180–184.
33. Cha RH, Kang SW, Park CW, Cha DR, Na KY, Kim SG, Yoon SA, Han SY, Chang JH, Park SK, et al. A randomized, controlled trial of oral intestinal sorbent AST-120 on renal function deterioration in patients with advanced renal dysfunction. *Clin J Am Soc Nephrol* 2016;11(4):559–567.
34. Sato E, Tanaka A, Oyama JI, Yamasaki A, Shimomura M, Hiwatashi A, Ueda Y, Amaha M, Nomura M, Matsumura D, et al. Long-term effects of AST-120 on the progression and prognosis of pre-dialysis chronic kidney disease: A 5-year retrospective study. *Heart Vessels* 2016;31(10):1625–1632.
35. Ellis EM. Reactive carbonyls and oxidative stress: Potential for therapeutic intervention. *Pharmacol Ther* 2007;115:13–24.
36. Negre-Salvayre A, Coatrieux C, Ingueneau C, Salvayre R. Advanced lipid peroxidation end products in oxidative damage to proteins. Potential role in diseases and therapeutic prospects for the inhibitors. *Br J Pharmacol* 2008;153:6–20.
37. Pamplona R. Advanced lipoxidation end-products. *Chem Biol Interact* 2011;192:14–20.
38. Baynes JW. The role of AGEs in aging: Causation or correlation. *Exp Gerontol* 2001;36:1527–1537.
39. Ahmed N. Advanced glycation endproducts—Role in pathology of diabetic complications. *Diabetes Res Clin Pract* 2005;67:3–21.
40. Vistoli G, Orioli M, Pedretti A, Regazzoni L, Canevotti R, Negrisoli G, Carini M, Aldini G. Design, synthesis, and evaluation of carnosine derivatives as selective and efficient sequestering agents of cytotoxic reactive carbonyl species. *ChemMedChem* 2009;4:967–975.
41. Orioli M, Vistoli G, Regazzoni L, Pedretti A, Lapolla A, Rossoni G, Canevotti R, Gamberoni L, Previtali M, Carini M, Aldini G. Design, synthesis, ADME properties, and pharmacological activities of beta-alanyl-D-histidine (D-carnosine) prodrugs with improved bioavailability. *ChemMedChem* 2011;6:1269–1282.
42. Menini S, Iacobini C, Ricci C, Scipioni A, Blasetti Fantauzzi C, Giaccari A, Salomone E, Canevotti R, Lapolla A, Orioli M, et al. D-Carnosine octylester attenuates atherosclerosis and renal disease in ApoE null mice fed a Western diet through reduction of carbonyl stress and inflammation. *Br J Pharmacol* 2012;166:1344–1356.
43. Menini S, Iacobini C, Ricci C, Blasetti Fantauzzi C, Pugliese G. Protection from diabetes-induced atherosclerosis and renal disease by D-carnosine-octylester: Effects of early vs late inhibition of advanced glycation end-products in Apoe-null mice. *Diabetologia* 2015;58:845–853.
44. Peters V, Riedl E, Braunagel M, Hoger S, Hauske S, Pfister F, Zschocke J, et al. Carnosine treatment in combination with ACE inhibition in diabetic rats. *Regul Pept* 2014;194–195:36–40.
45. Vistoli G, Carini M, Aldini G. Transforming dietary peptides in promising lead compounds: The case of bioavailable carnosine analogs. *Amino Acids* 2012;43:111–126.
46. Pfister F, Riedl E, Wang Q, vom Hagen F, Deinzer M, Harmsen MC, Molema G, Yard B, Feng Y, Hammes HP. Oral carnosine supplementation prevents vascular damage in experimental diabetic retinopathy. *Cell Physiol Biochem* 2011;28:125–136.

47. Riedl E, Pfister F, Braunagel M, Brinkkotter P, Sternik P, Deinzer M, Bakker SJ, et al. Carnosine prevents apoptosis of glomerular cells and podocyte loss in STZ diabetic rats. *Cell Physiol Biochem* 2011;28:279–288.
48. Pietkiewicz J, Bronowicka-Szydelko A, Dzierzba K, Danielewicz R, Gamian A. Glycation of the muscle-specific enolase by reactive carbonyls: Effect of temperature and the protection role of carnosine, pyridoxamine and phosphatidylserine. *Protein J* 2011;30:149–158.
49. Sebekova K, Gazdikova K, Syrova D, Blazicek P, Schinzel R, Heidland A, Spustova V, Dzurik R. Effects of ramipril in nondiabetic nephropathy: Improved parameters of oxidatives stress and potential modulation of advanced glycation end products. *J Hum Hypertens* 2003;17:265–270.
50. Komiya N, Hirose H, Saisho Y, Saito I, Itoh H. Effects of 12-month valsartan therapy on glycation and oxidative stress markers in type 2 diabetic subjects with hypertension. *Int Heart J* 2008;49:681–689.
51. Ono Y, Mizuno K, Takahashi M, Miura Y, Watanabe T. Suppression of advanced glycation and lipoxidation end products by angiotensin II type-1 receptor blocker candesartan in type 2 diabetic patients with essential hypertension. *Fukushima J Med Sci* 2013;59:69–75.
52. Saha SA, LaSalle BK, Clifton GD, Short RA, Tuttle KR. Modulation of advanced glycation end products by candesartan in patients with diabetic kidney disease—A dose-response relationship study. *Am J Ther* 2010;17:553–558.
53. Scharnagl H, Stojakovic T, Winkler K, Rosinger S, Marz W, Boehm BO. The HMG-CoA reductase inhibitor cerivastatin lowers advanced glycation end products in patients with type 2 diabetes. *Exp Clin Endocrinol Diabetes* 2007;115:372–375.
54. Cuccurullo C, Iezzi A, Fazia ML, De Cesare D, Di Francesco A, Muraro R, Bei R, et al. Suppression of RAGE as a basis of simvastatin-dependent plaque stabilization in type 2 diabetes. *Arterioscler Thromb Vasc Biol* 2006;26:2716–2723.
55. Nakamura T, Sato E, Fujiwara N, Kawagoe Y, Takeuchi M, Maeda S, Yamagishi S. Atorvastatin reduces proteinuria in non-diabetic chronic kidney disease patients partly via lowering serum levels of advanced glycation end products (AGEs). *Oxid Med Cell Longev* 2010;3:304–307.
56. Williams ME, Bolton WK, Khalifah RG, Degenhardt TP, Schotzinger RJ, McGill JB. Effects of pyridoxamine in combined phase 2 studies of patients with type 1 and type 2 diabetes and overt nephropathy. *Am J Nephrol* 2007;27:605–614.
57. Kass DA, Shapiro EP, Kawaguchi M, Capriotti AR, Scuteri A, deGroof RC, Lakatta EG. Improved arterial compliance by a novel advanced glycation end-product crosslink breaker. *Circulation* 2001;104:1464–1470.
58. Little WC, Zile MR, Kitzman DW, Hundley WG, O'Brien TX, Degroof RC. The effect of alagebrium chloride (ALT-711), a novel glucose cross-link breaker, in the treatment of elderly patients with diastolic heart failure. *J Card Fail* 2005;11:191–195.
59. Hartog JW, Willemsen S, van Veldhuisen DJ, Posma JL, van Wijk LM, Hummel YM, Hillege HL, Voors AA, Investigators B. Effects of alagebrium, an advanced glycation endproduct breaker, on exercise tolerance and cardiac function in patients with chronic heart failure. *Eur J Heart Fail* 2011;13:899–908.
60. Oudegeest-Sander MH, Olde Rikkert MG, Smits P, Thijssen DH, van Dijk AP, Levine BD, Hopman MT. The effect of an advanced glycation end-product crosslink breaker and exercise training on vascular function in older individuals: A randomized factorial design trial. *Exp Gerontol* 2013;48:1509–1517.
61. Tanaka Y, Uchino H, Shimizu T, Yoshii H, Niwa M, Ohmura C, Mitsuhashi N, Onuma T, Kawamori R. Effect of metformin on advanced glycation endproduct formation and peripheral nerve function in streptozotocin-induced diabetic rats. *Eur J Pharmacol* 1999;376:17–22.
62. Beisswenger PJ, Howell SK, Touchette AD, Lal S, Szwergold BS. Metformin reduces systemic methylglyoxal levels in type 2 diabetes. *Diabetes* 1999;48:198–202.
63. Kinsky OR, Hargraves TL, Anumol T, Jacobsen NE, Dai J, Snyder SA, Monks TJ, Lau SS. Metformin scavenges methylglyoxal to form a novel imidazolinone metabolite in humans. *Chem Res Toxicol* 2016;29:227–234.
64. Ruggiero-Lopez D, Lecomte M, Moinet G, Patereau G, Lagarde M, Wiernsperger N. Reaction of metformin with dicarbonyl compounds. Possible implication in the inhibition of advanced glycation end product formation. *Biochem Pharmacol* 1999;58:1765–1773.

30

Antagonizing the Effects of Dietary Advanced Glycation End Products on Endothelial Dysfunction

Ovidiu Alin Stirban
MVZ Sana Arztpraxen
Remscheid, Germany

CONTENTS

KEY POINTS

- Advanced glycation end products (AGEs) play a major role in the development of cardiovascular disease (CVD).
- Dietary AGEs acutely induce endothelial dysfunction (ED) in healthy subjects and in subjects with diabetes mellitus.
- Repeated postprandial AGE-induced ED might importantly contribute to the development of CVD.
- Changing the cooking method results not only in lower dietary AGE load but also in the reduction of postprandial ED.
- Dietary interventions might therefore represent a cheap and simple method to promote cardiovascular health.

30.1 Cardiovascular Complications in Diabetes

Cardiovascular disease (CVD) is the major cause for morbidity and mortality among people with diabetes mellitus (DM) [1]. Therefore, major efforts are done to develop strategies for primary and secondary prevention of CVD in this population. In primary prevention, the spectrum ranges from pharmacologic treatments to vitamin supplementation and dietetic interventions. Among the latter, we could include the reduction of ingested food toxins, like the advanced glycation end products (AGEs).

30.1.1 Cardiovascular Risk, Endothelial Dysfunction (ED), and Diabetes

The response-to-injury theory states that endothelial dysfunction (ED) is the first step toward atherosclerosis preceding it by decades [2]. Compared to their nondiabetic counterparts, subjects with DM show a markedly impaired endothelial function, which partly explains their increased cardiovascular risk [3].

ED is defined as an imbalance between relaxing and constricting factors, procoagulant and anticoagulant substances, and between proinflammatory and anti-inflammatory mediators produced by or acting on the endothelium. One of the main characteristics of ED is a decreased bioavailability of the endothelial nitric oxide (NO), a key mediator contributing to vascular health [4]. Thus, the vascular protective effects of NO, such as vasodilatation and its antiatherosclerotic, antioxidant, and antithrombotic properties, are impaired [3]. Such a defect is of special relevance in large vessels, where the vascular tone is mainly regulated by NO, whereas in small vessels, prostaglandins and other endothelial-derived factors are the main regulators [5]. Nitric oxide results from the transformation of L-arginine into citrulline and NO by the enzyme NO synthase (NOS). A detailed description of molecular mechanisms contributing to macrovascular disease in diabetes was detailed elsewhere [6].

ED accompanies conditions with a high CVD risk, such as smoking, dyslipidemia, arterial hypertension, erectile dysfunction, obesity, hyperhomocysteinemia, coronary artery disease (CAD), congestive heart failure, and type 1 and type 2 DM (6–8). In people with type 1 or type 2 DM, a large body of evidence associates ED with microvascular and macrovascular diseases [9]. Since the correction of ED has been suggested to prevent atherosclerosis [10], approaches aiming at ED prevention in people with DM might mitigate their CVD risk. As people with diabetes are prone to pronounced postprandial ED and humans spend most—approximately 2/3—of their daytime in the postprandial state, interventions aiming at reducing postprandial changes might be important for the prevention of CVD complications.

30.1.2 Postprandial Metabolic Changes in Diabetes-Induced ED and Trigger Cardiovascular Complications

There is a clear link between postprandial hyperglycemia and hyperlipidemia and cardiovascular risk [11–13]. Much attention has been paid lately to the link between increased postprandial oxidative stress (OS) and ED, and the hypothesis emerged that postprandial ED represents the mechanism linking postprandial metabolic changes to increased cardiovascular risk [14–16].

The postprandial state in people with DM is paralleled by hyperglycemia, hypertriglyceridemia, hyperinsulinemia and, as a consequence, increased OS and ED [16]. Distinctive and cumulative effects of hyperglycemia and hypertriglyceridemia on postprandial ED have been shown [17,18]. Sustained hyperinsulinemia also triggers ED [19]. On top of these effects, food toxins produced during cooking (e.g., AGEs) might supplementarily impair endothelial function [20]. Therefore, reduction of toxins production in food might represent a simple, cost-effective approach for preventing postprandial ED.

30.2 Pathogenetic Vascular Effects of AGEs

We have recently reviewed the molecular mechanisms mediating the AGEs effects on the vasculature [21]; therefore, only a brief description will be reproduced here.

Some of the mechanisms mediating the detrimental effects of AGEs on the vasculature are related to inflammation and OS [22], increased glycation of low-density and high-density lipoproteins (LDL, HDL) [23], activation of the proinflammatory iNOS [24], and decreased NO availability [25]. Further mechanisms comprise the increased production of cytokines, for example, insulin-like growth factor-1 (IGF-1) or the platelet-derived growth factor (PDGF), which modify the migration of monocytes and macrophages as well as the proliferation of vascular smooth muscle cells (VSMC) [26]. The AGE-induced effects can be classified according to their site of action or their receptor dependency.

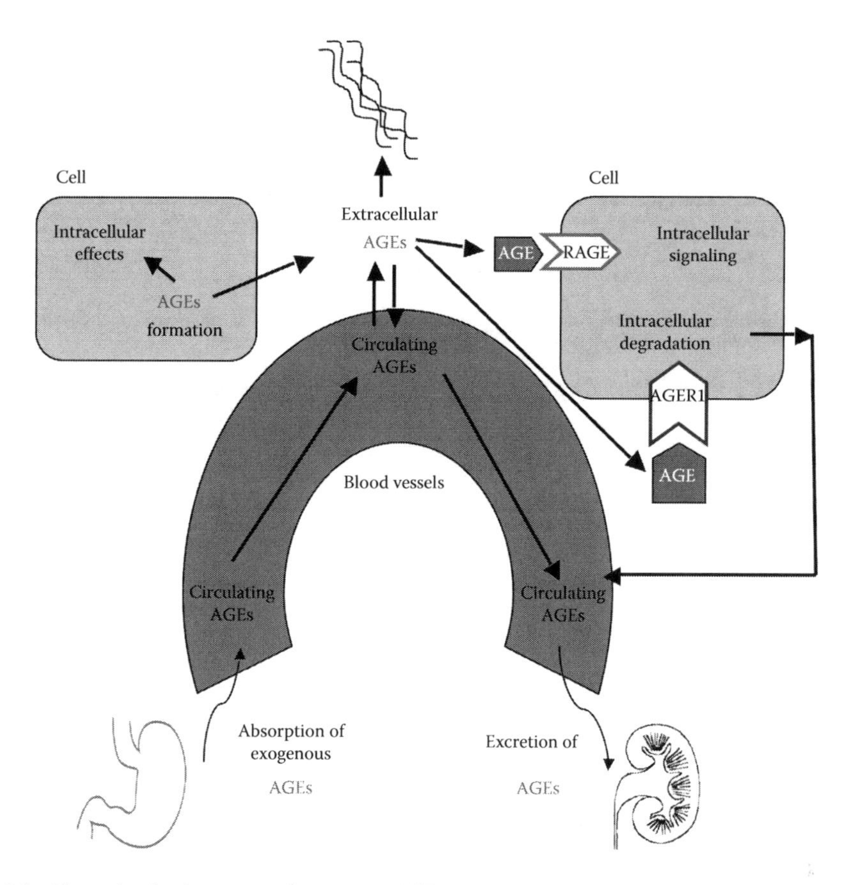

FIGURE 30.1 The cycle of endogenous and exogenous AGEs. Exogenous AGEs are partly absorbed, transported by the bloodstream to the peripheral tissues, or excreted through the kidney. Endogenously formed AGEs exert their effects in the vicinity, partly penetrate into the blood stream from where they are directed toward the kidneys or toward other tissues. (Adapted from Stirban, A., et al., *Mol. Metabol.*, 3(2), 94–108, 2013.)

AGE-induced damage can affect the vasculature structure and cells involved in vascular homeostasis via at least four mechanisms [6] (Figure 30.1).

1. AGEs modify intracellular proteins, including those involved in the regulation of gene transcription [27].
2. Precursors of AGEs leave the cells via diffusion and modify nearby extracellular matrix molecules, subsequently altering the signaling between matrix and cells and ultimately causing cellular dysfunction [28].
3. AGEs and their precursors modify circulating proteins in the bloodstream, thereby altering their function.
4. Circulating proteins modified by AGEs bind to and activate AGEs receptors, thereby altering the production of inflammatory cytokines and growth factors, which in turn drive cellular and tissue damage [26,29]. Indeed, the activation of certain receptors for AGEs (e.g., RAGE) promotes inflammatory response, mainly by the activation of nuclear factor-κB (NF-κB), apoptosis, prothrombotic activity, expression of adhesion molecules, and OS [30–32]. Furthermore, the AGEs-RAGE interaction can activate iNOS, potentially triggering nitrative stress.

More insights into receptor-dependent or receptor-independent effects of AGEs have been extensively given elsewhere [21].

The detection of AGEs and overexpressed RAGE in atheromatous plaques and lesions, as well as within lipid accumulations in VSMC and macrophages from diabetic patients, has narrowed the path between AGEs and atherosclerosis [33–35]. The fact that AGEs are not only bystanders but also contributors to CVD was first demonstrated in *in vitro* studies and then reproduced in animal and clinical studies.

In vitro studies and studies in animal models have shown that AGEs negatively impact on the function of different cell types involved in atherosclerosis: endothelial cells [26,36], platelets [37], monocytes/macrophages [38], or VSMC [39], thus explaining their association with vascular disease [21,40].

In genetically hypercholesterolemic apolipoprotein E-deficient (apoE[-/-]), streptozotocin-induced diabetic mice, a diet with a low-AGE (L-AGE) content compared with an isocaloric standard diet with a high-AGE (H-AGE) content resulted in >50% smaller lesions at the aortic root after 2 months. Only serum AGEs differed (by about 53%), while no differences were noted in plasma glucose, triglycerides, or cholesterol levels between both groups, suggesting dietary AGEs as responsible for the vascular changes seen [41].

In another mouse model of genetic hypercholesterolemia, Lin et al. [42] showed that lowering dietary AGEs reduces neointimal formation after arterial injury and suggested that dietary restriction of AGEs may play a in the prevention of restenosis after angioplasty.

Vlassara et al. [43] administered AGE-modified albumin to nondiabetic rats and rabbits, alone or in combination with the AGE cross-link inhibitor aminoguanidine. AGE treatment for 2–4 weeks led to a 6-fold higher AGE concentration in aortic tissue samples compared to untreated controls, which was accompanied by increased vascular permeability and markedly impaired vasodilatatory responses to acetylcholine and nitroglycerin. These effects were significantly reduced by combined treatment with aminoguanidine. Moreover, mononuclear cell migratory activity was enhanced in subendothelial and periarteriolar regions of various tissues from AGE-treated rats when compared to tissues from animals treated with aminoguanidine. Authors concluded that dietary AGEs can induce complex vascular alterations resembling those seen in diabetes or aging, independent of metabolic or genetic factors, and that these changes can be reversed by the AGE cross-link inhibitor aminoguanidine.

In rats, aminoguanidine administration was also effective in preventing diabetes-induced formation of fluorescent advanced nonenzymatic glycation products and cross-linking of arterial wall connective tissue protein *in vivo* [44]. Furthermore, aminoguanidine treatment for 18 months prevented increases in the AGE content in aged cardiac, aortic, and renal tissues, markedly inhibited age-related albuminuria and proteinuria as well as age-related cardiac hypertrophy, and preserved endothelium-dependent and endothelium-independent vascular function in nondiabetic, female Sprague-Dawley and Fischer 344 rats [45].

Soluble RAGE (sRAGE), composed of the extracellular ligand-binding domain of RAGE, binds AGEs and blocks their interaction with RAGE, thus partly reducing detrimental effects of AGEs. Treatment with sRAGE for approximately 6 weeks resulted in dose-dependent reduction of atherosclerotic lesion area and complexity, together with a decrease in AGEs, vascular inflammation, and OS in apoE-null mice, while plasma glucose, cholesterol, and triglyceride concentrations remained similar to vehicle-treated mice [46,47]. In another study, administration of sRAGE stabilized already existing atherosclerotic lesions [48]. Finally, Wendt et al. [49] bred apo E-/- mice into the db/db background and treated them with sRAGE. These animals had significantly reduced atherosclerotic lesion area independent of the prevailing glycemia and lipidemia, thereby highlighting an important role of AGEs-RAGE interaction in mediating proatherogenic mechanisms.

These studies showed that higher circulating concentrations of AGEs, particularly dietary-derived AGEs, can induce cross-linking of arterial wall connective tissue protein [44], aortic atherosclerotic lesions [41], and neointimal formation after arterial injury [42], increase vascular permeability, and markedly impair vascular vasodilatatory response [43]. On the contrary, inhibitors of AGEs such as aminoguanidine or sRAGE can counteract diabetes, or age-induced effects of AGEs on the vasculature, suggesting that dietary or therapeutic interventions can be effective—at least in animal models—in preventing some key proatherosclerotic mechanisms.

30.3 Vascular Effects of AGEs in Clinical Studies

In humans, several clinical studies have linked AGEs to CVD, particularly in patients with DM. Kiuchi and coworkers [50] reported higher serum AGEs concentrations in type 2 DM subjects with obstructive CAD than in patients without obstructive CAD and higher than in normoglycemic patients with and without obstructive CAD. Similar results were reported by Kilhovd et al. [51] and Aso et al. [52]. Moreover, serum AGEs were found to be associated with the degree of CAD in patients with type 2 DM and obstructive CAD. Of note, elevation of serum AGEs in patients undergoing percutaneous coronary interventions was identified as an independent risk factor for restenosis in subjects with DM [53].

Prospective studies also support the association of AGEs with CVD. In type 1 DM, circulating AGEs were associated with incident fatal and nonfatal CVD as well as all-cause mortality in a 12-years follow-up study [54].

In females, but not in males with type 2 DM, elevated serum AGEs predicted mortality due to CAD during a follow-up of more than 18 years [55]. Authors reported a similar gender-specific pattern, in that serum levels of AGEs predicted both total and CAD-induced mortality in normoglycemic women [56].

Studying patients with chronic heart failure (CHF) with only 9% having diabetes, Hartog et al. [57] demonstrated that carboxymethyllysine (CML), a major AGE, predicted a composite outcome (death, heart transplantation, ischemic cardiovascular events, and hospitalization due to heart failure) even after adjustment for age, gender, etiology of heart failure, and several other known predictors of CHF outcome.

Noninvasive measurements have shown that skin autofluorescence (SAF), as a measure of skin AGEs accumulation, is increased in people with increased cardiovascular risk such as those with carotid artery stenosis and peripheral artery disease independently of the presence of diabetes [58]. An association of SAF with the 1-year incidence of major adverse cardiac events has also been reported [59].

The above-mentioned studies linked high AGE concentrations to cardiac disease and its outcome, but these studies could not prove a causal relationship. Therefore, the question remained unsolved whether AGEs are innocent bystanders or contribute to the development of CVD. Our group has performed several studies demonstrating deleterious effects of dietary AGEs on endothelial function in subjects with DM, while at the same time demonstrating that these effects can be counteracted by changing the cooking method or by vitamin supplementation.

30.4 Acute Effects of AGEs on Vascular Function

While chronic dietary interventions provide valuable information about clinical implications of changing diet in a way or another, it is difficult to narrow the effects to a substance class like, for example, AGEs. During cooking, not only AGEs but also other food toxins with potentially deleterious vascular effects are generated, vitamins can be inactivated and substrates degraded, making it therefore difficult to demonstrate to what extent the vascular effects of changing the cooking method are attributable to AGEs alone. Therefore, acute interventions were designed to address these mechanistic aspects more specifically. Our group has performed several clinical studies to demonstrate the deleterious acute effect of food AGEs on endothelial function.

The first study was done to investigate the acute effects of food AGEs derived from an AGE-rich beverage on endothelial function in subjects with or without preexisting diabetes. The oral AGE challenge beverage (300 mL) contained 1.8 × 106 AGEs units, but neither carbohydrates nor lipids [60], and it was prepared from glucose and caffeine-free Coca-Cola light, which was concentrated 10 times by rotary evaporation at room temperature. The acute effects on arterial endothelial function were assessed by means of flow-mediated dilatation (FMD) measurements as well as measurements of circulating vascular cell adhesion molecule-1 (VCAM-1) and plasminogen activator inhibitor-1 (PAI-1) levels. We investigated 44 diabetic and 10 nondiabetic subjects. Diabetic subjects had higher baseline levels of serum AGEs ($p < 0.020$) and VCAM-1 ($p < 0.033$) and lower baseline values of FMD compared with nondiabetic subjects ($p < 0.032$). Ninety minutes after a single oral AGE challenge, serum AGEs and

PAI-1 levels increased and FMD decreased significantly in both healthy subjects (AGEs: 7.2 ± 0.5 to 9.3 ± 1.0 units/mL, $p < 0.014$; PAI-1: 5.4 ± 0.4 to 6.8 ± 0.4 ng/mL, $p < 0.007$; and FMD: 9.9 ± 0.7 to 7.4 ± 0.9%, $p < 0.019$) and diabetic subjects (AGEs: 10.5 ± 0.7 to 14.2 ± 1.0 units/mL, $p < 0.020$; PAI-1: 6.5 ± 1.0 to 10 ± 2 ng/mL, $p < 0.030$; and FMD: 5.4 ± 0.4 to 4.0 ± 0.3%, $p < 0.032$). Serum glucose and VCAM-1 levels remained unchanged after the beverage intake.

We concluded that in both diabetic and nondiabetic subjects following a single AGE-rich beverage, a significant increase in serum AGEs occurs, accompanied by altered endothelial function. Thus, repeated or chronic exposure to H-AGE diets might accelerate the development of vascular disease over time.

However, the study had some limitations [61]: as cola-derived AGEs are only present in low amounts and as small molecules, the results might not be representative for dietary AGEs derived from common foods. It also could not be excluded that other substances than AGEs contained in Coca-Cola might have influenced vascular function. Moreover, the study was not subject-blinded.

We therefore performed a randomized, double-blind, controlled, crossover study aimed at investigating the acute effects of dietary AGEs resulting from nonenzymatic glycation during heating of beta-lactoglobulins (BLG; a protein class frequently encountered in food) and comparing these effects to nonglycated, but heated BLG [62]. Thus, the sole difference between the two protein preparations was the advanced protein glycation.

A total of 19 subjects with type 2 DM received, on two different occasions, beverages containing either glycated, heat-treated BLG (AGEs-BLG) or as control nonglycated, heat-treated BLG (C-BLG). We measured macrovascular (FMD) and microvascular (laser-Doppler measurements of reactive hyperemia in hand, RH) functions at baseline (T_0), as well as 90 (T_{90}) and 180 (T_{180}) minutes after each beverage. Following the AGEs-BLG, FMD decreased at T_{90} by 80% ($p < 0.05$ vs. baseline, $p < 0.05$ vs. C-BLG) from baseline and remained decreased by 42% at T_{180} ($p < 0.05$ vs. baseline). In comparison, FMD decrease following C-BLG was lower, with a maximum decrease of 51% at T_{180}. A significant decrease in nitrite (T_{180}) and nitrate (T_{90} and T_{180}) as well as a significant increase in CML accompanied the changes following the AGEs-BLG. No change in microvascular function followed any of the two beverages.

We concluded that in patients with type 2 DM, an acute oral administration of AGEs from heat-treated, glycated BLG impairs macrovascular function transiently, but significantly. These effects were more pronounced than following administration of heat-treated, nonglycated BLG and were accompanied by an increase in circulating CML and a decrease in nitrate. We also suggested that the mechanisms leading to vascular dysfunction following AGE administration are related to a decrease in NO bioavailability, since nitrite and nitrate (metabolites of NO) were decreased after AGE intake.

Since detrimental effects of dietary AGEs were demonstrated, the next step was to develop strategies to reduce AGE formation in food and thus alleviate postprandial ED. Several therapeutic approaches have been suggested for the treatment of postprandial ED, including insulin, folic acid, tetrahydrobiopterin, vitamins C and E, benfotiamine, and statins. They aim at reducing postprandial OS (vitamins C and E, statins, and partly folic acid), postprandial hyperglycemia (insulin), and postprandial hypertriglyceridemia (statins) or have a direct effect on NO production (folic acid, insulin, and tetrahydrobiopterin) [21].

If deleterious effects of food AGEs are postulated, their detrimental effects can be counteracted by (1) decreasing AGE formation in foods by choosing appropriate cooking methods [63] and (2) counteracting their effects by means of anti-AGE interventions (e.g., with aminoguanidine or benfotiamine). Therefore, we investigated two AGE-related approaches to improve postprandial ED: changing the cooking method [64] and treatment with benfotiamine [65].

By changing the cooking method, we tested the hypothesis that a single "real-life" H-AGEs meal acutely induces more pronounced vascular dysfunction than does an L-AGEs meal [64]. We also tested whether the ED attributable to dietary AGEs exceeds the effects of postprandial hyperglycemia, hypertriglyceridemia, and hyperinsulinemia. Toward this aim, we compared the effects of two meals with identical ingredients, but different AGEs amounts, on microvascular and macrovascular functions, as well as on serum lipids, markers of inflammation, OS, and serum AGEs.

A total of twenty inpatients with type 2 DM, aged 55.4 ± 2.2 years and glycated hemoglobin (HbA1c) 8.8 ± 0.5% (values expressed as mean ± SEM), were investigated. In a randomized, crossover design, the effects of L-AGE and H-AGE meals on macrovascular (FMD) and microvascular (Laser-Doppler flowmetry) functions, serum markers of ED (E-selectin, intracellular adhesion molecule-1[ICAM-1], and VCAM-1), OS, and serum AGEs were assessed. The two meals were isocaloric, had identical ingredients, and differed only by the temperature and time of cooking. Each meal consisted of 200 g chicken breast, 250 g potatoes, 100 g carrots, 200 g tomatoes, and 15 g vegetable oil and provided 580 kcal, 54 g protein, 17 g fat, 48 g carbohydrates, 60 mg cholesterol, and 10 g fibers. The H-AGE meal (approximately 15.100 kU AGEs) was prepared by frying or broiling at 230°C for 20 minutes, whereas the L-AGE meal (approximately 2,750 kU AGEs) was prepared by steaming or boiling at 100°C for 10 minutes. Subjects were instructed to eat the test meal within 30 minutes. The measurements were performed at baseline and 2, 4, and 6 hours after each meal.

After the H-AGE meal, FMD decreased maximally by 36.2% from 5.77 ± 0.65% (baseline) to 3.93 ± 0.48 (2 hours), 3.70 ± 0.42 (4 hours), and 4.42 ± 0.54% (6 hours) ($p < 0.01$ for all compared with baseline). After the L-AGE meal, FMD decrease was reduced, the maximal postprandial reduction was 20.9%, from 6.04 ± 0.68% (baseline) to 4.75 ± 0.48% (2 hours), 4.69 ± 0.51% (4 hours), and 5.62 ± 0.63% (6 hours) ($p < 0.01$ for all compared with baseline; $p < 0.001$ for all compared with the H-AGE meal). This impairment of macrovascular function after the H-AGE meal was paralleled by an impairment of microvascular function (−67.2%) and increased concentrations of serum AGEs and markers of ED and OS. We concluded that in patients with T2DM, an H-AGE meal induces a more pronounced acute impairment of vascular function than does an otherwise identical L-AGE meal. Therefore, chemical modifications of food by means of cooking play a major role in influencing the extent of postprandial ED. The postprandial ED after ingestion of the H-AGE meal was accompanied by an increase in markers of ED (E-selectin, ICAM-1, and VCAM-1). The amplified postprandial OS in the present study was confirmed by the increase in serum thiobarbituric acid–reactive species, which was significantly higher after the H-AGE than after the L-AGE meal.

In line with our data, in type 2 DM subjects, an H-AGE diet over 6 weeks caused a significant increase in serum AGEs, markers of inflammation (C-reactive protein and tumor necrosis factor-α), and ED (VCAM-1), whereas an L-AGE diet led to suppression of all these markers [29]. Moreover, LDL pooled from patients on an H-AGE diet was more glycated and more oxidized and markedly stimulated NF-κB activity, thus enhancing LDL-mediated vascular toxicity [66].

A second approach to reduce postprandial ED was the administration of benfotiamine, a thiamine prodrug with much higher bioavailability than thiamine hydrochloride. Thiamine (vitamin B1) activates the intracellular enzyme transketolase and directs glucose substrates to the pentose phosphate pathway. Thus, it prevents the activation of four hyperglycemia-induced pathways: the polyol, hexosamine, and diacylglycerol—protein kinase C pathways, along with the endogenous AGEs formation [67]. Direct antioxidant effects have also been described for benfotiamine [68].

In a proof-of-principle study, Arora et al. [69] demonstrated in 10 healthy subjects, 10 subjects with impaired glucose tolerance and 10 patients with type 2 DM that a single intravenous administration of 100 mg thiamine reduced ED following a 75 g oral glucose challenge. Authors highlighted that protective effects of thiamine against hyperglycemia-induced ED were not related to glucose lowering. AGE-specific effects were not assessed in that study, but protective effects of thiamine on the endothelium were shown.

We therefore conducted a pilot study investigating whether benfotiamine counteracts postprandial microvascular and macrovascular ED in subjects with type 2 DM [65].

Thirteen subjects with type 2 DM were given a heat-processed test meal with H-AGE content (approximately 15.100 AGE kU, 580 kcal, 54 g protein, 17 g lipids, and 48 g carbohydrates as previously described [64]) before and after a 3-day therapy with benfotiamine (1,050 mg/day). Macrovascular FMD and microvascular reactive hyperemia (Laser-Doppler), along with serum markers of ED (E-selectin, VCAM-1 and ICAM-1), OS, and AGEs, were measured during both test-meal days after an overnight fast and then at 2, 4, and 6 hours postprandially. The H-AGE meal induced a maximum reactive hyperemia decrease of 60.0% after 2 hours and a maximum FMD impairment of 35.1% after 4 hours. The effects of an H-AGE meal on both FMD and reactive hyperemia were completely prevented by benfotiamine. Serum markers of ED and OS, as well as AGEs, increased after H-AGE meal and these effects were significantly reduced by benfotiamine. We concluded that in individuals with type 2 DM, microvascular and macrovascular ED accompanied by increased OS occur following a real-life, heat-processed, AGE-rich meal and suggest that these effects can be partly prevented by benfotiamine.

To strengthen these data, another study was designed to test in a larger population of subjects with type 2 DM and in a double-blind, placebo-controlled, randomized, crossover way, whether a 6-weeks treatment with high doses of benfotiamine (900 mg/day) can prevent the detrimental effects of an AGE-rich meal on postprandial FMD, as well as on microvascular and autonomic nervous function tests [70]. A total of 31 subjects with type 2 DM received 900 mg/day benfotiamine or placebo for 6 weeks (with a washout period of 6 weeks between). At the end of each treatment period, macrovascular and microvascular functions were assessed, together with variables of autonomic nervous function in fasting state, as well as 2, 4, and 6 hours following a heated, mixed test meal (H-AGE). Participants who had a high cardiovascular risk showed accordingly an impaired baseline FMD (2.63 ± 2.49%). Compared with the fasting state, neither variable changed postprandially following the placebo treatment. The 6-weeks treatment with high doses of benfotiamine did not alter this pattern, either in the fasting state or postprandially. These data were somehow surprising since we expected a postprandial decrease following the H-AGE meal, but our hypothesis is that these subjects at high risk had a markedly impaired endothelial function at baseline that could not further be impaired by the meal administration. Interestingly, among a subgroup of patients with the highest FMD following placebo treatment, there was (as seen in other studies) a significant postprandial FMD decrease and this effect was significantly attenuated by benfotiamine pretreatment.

We concluded that in subjects with type 2 DM and markedly impaired fasting FMD, a mixed test meal does not further deteriorate FMD or variables of microvascular or autonomic nervous function. Because no significant deterioration of postprandial FMD and microvascular or autonomic nervous function tests occurred after placebo treatment, prevention of the postprandial deterioration of these variables with benfotiamine could not be demonstrated.

The results of this study, together with the data of our previous pilot study [65], suggest that earlier interventions with benfotiamine or other agents with protective vascular effects could be more beneficial among patients with a less-pronounced impairment of FMD than in those with advanced vascular damage, where a "point-of-no-return" might be reached. Further studies are warranted to demonstrate this hypothesis.

30.5 Conclusions

The results of the DCCT-EDIC study have strengthened the role of the so-called glycemic memory, postulating that metabolic control over several years predicts the development of diabetic complications. The fact that glycated proteins form under hyperglycemic conditions and chronically accumulate within organs that are prone to diabetes-related complication suggests AGEs as ideal candidates mediating the "glycemic memory." Accumulation of AGEs within the body can result from increased endogenous production under conditions of hyperglycemia and from exogenous dietary sources. AGEs exert their deleterious effects on the vasculature by both receptor-dependent and receptor-independent mechanisms.

Indeed, we have recently demonstrated in subjects with type 2 DM that the acute administration of AGEs transiently impairs endothelial function and that this effect can be diminished by changing the cooking method alone (and thus changing the concentration of ingested AGEs). In line with our data, in further studies, the restriction of dietary AGEs in diabetic patients, in patients with renal failure, and in healthy subjects was accompanied by a significant fall in circulating AGEs and a decrease in markers of OS, inflammation, ED, and insulin resistance. Therefore, dietary interventions seem to be highly effective in reducing circulating AGEs and impact positively on factors of vascular homeostasis. Our data also suggest that benfotiamine could counteract detrimental effects of dietary AGEs on the vasculature of subjects with DM, but our data are preliminary, need to be confirmed, and do not suffice for clinical recommendations.

Overall, there is compelling evidence for a detrimental role of AGEs in driving vascular disease. We therefore believe that for the promotion of cardiovascular health, besides dietary recommendations regarding limitation in fat and carbohydrate intake, dietary recommendations should be made with regard to healthy cooking methods that reduce dietary AGEs load.

REFERENCES

1. Hobbs, F.D., 2006. Type-2 diabetes mellitus related cardiovascular risk: New options for interventions to reduce risk and treatment goals. *Atheroscler Suppl* 7:29–32.
2. Ross, R., 1993. The pathogenesis of atherosclerosis: A perspective for the 1990s. *Nature* 362:801–809.
3. Calles-Escandon, J. and Cipolla, M., 2001. Diabetes and ED: A clinical perspective. *Endocr Rev* 22:36–52.
4. Forstermann, U. and Munzel, T., 2006. Endothelial nitric oxide synthase in vascular disease: From marvel to menace. *Circulation* 113:1708–1714.
5. Holowatz, L.A., Thompson, C.S., Minson, C.T., and Kenney, W.L., 2005. Mechanisms of acetylcholine-mediated vasodilatation in young and aged human skin. *J Physiol* 563:965–973.
6. Stirban, A., Rosen, P., and Tschoepe, D., 2008. Complications of type 1 diabetes: New molecular findings. *Mt Sinai J Med* 75:328–351.
7. Clarkson, P., Celermajer, D.S., Donald, A.E., Sampson, M., Sorensen, K.E., Adams, M., Yue, D.K., Betteridge, D.J., and Deanfield, J.E., 1996. Impaired vascular reactivity in insulin-dependent diabetes mellitus is related to disease duration and low density lipoprotein cholesterol levels. *J Am Coll Cardiol* 28:573–579.
8. Tooke, J.E. and Goh, K.L., 1999. Vascular function in Type 2 diabetes mellitus and pre-diabetes: The case for intrinsic endotheiopathy. *Diabet Med* 16:710–715.
9. Cosentino, F. and Luscher, T.F., 1998. ED in diabetes mellitus. *J Cardiovasc Pharmacol* 32 Suppl 3:S54–S61.
10. Guerci, B., Kearney-Schwartz, A., Bohme, P., Zannad, F., and Drouin, P., 2001. ED and type 2 diabetes. Part 1: Physiology and methods for exploring the endothelial function. *Diabetes Metab* 27:425–434.
11. Cavalot, F., Petrelli, A., Traversa, M., Bonomo, K., Fiora, E., Conti, M., Anfossi, G., Costa, G., and Trovati, M., 2006. Postprandial blood glucose is a stronger predictor of cardiovascular events than fasting blood glucose in type 2 diabetes mellitus, particularly in women: Lessons from the San Luigi Gonzaga Diabetes Study. *J Clin Endocrinol Metab* 91:813–819.
12. Ceriello, A., 2000. The post-prandial state and cardiovascular disease: Relevance to diabetes mellitus. *Diabetes Metab Res Rev* 16:125–132.
13. O'Keefe, J.H. and Bell, D.S., 2007. Postprandial hyperglycemia/hyperlipidemia (postprandial dysmetabolism) is a cardiovascular risk factor. *Am J Cardiol* 100:899–904.
14. Ceriello, A., 2005. Postprandial hyperglycemia and diabetes complications: Is it time to treat? *Diabetes* 54:1–7.
15. Ceriello, A., Hanefeld, M., Leiter, L., Monnier, L., Moses, A., Owens, D., Tajima, N., and Tuomilehto, J., 2004. Postprandial glucose regulation and diabetic complications. *Arch Intern Med* 164:2090–2095.
16. Ceriello, A., Quagliaro, L., Piconi, L., Assaloni, R., Da, R.R., Maier, A., Esposito, K., and Giugliano, D., 2004. Effect of postprandial hypertriglyceridemia and hyperglycemia on circulating adhesion molecules and oxidative stress generation and the possible role of simvastatin treatment. *Diabetes* 53:701–710.
17. Lee, I.K., Kim, H.S., and Bae, J.H., 2002. ED: Its relationship with acute hyperglycaemia and hyperlipidemia. *Int J Clin Pract Suppl* 129:59–64.
18. Ceriello, A., Taboga, C., Tonutti, L., Quagliaro, L., Piconi, L., Bais, B., Da, R.R., and Motz, E., 2002. Evidence for an independent and cumulative effect of postprandial hypertriglyceridemia and hyperglycemia on ED and oxidative stress generation: Effects of short- and long-term simvastatin treatment. *Circulation* 106:1211–1218.
19. Campia, U., Sullivan, G., Bryant, M.B., Waclawiw, M.A., Quon, M.J., and Panza, J.A., 2004. Insulin impairs endothelium-dependent vasodilation independent of insulin sensitivity or lipid profile. *Am J Physiol Heart Circ Physiol* 286:H76–H82.
20. Vlassara, H., Fuh, H., Donnelly, T., and Cybulsky, M., 1995. Advanced glycation endproducts promote adhesion molecule (VCAM-1, ICAM-1) expression and atheroma formation in normal rabbits. *Mol Med* 1:447–456.
21. Stirban, A., Gawlowski, T., and Roden, M., 2013. Vascular effects of advanced glycation endproducts: Clinical effects and molecular mechanisms. *Mol Metabol* 3(2):94–108.
22. Cai, W., Gao, Q.D., Zhu, L., Peppa, M., He, C., and Vlassara, H., 2002. Oxidative stress-inducing carbonyl compounds from common foods: Novel mediators of cellular dysfunction. *Mol Med* 8:337–346.

23. Duell, P.B., Oram, J.F., and Bierman, E.L., 1991. Nonenzymatic glycosylation of HDL and impaired HDL-receptor-mediated cholesterol efflux. *Diabetes* 40:377–384.
24. Wever, R.M., Luscher, T.F., Cosentino, F., and Rabelink, T.J., 1998. Atherosclerosis and the two faces of endothelial nitric oxide synthase. *Circulation* 97:108–112.
25. Xu, B., Ji, Y., Yao, K., Cao, Y.X., and Ferro, A., 2005. Inhibition of human endothelial cell nitric oxide synthesis by advanced glycation end-products but not glucose: Relevance to diabetes. *Clin Sci (London)* 109:439–446.
26. Vlassara, H., 1996. Advanced glycation end-products and atherosclerosis. *Ann Med* 28:419–426.
27. Giardino, I., Edelstein, D., and Brownlee, M., 1994. Nonenzymatic glycosylation *in vitro* and in bovine endothelial cells alters basic fibroblast growth factor activity. A model for intracellular glycosylation in diabetes. *J Clin Invest* 94:110–117.
28. Charonis, A.S., Reger, L.A., Dege, J.E., Kouzi-Koliakos, K., Furcht, L.T., Wohlhueter, R.M., and Tsilibary, E.C., 1990. Laminin alterations after *in vitro* nonenzymatic glycosylation. *Diabetes* 39:807–814.
29. Vlassara, H., Cai, W., Crandall, J., Goldberg, T., Oberstein, R., Dardaine, V., Peppa, M., and Rayfield, E.J., 2002. Inflammatory mediators are induced by dietary glycotoxins, a major risk factor for diabetic angiopathy. *Proc Natl Acad Sci U S A* 99:15596–15601.
30. Rosen, P., Nawroth, P.P., King, G., Moller, W., Tritschler, H.J., and Packer, L., 2001. The role of oxidative stress in the onset and progression of diabetes and its complications: A summary of a Congress Series sponsored by UNESCO-MCBN, the American Diabetes Association and the German Diabetes Society. *Diabetes Metab Res Rev* 17:189–212.
31. Bierhaus, A., Humpert, P.M., Morcos, M., Wendt, T., Chavakis, T., Arnold, B., Stern, D.M., and Nawroth, P.P., 2005. Understanding RAGE, the receptor for advanced glycation end products. *J Mol Med* 83:876–886.
32. Ramasamy, R., Vannucci, S.J., Yan, S.S., Herold, K., Yan, S.F., and Schmidt, A.M., 2005. Advanced glycation end products and RAGE: A common thread in aging, diabetes, neurodegeneration, and inflammation. *Glycobiology* 15:16R–28R.
33. Stitt, A.W., He, C., Friedman, S., Scher, L., Rossi, P., Ong, L., Founds, H., Li, Y.M., Bucala, R., and Vlassara, H., 1997. Elevated AGE-modified ApoB in sera of euglycemic, normolipidemic patients with atherosclerosis: Relationship to tissue AGEs. *Mol Med* 3:617–627.
34. Nakamura, Y., Horii, Y., Nishino, T., Shiiki, H., Sakaguchi, Y., Kagoshima, T., Dohi, K., Makita, Z., Vlassara, H., and Bucala, R., 1993. Immunohistochemical localization of advanced glycosylation end products in coronary atheroma and cardiac tissue in diabetes mellitus. *Am J Pathol* 143:1649–1656.
35. Cipollone, F., Iezzi, A., Fazia, M., Zucchelli, M., Pini, B., Cuccurullo, C., De, C.D., et al., 2003. The receptor RAGE as a progression factor amplifying arachidonate-dependent inflammatory and proteolytic response in human atherosclerotic plaques: Role of glycemic control. *Circulation* 108:1070–1077.
36. Mamputu, J.C. and Renier,G., 2004. Advanced glycation end-products increase monocyte adhesion to retinal endothelial cells through vascular endothelial growth factor-induced ICAM-1 expression: Inhibitory effect of antioxidants. *J Leukoc Biol* 75:1062–1069.
37. Gawlowski, T., Stratmann, B., Ruetter, R., Buenting, C.E., Menart, B., Weiss, J., Vlassara, H., Koschinsky, T., and Tschoepe, D., 2009. Advanced glycation end products strongly activate platelets. *Eur J Nutr* 48:475–481.
38. Kirstein, M., Brett, J., Radoff, S., Ogawa, S., Stern, D., and Vlassara, H., 1990. Advanced protein glycosylation induces transendothelial human monocyte chemotaxis and secretion of platelet-derived growth factor: Role in vascular disease of diabetes and aging. *Proc Natl Acad Sci U S A* 87:9010–9014.
39. Yu, W., Liu-Bryan, R., Stevens, S., Damanahalli, J.K., and Terkeltaub, R., 2012. RAGE signaling mediates post-injury arterial neointima formation by suppression of liver kinase B1 and AMPK activity. *Atherosclerosis* 222:417–425.
40. Rojas, A. and Morales, M.A., 2004. Advanced glycation and endothelial functions: A link towards vascular complications in diabetes. *Life Sci* 76:715–730.
41. Lin, R.Y., Choudhury, R.P., Cai, W., Lu, M., Fallon, J.T., Fisher, E.A., and Vlassara, H., 2003. Dietary glycotoxins promote diabetic atherosclerosis in apolipoprotein E-deficient mice. *Atherosclerosis* 168:213–220.

42. Lin, R.Y., Reis, E.D., Dore, A.T., Lu, M., Ghodsi, N., Fallon, J.T., Fisher, E.A., and Vlassara, H., 2002. Lowering of dietary advanced glycation endproducts (AGE) reduces neointimal formation after arterial injury in genetically hypercholesterolemic mice. *Atherosclerosis* 163:303–311.
43. Vlassara, H., Fuh, H., Makita, Z., Krungkrai, S., Cerami, A., and Bucala, R., 1992. Exogenous advanced glycosylation end products induce complex vascular dysfunction in normal animals: A model for diabetic and aging complications. *Proc Natl Acad Sci U S A* 89:12043–12047.
44. Brownlee, M., Vlassara, H., Kooney, A., Ulrich, P., and Cerami, A., 1986. Aminoguanidine prevents diabetes-induced arterial wall protein cross-linking. *Science* 232:1629–1632.
45. Li, Y.M., Steffes, M., Donnelly, T., Liu, C., Fuh, H., Basgen, J., Bucala, R., and Vlassara, H., 1996. Prevention of cardiovascular and renal pathology of aging by the advanced glycation inhibitor aminoguanidine. *Proc Natl Acad Sci U S A* 93:3902–3907.
46. Park, L., Raman, K.G., Lee, K.J., Lu, Y., Ferran, L.J., Jr., Chow, W.S., Stern, D., and Schmidt, A.M., 1998. Suppression of accelerated diabetic atherosclerosis by the soluble receptor for advanced glycation endproducts. *Nat Med* 4:1025–1031.
47. Kislinger, T., Tanji, N., Wendt, T., Qu, W., Lu, Y., Ferran, L.J., Jr., Taguchi, A., et al., 2001. Receptor for advanced glycation end products mediates inflammation and enhanced expression of tissue factor in vasculature of diabetic apolipoprotein E-null mice. *Arterioscler Thromb Vasc Biol* 21:905–910.
48. Bucciarelli, L.G., Wendt, T., Qu, W., Lu, Y., Lalla, E., Rong, L.L., Goova, M.T., et al., 2002. RAGE blockade stabilizes established atherosclerosis in diabetic apolipoprotein E-null mice. *Circulation* 106:2827–2835.
49. Wendt, T., Harja, E., Bucciarelli, L., Qu, W., Lu, Y., Rong, L.L., Jenkins, D.G., Stein, G., Schmidt, A.M., and Yan, S.F., 2006. RAGE modulates vascular inflammation and atherosclerosis in a murine model of type 2 diabetes. *Atherosclerosis* 185:70–77.
50. Kiuchi, K., Nejima, J., Takano, T., Ohta, M., and Hashimoto, H., 2001. Increased serum concentrations of advanced glycation end products: A marker of coronary artery disease activity in type 2 diabetic patients. *Heart* 85:87–91.
51. Kilhovd, B.K., Berg, T.J., Birkeland, K.I., Thorsby, P., and Hanssen, K.F., 1999. Serum levels of advanced glycation end products are increased in patients with type 2 diabetes and coronary heart disease. *Diabetes Care* 22:1543–1548.
52. Aso, Y., Inukai, T., Tayama, K., and Takemura, Y., 2000. Serum concentrations of advanced glycation endproducts are associated with the development of atherosclerosis as well as diabetic microangiopathy in patients with type 2 diabetes. *Acta Diabetol* 37:87–92.
53. Choi, E.Y., Kwon, H.M., Ahn, C.W., Lee, G.T., Joung, B., Hong, B.K., Yoon, Y.W., et al., 2005. Serum levels of advanced glycation end products are associated with in-stent restenosis in diabetic patients. *Yonsei Med J* 46:78–85.
54. Nin, J.W., Jorsal, A., Ferreira, I., Schalkwijk, C.G., Prins, M.H., Parving, H.H., Tarnow, L., Rossing, P., and Stehouwer, C.D., 2011. Higher plasma levels of advanced glycation end products are associated with incident cardiovascular disease and all-cause mortality in type 1 diabetes: A 12-year follow-up study. *Diabetes Care* 34:442–447.
55. Kilhovd, B.K., Juutilainen, A., Lehto, S., Ronnemaa, T., Torjesen, P.A., Hanssen, K.F., and Laakso, M., 2007. Increased serum levels of advanced glycation endproducts predict total, cardiovascular and coronary mortality in women with type 2 diabetes: A population-based 18 year follow-up study. *Diabetologia* 50:1409–1417.
56. Kilhovd, B.K., Juutilainen, A., Lehto, S., Ronnemaa, T., Torjesen, P.A., Birkeland, K.I., Berg, T.J., Hanssen, K.F., and Laakso, M., 2005. High serum levels of advanced glycation end products predict increased coronary heart disease mortality in nondiabetic women but not in nondiabetic men: A population-based 18-year follow-up study. *Arterioscler Thromb Vasc Biol* 25:815–820.
57. Hartog, J.W., Voors, A.A., Schalkwijk, C.G., Scheijen, J., Smilde, T.D., Damman, K., Bakker, S.J., Smit, A.J., and Van Veldhuisen, D.J., 2007. Clinical and prognostic value of advanced glycation endproducts in chronic heart failure. *Eur Heart J* 28:2879–2885.
58. Noordzij, M.J., Lefrandt, J.D., Loeffen, E.A., Saleem, B.R., Meerwaldt, R., Lutgers, H.L., Smit, A.J., and Zeebregts, C.J., 2012. Skin autofluorescence is increased in patients with carotid artery stenosis and peripheral artery disease. *Int J Cardiovasc Imaging* 28:431–438.

59. Mulder, D.J., van Haelst, P.L., Graaff, R., Gans, R.O., Zijlstra, F., and Smit, A.J., 2009. Skin autofluorescence is elevated in acute myocardial infarction and is associated with the one-year incidence of major adverse cardiac events. *Neth Heart J* 17:162–168.
60. Uribarri, J., Stirban, A., Sander, D., Cai, W., Negrean, M., Buenting, C.E., Koschinsky, T., and Vlassara, H., 2007. Single oral challenge by advanced glycation end products acutely impairs endothelial function in diabetic and nondiabetic subjects. *Diabetes Care* 30:2579–2582.
61. Ahmed, N., Mirshekar-Syahkal, B., Kennish, L., Karachalias, N., Babaei-Jadidi, R., and Thornalley, P.J., 2005. Assay of advanced glycation endproducts in selected beverages and food by liquid chromatography with tandem mass spectrometric detection. *Mol Nutr Food Res* 49:691–699.
62. Stirban, A., Kotsi, P., Franke, K., Strijowski, U., Cai, W., Gotting, C., and Tschoepe, D., 2013. Acute macrovascular dysfunction in patients with type 2 diabetes induced by ingestion of advanced glycated beta-lactoglobulins. *Diabetes Care* 36:1278–1282.
63. Uribarri, J., Woodruff, S., Goodman, S., Cai, W., Chen, X., Pyzik, R., Yong, A., Striker, G.E., and Vlassara, H., 2010. Advanced glycation end products in foods and a practical guide to their reduction in the diet. *J Am Diet Assoc* 110:911–916.
64. Negrean, M., Stirban, A., Stratmann, B., Gawlowski, T., Horstmann, T., Gotting, C., Kleesiek, K., et al., 2007. Effects of low- and high-advanced glycation endproduct meals on macro- and microvascular endothelial function and oxidative stress in patients with type 2 diabetes mellitus. *Am J Clin Nutr* 85:1236–1243.
65. Stirban, A., Negrean, M., Stratmann, B., Gawlowski, T., Horstmann, T., Gotting, C., Kleesiek, K., et al., 2006. Benfotiamine prevents macro- and microvascular ED and oxidative stress following a meal rich in advanced glycation end products in individuals with type 2 diabetes. *Diabetes Care* 29:2064–2071.
66. Cai, W., He, J.C., Zhu, L., Peppa, M., Lu, C., Uribarri, J., and Vlassara, H., 2004. High levels of dietary advanced glycation end products transform low-density lipoprotein into a potent redox-sensitive mitogen-activated protein kinase stimulant in diabetic patients. *Circulation* 110:285–291.
67. Hammes, H.P., Du, X., Edelstein, D., Taguchi, T., Matsumura, T., Ju, Q., Lin, J., et al., 2003. Benfotiamine blocks three major pathways of hyperglycemic damage and prevents experimental diabetic retinopathy. *Nat Med* 9:294–299.
68. Schmid, U., Stopper, H., Heidland, A., and Schupp, N., 2008. Benfotiamine exhibits direct antioxidative capacity and prevents induction of DNA damage *in vitro*. *Diabetes Metab Res Rev* 24:371–377.
69. Arora, S., Lidor, A., Abularrage, C.J., Weiswasser, J.M., Nylen, E., Kellicut, D., and Sidawy, A.N., 2006. Thiamine (vitamin B1) improves endothelium-dependent vasodilatation in the presence of hyperglycemia. *Ann Vasc Surg* 20:653–658.
70. Stirban, A., Pop, A., and Tschoepe, D., 2013. A randomized, double-blind, crossover, placebo-controlled trial of 6 weeks benfotiamine treatment on postprandial vascular function and variables of autonomic nerve function in Type 2 diabetes. *Diabet Med* 30:1204–1208.

31

Methylglyoxal and Other AGEs: Good and Bad Dual Role in the Body

Mayuri Gogoi, Kapudeep Karmakar, Kasturi Chandra, and Dipshikha Chakravortty
Indian Institute of Science
Bangalore, India

CONTENTS

KEY POINTS

- Deleterious effects of methylglyoxal in various diseases.
- Therapeutic potentials of methylglyoxal against microbial disease and cancer.
- Dietary sources of methylglyoxal and other advanced glycation end products (AGEs).
- Various anti-AGE drugs and their ameliorative effects.

31.1 Introduction

Methylglyoxal [CH_3COCHO], also known as 2-oxopropanal or pyruvaldehyde, is a chemically reduced derivative of pyruvic acid [$CH_3COCOOH$]. Although early studies in 1930s (Case and Cook 1931) suggested methylglyoxal to be a glycolytic intermediate, not much work had been carried out till 1970s. Cooper and Anderson's discovery of methylglyoxal synthase–mediated methylglyoxal production resumed research in this field (Cooper and Anderson 1970). Methylglyoxal forms advanced glycation end products (AGEs) 20,000 times more efficiently than glucose (Angeloni et al. 2014) and has multiple cytotoxic effects such as cell cycle inhibition, mutagenesis, apoptosis (Antognelli et al. 2013), inhibition of enzymatic activity, protein cross-linking (Oya et al. 1999), and DNA damage (Kang 2003).

31.2 Methylglyoxal and AGE Metabolism

In biological systems, many metabolic pathways such as glycolysis, threonine catabolism, metabolism of ketone bodies, lipid peroxidation, and degradation of glycated proteins produce methylglyoxal as a by-product. It is formed from nonenzymatic removal of phosphate from glycolytic intermediates, glyceraldehyde-3-phosphate (GAP) anddihydroxyacetone-3-phosphate(DHAP) (Dhar et al. 2008). Food items such as alcoholic beverages and coffee also serve as exogenous sources of methylglyoxal.

Methylglyoxal is mainly synthesized from glucose, triglycerols, and amino acid precursors with the help of methylglyoxal synthase (MG synthase) and amine oxidases. Glycolytic intermediate dihydroxyacetone-3-phosphate gives rise to methylglyoxal directly when acted upon by methylglyoxal synthase. The conversion of acetone to methylglyoxal is mediated by NADPH via acetol intermediates. Aminoacetone, which is a threonine and glycine metabolism intermediate, is converted to methylglyoxal by the action of amine oxidase (Dhar et al. 2008) (Figure 31.1). Xenobiotic like 2-(*p*-methoxyphenyl)-4-methylthiazole also produce methylglyoxal inside the cells as they undergo epoxidation (Mizutani et al. 1994).

Apart from its direct cytotoxic effects, methylglyoxal can cause nonenzymatic glycation of protein or lipid, resulting in formation of AGEs format ion. This nonenzymatic glycation reaction is called Maillard reaction. Early glycation of protein results in the formation of a Schiff base that undergoes rearrangement to form Amadori intermediates. Further oxidation finally leads to the formation of AGEs (Luevano-Contreras and Chapman-Novakofski 2010).

Other pathways that give rise to AGEs are autoxidation of glucose and lipid peroxidation. In these pathways, α-oxaldehydes (e.g., glyoxals, 3-deoxyglucosone, and methylglyoxal) interact with monoacids to form AGEs. Another well-explored pathway of AGE production is the polyol pathway (Dhar et al. 2008). Aldose reductase converts glucose to sorbitol, which is then converted to fructose by the action of sorbitol dehydrogenase. Fructose is further metabolized to α-oxaldehyde, which in turn forms AGEs (Figure 31.2) (Luevano-Contreras and Chapman-Novakofski 2010).

According to their characteristics, AGEs have been divided into three categories: fluorescent cross-linking, for example, pentosidine; nonfluorescent cross-linking, for example, imidazolium di-lysine cross-links; and nonfluorescent non-crosslinking AGEs, for example, N-carboxy-methyl-lysine (CML) (Stirban et al. 2014).

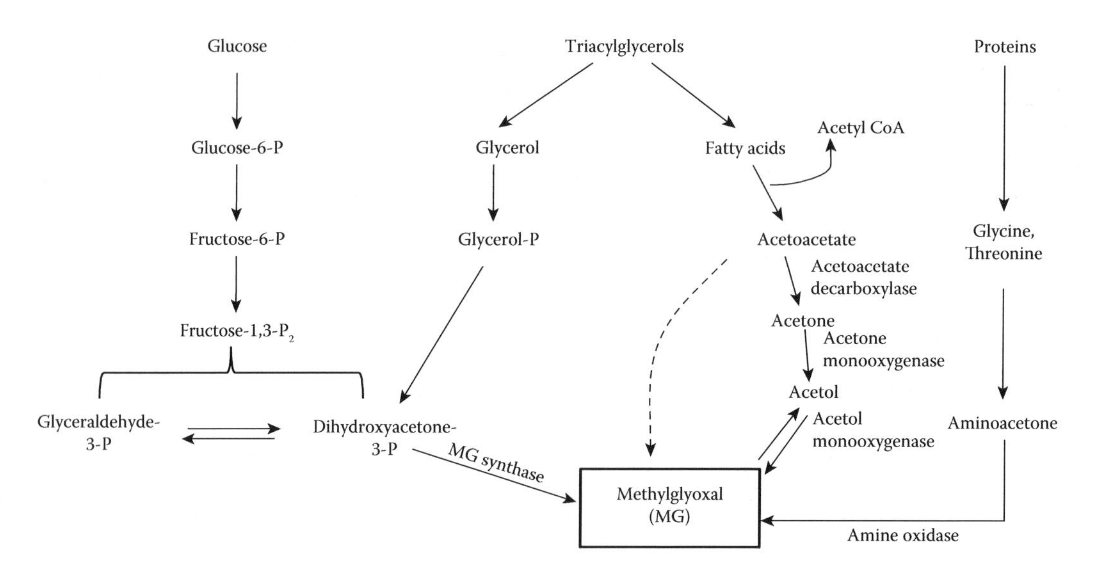

FIGURE 31.1 Pathways for methylglyoxal generation.

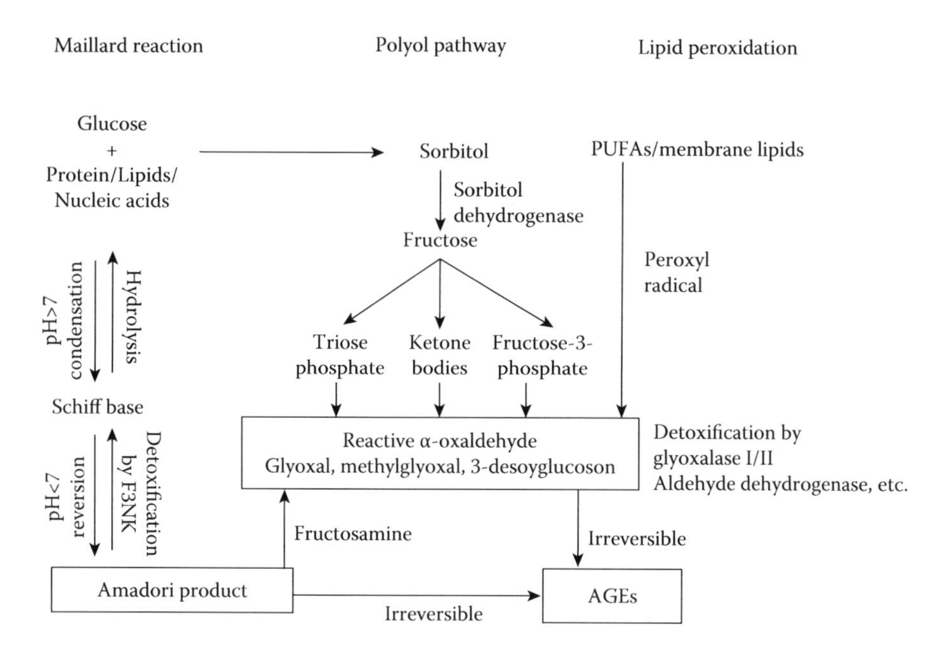

FIGURE 31.2 Pathways for AGE generation.

31.3 AGE Signaling

AGEs affect the intracellular signaling in various cells. For example, circulating AGEs activate different intracellular signaling pathways by interacting with RAGE (receptor for AGEs) present on endothelial cells. There are also some non-RAGE receptors for AGEs like AGE-R1/OST-48, AGE-R2/80K-H, and AGE-R3/galectin-3, which have been extensively studied (Kierdorf and Fritz 2013). RAGE recognizes a vast array of ligands such as AGEs, amyloid β-peptides, and LPS. The ligand-binding results in downstream upregulation of NF-κB-mediated cellular signaling pathways (Kierdorf and Fritz 2013). In response to AGE–RAGE interaction, reactive oxygen species (ROS) production and inflammatory responses are upregulated. This in turn translocates interferon regulatory factor (IRF-1) into the nucleus and induces cytokine response (Kierdorf and Fritz 2013).

Another intracellular signaling pathway utilizes a type-I transmembrane protein called AGER1 that interferes via NAD-dependent deacetylase SIRT1 (sirtuin-1) (Cai et al. 2012). AGER1 facilitates turnover of AGEs by modulating their uptake, metabolism, and clearance and has regulatory effect on insulin signaling and some anti-inflammatory pathways. AGER1 also negatively regulates AGE–RAGE signaling by suppressing MAPK phosphorylation and NF-κB activation, thus helping in detoxification of AGEs (Figure 31.3) (Cai et al. 2012).

31.4 Methylglyoxal and AGE Clearance

The body has developed mechanisms to counteract the adverse effects of methylglyoxal and AGEs. The major detoxification route is the glyoxalase pathway, where methylglyoxal reacts with glutathione to form hemithioacetal, which is further metabolized into the nontoxic product D-lactate. This pathway involves two enzymes, namely glyoxalase I (GLO1) and glyoxalase II (GLO2), and reduced glutathione (GSH) as cofactors. GLO1 is present in cytoplasm and endoplasmic reticulum, whereas GLO2 is present in the mitochondria. Glyoxalase system is present in both prokaryotes and eukaryotes (Chakraborty et al. 2014). Other detoxification pathways include aldose reductase (also known as ketose reductase) that reduces methylglyoxal to L-lactaldehyde using NADPH as cofactor. Methylglyoxal reductase catalyzes

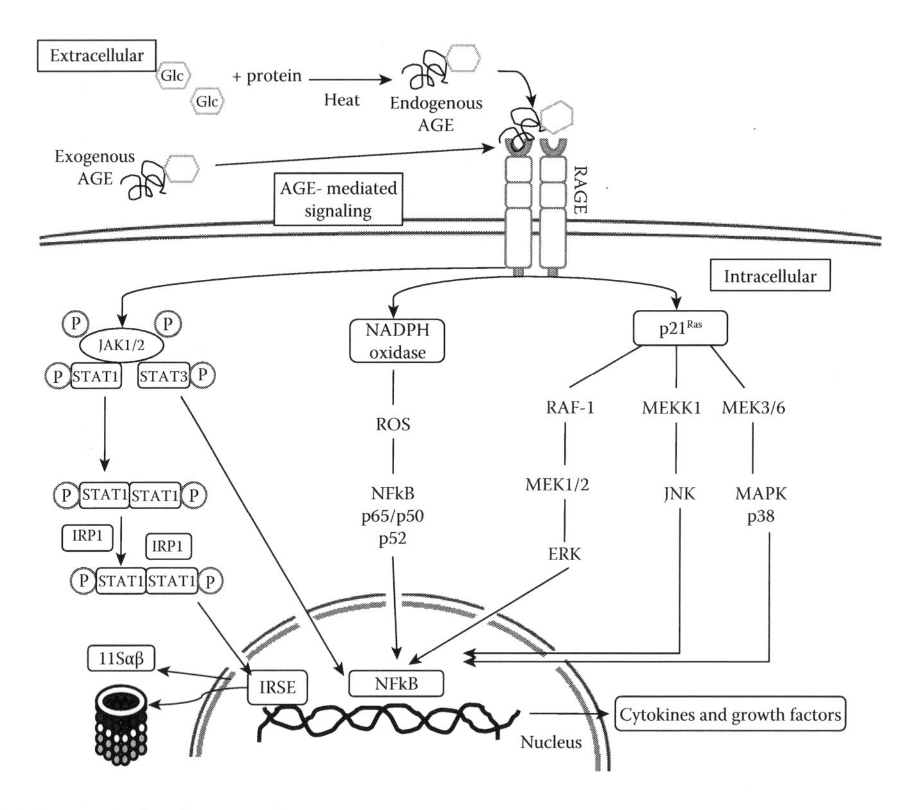

FIGURE 31.3 AGE signaling network.

this reaction to produce pyruvate which is converted to acetyl-coA by pyruvate dehydrogenase enzyme (Kalapos 1999) (Figure 31.4). Besides the above mechanisms, other pathways to clear accumulated AGEs also exist. The major one involves proteolytic cleavage of AGEs, which results in the production of AGE peptides and free AGE-adducts. These are then excreted in urine (Kalapos 1999). However, this clearance method is not applicable for AGE-modified extracellular matrix proteins. Epithelial cells of proximal convoluted tubules endocytose AGE peptides and degrade them by lysosomal degradation pathways, releasing AGE amino acids (Kalapos 1999).

31.5 Methylglyoxal: A Hidden Enemy

AGEs are associated with many age- and lifestyle-related diseases such as Alzheimer's disease, cardiovascular diseases, and diabetes. Methylglyoxal damages the target cells by modifying proteins and extracellular matrix components, and by inducing receptor-mediated ROS production (Brownlee 2001).

The effects of methylglyoxal in diabetes-related complications like retinopathy, nephropathy, and cardiovascular complications have been well documented. Increase in the production of AGEs is associated with diabetes, atherosclerosis, hypertension, diabetic cardiomyopathy, and arterial stiffness (Brownlee 2001). Kiuchi *et al.* have reported elevated concentration of serum AGEs in coronary artery disease (CAD) patients with type 2 diabetes (Kiuchi et al. 2001). AGE modification of extracellular matrix interferes with matrix–cell interaction and protein–protein interaction. AGE deposition on laminin blocks its self-assembly and polymerization, which in turn affects its interaction with type-IV collagen and heparin-sulfate proteoglycan (Charonis et al. 1988). Modification of collagen type-IV by AGEs interferes with intermolecular noncollagenous1 (NC1) and helix-rich domain's interaction (Tsilibary et al. 1988). AGE-mediated intermolecular cross-linking of type-I collagen and elastin disrupts the molecular packaging and affects vascular elasticity (Tanaka et al. 1988). Huijberts et al. demonstrated that hyperglycemic rats,

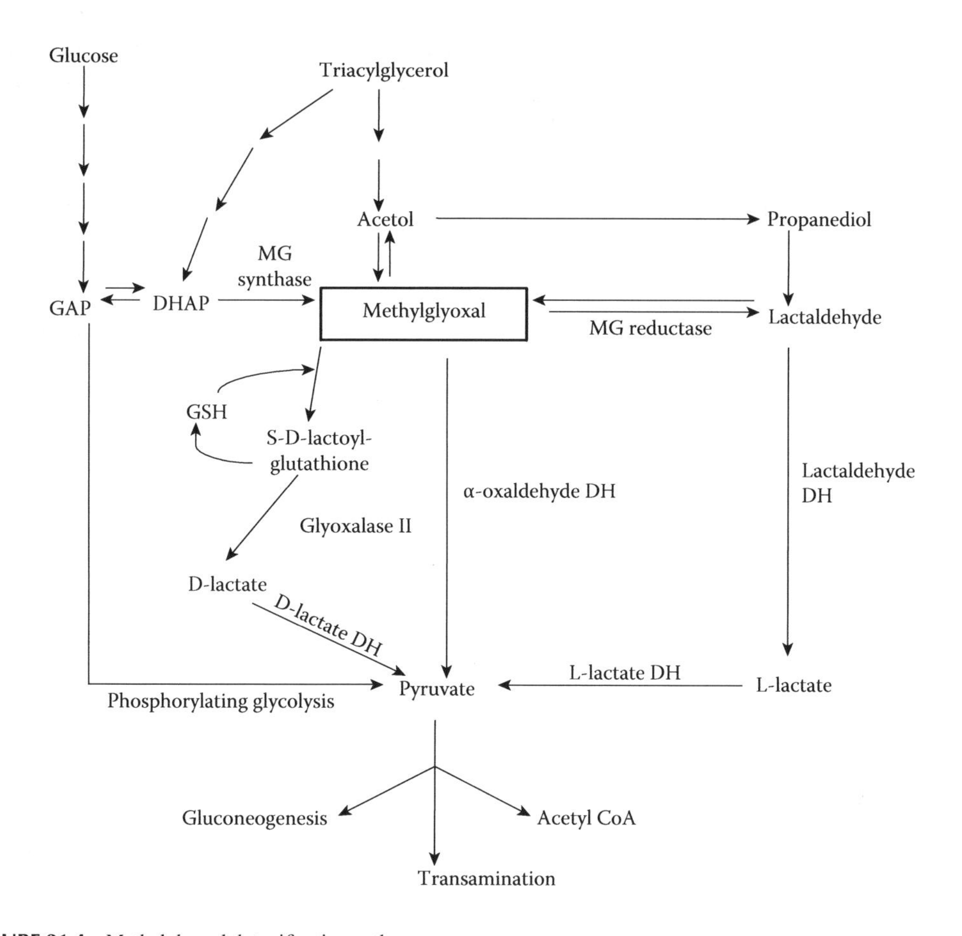

FIGURE 31.4 Methylglyoxal detoxification pathway.

which produce more AGEs, show loss of blood vessel elasticity and decreased fluid filtration across the carotid artery (Huijberts et al. 1993).

Methylglyoxal is also implicated in hypertension as it (Chang and Wu 2006) increases the resistance of peripheral blood vessels by decreasing the bioavailability of NO, which is a vasodilator (Sena et al. 2012). This effect of AGEs on NO is in part due to quenching of the molecule itself by AGEs and by inducing reduction in the half-life of the endothelial NO synthase (eNOS) mRNA. In addition, binding of CML residues to RAGE present on endothelial cells deactivates NOS by decreasing its phosphorylation (Dhar et al. 2010). AGE–RAGE binding enhances oxidative stress (ROS) by increasing NADPH oxidase activity and downregulates reduced glutathione (GSH). Furthermore, increase in ROS level activates NF-κB, resulting in the activation of VCA1, ICAM1, E-selectin, IL-1, IL- 6, IL-8, and IFN-γ (Kalapos et al. 1991).

Increase in methylglyoxal and AGEs are often linked to diabetes. This increase in methylglyoxal is explained by both an increase in glucose flux and decreased expression of glyoxalase (Rabbani and Thornalley 2011). Enhanced level of methylglyoxal disturbs the function of pancreatic β-cell. Methylglyoxal covalently modifies insulin, thereby blocking the activation of PI3 kinase pathway and expression of Ins1, Gck, and Pdx1 (Campbell et al. 2010; Fiory et al. 2011). High levels of methylglyoxal under diabetic conditions can lead to insulin resistance, platelet aggregation, and thrombus formation by induction of ROS and RNS (Hadas et al. 2013). One of the signaling molecules like Hog1 is upregulated in type 2 diabetes due to constitutive exposure to methylglyoxal (Maeta et al. 2005). Methylglyoxal-mediated signaling cascade eventually results in the activation of various stress tolerance pathways (Maeta et al. 2004).

A frequent complication associated with diabetes is retinopathy. AGEs are one of the major causes of retinal damage (Berner et al. 2012). *In vitro* studies have indicated that in hyperglycemia, the concentration of ROS is elevated in retinal cells but the concentration of antioxidant remains unchanged. This imbalance between the ROS and antioxidants in cellular system further enhances the level of methylglyoxal causing AGE accumulation (Stitt 2010). The oxidative stress created by AGEs can cause loss of integrin signaling and apoptosis of retinal pericytes cells (Liu et al. 2004). The pathophysiology of retinal pericyte growing on an AGE cross-linked matrix can be attributed to attenuation of endothelin-1 induced Ca^{2+} signaling (Hughes et al. 2004). Retinal pericyte cells also undergo calcification due to methylglyoxal-mediated activation of alkaline phosphatase (Yamagishi et al. 1999). Methylglyoxal-derived AGE-adducts like hydroimidazolone-1 and argpyrimidine result in the closure of blood capillaries (Padayatti et al. 2001; Berner et al. 2012). Nondiabetic mice show dysfunction of blood–retinal barrier when exposed to AGE–albumin, which is ascribed to increased retinal expression of VEGF and ICAM (Moore et al. 2003; Canning et al. 2007).

Many diabetic patients develop kidney malfunction as a long-term complication. AGEs cause upregulation of extracellular matrix proteins in glomerulus mesangium and tubulointerstitium (Forbes et al. 2003), which is a hallmark of diabetic nephropathy (Mason and Wahab 2003). Expression of type-IV collagen and laminin mice is found to be higher after AGE injection (Yang et al. 1994). AGE-mediated cross-linking of matrix protein changes the packing density (Bai et al. 1992) and reduces its susceptibility to pepsin degradation (Nyengaard et al. 1997). AGEs upregulate expression of proinflammatory and profibrotic chemokines such as CTGF, TGF-β, and VEGF in tubular epithelial cells. TGF-β, in particular, is implicated in fibrosis and epithelial to mesenchymal transition in renal tubular cells (Lan 2003).

Induction of oxidative stress by methylglyoxal interferes with the anabolic functions of osteoblasts. This leads to severe decrease in the rate of bone mineral deposition. This condition can lead to reduction in bone strength causing diabetic osteopathy (Mori et al. 2014).

Diabetic patients show increased susceptibility to infection, which is often attributed to the elevated glucose level. This increased glucose flux is accompanied by reduced glyoxalase expression, resulting in increased methylglyoxal levels (Skapare et al. 2013). However, the immune compromised state of diabetic patients with respect to methylglyoxal is not established. Recent reports show that treatment of myeloid cell with exogenous methylglyoxal interferes with CD83 upregulation (Price et al. 2010) and T-cell stimulation, and increases the propensity for apoptosis (Du et al. 2000). Methylglyoxal is also associated with reduced surface expression of MHC class I and decrease in IL-10 and IFN-γ in myeloid cells, and reduced TNF-γ levels in T-cells (Price et al. 2010). Diabetic hyperalgesia has been linked to methylglyoxal-mediated modification of sodium ion channel (Nav1.8) in neurons. This condition can be improved by providing alternate substrate (Gly-Glu-Arg-Pro $(GERP)_{10}$) for methylglyoxal reaction (Bierhaus et al. 2012).

Methylglyoxal toxicity is also implicated in age-related neurodegenerative diseases like Alzheimer's disease and Parkinson's disease. Alzheimer's disease is a fatal neurodegenerative disease, which leads to progressive decline in cognitive ability and memory. A hallmark of Alzheimer's disease pathology is extracellular amyloid β (Aβ 40-42) plaques accumulation and formation of neurofibrillary tangles which contains hyperphosphorylated τ protein. High dietary intake of AGEs and serum methylglyoxal level has been correlated with the decline in cognitive ability. Methylglyoxal has been reported to enhance the size of amyloid β plaque. In SH-SY5Yneuroblastoma cells, methylglyoxal treatment induces GSK 3β and P38 dependent phosphorylation of τ protein and downregulates protein phosphatase expression, thus resulting in increased hyperphosphorylated τ protein level (Angeloni et al. 2014). An *in vitro* study in Neuro 2A cell has shown that methylglyoxal treatment induces apoptosis via decreasing both bcl2/bax ratio and mitochondrial membrane potential. Similarly, methylglyoxal treatment of primary rat hippocampal culture upregulates caspase 3 cleavage and induces proapoptotic MAPK pathway (Huang et al. 2008). In accordance with these *in vitro* data, patient brain samples show an increase in caspase 3 activity and its colocalization with neurofibrillary tangles (Angeloni et al. 2014). Older mice fed with either methylglyoxal supplemented diet or sucrose-sweetened water shows symptoms of type 2 diabetes and increase in amyloid β levels. Methylglyoxal has also been linked to sirtuin1 suppression in Alzheimer's disease and type 2 diabetes (Cai et al. 2014).

The role of methylglyoxal has been implicated in Parkinson's disease (PD). In the case of humans, low glycemic index diet reduces the risk for PD. Animals fed with high glycemic diet exhibit increased methylglyoxal-modified proteins in substantia nigra. Reaction between methylglyoxal and dopamine forms 1-acetyl-6,7 -dihydroxy-1,2,3,4-tetrahydroisoquinoline (ADTIQ), a toxic by-product which accumulates in the brain. ADTIQ structurally resembles MPTP (1-methyl-4-phenyl-1,2,3,6-tetrahydropyridine) (Deng et al. 2012). MPTP is implicated in PD-related mitochondrial dysfunction as it inhibits complex I of electron transport chain (Winklhofer and Haass 2010). One of the signatures of PD is the aggregation of α-synuclein, which is highly susceptible to glycation. Methylglyoxal is known to induce protein glycation and transglutaminase in porcine tenocyte; hence, it might contribute to the formation of Lewy bodies (Verhaar et al. 2012; Wan and Chung 2012). Moreover, Uchiki *et al.* have reported that glycated proteins are more resistant to proteosomal degradation. Reaction of methylglyoxal with ubiquitin compromises its function (Jung et al. 2013). Genetic correlation between PD and methylglyoxal can be extrapolated from the fact that a defect in DJ-1 gene, a novel form of glyoxalase, is related to early onset of PD (Lee et al. 2012). DJ-1 also controls the expression of transcription factor Nfr2, which regulates glyoxalase 1 expression in response to oxidative stress and thus perturbs methylglyoxal detoxification (Xue et al. 2012). Methylglyoxal also elevates tyrosine hydroxylase and dopamine transporter expression in SH-SY5Y cells which leads to higher ROS levels (Xie et al. 2014).

Methylglyoxal has been reported to induce diarrhea, visceral hypersensitivity, headache, and depression in rats (Zhang et al. 2014). Activation of Ca^{2+} channels in gut bacteria by methylglyoxal during lactose intolerance can worsen the disease condition. High external methylglyoxal can affect the growth of the commensal microbes (Campbell et al. 2007). The altered microflora in gut is implicated to cause irritable bowel syndrome (Campbell et al. 2010). AGEs are also found to be associated with end-stage renal disease, sarcopenia, rheumatoid arthritis, vascular dementia, cataracts, and other ophthalmic diseases (Shuvaev et al. 2001; Jakus and Rietbrock 2004).

31.6 Methylglyoxal: A Blessing in Disguise

Most of the studies on methylglyoxal have focused on its deleterious role. However, a few studies have tried to understand the antimicrobial and anticancer potential of methylglyoxal.

Methylglyoxal shows antiproliferative activity against malarial parasite *Plasmodium falciparum*. Treatment of uninfected red blood cells with methylglyoxal does not show any morphological defect, but in infected host cells, it inhibits glyceraldehyde-3-phosphate dehydrogenase (GAPDH). Hence, methylglyoxal probably affects the energy source of the parasite. The antimalarial activity of methylglyoxal corroborates with the antimalarial effect of glyoxalase I inhibitor, S-p-bromobenzyl glutathione (Iozef et al. 2003). Methylglyoxal can also enter the parasite cell via the aqua glycoporin channel, which blocks proliferation by inhibiting GAPDH function. In infected erythrocytes, the lactate pool has been found to be higher as malarial parasites convert methylglyoxal to D-lactate to escape methylglyoxal assault (Vander Jagt et al. 1990).

Methylglyoxal plays a role in bacterial pathogenesis. Mycobacterial infection elevates methylglyoxal production in mouse alveolar macrophage, resulting in both activation and apoptosis of infected macrophages. Methylglyoxal-induced apoptosis of macrophages is either JNK dependent or oxidative stress mediated. The latter can be prevented by pre-treatment with reduced glutathione (Rachman et al. 2006). Patient samples isolated from tuberculoid lesions show an abundance of AGEs (Rachman et al. 2006). Besides, methylglyoxal plays a pivotal role in anti-TB immunity by inducing macrophage activation genes such as TNF-α, CXCL2, and CXCL10 (Rachman et al. 2006).

Methylglyoxal is reported to show antiviral activity against certain strains of influenza virus (Charyasriwong et al. 2015) and foot and mouth disease virus (Ghizatullina 1976). Methylglyoxal bis-(guanylhydrazone) inhibits vaccinia virus proliferation by inhibiting S-adenosyl-L-methionine decarboxylase in HeLa cells (Williamson 1976).

Various groups have demonstrated the anticancer property of methylglyoxal. Apple *et al.* have reported that a daily dose of 80 mg/kg body weight methylglyoxalcan can significantly inhibit leukemia, lymphosarcoma, and carcinoma in mice (Apple and Greenberg 1967; Egyud and Szent-Gyorgyi 1968). Methylglyoxal is also toxic to neuroblastoma cells, breast cancer cells, colon cancer cells (Ayoub et al. 1993; Webster et al. 2005), and human prostate cancer cells (Davidson et al. 2002). These data are supported by the protection offered by overexpression of glyoxalase II against methylglyoxal-induced apoptosis. In the case of prostate cancer, glyoxalase I function is critical to evade methylglyoxal-mediated death (Davidson et al. 2002).

In fact, methylglyoxal present in Manuka honey renders antibacterial properties against *Clostridium difficile, Staphylococcus aureus, Staphylococcus epidermidis, Enterococcus faecium, Enterobacter cloacae, Escherichia coli, Klebsiella oxytoca and,* and *Pseudomonas aeruginosa* (Kwakman et al. 2008; Jervis-Bardy et al. 2011).

31.7 Dietary AGEs

Exogenous AGEs arise when sugars are cooked with proteins or fats in food which is ingested and they are partially absorbed during digestion. Many lifestyle and dietary components can induce AGE formation in the body. Various food items contain AGEs as flavor enhancers and colorants.

AGEs are formed during curing of tobacco leaves. During smoking, these AGEs are absorbed by alveolar cells and subsequently transported to the circulation where they interact with other glycation products (Vlassara and Palace 2002). Dietary intake of preformed (exogenous) AGEs increases total oxidative and peroxidative stress on the body. Glycation may often result in production of acrylamide (a potent carcinogen) in cooked food items (Vlassara and Palace 2002). Food items of animal origin, that are high in fats and proteins, are more prone to AGE formation during cooking. Sugary items such as candies and cookies, barbecued meat, oils, margarine, and butter contain high levels of AGEs. AGEs can also form during high-temperature cooking methods such as frying, grilling, baking, and roasting (Uribarri et al. 2010). Nearly 30% of the arginine is modified while roasting coffee beans (Henle et al. 1994). Carbohydrate-rich foods, that is, whole grains, vegetables, and fruits maintain low AGE profile even after cooking. Shorter cooking time, lower temperature, and acidic ingredients such as lemon juice or vinegar produce least amount of AGEs. To reduce the risk of type 2 and insulin-resistance diabetes, foods containing low AGE levels should be consumed. Uribarri et al. had shown that dry heat facilitated 10–100-folds greater AGE formation as compared to uncooked food (Uribarri et al. 2010). A controlled intake of high protein and fat containing diet and avoidance of grilling and fried items can also help in reducing AGE accumulation in the body.

31.8 Anti-AGE Therapy

Methylglyoxal and other AGE-mediated toxicity can be treated with various carbonyl scavenger compounds like aminoguanidine (AG) and metformin (Desai and Wu 2008). Aminoguanidine treatment is successful in increasing arterial elasticity and reduces the severity of diabetic complications such as micro aneurysms, diabetic retinopathy, diabetic nephropathy, and atherosclerosis in diabetic rats (Forbes et al. 2004). However, its short half-life and nonspecific nature make it an unsuitable drug of choice. In addition, aminoguanidine treatment in type 1 diabetes patients during the clinical trial generated antinuclear antibodies along with signs of anemia, compromised liver function, and interference with vitamin B6 metabolism.

Oral hypoglycemic drugs like metformin (dimethyl-biguanide) inhibits glycation of proteins in post-Amadori step (Beisswenger and Ruggiero-Lopez 2003). Metformin treatment in type 2 diabetes reduces the serum methylglyoxal level and AGE build-up in renal cortex and lens in diabetes-induced rats (Beisswenger et al. 1999). Pioglitazone, which is a thiazolidinedione type 2 antidiabetic drug, also shows a similar scavenging property (Yuan and Liu 2011; Puddu et al. 2012).

Another methylglyoxal scavenging compound is Gly-Glu-X-Pro $(GEXP)_n$ where X is either lysine or arginine. It prevents binding of methylglyoxal to a lysine- or arginine-containing cellular protein, thus diverting the substrate from methylglyoxal modification. $GERP_{10}$ is effective against diabetic hyperalgesia *in vitro* (Bierhaus et al. 2012). Apart from GEXP, carnosine(β-alanyl-L-histidine), an endogenous human protein can also suppress hyperalgesia in diabetic mice. Its resistance to digestive enzymes and the ability to cross the blood–brain barrier makes it a potential candidate for AGE-mediated neurodegenerative disease treatment (Hipkiss and Chana 1998).

Another class of anti-AGE treatment is a cross-link breaker such as N-phenacylthiazolium bromide (PTB), OPB 9195 [(±)-2-isopropylidenhydrazono-4-oxo-thiazolidin-5-ylacetalinide], N-(2-Acetamidoethyl) hydrozine carboximidamide hydrochloride (ALT-946), and alagebrium (3-phenacyl-4,5-dimethylthiazolium chloride, 4,5-Dimethyl-3-(2-oxo-2-phenylethyl)-1,3-thiazol-3-ium chloride and ALT-711 is its former name). PTB and OPB 9195 are cross-linking breaker, but they are unstable in aqueous solution. However, alagebrium shows better stability in aqueous solution and is effective in reducing the severity of heart failure and atherosclerosis; decreases cardiovascular stiffness, pulse pressure, and nephropathy; and improves ventricular diastolic function in diabetic rats. It also prevents collagen cross-linking (Kiland et al. 2009).

Pyridoxamine, an antioxidant, blocks AGE formation. Pyridoxamine treatment in rats results in a decrease in plasma levels of methylglyoxal and AGE-collagen. It shows promising results in diabetic rats, suffering from nephropathy, retinopathy, peripheral neuropathy, and vascular complications without any adverse effects (Voziyan and Hudson 2005). Another thiamine derivative benfotiamine also inhibits AGE formation (Alkhalaf et al. 2012).

Lalezari-Rahbar et al. have developed another class of anti-AGE compounds. These LR aromatic compounds, designated as LR 90, LR 9, and LR 74, contain ureido and carboxamide functional groups. They inhibit AGE formation by chelating metal ions (Rahbar and Figarola 2003). Although these compounds are more efficient than aminoguanidine and pyridoxamine in encountering AGE toxicity, they affect the expression of NF-κB and hence affect immune response (Rahbar and Figarola 2003; Nagai et al. 2012).

The soluble extracellular domain of RAGE (sRAGE) can prevent AGE–RAGE interaction and hence can inhibit RAGE signaling pathway. sRAGE treatment in atherosclerosis shows favorable results (Goldin et al. 2006). Newer therapies against AGE-mediated toxicity are being developed which may aid in the treatment of disorders such as diabetes, Alzheimer's disease, and PD.

31.9 Conclusions

Methylglyoxal is a highly reactive by-product of various biological pathways. Due to the presence of two carbonyl groups, it often reacts with a large number of macromolecules like protein, lipids, and nucleic acid, resulting in aberrant change in their properties. Its interaction with structural proteins forms irreversible adducts, leading to AGE formation. AGE-mediated cross-linking of these modified proteins can cause various adverse effects like blockage of blood vessels, malfunction in glomerular ultrafiltration, and enhanced neurodegeneration. However, the protective role of methylglyoxal against various microbial diseases and certain cancers cannot be ignored. Thus, methylglyoxal exhibits both detrimental and ameliorative effects. Current research has provided novel molecules which can counteract toxic effects of AGEs either by breaking cross-linking or by scavenging reactive carbonyl compounds. Many antioxidants and metal ion chelators can also reduce AGE formation and hence be used as anti-AGE therapy. However, further research is required to increase the half-life and to eliminate the side effects of these drugs. This chapter also discusses about the adverse effects of dietary AGEs on human physiology. However, these effects can be avoided by making modifications in our lifestyle and food habits.

REFERENCES

Alkhalaf, A., N. Kleefstra, K. H. Groenier, H. J. Bilo, R. O. Gans, P. Heeringa, J. L. Scheijen, C. G. Schalkwijk, G. J. Navis, and S. J. Bakker. 2012. Effect of benfotiamine on advanced glycation endproducts and markers of endothelial dysfunction and inflammation in diabetic nephropathy. *PLoS One* 7 (7):e40427. doi: 10.1371/journal.pone.0040427.

Angeloni, C., L. Zambonin, and S. Hrelia. 2014. Role of methylglyoxal in Alzheimer's disease. *Biomed Res Int* 2014:238485. doi: 10.1155/2014/238485.

Antognelli, C., L. Mezzasoma, K. Fettucciari, and V. N. Talesa. 2013. A novel mechanism of methylglyoxal cytotoxicity in prostate cancer cells. *Int J Biochem Cell Biol* 45 (4):836–44. doi: 10.1016/j.biocel.2013.01.003.

Apple, M. A., and D. M. Greenberg. 1967. Inhibition of cancer growth in mice by a normal metabolite. *Life Sci* 6 (20):2157–60.

Ayoub, F. M., R. E. Allen, and P. J. Thornalley. 1993. Inhibition of proliferation of human leukaemia 60 cells by methylglyoxal *in vitro*. *Leuk Res* 17 (5):397–401.

Bai, P., K. Phua, T. Hardt, M. Cernadas, and B. Brodsky. 1992. Glycation alters collagen fibril organization. *Connect Tissue Res* 28 (1–2):1–12.

Beisswenger, P., and D. Ruggiero-Lopez. 2003. Metformin inhibition of glycation processes. *Diabetes Metab* 29 (4 Pt 2):6S95–103.

Beisswenger, P. J., S. K. Howell, A. D. Touchette, S. Lal, and B. S. Szwergold. 1999. Metformin reduces systemic methylglyoxal levels in type 2 diabetes. *Diabetes* 48 (1):198–202.

Berner, A. K., O. Brouwers, R. Pringle, I. Klaassen, L. Colhoun, C. McVicar, S. Brockbank, et al. 2012. Protection against methylglyoxal-derived AGEs by regulation of glyoxalase 1 prevents retinal neuroglial and vasodegenerative pathology. *Diabetologia* 55 (3):845–54. doi: 10.1007/s00125-011-2393-0.

Bierhaus, A., T. Fleming, S. Stoyanov, A. Leffler, A. Babes, C. Neacsu, S. K. Sauer, et al. 2012. Methylglyoxal modification of Nav1.8 facilitates nociceptive neuron firing and causes hyperalgesia in diabetic neuropathy. *Nat Med* 18 (6):926–33. doi: 10.1038/nm.2750.

Brownlee, M. 2001. Biochemistry and molecular cell biology of diabetic complications. *Nature* 414 (6865):813–20. doi: 10.1038/414813a.

Cai, W., M. Ramdas, L. Zhu, X. Chen, G. E. Striker, and H. Vlassara. 2012. Oral advanced glycation end-products (AGEs) promote insulin resistance and diabetes by depleting the antioxidant defenses AGE receptor-1 and sirtuin 1. *Proc Natl Acad Sci U S A* 109 (39):15888–93. doi: 10.1073/pnas.1205847109.

Cai, W., J. Uribarri, L. Zhu, X. Chen, S. Swamy, Z. Zhao, F. Grosjean, et al. 2014. Oral glycotoxins are a modifiable cause of dementia and the metabolic syndrome in mice and humans. *Proc Natl Acad Sci U S A* 111 (13):4940–5. doi: 10.1073/pnas.1316013111.

Campbell, A. K., S. B. Matthews, N. Vassel, C. D. Cox, R. Naseem, J. Chaichi, I. B. Holland, J. Green, and K. T. Wann. 2010. Bacterial metabolic 'toxins': A new mechanism for lactose and food intolerance, and irritable bowel syndrome. *Toxicology* 278 (3):268–76. doi: 10.1016/j.tox.2010.09.001.

Campbell, A. K., R. Naseem, I. B. Holland, S. B. Matthews, and K. T. Wann. 2007. Methylglyoxal and other carbohydrate metabolites induce lanthanum-sensitive Ca^{2+} transients and inhibit growth in *E. coli*. *Arch Biochem Biophys* 468 (1):107–13. doi: 10.1016/j.abb.2007.09.006.

Canning, P., J. V. Glenn, D. K. Hsu, F. T. Liu, T. A. Gardiner, and A. W. Stitt. 2007. Inhibition of advanced glycation and absence of galectin-3 prevent blood-retinal barrier dysfunction during short-term diabetes. *Exp Diabetes Res* 2007:51837. doi: 10.1155/2007/51837.

Case, E. M., and R. P. Cook. 1931. The occurrence of pyruvic acid and methylglyoxal in muscle metabolism. *Biochem J* 25 (4):1319–35.

Chakraborty, S., K. Karmakar, and D. Chakravortty. 2014. Cells producing their own nemesis: Understanding methylglyoxal metabolism. *IUBMB Life* 66 (10):667–78. doi: 10.1002/iub.1324.

Chang, T., and L. Wu. 2006. Methylglyoxal, oxidative stress, and hypertension. *Can J Physiol Pharmacol* 84 (12):1229–38. doi: 10.1139/y06-077.

Charonis, A. S., A. P. Skubitz, G. G. Koliakos, L. A. Reger, J. Dege, A. M. Vogel, R. Wohlhueter, and L. T. Furcht. 1988. A novel synthetic peptide from the B1 chain of laminin with heparin-binding and cell adhesion-promoting activities. *J Cell Biol* 107 (3):1253–60.

Charyasriwong, S., K. Watanabe, R. Rahmasari, A. Matsunaga, T. Haruyama, and N. Kobayashi. 2015. *In vitro* evaluation of synergistic inhibitory effects of neuraminidase inhibitors and methylglyoxal against influenza virus infection. *Arch Med Res* 46 (1):8–16. doi: 10.1016/j.arcmed.2014.12.002.

Cooper, R. A., and A. Anderson. 1970. The formation and catabolism of methylglyoxal during glycolysis in Escherichia coli. *FEBS Lett* 11 (4):273–276.

Davidson, S. D., D. M. Milanesa, C. Mallouh, M. S. Choudhury, H. Tazaki, and S. Konno. 2002. A possible regulatory role of glyoxalase I in cell viability of human prostate cancer. *Urol Res* 30 (2):116–21.

Deng, Y., Y. Zhang, Y. Li, S. Xiao, D. Song, H. Qing, Q. Li, and A. H. Rajput. 2012. Occurrence and distribution of salsolinol-like compound, 1-acetyl-6,7-dihydroxy-1,2,3,4-tetrahydroisoquinoline (ADTIQ) in parkinsonian brains. *J Neural Transm (Vienna)* 119 (4):435–41. doi: 10.1007/s00702-011-0724-4.

Desai, K. M., and L. Wu. 2008. Free radical generation by methylglyoxal in tissues. *Drug Metabol Drug Interact* 23 (1–2):151–73.

Dhar, A., K. Desai, M. Kazachmov, P. Yu, and L. Wu. 2008. Methylglyoxal production in vascular smooth muscle cells from different metabolic precursors. *Metabolism* 57 (9):1211–20. doi: 10.1016/j.metabol.2008.04.014.

Dhar, A., I. Dhar, K. M. Desai, and L. Wu. 2010. Methylglyoxal scavengers attenuate endothelial dysfunction induced by methylglyoxal and high concentrations of glucose. *Br J Pharmacol* 161 (8):1843–56. doi: 10.1111/j.1476-5381.2010.01017.x.

Du, J., H. Suzuki, F. Nagase, A. A. Akhand, T. Yokoyama, T. Miyata, K. Kurokawa, and I. Nakashima. 2000. Methylglyoxal induces apoptosis in Jurkat leukemia T cells by activating c-Jun N-terminal kinase. *J Cell Biochem* 77 (2):333–44.

Egyud, L. G., and A. Szent-Gyorgyi. 1968. Cancerostatic action of methylglyoxal. *Science* 160 (3832):1140.

Fiory, F., A. Lombardi, C. Miele, J. Giudicelli, F. Beguinot, and E. Van Obberghen. 2011. Methylglyoxal impairs insulin signalling and insulin action on glucose-induced insulin secretion in the pancreatic beta cell line INS-1E. *Diabetologia* 54 (11):2941–52. doi: 10.1007/s00125-011-2280-8.

Forbes, J. M., M. E. Cooper, M. D. Oldfield, and M. C. Thomas. 2003. Role of advanced glycation end products in diabetic nephropathy. *J Am Soc Nephrol* 14 (8 Suppl 3):S254–8.

Forbes, J. M., L. T. Yee, V. Thallas, M. Lassila, R. Candido, K. A. Jandeleit-Dahm, M. C. Thomas, et al. 2004. Advanced glycation end product interventions reduce diabetes-accelerated atherosclerosis. *Diabetes* 53 (7):1813–23.

Ghizatullina, N. K. 1976. Effect of methyl glyoxal on infectivity and antigenicity of foot-and-mouth disease virus. *Acta Virol* 20 (5):380–6.

Goldin, A., J. A. Beckman, A. M. Schmidt, and M. A. Creager. 2006. Advanced glycation end products: Sparking the development of diabetic vascular injury. *Circulation* 114 (6):597–605. doi: 10.1161/CIRCULATIONAHA.106.621854.

Hadas, K., V. Randriamboavonjy, A. Elgheznawy, A. Mann, and I. Fleming. 2013. Methylglyoxal induces platelet hyperaggregation and reduces thrombus stability by activating PKC and inhibiting PI3K/Akt pathway. *PLoS One* 8 (9):e74401. doi: 10.1371/journal.pone.0074401.

Henle, T., A. W. Walter, R. Haessner, and H. Klostermeyer. 1994. Detection and identification of a protein-bound imidazolone resulting from the reaction of arginine residues and methylglyoxal. *Zeitschrift Fur Lebensmittel-Untersuchung Und-Forschung* 199 (1):55–8. doi: 10.1007/Bf01192954.

Hipkiss, A. R., and H. Chana. 1998. Carnosine protects proteins against methylglyoxal-mediated modifications. *Biochem Biophys Res Commun* 248 (1):28–32. doi: 10.1006/bbrc.1998.8806.

Huang, S. M., H. C. Chuang, C. H. Wu, and G. C. Yen. 2008. Cytoprotective effects of phenolic acids on methylglyoxal-induced apoptosis in Neuro-2A cells. *Mol Nutr Food Res* 52 (8):940–9. doi: 10.1002/mnfr.200700360.

Hughes, S. J., N. Wall, C. N. Scholfield, J. G. McGeown, T. A. Gardiner, A. W. Stitt, and T. M. Curtis. 2004. Advanced glycation endproduct modified basement membrane attenuates endothelin-1 induced $[Ca^{2+}]i$ signalling and contraction in retinal microvascular pericytes. *Mol Vis* 10:996–1004.

Huijberts, M. S., B. H. Wolffenbuttel, H. A. Boudier, F. R. Crijns, A. C. Kruseman, P. Poitevin, and B. I. Levy. 1993. Aminoguanidine treatment increases elasticity and decreases fluid filtration of large arteries from diabetic rats. *J Clin Invest* 92 (3):1407–11. doi: 10.1172/JCI116716.

Iozef, R., S. Rahlfs, T. Chang, H. Schirmer, and K. Becker. 2003. Glyoxalase I of the malarial parasite Plasmodium falciparum: Evidence for subunit fusion. *FEBS Lett* 554 (3):284–8.

Jakus, V., and N. Rietbrock. 2004. Advanced glycation end-products and the progress of diabetic vascular complications. *Physiol Res* 53 (2):131–42.

Jervis-Bardy, J., A. Foreman, S. Bray, L. Tan, and P. J. Wormald. 2011. Methylglyoxal-infused honey mimics the anti-Staphylococcus aureus biofilm activity of manuka honey: Potential implication in chronic rhinosinusitis. *Laryngoscope* 121 (5):1104–7. doi: 10.1002/lary.21717.

Jung, T., A. Hohn, and T. Grune. 2013. The proteasome and the degradation of oxidized proteins: Part II—Protein oxidation and proteasomal degradation. *Redox Biol* 2C:99–104. doi: 10.1016/j.redox.2013.12.008.

Kalapos, M. P. 1999. Methylglyoxal in living organisms: Chemistry, biochemistry, toxicology and biological implications. *Toxicol Lett* 110 (3):145–75.

Kalapos, M. P., T. Garzo, F. Antoni, and J. Mandl. 1991. Effect of methylglyoxal on glucose formation, drug oxidation and glutathione content in isolated murine hepatocytes. *Biochim Biophys Acta* 1092 (3):284–90.

Kang, J. H. 2003. Oxidative damage of DNA induced by methylglyoxal *in vitro*. *Toxicol Lett* 145 (2):181–7.

Kierdorf, K., and G. Fritz. 2013. RAGE regulation and signaling in inflammation and beyond. *J Leukoc Biol* 94 (1):55–68. doi: 10.1189/jlb.1012519.

Kiland, J. A., B. T. Gabelt, G. Tezel, E. Lutjen-Drecoll, and P. L. Kaufman. 2009. Effect of the age cross-link breaker alagebrium on anterior segment physiology, morphology, and ocular age and rage. *Trans Am Ophthalmol Soc* 107:146–58.

Kiuchi, K., J. Nejima, T. Takano, M. Ohta, and H. Hashimoto. 2001. Increased serum concentrations of advanced glycation end products: A marker of coronary artery disease activity in type 2 diabetic patients. *Heart* 85 (1):87–91.

Kwakman, P. H., J. P. Van den Akker, A. Guclu, H. Aslami, J. M. Binnekade, L. de Boer, L. Boszhard, et al. 2008. Medical-grade honey kills antibiotic-resistant bacteria *in vitro* and eradicates skin colonization. *Clin Infect Dis* 46 (11):1677–82. doi: 10.1086/587892.

Lan, H. Y. 2003. Tubular epithelial-myofibroblast transdifferentiation mechanisms in proximal tubule cells. *Curr Opin Nephrol Hypertens* 12 (1):25–9. doi: 10.1097/01.mnh.0000049812.98789.97.

Lee, J. Y., J. Song, K. Kwon, S. Jang, C. Kim, K. Baek, J. Kim, and C. Park. 2012. Human DJ-1 and its homologs are novel glyoxalases. *Hum Mol Genet* 21 (14):3215–25. doi: 10.1093/hmg/dds155.

Liu, B., M. Bhat, A. K. Padival, D. G. Smith, and R. H. Nagaraj. 2004. Effect of dicarbonyl modification of fibronectin on retinal capillary pericytes. *Invest Ophthalmol Vis Sci* 45 (6):1983–95.

Luevano-Contreras, C., and K. Chapman-Novakofski. 2010. Dietary advanced glycation end products and aging. *Nutrients* 2 (12):1247–65. doi: 10.3390/nu2121247.

Maeta, K., S. Izawa, and Y. Inoue. 2005. Methylglyoxal, a metabolite derived from glycolysis, functions as a signal initiator of the high osmolarity glycerol-mitogen-activated protein kinase cascade and calcineurin/Crz1-mediated pathway in Saccharomyces cerevisiae. *J Biol Chem* 280 (1):253–60. doi: 10.1074/jbc.M408061200.

Maeta, K., S. Izawa, S. Okazaki, S. Kuge, and Y. Inoue. 2004. Activity of the Yap1 transcription factor in Saccharomyces cerevisiae is modulated by methylglyoxal, a metabolite derived from glycolysis. *Mol Cell Biol* 24 (19):8753–64. doi: 10.1128/MCB.24.19.8753-8764.2004.

Mason, R. M., and N. A. Wahab. 2003. Extracellular matrix metabolism in diabetic nephropathy. *J Am Soc Nephrol* 14 (5):1358–73.

Mizutani, T., K. Yoshida, and S. Kawazoe. 1994. Formation of toxic metabolites from thiabendazole and other thiazoles in mice. Identification of thioamides as ring cleavage products. *Drug Metab Dispos* 22 (5):750–5.

Moore, T. C., J. E. Moore, Y. Kaji, N. Frizzell, T. Usui, V. Poulaki, I. L. Campbell, et al. 2003. The role of advanced glycation end products in retinal microvascular leukostasis. *Invest Ophthalmol Vis Sci* 44 (10):4457–64.

Mori, K., R. Kitazawa, T. Kondo, M. Mori, Y. Hamada, M. Nishida, Y. Minami, R. Haraguchi, Y. Takahashi, and S. Kitazawa. 2014. Diabetic osteopenia by decreased beta-catenin signaling is partly induced by epigenetic derepression of sFRP-4 gene. *PLoS One* 9 (7):e102797. doi: 10.1371/journal.pone.0102797.

Nagai, R., D. B. Murray, T. O. Metz, and J. W. Baynes. 2012. Chelation: A fundamental mechanism of action of AGE inhibitors, AGE breakers, and other inhibitors of diabetes complications. *Diabetes* 61 (3):549–59. doi: 10.2337/db11-1120.

Nyengaard, J. R., K. Chang, S. Berhorst, K. M. Reiser, J. R. Williamson, and R. G. Tilton. 1997. Discordant effects of guanidines on renal structure and function and on regional vascular dysfunction and collagen changes in diabetic rats. *Diabetes* 46 (1):94–106.

Oya, T., N. Hattori, Y. Mizuno, S. Miyata, S. Maeda, T. Osawa, and K. Uchida. 1999. Methylglyoxal modification of protein. Chemical and immunochemical characterization of methylglyoxal-arginine adducts. *J Biol Chem* 274 (26):18492–502.

Padayatti, P. S., C. Jiang, M. A. Glomb, K. Uchida, and R. H. Nagaraj. 2001. High concentrations of glucose induce synthesis of argpyrimidine in retinal endothelial cells. *Curr Eye Res* 23 (2):106–15.

Price, C. L., H. O. Hassi, N. R. English, A. I. Blakemore, A. J. Stagg, and S. C. Knight. 2010. Methylglyoxal modulates immune responses: Relevance to diabetes. *J Cell Mol Med* 14 (6B):1806–15. doi: 10.1111/j.1582-4934.2009.00803.x.

Puddu, A., R. Sanguineti, A. Durante, and G. L. Viviani. 2012. Pioglitazone attenuates the detrimental effects of advanced glycation end-products in the pancreatic beta cell line HIT-T15. *Regul Pept* 177 (1–3):79–84. doi: 10.1016/j.regpep.2012.05.089.

Rabbani, N., and P. J. Thornalley. 2011. Glyoxalase in diabetes, obesity and related disorders. *Semin Cell Dev Biol* 22 (3):309–17. doi: 10.1016/j.semcdb.2011.02.015.

Rachman, H., N. Kim, T. Ulrichs, S. Baumann, L. Pradl, A. Nasser Eddine, M. Bild, et al. 2006. Critical role of methylglyoxal and AGE in mycobacteria-induced macrophage apoptosis and activation. *PLoS One* 1:e29. doi: 10.1371/journal.pone.0000029.

Rahbar, S., and J. L. Figarola. 2003. Novel inhibitors of advanced glycation endproducts. *Arch Biochem Biophys* 419 (1):63–79.

Sena, C. M., P. Matafome, J. Crisostomo, L. Rodrigues, R. Fernandes, P. Pereira, and R. M. Seica. 2012. Methylglyoxal promotes oxidative stress and endothelial dysfunction. *Pharmacol Res* 65 (5):497–506. doi: 10.1016/j.phrs.2012.03.004.

Shuvaev, V. V., I. Laffont, J. M. Serot, J. Fujii, N. Taniguchi, and G. Siest. 2001. Increased protein glycation in cerebrospinal fluid of Alzheimer's disease. *Neurobiol Aging* 22 (3):397–402.

Skapare, E., I. Konrade, E. Liepinsh, I. Strele, M. Makrecka, A. Bierhaus, A. Lejnieks, V. Pirags, and M. Dambrova. 2013. Association of reduced glyoxalase 1 activity and painful peripheral diabetic neuropathy in type 1 and 2 diabetes mellitus patients. *J Diabetes Complications* 27 (3):262–7. doi: 10.1016/j.jdiacomp.2012.12.002.

Stirban, A., T. Gawlowski, and M. Roden. 2014. Vascular effects of advanced glycation endproducts: Clinical effects and molecular mechanisms. *Mol Metab* 3 (2):94–108. doi: 10.1016/j.molmet.2013.11.006.

Stitt, A. W. 2010. AGEs and diabetic retinopathy. *Invest Ophthalmol Vis Sci* 51 (10):4867–74. doi: 10.1167/iovs.10-5881.

Tanaka, S., G. Avigad, B. Brodsky, and E. F. Eikenberry. 1988. Glycation induces expansion of the molecular packing of collagen. *J Mol Biol* 203 (2):495–505.

Tsilibary, E. C., A. S. Charonis, L. A. Reger, R. M. Wohlhueter, and L. T. Furcht. 1988. The effect of nonenzymatic glucosylation on the binding of the main noncollagenous NC1 domain to type IV collagen. *J Biol Chem* 263 (9):4302–8.

Uribarri, J., S. Woodruff, S. Goodman, W. Cai, X. Chen, R. Pyzik, A. Yong, G. E. Striker, and H. Vlassara. 2010. Advanced glycation end products in foods and a practical guide to their reduction in the diet. *J Am Diet Assoc* 110 (6):911–16 e12. doi: 10.1016/j.jada.2010.03.018.

Vander Jagt, D. L., L. A. Hunsaker, N. M. Campos, and B. R. Baack. 1990. D-lactate production in erythrocytes infected with Plasmodium falciparum. *Mol Biochem Parasitol* 42 (2):277–84.

Verhaar, R., B. Drukarch, J. G. Bol, C. A. Jongenelen, R. J. Musters, and M. M. Wilhelmus. 2012. Increase in endoplasmic reticulum-associated tissue transglutaminase and enzymatic activation in a cellular model of Parkinson's disease. *Neurobiol Dis* 45 (3):839–50. doi: 10.1016/j.nbd.2011.10.012.

Vlassara, H., and M. R. Palace. 2002. Diabetes and advanced glycation endproducts. *J Intern Med* 251 (2):87–101.

Voziyan, P. A., and B. G. Hudson. 2005. Pyridoxamine as a multifunctional pharmaceutical: Targeting pathogenic glycation and oxidative damage. *Cell Mol Life Sci* 62 (15):1671–81. doi: 10.1007/s00018-005-5082-7.

Wan, O. W., and K. K. Chung. 2012. The role of alpha-synuclein oligomerization and aggregation in cellular and animal models of Parkinson's disease. *PLoS One* 7 (6):e38545. doi: 10.1371/journal.pone.0038545.

Webster, J., C. Urban, K. Berbaum, C. Loske, A. Alpar, U. Gartner, S. G. de Arriba, T. Arendt, and G. Munch. 2005. The carbonyl scavengers aminoguanidine and tenilsetam protect against the neurotoxic effects of methylglyoxal. *Neurotox Res* 7 (1–2):95–101.

Williamson, J. D. 1976. The effect of methylglyoxal bis(guanylhydrazone) on vaccinia virus replication. *Biochem Biophys Res Commun* 73 (1):120–6.

Winklhofer, K. F., and C. Haass. 2010. Mitochondrial dysfunction in Parkinson's disease. *Biochim Biophys Acta* 1802 (1):29–44. doi: 10.1016/j.bbadis.2009.08.013.

Xie, B., F. Lin, L. Peng, K. Ullah, H. Wu, H. Qing, and Y. Deng. 2014. Methylglyoxal increases dopamine level and leads to oxidative stress in SH-SY5Y cells. *Acta Biochim Biophys Sin (Shanghai)* 46 (11):950–6. doi: 10.1093/abbs/gmu094.

Xue, M., N. Rabbani, H. Momiji, P. Imbasi, M. M. Anwar, N. Kitteringham, B. K. Park, et al. 2012. Transcriptional control of glyoxalase 1 by Nrf2 provides a stress-responsive defence against dicarbonyl glycation. *Biochem J* 443 (1):213–22. doi: 10.1042/BJ20111648.

Yamagishi, S., H. Fujimori, H. Yonekura, N. Tanaka, and H. Yamamoto. 1999. Advanced glycation endproducts accelerate calcification in microvascular pericytes. *Biochem Biophys Res Commun* 258 (2):353–7.

Yang, C. W., H. Vlassara, E. P. Peten, C. J. He, G. E. Striker, and L. J. Striker. 1994. Advanced glycation end products up-regulate gene expression found in diabetic glomerular disease. *Proc Natl Acad Sci U S A* 91 (20):9436–40.

Yuan, X., and N. Liu. 2011. Pioglitazone suppresses advanced glycation end product-induced expression of plasminogen activator inhibitor-1 in vascular smooth muscle cells. *J Genet Genomics* 38 (5):193–200. doi: 10.1016/j.jgg.2011.04.001.

Zhang, S., T. Jiao, Y. Chen, N. Gao, L. Zhang, and M. Jiang. 2014. Methylglyoxal induces systemic symptoms of irritable bowel syndrome. *PLoS One* 9 (8):e105307. doi: 10.1371/journal.pone.0105307.

Index

D

E

Q

R

S

T

U

V

W